AF666116

Emerging Zoonotic Threats from Swine

Rajib Deb
Jitendrakumar Nayak
Gyanendra Singh Sengar
Vivek Kumar Gupta
Editors

Emerging Zoonotic Threats from Swine

A Public Health Perspective

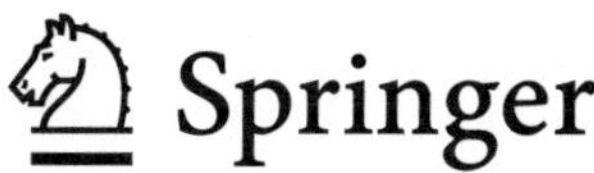

Editors
Rajib Deb
National Research Centre on Pig
Indian Council of Agricultural Research
Guwahati, Assam, India

Gyanendra Singh Sengar
National Research Centre on Pig
Indian Council of Agricultural Research
Guwahati, Assam, India

Jitendrakumar Nayak
Department of Veterinary Public Health
and Epidemiology
College of Veterinary Science
and Animal Husbandry
Kamdhenu University
Anand, Gujarat, India

Vivek Kumar Gupta
National Research Centre on Pig
Indian Council of Agricultural Research
Guwahati, Assam, India

ISBN 978-981-96-7406-0 ISBN 978-981-96-7407-7 (eBook)
https://doi.org/10.1007/978-981-96-7407-7

This Springer imprint is published by the registered company Springer Nature Singapore Pte Ltd.
The registered company address is: 152 Beach Road, #21-01/04 Gateway East, Singapore 189721, Singapore

To all researchers, veterinarians, public health professionals, and frontline workers who tirelessly strive to protect human and animal health.
And to the families and communities impacted by zoonotic diseases—may this book serve as a step toward a safer and healthier future for all.

Preface

The intricate interplay between animal health, human health, and environmental sustainability is becoming increasingly evident in today's interconnected world. Swine, as one of the most economically significant livestock species, play a pivotal role in the agricultural sector. However, their role as reservoirs or amplifiers of zoonotic pathogens presents a pressing challenge to public health. The dynamic relationship between swine farming practices, pathogen evolution, and disease transmission underscores the importance of a holistic approach to understanding and mitigating emerging zoonotic threats.

This book, *Emerging Zoonotic Threats from Swine*, is a collaborative effort by leading experts in the field to address the multifaceted challenges posed by swine-related zoonoses. It brings together a wealth of knowledge and insights across a broad spectrum of topics, ranging from swine farming practices and disease surveillance to specific zoonotic pathogens and prevention strategies. By examining these issues through the lens of the One Health approach, this book highlights the interconnectedness of human, animal, and environmental health.

The chapters included in this volume provide a comprehensive exploration of emerging zoonotic threats, with contributions from esteemed researchers and practitioners who offer in-depth analyses and evidence-based recommendations. Readers will gain insights into key areas such as the impact of swine farming on public health, surveillance, and monitoring of zoonotic diseases, the role of vaccination, biosecurity measures, and risk communication. Furthermore, this book delves into specific pathogens of significant concern, including swine influenza, Nipah virus, *Streptococcus suis*, Hepatitis E virus, and emerging coronaviruses, among others.

Our aim is to provide a valuable resource for researchers, veterinarians, public health officials, policymakers, and students who are keen to understand and address the zoonotic risks associated with swine. By fostering a deeper understanding of these threats and their control, we hope this book will contribute to the development of integrated strategies for safeguarding public health and promoting sustainable livestock farming practices.

We extend our heartfelt gratitude to all contributors for their dedication and expertise, which have enriched this volume. We also thank the editorial team at Springer for their support in bringing this project to fruition. It is our hope that this book will serve as a foundation for further research and collaboration in addressing zoonotic diseases at the interface of swine and human health.

Guwahati, Assam, India Rajib Deb
Anand, Gujarat, India Jitendrakumar Nayak
Guwahati, Assam, India Gyanendra Singh Sengar
Guwahati, Assam, India Vivek Kumar Gupta

Acknowledgments

The editors extend their heartfelt gratitude to all the chapter authors for their valuable contributions, which have enriched this book immensely. We also express our sincere appreciation to Dr. Pranav Anjaria from the College of Veterinary Science & Animal Husbandry, Kamdhenu University, Anand, Gujarat, for his unwavering support and technical expertise throughout the process. From the initial ideation and conceptualization to the finalization of the book, his guidance and assistance have been indispensable. This endeavor would not have been possible without his dedication and efforts.

Contents

Editors and Contributors

About the Editors

Rajib Deb, PhD, is currently serving as a Senior Scientist at the ICAR-National Research Centre on Pig, Guwahati, Assam, India. He completed his postgraduate and doctoral studies in Animal Biotechnology at the Indian Veterinary Research Institute, Uttar Pradesh, India.

He has authored over 40 research papers in peer-reviewed journals and is the recipient of several prestigious national and international awards, including the TWAS Fellowship (Italy), the ICMR-DHR International Fellowship, and recognition as an Associate of the National Academy of Agricultural Sciences, India. He is also a member of the National Academy of Sciences, India, and the Indian National Young Academy of Sciences.

He has filed nine Indian patents, of which three have been granted, and has developed several innovative technologies. His current research focuses on the development of diagnostics and vaccines for porcine diseases.

Jitendrakumar Nayak, Associate Professor at Kamdhenu University, Anand, is a distinguished expert in veterinary public health and epidemiology with over 30 years of experience. He holds a BVSc and AH (1993), MVSc (2004), and PhD (2009) and has been actively involved in teaching, research, and guiding 17 postgraduate students, including three currently under his mentorship.

He has made significant contributions to zoonotic disease research, particularly in the molecular epidemiology of foodborne pathogens such as *Campylobacter* spp., ESKAPE pathogens, *Brucella*, and *Mycobacterium*. His work includes advanced diagnostic techniques like PCR-RFLP and multilocus sequence typing, with several gene sequences submitted to the NCBI database.

Recognized for his excellence, he has received numerous awards, including the Best Ph.D. Thesis Award (2011), Best Teacher Award (2015), and Prof. Ram Raksha Kiran Shukla Award (2023). His students have also earned prestigious accolades under his guidance. Beyond academia, he has contributed to state-level committees on zoonotic disease surveillance and veterinary recruitment, as well as public education initiatives reaching rural Gujarat.

A prolific author with over 50 research papers, 5 book chapters, and numerous editorial roles, Dr. Nayak is committed to advancing epidemiological surveillance and developing innovative diagnostic tools for zoonotic diseases. His dedication to teaching, research, and community outreach continues to make a significant impact on veterinary public health and the broader One Health framework.

Gyanendra Singh Sengar, PhD, is currently working as a National Post-Doctoral Fellow at the ICAR-National Research Centre on Pig, Guwahati, Assam, India. He obtained his doctoral degree in Biotechnology (Animal Sciences) at the Sam Higginbottom University of Agriculture, Technology and Sciences, Prayagraj, Uttar Pradesh, India. His current research focuses on the development of diagnostics and vaccines for livestock diseases.

His present work is based on development of bilateral immune assay for the simultaneous detection of African swine fever and classical swine fever virus. For this work he got the financial support from Anusandhan National Research Foundation, Government of India, New Delhi.

He has published 30 research papers in peer reviewed journals and also filed seven Indian patents, of which two have been granted. He also developed several innovative technologies. He has presented his research finding on various international conferences in Bangkok, Germany, and Vietnam. He is also peer reviewer of many reputed journals and given invited talk and acted as resource person in many universities and colleges.

Vivek Kumar Gupta, PhD, currently serves as the Director of the ICAR-National Research Centre on Pig, Guwahati, Assam, a position he has held since January 19, 2021. With over 32 years of experience in the Indian Council of Agricultural Research (ICAR), He has held various key roles, including Joint Director (CADRAD) at ICAR-IVRI, Izatnagar (2015–2021), and Principal Scientist of Veterinary Microbiology at ICAR-Central Institute for Research on Goats, Makhdoom, Uttar Pradesh, India.

He completed his BVSc & AH from Veterinary College, Mathura, Uttar Pradesh, and his MVSc and PhD in Veterinary Immunology from ICAR-Indian Veterinary Research Institute, Izatnagar. He also holds a PGD-TMA from the University of Hyderabad-NAARM and pursued postdoctoral research at the University of Wisconsin, Madison, USA. His contributions to veterinary science and livestock health are substantial, with a focus on small ruminants and pigs. He has authored over 200 research papers, 28 lead papers, and 7 books/manuals, in addition to numerous popular articles. He has led several national projects, including the All India Coordinated Research Project (AICRP) on Pig and two All India Network Programs on Bluetongue and Haemorrhagic Septicaemia, serving as Project Coordinator.

He has handled approximately 30 research projects, developed 19 technologies (three of which are commercialized), and holds 4 granted patents, 2 trademarks, 1 copyright, and 2 registered designs. He has mentored 5 PhD and 6 MVSc/MSc students and has served as a referee for more than 13 peer-reviewed journals and as an examiner for 6 academic institutions.

He has contributed significantly to institutional and livestock sector development through infrastructure creation, strengthening research linkages, supporting start-ups/Farmer Producer Organizations (FPOs), and providing incubation support, human resource development, and policy advisory for state governments and the Government of India.

His expertise has been recognized with prestigious fellowships, including the National Academy of Veterinary Sciences and the Indian Association of Veterinary Microbiologists, Immunologists, and Specialists in Infectious Diseases (IAVMI). Additionally, he has served as a member of scientific selection boards for State Agricultural Universities (SAUs) and Indian Council of Medical Research (ICMR), participated in several national committees of importance, and contributed to national-level examinations conducted by Agricultural Scientist Recruitment Board (ASRB).

Contributors

Surakaram Abhilash Department of Veterinary Microbiology, ICAR-Indian Veterinary Research Institute (ICAR-IVRI), Bareilly, Uttar Pradesh, India

Fatema Akter Department of Veterinary Microbiology, ICAR-Indian Veterinary Research Institute, Bareilly, Uttar Pradesh, India

Pranav Anjaria Kamdhenu University, Anand, Gujarat, India

College of Veterinary Science & Animal Husbandry, Kamdhenu University, Anand, Gujarat, India

Sejal Antiya Department of Veterinary Microbiology, College of Veterinary Science and Animal Husbandry at Kamdhenu University (KU), Anand, Gujarat, India

S. Arutkumaran ICAR-Indian Veterinary Research Institute, Bareilly, Uttar Pradesh, India

Varun Asediya M.B. Veterinary College, Dungarpur, Rajasthan, India

Nitin M. Attupuram National Research Centre on Pig, Indian Council of Agricultural Research, Guwahati, Assam, India

Taruna Bhati Department of Veterinary Microbiology and Biotechnology, College of Veterinary and Animal Science, Bikaner, Rajasthan, India

Indu Reddy Bode JRF, DBT-One Health Project, ICAR-National Meat Research Institute, Hyderabad, Telangana, India

M. S. Chandana Division of Biological Standardization, ICAR- Indian Veterinary Research Institute, Bareilly, Uttar Pradesh, India

Ravi Dabas Division of Medicine, ICAR-Indian Veterinary Research Institute, Bareilly, India

Rajib Deb National Research Centre on Pig, Indian Council of Agricultural Research, Guwahati, Assam, India

Dhruv Desai University of Pennsylvania, Philadelphia, PA, USA

Kritika Dhial Department of Veterinary Microbiology, Apollo College of Veterinary Medicine, Jaipur, Rajasthan, India

Apollo College of Veterinary Medicine, Jaipur, Rajasthan, India

Tapan Kumar Dutta Department of Veterinary Microbiology, CVSc&AH, Central Agricultural University, Aizawl, Mizoram, India

Department of Veterinary Microbiology, College of Veterinary Sciences and Animal Husbandry, Central Agricultural University, Selesih, Mizoram, India

Ashok Gaur Department of Veterinary Pharmacology and Toxicology, College of Veterinary and Animal Science, Bikaner, Rajasthan, India

Rajasthan University of Veterinary and Animal Sciences, Bikaner, Rajasthan, India

P. Manoj Kumar Goud ICAR-Indian Veterinary Research Institute (ICAR-IVRI), Bareilly, India

Surakaram Abhilash Goud Division of Veterinary Microbiology, ICAR-IVRI, Bareilly, Uttar Pradesh, India

M. Gowtham Division of Veterinary Microbiology, ICAR-IVRI, Bareilly, Uttar Pradesh, India

Vivek Kumar Gupta National Research Centre on Pig, Indian Council of Agricultural Research, Guwahati, Assam, India

A. Hemavathi ICAR-Indian Veterinary Research Institute, Bareilly, Uttar Pradesh, India

Prabodh Kumar Hembram Animal Resources Development Department, Government of West Bengal, Kolkata, West Bengal, India

Lakshmi Kant Department of Veterinary Pharmacology and Toxicology, College of Veterinary and Animal Science, Bikaner, Rajasthan, India

Rajasthan University of Veterinary and Animal Sciences, Bikaner, Rajasthan, India

Shivali Khandelwal ICAR-Indian Veterinary Research Institute (ICAR-IVRI), Izatnagar, Bareilly, Uttar Pradesh, India

D. Mohan Krishna Division of Animal Biotechnology, ICAR-NDRI, Karnal, Haryana, India

Gatchanda Shravan Kumar Department of Veterinary Parasitology, Shourabh College of Veterinary Science, Hindaun, Rajasthan, India

Pankaj Kumar Department of Veterinary Physiology, College of Veterinary and Animal Science, Bikaner, Rajasthan, India

Prem Kumar Division of Physiology and Climatology, ICAR-Indian Veterinary Research Institute, Izatnagar, Bareilly, India

Sanjeev Kumar Department of Veterinary Microbiology, Institute of Veterinary Science and Animal Husbandry, Siksha 'O' Anusandhan (Deemed to be University), Bhubaneswar, Odisha, India

Tapan R. Kumbhani Department of Veterinary Pathology, College of Veterinary Science and Animal Husbandry at Kamdhenu University (KU), Anand, Gujarat, India

Reddi Lokeswari ICAR-Indian Veterinary Research Institute (ICAR-IVRI), Bareilly, Uttar Pradesh, India

Bavadharani Mani ICAR-Indian Veterinary Research Institute (ICAR-IVRI), Hebbal,, Bengaluru, Karnataka, India

Belore Balaji Manoher Department of Veterinary Microbiology, ICAR-Indian Veterinary Research Institute (ICAR-IVRI), Bareilly, Uttar Pradesh, India

Irtiqa Manzoor Department of Veterinary Medicine, College of Veterinary & Animal Sciences, G.B. Pant University of Agriculture and Technology, Pantnagar, Uttarakhand, India

K. Meera National Research Centre on Pig, Indian Council of Agricultural Research, Guwahati, Assam, India

R. J. Modi Livestock Farm Complex, Collage of Veterinary Science and Animal Husbandry, Kamdhenu University, Anand, Gujarat, India

Mukul Department of Veterinary Public Health, ndian Veterinary Research Institute (IVRI), Izatnagar, Bareilly, Uttar Pradesh, India

Dumala Naveen ICAR-Indian Veterinary Research Institute (ICAR-IVRI), Izatnagar, Bareilly, Uttar Pradesh, India

J. B. Nayak Department of Veterinary Public Health and Epidemiology, College of Veterinary Science and Animal Husbandry, Kamdhenu University, Anand, Gujarat, India

Santanu Pal ICAR-Indian Veterinary Research Institute (ICAR-IVRI), Bareilly, Uttar Pradesh, India

J. H. Patel Livestock Farm Complex, Collage of Veterinary Science and Animal Husbandry, Kamdhenu University, Anand, Gujarat, India

N. M. Patel Department of Veterinary Public Health and Epidemiology, College of Veterinary Science and Animal Husbandry, Kamdhenu University, Anand, Gujarat, India

Y. G. Patel Department of Livestock Production Management, College of Veterinary Science and Animal Husbandry, Kamdhenu University, Anand, Gujarat, India

Abhishek Pathak Department of Veterinary Pharmacology & Toxicology, MJF College of Veterinary & Animal Sciences, Jaipur, Rajasthan, India

Department of Veterinary Pharmacology & Toxicology, Apollo College of Veterinary Medicine, Jaipur, Rajasthan, India

Seema Rani Pegu National Research Centre on Pig, Indian Council of Agricultural Research, Guwahati, Assam, India

N. Ratnamrutha Division of Biological Standardization, ICAR- Indian Veterinary Research Institute, Bareilly, Uttar Pradesh, India

Annepu Revathi Division of Biological Products, ICAR- Indian Veterinary Research Institute, Bareilly, Uttar Pradesh, India

Ravi Saraf M. B. Veterinary College, Rajasthan, India

Gyanendra Singh Sengar National Research Centre on Pig, Indian Council of Agricultural Research, Guwahati, Assam, India

S. Shanmathi ICAR-Indian Veterinary Research Institute, Bareilly, Uttar Pradesh, India

Pratishtha Sharma Department of Veterinary Pharmacology and Toxicology, College of Veterinary and Animal Science, Bikaner, Rajasthan, India

Rajasthan University of Veterinary and Animal Sciences, Bikaner, Rajasthan, India

Shruti Shaurya Division of Medicine, ICAR-Indian Veterinary Research Institute, Izatnagar, UP, India

Devendra Singh Department of Veterinary Pharmacology and Toxicology, College of Veterinary and Animal Science, Bikaner, Rajasthan, India

Rajasthan University of Veterinary and Animal Sciences, Bikaner, Rajasthan, India

J. L. Singh Department of Veterinary Medicine, College of Veterinary & Animal Sciences, G.B. Pant University of Agriculture and Technology, Pantnagar, Uttarakhand, India

Prachand Pratap Singh Division of Parasitology, ICAR-Indian Veterinary Research Institute, Izatnagar, Bareilly, India

E. N. P. Sneha Department of Veterinary Microbiology, ICAR-Indian Veterinary Research Institute (ICAR-IVRI), Bareilly, Uttar Pradesh, India

Tejpal ICAR-Indian Veterinary Research Institute (ICAR-IVRI), Bareilly, Uttar Pradesh, India

Sanjay Vaghela Kamdhenu University, Anand, Gujarat, India

Priyanshi Yadav ICAR-Indian Veterinary Research Institute (ICAR-IVRI), Izatnagar, Bareilly, Uttar Pradesh, India

Vishal Yadav ICAR-National Dairy Research Institute (ICAR-NDRI), Karnal, Haryana, India

Swine Farming Practices and Their Impact on Public Health

N. M. Patel, Y. G. Patel, R. J. Modi, J. H. Patel, and J. B. Nayak

Abstract

Intensive pig farming (IPF), characterized by high stocking densities and reliance on antibiotics, presents significant public health concerns. The excessive use of antibiotics in livestock contributes to the rise of antimicrobial resistance (AMR), limiting treatment options for human infections. IPF can also facilitate the emergence and spread of zoonotic diseases, such as influenza and African swine fever (ASF), posing a direct threat to human health. Furthermore, environmental pollution from IPF, including the release of greenhouse gases and organic waste, can degrade air and water quality, impacting human health and ecosystems. Occupational health risks for farm workers, including exposure to pathogens and hazardous working conditions, are also prevalent in this sector. Food safety concerns arise from potential contamination of pork products with bacteria like Salmonella and Campylobacter, increasing the risk of foodborne illnesses. Addressing these challenges requires a multifaceted approach, including promoting responsible antibiotic use, strengthening surveillance systems for zoonotic diseases and AMR, improving farm worker safety, and encouraging

N. M. Patel · J. B. Nayak
Department of Veterinary Public Health and Epidemiology, College of Veterinary Science and Animal Husbandry, Kamdhenu University, Anand, Gujarat, India
e-mail: jbnayak69@kamdhenuuni.edu.in

Y. G. Patel (✉)
Department of Livestock Production Management, College of Veterinary Science and Animal Husbandry, Kamdhenu University, Anand, Gujarat, India
e-mail: ygpatel89@kamdhenuuni.edu.in

R. J. Modi · J. H. Patel
Livestock Farm Complex, Collage of Veterinary Science and Animal Husbandry, Kamdhenu University, Anand, Gujarat, India
e-mail: rjmodi@kamdhenuuni.edu.in; jigarpatel@kamdhenuuni.edu.in

R. Deb et al. (eds.), *Emerging Zoonotic Threats from Swine*,
https://doi.org/10.1007/978-981-96-7407-7_1

theadoption of more sustainable farming practices. By implementing these measures, the swine farming industry can contribute to food security while minimizing its negative impacts on public health and the environment.

Keywords

Intensive pig farming · Antimicrobial resistance · Zoonotic diseases · Environmental pollution · Occupational health · Food safety

Introduction

Swine farming, an essential component of global agriculture, embodies a sophisticated amalgamation of management strategies and practices meticulously designed to rear and optimize the lifecycle of domestic pigs (Cole et al., 2000). This intricate domain traverses diverse aspects spanning housing and facilities, feeding and nutrition, health and disease management, breeding and reproduction, waste management, ethical considerations, technological integration, economic management, and sustainability efforts (Osterberg & Wallinga, 2004).

Type of Swine Farming

In a pig farming system, pigs are raised for meat using a variety of techniques and strategies. There are a lot of factors to consider, like effectiveness, animal well-being, environmental consequences, and economics. Depending on their characteristics and techniques, these systems can be classified as extended, semi-intensive, and intense (Davies, 2011).

A. **Extensive Swine Farming:**
   1. **Free-Range Systems:** Pigs in free-range systems frequently go foraging, rooting, and socializing. Besides providing shelter and food, farmers let pigs roam and exhibit their innate characteristics (Bench et al., 2013). The system increases animal comfort by giving pigs more autonomy and opportunities to do what they're naturally inclined to do. Usually found in small-scale or traditional agriculture (Hötzel et al., 2011).
   2. **Pasture-Based Systems:** Within specifically defined outdoor areas, pigs graze, consuming grass and forage crops (Garcia et al., 2015). By rotating paddocks, farmers can keep grazing areas under control and maximize forage production. To apply this technique, pigs must be capable of converting grass and fodder into meat. Compared to intensive systems, it enhances the health of the soil, has environmental advantages, and is more economical (Cole et al., 2000).

B. **Semi-Intensive Swine Farming:**
   1. **Outdoor/Indoor Systems:** It is possible for pigs to choose between indoor shelters and outside areas, allowing them to determine which environment they would prefer to live in (Mahfuz et al., 2022). Farmers provide their animals with cover, feeding spaces, and additional feed and they also ensure that the animals have access to the outdoors for physical activity and foraging. With the help of this system, a harmony can be achieved between the inherent behaviors of outdoor systems and the regulated conditions of interior systems (Stygar et al., 2020).
   2. **Deep-Bedded Systems:** Indoors, pigs are kept in permanent cages, typically in straw or wood shaving bedding that is covered with a substantial layer of bedding material. With the help of the bedding, the pigs are able to experience a variety of benefits, including comfort (Albernaz-Gonçalves et al., 2021), an absorption of waste, and the ability to display their natural behaviors and root. There is no doubt that farmers are making use of updated bedding and handling waste effectively, thereby creating a more comfortable and sanitary environment than slatted flooring (Sarrazin et al., 2019).

C. **Intensive Swine Farming:**
   1. **Confined Housing Systems:** In addition to being confined to indoor facilities, pigs have limited mobility. Specifically designed facilities cater to the optimization of feeding, the effective handling of waste, and the prevention of disease transmission (Mencía-Ares et al., 2021). Despite their ability to facilitate waste removal for enhanced cleanliness, fully slatted floors restrict pigs' ability to engage in innate behaviors. Due to superior productivity and environmental management, this is commonly observed in large commercial enterprises (Bellini et al., 2016).
   2. **Controlled Environment Systems:** Implementing cutting-edge technologies to control interior building temperatures, humidity, ventilation, and lighting. The purpose of this program is to increase pigs' growth rates, feed conversion efficiency, and stress factors. Precision agriculture techniques are commonly used on contemporary, technologically advanced commercial farms (Albernaz-Gonçalves et al., 2022).

D. **Integrated Farming Systems:**
   1. **Mixed Farming:** In addition to crops, livestock, and aquaculture, pigs are integrated into a multifaceted agricultural system. A closed-loop system can be achieved by using pig manure as a fertilizer for crops, thus improving sustainability. Economic stability and market resistance can be achieved through diversity within a system (Mahfuz et al., 2022).
   2. **Organic Farming:** Limit the use of synthetic chemicals, antibiotics, and genetically modified organisms in accordance with organic principles (Cole et al., 2000). During the rearing process, pigs are fed organic feed and are allowed to access the outdoors, adhering to strict welfare guidelines. Maintains a high level of concern for the responsible management of the environment, the preservation of a wide range of species, and the welfare of animals (Herskin & Di Giminiani, 2018).

E. **Considerations Across Systems:**
   (a) **Animal Welfare:** The level of animal welfare offered by different systems varies from one to another. There is no doubt that extensive systems allow pigs to display more natural behaviors compared to intensive systems (Grunert et al., 2018).
   (b) **Environmental Impact:** In intensive systems, waste and resources are concentrated, resulting in a larger environmental footprint. Extensive systems, on the other hand, may have less impact, but they require a greater amount of land (Mellor, 2016).
   (c) **Disease Management:** Biosecurity measures are often strictly implemented in intensive systems, while those in outdoor systems are less strict (Moberg & Mench, 2000).
   (d) **Feed Efficiency and Productivity:** Pig production is generally maximized in intensive systems as well. The opposite may be true for extensive systems, in which input costs are lower, but growth rates are slower (Garcia Pinillos et al., 2016).

Pig meat production systems vary considerably, offering a variety of approaches. There are many factors to consider when choosing a farming system, including the scale of operation, resources available, market demands, and animal welfare concerns (Baxter et al., 2013). The challenge of balancing productivity, sustainability, animal welfare, and profitability continues to spur research and innovation (von Keyserlingk & Hötzel, 2015).

Zoonotic Diseases Transmission from Swine to Humans

The term zoonotic disease refers to diseases that can be transmitted between animals and humans because of their infectious nature (Miyoshi et al., 2017). Because pigs have close contact with humans, whether in farming, consumption, or residential settings, it is now recognized that they are reservoirs for several zoonotic infections. It is important to note that these diseases pose significant public health challenges around the world (Uemoto et al., 2021). Here is an in-depth exploration of some prominent zoonotic diseases transmitted from pigs to humans:

1. **Influenza (Swine Flu)** (Woods, 2019)**:**
   - **Pathogen:** Influenza A virus, primarily subtype H1N1.
   - **Transmission:** Direct contact with infected pigs, inhalation of respiratory droplets, or contact with contaminated surfaces.
   - **Symptoms:** Fever, cough, sore throat, body aches, fatigue, and sometimes vomiting and diarrhea.
   - **Severity:** Can range from mild to severe, leading to hospitalization and even death in vulnerable populations.
   - **Pandemic Concerns:** Certain strains have caused global pandemics, with the potential to rapidly spread among humans.

2. **Salmonellosis** (Davies, 2011)**:**
    - **Pathogen:** Salmonella bacteria (mainly *Salmonella enterica*).
    - **Transmission:** Ingestion of contaminated pork or products, especially undercooked meat, as well as contact with infected animals or their feces.
    - **Symptoms:** Diarrhea, abdominal pain, fever, nausea, vomiting, and occasionally severe symptoms in vulnerable individuals.
    - **Prevention:** Thorough cooking of pork, proper hygiene, and sanitation practices in handling raw meat.
3. **Campylobacteriosis** (VanderWaal & Deen, 2018)**:**
    - **Pathogen:** Campylobacter bacteria (commonly *Campylobacter jejuni*).
    - **Transmission:** Ingestion of undercooked pork or contaminated food, water, or contact with infected animals or their feces.
    - **Symptoms:** Diarrhea (often bloody), abdominal pain, fever, and occasionally complications like Guillain-Barré syndrome.
    - **Prevention:** Cooking meat thoroughly, practicing good hygiene, and avoiding cross-contamination.
4. **Toxoplasmosis** (Drolet et al., 2019)**:**
    - **Pathogen:** *Toxoplasma gondii* parasite.
    - **Transmission:** Consumption of undercooked pork containing T. gondii cysts or contact with contaminated soil, water, or cat feces.
    - **Symptoms:** Often asymptomatic in healthy individuals but can cause flu-like symptoms or severe complications in pregnant women and immunocompromised individuals.
    - **Prevention:** Cooking meat thoroughly, washing hands and surfaces, and avoiding contact with cat feces.
5. **Hepatitis E** (Obregon-Gutierrez et al., 2021)**:**
    - **Pathogen:** Hepatitis E virus (HEV).
    - **Transmission:** Consumption of undercooked pork or contaminated water.
    - **Symptoms:** Like other forms of viral hepatitis, including jaundice, fatigue, abdominal pain, nausea, and fever.
    - **Risk Groups:** Pregnant women and those with underlying liver disease face higher risks of severe complications.
6. **Methicillin-Resistant Staphylococcus Aureus (MRSA)** (Rhouma et al., 2016)**:**
    - **Pathogen:** *Staphylococcus aureus* bacteria resistant to certain antibiotics.
    - **Transmission:** Contact with contaminated surfaces, including pork products, or direct contact with infected pigs or humans.
    - **Symptoms:** Skin infections, abscesses, pneumonia, and in severe cases, bloodstream infections.
    - **Prevention:** Strict hygiene measures, proper wound care, and antibiotic stewardship to reduce antibiotic resistance.
7. **Brucellosis** (Herskin & Di Giminiani, 2018)**:**
    - **Pathogen:** Brucella bacteria (e.g., *Brucella suis*).
    - **Transmission:** Direct contact with infected pigs, consumption of unpasteurized dairy products, or inhalation of aerosols.

- **Symptoms:** Fever, joint pain, fatigue, and potentially severe complications affecting the heart, liver, or nervous system.
- **Prevention:** Vaccination of animals, pasteurization of dairy products, and protective measures for those in contact with pigs.

8. **Trichinellosis** (Hötzel et al., 2018)**:**
   - **Pathogen:** Trichinella spiralis parasite.
   - **Transmission:** Consumption of undercooked pork containing encysted larvae.
   - **Symptoms:** Initially gastrointestinal issues followed by muscle pain, fever, swelling, and potentially serious complications affecting the heart, lungs, or nervous system.
   - **Prevention:** Thorough cooking and freezing of pork to kill larvae.
9. **Cryptosporidiosis** (Garcia Pinillos et al., 2016)**:**
   - **Pathogen:** Cryptosporidium parasite (e.g., *Cryptosporidium hominis*, *Cryptosporidium parvum*).
   - **Transmission:** Ingestion of contaminated water, food, or contact with infected animals or their feces.
   - **Symptoms:** Watery diarrhea, stomach cramps, nausea, and fever, which can be severe in immunocompromised individuals.
   - **Prevention:** Proper hygiene, avoiding contaminated water sources, and safe food handling practices.

Since these zoonotic diseases are transmitted from pigs to humans, it is important to practice basic hygiene, safe food handling, and thorough cooking practices to avoid infection (Wisener et al., 2021). Furthermore, by implementing rigorous biosecurity protocols in pig farming and veterinary care, this disease can be effectively mitigated. Both humans and animals will benefit from this action. To reduce the risks associated with zoonotic diseases, public awareness, education, and coordination are essential (Pedersen, 2018).

Antibiotic Resistance Concerns to Swine Farm Farming

It is important to recognize that antibiotic resistance in swine farming is a major issue that has a substantial impact on both animal health and human health (Mutua et al., 2020). Bacteria that exhibit antimicrobial resistance can survive the effects of antibiotics, thereby reducing their efficacy in combating bacterial infections. In the swine industry, antibiotics are widely used to prevent illness, enhance growth, and treat medical conditions, which has contributed to the creation and spread of antibiotic-resistant bacteria (Holman & Chénier, 2015). Here's an in-depth exploration of the concerns associated with antibiotic resistance in swine farming:

Antibiotic Use in Swine Farming:

1. **Disease Prevention and Treatment:** Pigs are commonly treated with antibiotics to prevent and treat bacterial infections. It is common for diseases to spread rapidly in crowded and intensive farming systems where animals are close to one

another, leading to the widespread use of antibiotics to control disease (Vishnuraj et al., 2016).
2. **Growth Promotion:** Swine farming uses antibiotics to promote growth. As a means of enhancing growth and improving feed efficiency, pigs were given sub-therapeutic doses of antibiotics (Rhouma et al., 2016).

Factors Contributing to Antibiotic Resistance:

- **Overuse and Misuse of Antibiotics:** In some cases, antibiotics are used indiscriminately or inappropriately, such as using them without proper diagnosis or prescription, leading to increased selective pressure on bacteria (Taneja & Sharma, 2019).
- **Sub-therapeutic Use:** Continuous administration of antibiotics at low doses for growth promotion purposes can promote the development of resistance among bacteria (Manyi-Loh et al., 2018).
- **Environmental Factors:** Antibiotics and resistant bacteria from swine farms can enter the environment through manure runoff, contaminating soil and water sources and potentially spreading resistance genes to other bacteria (Dowarah et al., 2018).
- **Transmission Pathways:** Resistant bacteria can spread from pigs to humans through direct contact, consumption of contaminated meat or products, or exposure to contaminated environments (Kahn, 2017).

Implications of Antibiotic Resistance in Swine Farming:

1. **Animal Health:** Antibiotic resistance compromises the effectiveness of antibiotics in treating bacterial infections in pigs, leading to prolonged illnesses, decreased welfare, and economic losses for farmers (Cheng et al., 2020).
2. **Public Health Concerns:** Resistant bacteria and antibiotic resistance genes can be transmitted from pigs to humans, potentially causing difficult-to-treat infections. People working in or living near swine farms are at a higher risk of exposure to resistant bacteria (Lekagul et al., 2019).
3. **Reduced Treatment Options:** Antibiotic resistance limits the effectiveness of antibiotics, reducing the number of available treatment options for both animal and human infections (Albernaz-Gonçalves et al., 2022).
4. **Increased Healthcare Costs and Risks:** Treating infections caused by antibiotic-resistant bacteria can be more challenging, leading to prolonged illnesses, increased healthcare costs, and a higher risk of treatment failure (Cuong et al., 2018).

Measures to Address Antibiotic Resistance in Swine Farming:

- **Regulation and Policy Changes:** Implementing regulations and policies to restrict the use of antibiotics as growth promoters and promote responsible antibiotic use in farming practices. Some countries have banned or restricted the use

of certain antibiotics for non-therapeutic purposes in animal agriculture (Waluszewski et al., 2021).
- **Veterinary Oversight and Prescription Control:** Encouraging veterinary oversight and requiring prescriptions for antibiotic use in swine farming to ensure proper diagnosis, dosage, and duration of treatment (Tiseo et al., 2020).
- **Alternative Strategies:** Exploring alternative strategies to antibiotics, such as probiotics, prebiotics, immunomodulators, and vaccines, to promote animal health and reduce the reliance on antibiotics (Wisener et al., 2021).
- **Improved Farm Management Practices:** Implementing better hygiene and biosecurity measures on farms to reduce the spread of infections and minimize the need for antibiotics (Centner, 2016).
- **Surveillance and Research:** Conducting surveillance programs to monitor antibiotic use, antibiotic resistance patterns, and the transmission of resistant bacteria from pigs to humans. Investing in research to develop new antibiotics, diagnostic tools, and alternative strategies to combat antibiotic resistance (Raasch et al., 2018).

Antibiotic resistance in swine farming poses significant challenges to both animal and human health. Addressing this issue requires a multifaceted approach that involves collaboration between the agricultural, veterinary, and healthcare sectors. Implementing stricter regulations, promoting responsible antibiotic use, exploring alternative strategies, and conducting surveillance and research are crucial steps in mitigating antibiotic resistance in swine farming (Van Boeckel et al., 2015). It's essential to prioritize prudent antibiotic use to safeguard animal welfare, public health, and the effectiveness of antibiotics for both veterinary and human medicine (Minssen et al., 2020).

Environmental Pollution and Its Health Implications for Swine Farm Farming

Environmental pollution can be caused by swine farming as well as other types of concentrated animal farming. A significant amount of waste is generated in swine farming; chemicals are used, and noxious gases can be released (Cole et al., 2000). As a result of these concerns, not only do they have an impact on the immediate surroundings, but they also have broader implications for the well-being of individuals. Environmental contamination in swine farming and its health consequences will be the focus of this comprehensive study (Osterberg & Wallinga, 2004).

Waste Management and Runoff:

1. **Manure Production:** Manure generated by swine farms contains nutrients, pathogens, and organic matter. A high concentration of manure is produced in intensive agricultural systems due to the enclosure of animals (Grunert et al., 2018).

2. **Nutrient Runoff:** A lack of proper handling of pig waste can result in the release of nutrients into water bodies, thereby causing water contamination. Manure-containing nutrients, such as nitrogen and phosphorus, can contaminate water bodies, resulting in eutrophication and altered aquatic ecosystems (Taneja & Sharma, 2019).
3. **Water Contamination:** Both surface and groundwater can be polluted by manure discharge. Pathogenic microorganisms like bacteria and viruses that are present in swine manure can cause waterborne illnesses (Penakalapati et al., 2017).

Air Quality and Emissions:

1. **Ammonia and Hydrogen Sulfide:** In the process of decomposing pig manure, pig farms release gases, such as ammonia (NH3) and hydrogen sulfide (H2S), which are harmful to humans. Particularly near swine farms, these gases can cause respiratory ailments, discomfort in the eyes, and other health complications in people, which may have serious health consequences (Shi et al., 2022).
2. **Particulate Matter:** In a pig farm, if the housing system is restricted, there are likely to be allergens, endotoxins, and other contaminants present. There are several respiratory illnesses that can be caused by breathing these particles into the lungs (Centner, 2016).
3. **Volatile Organic Compounds (VOCs):** Manure storage and treatment facilities can emit volatile organic compounds (VOCs), such as methane, as well as other organic compounds, when they store and treat manure. When people are exposed to volatile organic compounds (VOCs) for an extended period of time, the effects on their respiratory health are adverse, and ozone at ground level can worsen with prolonged exposure (Woolhouse et al., 2015).

Soil Quality:

1. **Nutrient Overloading:** As a result of improper management of swine manure as a fertilizer, soil nitrogen levels can be too high, leading to the accumulation of excess nutrients in the soil. Overabundances of nutrients in the soil can disrupt its inherent equilibrium, resulting in unfavorable effects on plant growth and the possibility of these nutrients migrating into the groundwater (Resuggen et al., 2019).
2. **Soil Erosion:** In addition to deforestation, land conversion to swine farming can exacerbate soil erosion in the area. Agricultural land productivity can be negatively impacted by soil erosion, which can in turn lead to the accumulation of sediment in water bodies, resulting in further deterioration of the quality of the water in these bodies (Bracke & Hopster, 2006).

Health Implications for Humans:

1. **Respiratory Issues:** Pig farms emit gases such as ammonia and hydrogen sulfide, which can cause irritation to the respiratory system because of the respiratory gases they emit. It has been reported that residents living near swine farms are more prone to coughing, wheezing, and heightened susceptibility to respiratory diseases due to their proximity to these farms (von Keyserlingk et al., 2015).
2. **Waterborne Diseases:** In some cases, the presence of pathogens from swine dung in water sources may be responsible for causing waterborne diseases. It is possible to contract viral and bacterial diseases such as gastroenteritis by either consuming or encountering contaminated water (Hötzel et al., 2011).
3. **Allergies and Asthma:** Pig farms emit particulate matter and allergens that cause allergies and asthma to worsen as they emit particulates and allergens. When there is a high level of airborne pollution in places where there are people with respiratory disorders, the symptoms may be more severe (Wen et al., 2021).
4. **Zoonotic Diseases:** Swine's serve as reservoirs for several zoonotic diseases, and, due to their proximity to swine farms, there is an increased chance that they may be transmitted to humans. Public health has been adversely affected because of bacterial infections that are resistant to antibiotics, flu, and other illnesses that pose a threat to public health (Zhang et al., 2020).

Regulatory Measures and Best Practices:

1. **Waste Management Plans:** Implementing comprehensive waste management strategies to effectively manage, process, and eliminate swine dung from a production system. In accordance with the principles of effective nutrient management, it is important to promote techniques such as the proper storage, treatment, and use of manure (Tatemoto et al., 2019).
2. **Emission Controls:** Emission control measures require the installation and regular maintenance of technologies such as biofilters and manure covers. Gases and particulates are effectively minimized. It would be advantageous if pig farms were located and configured in such a way as to mitigate adverse effects on air quality (Cheng et al., 2020).
3. **Buffer Zones:** In addition, by creating designated areas between swine farms and residential areas to mitigate the direct impact of emissions on human health, buffer zones will be established to mitigate emissions' direct impact on human health. It is possible to plant vegetation in these areas in order to absorb and purify pollutants in a human-friendly manner (Wisener et al., 2021).
4. **Nutrient Management:** Utilization of precision farming techniques and implementation of strategies to maximize nutrient efficiency from swine manure fertilizer can also be utilized in this process. It is imperative that excess manure is not applied to water bodies in order to reduce nutrient runoff (Dowarah et al., 2018).
5. **Sustainable Practices:** There is also a need to promote sustainable farming practices such as rotational grazing, agroforestry, and organic farming in order to minimize the impact on the environment. In order to improve soil health, it is

important to introduce a variety of farming techniques in order to reduce the dependence on intensive operations (Doster, 2000).

Environmental contamination caused by swine farming affects both ecosystems and human health. Sustainable farming methods, regulatory interventions, and technical advancements are needed to tackle these challenges (Marchant-Forde et al., 2014). Implementing emission control technology, improving waste management, and adopting optimal management practices reduce swine farming's environmental impact. Sustainable agriculture is possible while mitigating health hazards for neighboring towns and the wider population through ecologically conscious practices (Herskin et al., 2016).

Dynamics of Disease Transmission and Disease Outbreaks in Swine Farming

Swine farming is a critical component of global agriculture, providing a significant source of meat production. However, the industry faces constant challenges related to disease transmission, which can lead to devastating outbreaks (Mur et al., 2018). The dynamics of disease transmission in swine farming are influenced by various factors, including the concentration of animals, biosecurity measures, environmental conditions, and the movement of livestock (Zhang et al., 2021). This comprehensive exploration will delve into the intricate dynamics of disease transmission, common swine diseases, factors influencing outbreaks, and strategies for prevention and control (Meester et al., 2021).

I. Dynamics of Disease Transmission in Swine Farming
   1. **Direct Transmission:**
      (a) **Contact Transmission:** Direct physical contact between infected and susceptible pigs is a primary mode of transmission. This can occur during common behaviors such as mating, feeding, or fighting. Pathogens can be transferred through bodily fluids, skin contact, or mucous membrane exposure. For example, respiratory viruses, bacteria causing skin infections (Lindström et al., 2012).
      (b) **Aerosol Transmission:** Airborne transmission involves the spread of pathogens through respiratory droplets, creating a risk for susceptible pigs in close proximity. Infected pigs expel respiratory droplets containing pathogens during coughing or sneezing. For example, influenza viruses, mycoplasma bacteria (Chauhan & Gordon, 2022).
   2. **Indirect Transmission:**
      (a) **Fomite Transmission**: Inanimate objects or surfaces, such as equipment, feed, or clothing, can become contaminated and act as carriers for pathogens. Pigs come into contact with contaminated fomites, facilitating the transmission of pathogens. For example, Feed-borne diseases, pathogens on equipment (Rossi et al., 2017).

   (b) **Vector-Borne Transmission:** Arthropod vectors, such as ticks or mosquitoes, can transmit diseases by carrying pathogens from infected to susceptible pigs. Infected vectors introduce pathogens into the pig population through bites or contact. For examples, African swine fever (ASF) transmitted by ticks (Reynolds et al., 2014).

3. **Vertical Transmission:**
   (a) **Mother-to-Offspring Transmission:** Vertical transmission involves the passage of pathogens from a sow to her offspring during pregnancy, birth, or through infected milk. Infected sows transmit pathogens to piglets through the placenta, birth canal, or suckling. For examples, Transplacental transmission of viruses, bacterial infections through colostrum (Vijaykrishna et al., 2011).
4. **Environmental Transmission**:
   (a) **Fecal-Oral Transmission:** Contaminated water and feed present opportunities for pigs to ingest pathogens, leading to infections. Pigs consume water or feed contaminated with fecal material containing pathogens. For examples, Diseases caused by Salmonella, *E. coli* (Neumann, 2012).

II. **Common Swine Diseases and Their Dynamics:**

1. **African Swine Fever (ASF)** (Lehmann et al., 2003)**:**
   (a) **Virus:** African swine fever virus (ASFV).
   (b) **Hosts:** Domestic pigs and wild boars.
   (c) **Transmission Dynamics:**
      - **Direct Contact:** Close contact between infected and susceptible pigs.
      - **Contaminated Fomites:** Spread through contaminated objects or materials.
      - **Vector-Borne:** Transmission by arthropod vectors, especially soft ticks (*Ornithodoros* spp.).
      - **Airborne:** Limited but possible through aerosol transmission.
   (d) **Global Impact:**
      - ASF has a significant global impact due to its rapid spread, high mortality rates, and economic consequences.
      - The disease has been reported in Africa, Europe, Asia, and beyond, affecting both domestic and wild pig populations.
2. **Porcine Reproductive and Respiratory Syndrome (PRRS)** (Crombé et al., 2013)**:**
   (a) **Virus:** Porcine reproductive and respiratory syndrome virus (PRRSV).
   (b) **Hosts:** Domestic pigs and wild boars.
   (c) **Transmission Dynamics:**
      - **Direct Contact:** Mainly through direct pig-to-pig contact.
      - **Contaminated Fomites:** Spread via contaminated objects or equipment.
      - **Vertical Transmission:** Transmission from sow to piglet during pregnancy.
      - **Aerosol Transmission:** Airborne transmission of the virus.

(d) **Global Impact:**
- PRRS causes reproductive failure in sows, respiratory issues in pigs, and has significant economic implications due to decreased production efficiency.

3. **Swine Influenza** (Dietze et al., 2012):
   (a) **Viruses:** Influenza A viruses, including H1N1, H1N2, and H3N2 subtypes.
   (b) **Transmission Dynamics:**
   - **Respiratory Droplets:** Spread through respiratory droplets released by infected pigs.
   - **Direct Contact:** Close contact between infected and susceptible pigs.

   (c) **Zoonotic Potential:** Swine influenza viruses have been known to infect humans, especially those in close contact with infected pigs. Monitoring and surveillance are crucial to prevent potential pandemics. Certain strains of swine influenza have zoonotic potential, posing risks to human health.
4. **Classical Swine Fever (CSF)** (Thakur et al., 2016):
   (a) **Viruses:** Classical swine fever virus.
   (b) **Transmission Dynamics:**
   - **Direct Contact: Transmission through direct pig-to-pig contact.**
   - **Contaminated Fomites: Spread via contaminated objects or materials.**
   - **Wild Boars as Reservoirs:** Wild boars can act as reservoirs for the virus, contributing to the persistence of the disease.

   (c) **Economic Impact:** CSF causes high fever, hemorrhages, and high mortality rates. The economic impact is significant due to trade restrictions and control measures.
5. **Foot-and-Mouth Disease (FMD)** (Das et al., 2020):
   (a) **Viruses:** Foot-and-mouth disease virus.
   (b) **Transmission Dynamics:**
   - **Direct Contact:** Transmission through direct pig-to-pig contact.
   - **Aerosol Transmission: Airborne transmission of the virus.**
   - **Contaminated Fomites:** Spread via contaminated objects or materials.

   (c) **Economic Impact:** FMD results in fever, blisters, and lameness in pigs. The economic impact is severe due to trade restrictions and the culling of affected animals.

III. **Factors Influencing Disease Outbreaks** (Wang & Hu, 2023):
- **Confinement and Density:**
  - **Intensive Farming:** Concentrating large numbers of pigs in intensive farming systems increases the risk of disease transmission.
    - **Factors:** Close contact, shared environments, high density.
  - **Overcrowding:** High stocking density in confined spaces creates an environment conducive to rapid disease spread.

        - **Factors:** Limited space, increased stress, compromised biosecurity.
    - **Biosecurity Measures:**
      - **Inadequate Biosecurity:** Poor biosecurity practices contribute to the introduction and spread of diseases on swine farms.
        - **Factors:** Uncontrolled human and equipment movements, lax sanitation.
      - **Contaminated Vehicles:** Vehicles entering and leaving farms can act as vectors for pathogen introduction if not properly disinfected.
        - **Factors:** Limited space, increased stress, compromised biosecurity.
    - **Global Trade and Movements** (Whitaker et al., 2024)**:**
      - **International Movements:** The global trade of live pigs, pork products, and genetic materials increases the risk of introducing exotic diseases to new regions**.**
        - **Factors:** Movement across borders, insufficient quarantine measures.
      - **Local Movements:** The movement of pigs between farms or regions within a country can facilitate the spread of diseases.
        - **Factors:** Poor quarantine practices, inadequate monitoring.
    - **Wildlife Interactions** (Wang & Yang, 2022)**:**
      - **Contact with Wild Animals:** Interaction between domestic pigs and wildlife can introduce and spread diseases.
        - **Factors:** Shared environments, lack of barriers.
    - **Disease Reservoirs:**
      - **Carrier Pigs:** Some pigs may carry pathogens without exhibiting clinical signs, serving as reservoirs for diseases.
        - **Factors:** Challenges in identifying carriers, inadequate testing.
    - **Environmental Factors** (Wang et al., 2023)**:**
      - **Climate Conditions:** Weather conditions, such as temperature and humidity, can influence the survival and transmission of certain pathogens.
        - **Factors:** Seasonal variations, impact on pathogen stability.
    - **Introduction of New Animals** (Garforth et al., 2013)**:**
      - **Poor Quarantine Practices:** The introduction of new pigs to a farm without proper quarantine measures can lead to the introduction of diseases.
        - **Factors:** Inadequate isolation, insufficient health monitoring.
    - **Genetic Susceptibility** (Bergmann et al., 2021)**:**
      - **Variability in Susceptibility:** Genetic factors can influence the susceptibility of pigs to specific diseases.
        - **Factors:** Breeding for resistance, selecting stock with a history of good health.

IV. **Strategies for Disease Prevention and Control:**
    - **Biosecurity Measures** (VanderWaal & Deen, 2018)**:**
      - **Restricted Access:** Implement strict access controls to farms, limiting human and vehicle movement.
        - **Implementation:** Controlled entry points, visitor protocols.

- **Quarantine Practices** (De Lucia & Ostanello, 2020)**:**
  - **Restricted Access:** Quarantine new animals and closely monitor their health before integrating them into existing herds.
    - **Implementation:** Isolation facilities, health assessments.
- **Vaccination Programs** (Nöremark et al., 2009)**:**
  - **Routine Vaccination:** Implement routine vaccination programs to protect against common swine diseases.
    - **Implementation:** Timely vaccination schedules, collaboration with veterinarians.
  - **Disease-Specific Vaccines:** Use vaccines tailored to the prevalent diseases in a particular region or farm.
    - **Implementation:** Periodic reviews of vaccine efficacy, adjustments based on disease trends.
- **Surveillance and Monitoring** (Davies, 2011)**:**
  - **Early Detection:** Implement surveillance programs to detect diseases at an early stage.
    - **Implementation:** Regular health monitoring, diagnostic testing.
  - **Diagnostic Testing:** Regularly test animals for common diseases, especially when introducing new animals or during periods of increased risk.
    - **Implementation:** Laboratory partnerships, rapid testing technologies.
- **Education and Training** (Bellini et al., 2016)**:**
  - **Farm Personnel Training:** Educate farm personnel about disease prevention, recognition of clinical signs, and the importance of biosecurity measures.
    - **Implementation:** Training programs, informational resources.
  - **Communication:** Establish communication channels with veterinary authorities to stay informed about disease trends and outbreaks.
    - **Implementation:** Reporting mechanisms, collaborative networks.
- **Environmental Management** (Ebata et al., 2020)**:**
  - **Waste Management:** Properly manage swine manure to minimize the risk of disease transmission.
    - **Implementation:** Adequate storage, treatment, and disposal procedures.
  - **Vector Control:** Implement measures to control vectors such as insects and rodents that can contribute to disease spread.
    - **Implementation:** Environmental modifications, targeted control strategies.
- **Genetic Selection** (Fablet, 2009)**:**
  - **Breeding for Resistance:** Incorporate genetic selection for disease resistance in breeding programs.
    - **Implementation:** Collaborate with geneticists, ongoing evaluation of resistance traits.
  - **Improved Stock:** Select breeding stock with a history of good health and resistance to prevalent diseases.

  - **Implementation:** Regular health assessments, collaboration with breeding programs.
- **International Collaboration** (Hsu et al., 2023):
  - **Surveillance Sharing:** Collaborate internationally to share information on disease surveillance, outbreaks, and control measures.
    - **Implementation:** Global health organizations coordinated efforts.
  - **Trade Regulations:** Establish and adhere to international trade regulations to prevent the spread of diseases across borders.
    - **Implementation:** Compliance with global standards, transparent reporting.

It is complex and multidimensional to transmit diseases and prepare for outbreaks in swine husbandry. Effective preventative and control techniques require an understanding of these processes (Straw et al., 2013). Vaccination programs, surveillance, and international coordination are key components for effective disease control in swine herds. With a comprehensive and integrated approach, the swine industry can strengthen its resilience, safeguard animal health, and maintain sustainable production of high-quality pork despite challenges posed by disease transmission dynamics in a world of interconnected swine farming (Delsart et al., 2020).

Health Effects on Workers and Nearby Communities Associated with Swine Farming

Swine farming, a crucial aspect of global agriculture, plays a significant role in providing meat products for human consumption. While it contributes to food security and economic development, the industry is not without challenges (Donham, 2010). One of the key concerns is the potential health effects on both workers directly involved in swine farming and nearby communities. This comprehensive exploration will delve into the various health risks associated with swine farming, examining both occupational hazards for workers and the potential impact on the health of individuals living in proximity to swine farms (Villeneuve et al., 2009).

I. **Occupational Health Risks for Swine Farm Workers:**

  A. **Respiratory Health** (Donham et al., 2007):

  - **Exposure to Airborne Particulates:** Swine farming operations generate airborne particulates, including dust, dander, and microbial agents, which can pose respiratory risks to workers.
    - **Health effects:** Increased risk of respiratory issues such as asthma, chronic bronchitis, and exacerbation of pre-existing conditions.
  - **Inhalation of Harmful Gases:** Swine manure produces gases like ammonia and hydrogen sulfide, which, when inhaled, can lead to respiratory irritation and compromise lung function.
    - **Health effects:** Respiratory symptoms, irritation of the eyes and throat, exacerbation of respiratory diseases.

B. **Zoonotic Infections** (Von Essen & Auvermann, 2005)**:**
- **Direct Contact with Pigs:** Swine workers are at risk of zoonotic infections through direct contact with pigs, which can transmit diseases such as influenza, Salmonella, and Escherichia coli.
  - **Health effects:** Influenza-like illnesses, gastrointestinal infections, and potential for antibiotic-resistant strains.

C. **Skin and Allergies** (Casey et al., 2015)**:**
- **Contact with Allergens:** Handling pigs, manure, and feed exposes workers to allergens and irritants, leading to skin conditions and allergies.
  - **Health effects:** Dermatitis, skin rashes, and respiratory allergies.

D. **Musculoskeletal Issues** (Hu et al., 2017)**:**
- **Manual Labor and Repetitive Movements:** Swine farming often involves manual labor and repetitive movements, leading to musculoskeletal problems.
  - **Health effects:** Back pain, joint issues, and musculoskeletal strains.

E. **Noise-Related Health Risks:** Swine farms can be noisy environments due to equipment, ventilation systems, and pig vocalizations, leading to potential hearing damage.
- **Health effects**: Noise-induced hearing loss and related stress.

II. **Health Impact on Nearby Communities:**

1. Air Quality Concerns (Benjamin & Yik, 2019):	**Health effects**
(a) **Odor emissions:** Swine farming operations can release odorous compounds, including ammonia and sulfur compounds, affecting air quality in nearby communities	Respiratory irritation, nausea, and stress-related symptoms
(b) **Airborne particulate matter:** Particulate matter from swine farms can be carried by the wind, impacting air quality and potentially causing respiratory issues	Exacerbation of respiratory conditions, cardiovascular effects
2. Water Quality and Contamination (Nadimpalli et al., 2018):	
(a) **Runoff from swine manure:** Improper management of swine manure can lead to nutrient runoff, contaminating water sources with pathogens and pollutants	Waterborne diseases, gastrointestinal infections, and potential exposure to antibiotic-resistant bacteria
3. Zoonotic Disease Transmission (Borlée et al., 2017):	
(a) **Spread of diseases to humans:** Zoonotic diseases from swine farms can be transmitted to nearby communities through various pathways, including direct contact, contaminated water, or airborne transmission	Potential outbreaks of zoonotic infections, including influenza and antibiotic-resistant bacterial strains
4. Mental Health Impact (Dutkiewicz et al., 2017):	
(a) **Odor-related stress:** Odor emissions from swine farms can lead to stress and mental health issues among nearby residents	Increased stress levels, anxiety, and decreased quality of life

5. Socioeconomic Impact (Townsend, 2017):	
(a) **Property values and livelihoods:** The presence of swine farms in the vicinity can impact property values and affect the livelihoods of nearby residents	Stress-related health issues due to concerns about property values and community well-being

III. Strategies for Mitigation and Improvement:

1. Occupational Health Measures (Weiss, 2016):	**Implementation**
(a) **Personal protective equipment (PPE):** Providing workers with appropriate PPE, including respiratory masks, gloves, and coveralls, to minimize exposure to airborne particulates and pathogens	Mandatory use of PPE, regular training programs
(b) **Improved ventilation systems:** Upgrading ventilation systems in swine barns to reduce the concentration of airborne pollutants and improve air quality for workers	Installation of efficient ventilation systems, regular maintenance
2. Enhanced Biosecurity Practices: (Jensen et al., 2018)	
(a) **Hygiene protocols:** Implementing strict hygiene protocols to reduce the risk of zoonotic infections among swine workers	Regular handwashing, use of disinfectants, and proper sanitation measures
3. Sustainable Manure Management (Blanchette, 2020):	
(a) **Manure treatment and storage:** Adopting sustainable manure management practices, including proper treatment and storage, to reduce odor emissions and water contamination	Use of anaerobic digesters, manure lagoons, and innovative treatment technologies
4. Technology and Innovation (Gržinić et al., 2023):	
(a) **Air quality monitoring systems:** Installing air quality monitoring systems to assess and mitigate the impact of airborne pollutants on both workers and nearby communities	Continuous monitoring, data analysis, and real-time reporting
5. Community Engagement (Molnár & Fraser, 2020):	
(a) **Communication and education:** Engaging with nearby communities through effective communication and education programs to address concerns, disseminate information, and build awareness	Town hall meetings, informational campaigns, community workshops
6. Regulatory Measures (Clark et al., 2017):	
(a) **Stringent regulations:** Implementing and enforcing stringent regulations on swine farming practices to ensure compliance with health and environmental standards	Regular inspections, penalties for non-compliance, and continuous improvement of regulatory frameworks
7. Sustainable Practices (Alonso et al., 2020):	
(a) **Transition to sustainable farming:** Encouraging the adoption of sustainable swine farming practices, including organic farming, rotational grazing, and agroforestry	Incentives for sustainable practices, awareness campaigns

IV. Future Considerations and Research:

1. Long-Term Health Studies (Menchaca, 2021):	**Implementation**
(a) Epidemiological studies: Conducting long-term epidemiological studies to assess the health effects on both swine farm workers and nearby communities	Collaborative research initiatives, involvement of public health institutions
2. Technological Innovations (Andersson et al., 2020):	
(a) Advancements in farming technology: Investing in and adopting technological innovations that reduce environmental impact, minimize odors, and enhance overall sustainability	Research and development partnerships, technology transfer initiatives
3. Community-Driven Solutions (De Oliveira et al., 2019):	
(a) Participatory approaches: Engaging communities in the development of solutions and mitigation strategies to address their specific concerns related to swine farming	Community forums, participatory decision-making processes
4. Policy Advocacy (Meyer et al., 2020):	
(a) Stakeholder engagement: Advocating for policies that prioritize the health and Well-being of both swine workers and nearby communities	Collaboration with policymakers, advocacy groups, and industry stakeholders

People living near swine farms and personnel directly involved in farming face health hazards. This problem requires a comprehensive approach, which includes implementing better health protection measures, enforcing stricter regulations, creating sustainable manure management methods, involving the community, and developing new technologies (Rault et al., 2020). Since swine farming is continuing to grow, it is vital to emphasize the physical and mental health of individuals and the community (Lange et al., 2020). To reduce its impact on public health, the swine farming sector should conduct cooperative endeavors, conduct research, and implement sustainable methods. As a result, it will allow the agricultural industry to become more efficient and robust (Wen et al., 2021).

References

Albernaz-Gonçalves, R., Olmos, G., & Hötzel, M. J. (2021). My pigs are ok, why change? – Animal welfare accounts of pig farmers. *Animal: An International Journal of Animal Bioscience, 15*(3), 100154.

Albernaz-Gonçalves, R., Olmos Antillón, G., & Hötzel, M. J. (2022). Linking animal welfare and antibiotic use in pig farming—A review. *Animals, 12*(2), 216.

Alonso, M. E., González-Montaña, J. R., & Lomillos, J. M. (2020). Consumers' concerns and perceptions of farm animal welfare. *Animals: An Open Access Journal from MDPI, 10*(3), 385.

Andersson, E., Frössling, J., Westin, R., Algers, B., & Gunnarsson, S. (2020). Associations between litter size and medical treatment of sows during farrowing and lactation. *Acta Agriculturae Scandinavica. Section A, Animal Science, 69*(3), 176–182.

Baxter, E. M., Rutherford, K. M. D., D'Eath, R. B., Arnott, G., Turner, S. P., Sandøe, P., et al. (2013). The welfare implications of large litter size in the domestic pig II: Management factors. *Animal Welfare (South Mimms, England), 22*(2), 219–238.

Bellini, S., Rutili, D., & Guberti, V. (2016). Preventive measures aimed at minimizing the risk of African swine fever virus spread in pig farming systems. *Acta Veterinaria Scandinavica, 58*(1), 82.

Bench, C. J., Rioja-Lang, F. C., Hayne, S. M., & Gonyou, H. W. (2013). Group gestation housing with individual feeding—I: How feeding regime, resource allocation, and genetic factors affect sow welfare. *Livestock Science, 152*(2–3), 208–217.

Benjamin, M., & Yik, S. (2019). Precision livestock farming in swine welfare: A review for swine practitioners. *Animals, 9*(4), 133.

Bergmann, H., Schulz, K., Conraths, F. J., & Sauter-Louis, C. (2021). A review of environmental risk factors for African swine fever in European wild boar. *Animals, 11*(9), 2692.

Blanchette, A. (2020). *Porkopolis: American animality, standardized life, and the factory farm*. Duke University Press.

Borlée, F., Yzermans, C. J., Aalders, B., Rooijackers, J., Krop, E., Maassen, C. B., et al. (2017). Air pollution from livestock farms is associated with airway obstruction in neighboring residents. *American Journal of Respiratory and Critical Care Medicine, 196*(9), 1152–1161.

Bracke, M. B. M., & Hopster, H. (2006). Assessing the importance of natural behavior for animal welfare. *Journal of Agricultural & Environmental Ethics, 19*(1), 77–89.

Casey, J. A., Kim, B. F., Larsen, J., Price, L. B., & Nachman, K. E. (2015). Industrial food animal production and community health. *Current Environmental Health Reports, 2*, 259–271.

Centner, T. J. (2016). Recent government regulations in the United States seek to ensure the effectiveness of antibiotics by limiting their agricultural use. *Environment International, 94*, 1–7.

Chauhan, R. P., & Gordon, M. L. (2022). A systematic review of influenza a virus prevalence and transmission dynamics in backyard swine populations globally. *Porcine Health Management, 8*(1), 10.

Cheng, D., Ngo, H. H., Guo, W., Chang, S. W., Nguyen, D. D., Liu, Y., et al. (2020). A critical review on antibiotics and hormones in swine wastewater: Water pollution problems and control approaches. *Journal of Hazardous Materials, 387*, 121682.

Clark, B., Stewart, G. B., Panzone, L. A., Kyriazakis, I., & Frewer, L. J. (2017). Citizens, consumers and farm animal welfare: A meta-analysis of willingness-to-pay studies. *Food Policy, 68*, 112–127.

Cole, D., Todd, L., & Wing, S. (2000). Concentrated swine feeding operations and public health: A review of occupational and community health effects. *Environmental Health Perspectives, 108*(8), 685–699.

Crombé, F., Argudín, M. A., Vanderhaeghen, W., Hermans, K., Haesebrouck, F., & Butaye, P. (2013). Transmission dynamics of methicillin-resistant Staphylococcus aureus in pigs. *Frontiers in Microbiology, 4*, 57.

Cuong, N. V., Padungtod, P., Thwaites, G., & Carrique-Mas, J. J. (2018). Antimicrobial usage in animal production: A review of the literature with a focus on low-and middle-income countries. *Antibiotics, 7*(3), 75.

Das, S., Das, P., & Das, P. (2020). Control of Nipah virus outbreak in commercial pig-farm with biosecurity and culling. *Mathematical Modelling of Natural Phenomena, 15*, 64.

Davies, P. R. (2011). Intensive swine production and pork safety. *Foodborne Pathogens and Disease, 8*(2), 189–201.

De Lucia, A., & Ostanello, F. (2020). On-farm risk factors associated with salmonella in pig herds. *Large Animals Review, 26*, 133–140.

De Oliveira, D., Keeling, L. J., & Da Costa, M. J. R. P. (2019). Individual variation over time in piglet's reactions to early handling and its association to weight gain. *Applied Animal Behaviour Science, 215*, 7–12.

Delsart, M., Pol, F., Dufour, B., Rose, N., & Fablet, C. (2020). Pig farming in alternative systems: strengths and challenges in terms of animal welfare, biosecurity, animal health and pork safety. *Agriculture, 10*(7), 261.

Dietze, K., Beltran-Alcrudo, D., Pinto, J., Khomenko, S., Slingenbergh, J., & Lubroth, J. (2012). Factors affecting emergence of diseases in swine. In *IPVS 2012 Korea 22nd International Pig Veterinary Society congress; IPVS: Jeju, Korea* (pp. 11–15).

Donham, K. J. (2010). Community and occupational health concerns in pork production: A review. *Journal of Animal Science, 88*(suppl_13), E102–E111.

Donham, K. J., Wing, S., Osterberg, D., Flora, J. L., Hodne, C., Thu, K. M., & Thorne, P. S. (2007). Community health and socioeconomic issues surrounding concentrated animal feeding operations. *Environmental Health Perspectives, 115*(2), 317–320.

Doster, A. R. (2000). Porcine gastric ulcer. *The Veterinary Clinics of North America. Food Animal Practice, 16*(1), 163–174.

Dowarah, R., Verma, A. K., Agarwal, N., Singh, P., & Singh, B. R. (2018). Selection and characterization of probiotic lactic acid bacteria and its impact on growth, nutrient digestibility, health and antioxidant status in weaned piglets. *PLoS One, 13*(3), e0192978.

Drolet, R., System Zimmerman, J. J., Karriker, L. A., Ramirez, A., Schwartz, K. J., Stevenson, G. W., & Zhang, J. (2019). *Diseases of swine* (pp. 408–424). Wiley.

Dutkiewicz, J., Sroka, J., Zając, V., Wasiński, B., Cisak, E., Sawczyn, A., et al. (2017). Streptococcus suis: A re-emerging pathogen associated with occupational exposure to pigs or pork products. Part I – Epidemiology. *Annals of Agricultural and Environmental Medicine, 24*(4), 683–695.

Ebata, A., MacGregor, H., Loevinsohn, M., & Win, K. S. (2020). Why behaviours do not change: Structural constraints that influence household decisions to control pig diseases in Myanmar. *Preventive Veterinary Medicine, 183*, 105138.

Fablet, C. (2009). An overview of the impact of the environment on enzootic respiratory diseases in pigs. *Sustainable Animal Production*, 239–260. https://doi.org/10.3920/9789086866854_019

Garcia, A., Pirner, G., Picinin, G., May, M., Guay, K., Backus, B., et al. (2015). Effect of provision of feed and water during transport on the welfare of weaned pigs. *Animals: An Open Access Journal from MDPI, 5*(2), 407–425.

Garforth, C. J., Bailey, A. P., & Tranter, R. B. (2013). Farmers' attitudes to disease risk management in England: A comparative analysis of sheep and pig farmers. *Preventive Veterinary Medicine, 110*(3–4), 456–466.

Grunert, K. G., Sonntag, W. I., Glanz-Chanos, V., & Forum, S. (2018). Consumer interest in environmental impact, safety, health and animal welfare aspects of modern pig production: Results of a cross-national choice experiment. *Meat Science, 137*, 123–129.

Gržinić, G., Piotrowicz-Cieślak, A., Klimkowicz-Pawlas, A., Górny, R. L., Ławniczek-Wałczyk, A., Piechowicz, L., et al. (2023). Intensive poultry farming: A review of the impact on the environment and human health. *Science of the Total Environment, 858*, 160014.

Herskin, M. S., & Di Giminiani, P. (2018). Pain in pigs: Characterisation, mechanisms and indicators. In *Advances in pig welfare* (pp. 325–355). Elsevier.

Herskin, M. S., Jensen, H. E., Jespersen, A., Forkman, B., Jensen, M. B., Canibe, N., & Pedersen, L. J. (2016). Impact of the amount of straw provided to pigs kept in intensive production conditions on the occurrence and severity of gastric ulceration at slaughter. *Research in Veterinary Science, 104*, 200–206.

Holman, D. B., & Chénier, M. R. (2015). Antimicrobial use in swine production and its effect on the swine gut microbiota and antimicrobial resistance. *Canadian Journal of Microbiology, 61*(11), 785–798.

Hötzel, M. J., de Souza, G. P. P., Costa, O. A. D., & Machado Filho, L. C. P. (2011). Disentangling the effects of weaning stressors on piglets' behaviour and feed intake: Changing the housing and social environment. *Applied Animal Behaviour Science, 135*(1–2), 44–50.

Hötzel, M. J., Mota, S. M., Ludtke, C. B., & Poletto, R. (2018). Knowledge and attitudes of official inspectors at slaughterhouses in southern Brazil regarding animal welfare. *Revista Brasileira de Zootecnia, 47*. https://doi.org/10.1590/rbz4720170065

Hsu, C. H., Schambow, R., Montenegro, M., Miclat-Sonaco, R., & Perez, A. (2023). Factors affecting the spread, diagnosis, and control of African swine fever in The Philippines. *Pathogens, 12*(8), 1068.

Hu, Y., Cheng, H., & Tao, S. (2017). Environmental and human health challenges of industrial livestock and poultry farming in China and their mitigation. *Environment International, 107*, 111–130.

Jensen, J., Kyvsgaard, N. C., Battisti, A., & Baptiste, K. E. (2018). Environmental and public health related risk of veterinary zinc in pig production-using Denmark as an example. *Environment International, 114*, 181–190.

Kahn, L. H. (2017). Antimicrobial resistance: A One Health perspective. *Transactions of the Royal Society of Tropical Medicine and Hygiene, 111*(6), 255–260.

Lange, A., Gentz, M., Hahne, M., Lambertz, C., Gauly, M., Burfeind, O., & Traulsen, I. (2020). Effects of different farrowing and rearing systems on post-weaning stress in piglets. *Agriculture, 10*(6), 230.

Lehmann, T., Graham, D. H., Dahl, E., Sreekumar, C., Launer, F., Corn, J. L., et al. (2003). Transmission dynamics of toxoplasma gondii on a pig farm. *Infection, Genetics and Evolution, 3*(2), 135–141.

Lekagul, A., Tangcharoensathien, V., & Yeung, S. (2019). Patterns of antibiotic use in global pig production: A systematic review. *Veterinary and Animal Science, 7*, 100058.

Lindström, T., Lewerin, S. S., & Wennergren, U. (2012). Influence on disease spread dynamics of herd characteristics in a structured livestock industry. *Journal of the Royal Society Interface, 9*(71), 1287–1294.

Mahfuz, S., Mun, H. S., Dilawar, M. A., & Yang, C. J. (2022). Applications of smart technology as a sustainable strategy in modern swine farming. *Sustainability, 14*(5), 2607.

Manyi-Loh, C., Mamphweli, S., Meyer, E., & Okoh, A. (2018). Antibiotic use in agriculture and its consequential resistance in environmental sources: Potential public health implications. *Molecules, 23*(4), 795.

Marchant-Forde, J. N., Lay, D. C., Jr., McMunn, K. A., Cheng, H. W., Pajor, E. A., & Marchant-Forde, R. M. (2014). Postnatal piglet husbandry practices and well-being: The effects of alternative techniques delivered in combination. *Journal of Animal Science, 92*(3), 1150–1160.

Meester, M., Tobias, T. J., Bouwknegt, M., Kusters, N. E., Stegeman, J. A., & van der Poel, W. H. (2021). Infection dynamics and persistence of hepatitis E virus on pig farms – A review. *Porcine Health Management, 7*, 1–16.

Mellor, D. J. (2016). Updating animal welfare thinking: Moving beyond the "five freedoms" towards "a life worth living". *Animals, 6*(3), 21.

Menchaca, A. (2021). Sustainable food production: The contribution of genome editing in livestock. *Sustainability, 13*(12), 6788.

Mencía-Ares, O., Argüello, H., Puente, H., Gómez-García, M., Manzanilla, E. G., Álvarez-Ordóñez, A., et al. (2021). Antimicrobial resistance in commensal Escherichia coli and Enterococcus spp. is influenced by production system, antimicrobial use, and biosecurity measures on Spanish pig farms. *Porcine Health Management, 7*(1), 27.

Meyer, D., Amalraj, D., Van Limbergen, A., Fockedey, T., Edwards, M., Moustsen, S., et al. (2020). Short communication: Effect of positive handling of sows on litter performance and pre-weaning piglet mortality. *Animal, 14*, 1733–1739.

Minssen, T., Outterson, K., Van Katwyk, S. R., Batista, P. H. D., Chandler, C. I., Ciabuschi, F., et al. (2020). Social, cultural and economic aspects of antimicrobial resistance. *Bulletin of the World Health Organization, 98*(12), 823.

Miyoshi, J., Bobe, A. M., Miyoshi, S., Huang, Y., Hubert, N., Delmont, T. O., et al. (2017). Peripartum antibiotics promote gut dysbiosis, loss of immune tolerance, and inflammatory bowel disease in genetically prone offspring. *Cell Reports, 20*(2), 491–504.

Moberg, G. P., & Mench, J. A. (Eds.). (2000). *The biology of animal stress: Basic principles and implications for animal welfare*. CABI.

Molnár, M., & Fraser, D. (2020). Protecting farm animal welfare during intensification: Farmer perceptions of economic and regulatory pressures. *Animal Welfare (South Mimms, England), 29*(2), 133–141.

Mur, L., Sánchez-Vizcaíno, J. M., Fernández-Carrión, E., Jurado, C., Rolesu, S., Feliziani, F., et al. (2018). Understanding African swine fever infection dynamics in Sardinia using a spatially explicit transmission model in domestic pig farms. *Transboundary and Emerging Diseases, 65*(1), 123–134.

Mutua, F., Sharma, G., Grace, D., Bandyopadhyay, S., Shome, B., & Lindahl, J. (2020). A review of animal health and drug use practices in India, and their possible link to antimicrobial resistance. *Antimicrobial Resistance & Infection Control, 9*, 1–13.

Nadimpalli, M. L., Stewart, J. R., Pierce, E., Pisanic, N., Love, D. C., Hall, D., et al. (2018). Face mask use and persistence of livestock-associated Staphylococcus aureus nasal carriage among industrial hog operation workers and household contacts, USA. *Environmental Health Perspectives, 126*(12), 127005.

Neumann, E. J. (2012). Disease transmission and biosecurity. In *Diseases of swine* (10th ed., pp. 141–164). Wiley.

Nöremark, M., Lindberg, A., Vågsholm, I., & Lewerin, S. S. (2009). Disease awareness, information retrieval and change in biosecurity routines among pig farmers in association with the first PRRS outbreak in Sweden. *Preventive Veterinary Medicine, 90*(1–2), 1–9.

Obregon-Gutierrez, P., Aragon, V., & Correa-Fiz, F. (2021). Sow contact is a major driver in the development of the nasal microbiota of piglets. *Pathogens, 10*(6), 697.

Osterberg, D., & Wallinga, D. (2004). Addressing externalities from swine production to reduce public health and environmental impacts. *American Journal of Public Health, 94*(10), 1703–1708.

Pedersen, L. J. (2018). Overview of commercial pig production systems and their main welfare challenges. In *Advances in pig welfare* (pp. 3–25). Elsevier.

Penakalapati, G., Swarthout, J., Delahoy, M. J., McAliley, L., Wodnik, B., Levy, K., & Freeman, M. C. (2017). Exposure to animal feces and human health: A systematic review and proposed research priorities. *Environmental Science & Technology, 51*(20), 11537–11552.

Pinillos, R. G., Appleby, M. C., Manteca, X., Scott-Park, F., Smith, C., & Velarde, A. (2016). One Welfare–a platform for improving human and animal welfare. *Veterinary Record, 179*(16), 412–413.

Raasch, S., Postma, M., Dewulf, J., Stärk, K. D. C., & grosse Beilage, E. (2018). Association between antimicrobial usage, biosecurity measures as well as farm performance in German farrow-to-finish farms. *Porcine Health Management, 4*, 1–14.

Rault, J.-L., Waiblinger, S., Boivin, X., & Hemsworth, P. (2020). The power of a positive human-animal relationship for animal welfare. *Frontiers in Veterinary Science, 7*, 590867.

Reynolds, J. J., Torremorell, M., & Craft, M. E. (2014). Mathematical modeling of influenza A virus dynamics within swine farms and the effects of vaccination. *PLoS One, 9*(8), e106177.

Rhouma, M., Beaudry, F., Thériault, W., & Letellier, A. (2016). Colistin in pig production: Chemistry, mechanism of antibacterial action, microbial resistance emergence, and one health perspectives. *Frontiers in Microbiology, 7*, 1789.

Rossi, G., Smith, R. L., Pongolini, S., & Bolzoni, L. (2017). Modelling farm-to-farm disease transmission through personnel movements: From visits to contacts, and back. *Scientific Reports, 7*(1), 2375.

Sarrazin, S., Joosten, P., Van Gompel, L., Luiken, R. E. C., Mevius, D. J., Wagenaar, J. A., et al. (2019). Quantitative and qualitative analysis of antimicrobial usage patterns in 180 selected farrow-to-finish pig farms from nine European countries based on single batch and purchase data. *The Journal of Antimicrobial Chemotherapy, 74*(3), 807–816.

Shi, R., Irfan, M., Liu, G., Yang, X., & Su, X. (2022). Analysis of the impact of livestock structure on carbon emissions of animal husbandry: A sustainable way to improving public health and green environment. *Frontiers in Public Health, 10*, 835210.

Straw, B. E., Zimmerman, J. J., D'Allaire, S., & Taylor, D. J. (Eds.). (2013). Diseases of swine. John Wiley & Sons.

Stygar, A. H., Chantziaras, I., Toppari, I., Maes, D., & Niemi, J. K. (2020). High biosecurity and welfare standards in fattening pig farms are associated with reduced antimicrobial use. *Animal: An International Journal of Animal Bioscience, 14*(10), 2178–2186.

Taneja, N., & Sharma, M. (2019). Antimicrobial resistance in the environment: The Indian scenario. *Indian Journal of Medical Research, 149*(2), 119–128.

Tatemoto, P., Bernardino, T., Alves, L., de Oliveira, C., Souza, A., Palme, R., & José Zanella, A. (2019). Environmental enrichment for pregnant sows modulates HPA-axis and behavior in the offspring. *Applied Animal Behaviour Science, 220*(104854), 104854.

Thakur, K. K., Revie, C. W., Hurnik, D., Poljak, Z., & Sanchez, J. (2016). Analysis of swine movement in four Canadian regions: Network structure and implications for disease spread. *Transboundary and Emerging Diseases, 63*(1), e14–e26.

Tiseo, K., Huber, L., Gilbert, M., Robinson, T. P., & Van Boeckel, T. P. (2020). Global trends in antimicrobial use in food animals from 2017 to 2030. *Antibiotics, 9*(12), 918.

Townsend, P. K. (2017). *Environmental anthropology: From pigs to policies*. Waveland Press.

Uemoto, Y., Ichinoseki, K., Matsumoto, T., Oka, N., Takamori, H., Kadowaki, H., et al. (2021). Genome-wide association studies for production, respiratory disease, and immune-related traits in landrace pigs. *Scientific Reports, 11*(1), 15823.

Van Boeckel, T. P., Brower, C., Gilbert, M., Grenfell, B. T., Levin, S. A., Robinson, T. P., et al. (2015). Global trends in antimicrobial use in food animals. *Proceedings of the National Academy of Sciences, 112*(18), 5649–5654.

VanderWaal, K., & Deen, J. (2018). Global trends in infectious diseases of swine. *Proceedings of the National Academy of Sciences, 115*(45), 11495–11500.

Vijaykrishna, D., Smith, G. J., Pybus, O. G., Zhu, H., Bhatt, S., Poon, L. L., et al. (2011). Long-term evolution and transmission dynamics of swine influenza A virus. *Nature, 473*(7348), 519–522.

Villeneuve, P. J., Ali, A., Challacombe, L., & Hebert, S. (2009). Intensive hog farming operations and self-reported health among nearby rural residents in Ottawa, Canada. *BMC Public Health, 9*, 1–10.

Vishnuraj, M. R., Kandeepan, G., Rao, K. H., Chand, S., & Kumbhar, V. (2016). Occurrence, public health hazards and detection methods of antibiotic residues in foods of animal origin: A comprehensive review. *Cogent Food & Agriculture, 2*(1), 1235458.

Von Essen, S. G., & Auvermann, B. W. (2005). Health effects from breathing air near CAFOs for feeder cattle or hogs. *Journal of Agromedicine, 10*(4), 55–64.

von Keyserlingk, M. A. G., & Hötzel, M. J. (2015). The ticking clock: Addressing farm animal welfare in emerging countries. *Journal of Agricultural & Environmental Ethics, 28*(1), 179–195.

Waluszewski, A., Cinti, A., & Perna, A. (2021). Antibiotics in pig meat production: Restrictions as the odd case and overuse as normality? Experiences from Sweden and Italy. *Humanities and Social Sciences Communications, 8*(1), 1–12.

Wang, J., & Hu, X. (2023). Factors influencing disease prevention and control behaviours of hog farmers. *Animals, 13*(5), 787.

Wang, L., & Yang, Z. G. (2022). Analysis on risk avoidance behaviors and influential factors of epidemic disease among pig farmers. *African and Asian Studies, 21*(1–2), 90–111.

Wang, H., Chen, M., Guo, Z., Shen, Y., Chen, Y., Luo, T., et al. (2023). The influencing factors of "post-African swine fever" pig farm biosecurity: Evidence from Sichuan Province, China. *Animals, 13*(19), 3053.

Weiss, B. (2016). *Real pigs: Shifting values in the field of local pork*. Duke University Press.

Wen, C., van Dixhoorn, I., Schokker, D., Woelders, H., Stockhofe-Zurwieden, N., Rebel, J. M. J., & Smidt, H. (2021). Environmentally enriched housing conditions affect pig welfare, immune system and gut microbiota in early life. *Animal Microbiome, 3*(1), 52.

Whitaker, S. H., Mannelli, A., Kitron, U., & Bellini, S. (2024). An analysis of the social, cultural, and ecological factors that affect the implementation of biosecurity measures on smallholder commercial swine farms in Italy in the context of an emerging African swine fever outbreak. *Preventive Veterinary Medicine, 229*, 106238.

Wisener, L. V., Sargeant, J. M., O'Sullivan, T. L., O'Connor, A. M., McEwen, S. A., Reist, M., & Churchill, K. J. (2021). Non-antibiotic approaches for disease prevention and control in nursery pigs: A scoping review. *Frontiers in Veterinary Science, 8*, 620347.

Woods, A. (2019). Decentring antibiotics: UK responses to the diseases of intensive pig production (ca. 1925–1965). *Palgrave Commun, 5*, 41.

Woolhouse, M., Ward, M., van Bunnik, B., & Farrar, J. (2015). Antimicrobial resistance in humans, livestock and the wider environment. *Philosophical Transactions of the Royal Society of London. Series B, Biological Sciences, 370*(1670), 20140083.

Zhang, X., Li, C., Hao, Y., & Gu, X. (2020). Effects of different farrowing environments on the behavior of sows and piglets. *Animals: An Open Access Journal from MDPI, 10*(2), 320.

Zhang, X., Rong, X., Li, J., Fan, M., Wang, Y., Sun, X., et al. (2021). Modeling the outbreak and control of African swine fever virus in large-scale pig farms. *Journal of Theoretical Biology, 526*, 110798.

One Health Approach: Integrating Swine, Humans, and the Environment

Varun Asediya, Dhruv Desai, Pranav Anjaria, and Ravindra Saraf

Abstract

This chapter presents a comprehensive examination of the One Health paradigm, utilizing a synthesis of philosophical discourse, scientific inquiry, and prospective modeling to expound upon the intricate interrelationships among swine, humans, and the environment. Commencing as an homage to the holistic tenets of Hippocrates, the narrative navigates through the intricate web of ecological dynamics, socio-economic determinants, and ethical considerations with meticulous scholarly rigor. Each section rigorously scrutinizes its respective theme, ranging from epidemiological surveillance and ethical quandaries to ecosystem services and technological advancements. As the chapter unfolds, it transcends disciplinary confines, offering scholarly insights that reverberate across diverse academic domains. Through scenario planning and forward-looking projections, it provides a glimpse into the evolving landscape of One Health, guided by principles of innovation, ethical stewardship, and collective engagement. In conclusion, the chapter advocates for a vision of One Health that transcends individual interests, nurturing a future where the health and well-being of all entities are intricately interwoven in a symphony of mutual flourishing and resilience.

V. Asediya (✉) · R. Saraf
M. B. Veterinary College, Dungarpur, Rajasthan, India

D. Desai
University of Pennsylvania, Philadelphia, PA, USA

P. Anjaria
Kamdhenu University, Anand, Gujarat, India

R. Deb et al. (eds.), *Emerging Zoonotic Threats from Swine*,
https://doi.org/10.1007/978-981-96-7407-7_2

Keywords

Ecological dynamics · Ethical considerations · Epidemiological surveillance · Innovation · One Health paradigm · Philosophical discourse · Prospective modeling · Scientific inquiry · Socio-economic determinants · Swine-human-environment interactions

Introduction

The discipline of One Health is an integrative field of inquiry that scrutinizes the intricate confluence of human health, animal health, and environmental health, thereby challenging conventional disciplinary boundaries (Cunningham et al., 2017). This discipline compels us to comprehend the profound symbiosis inherent within the fabric of life. Echoes of historical wisdom permeate this field, with ancient scholars such as Hippocrates advocating for a view of health that encompasses the physical body, the mind, and the environment. This principle serves as a beacon for the holistic ethos of One Health, underscoring the inseparable linkage between individual health and the broader ecological context (Gebreyes et al., 2014).

The trajectory of human thought has witnessed a paradigm shift from reductionist perspectives, as proposed by Descartes, toward a more holistic, systems-based approach. This transition is mirrored in the evolution of One Health (Mackenzie et al., 2013). Pioneers such as Aldo Leopold and Rachel Carson were at the forefront of this transition, advocating for a biocentric ethical framework and emphasizing our interconnectedness with the broader web of life. Their teachings form the bedrock of One Health, prompting us to perceive health as a complex network of mutualistic relationships. At the core of One Health lie numerous ethical dilemmas, leading us into a labyrinth of moral complexities. The challenge of harmonizing human aspirations with the welfare of animals and ecosystems is formidable. This convergence of bioethical, ecoethical, and zoethical discourses prompts us to construct an ethical framework that respects the sanctity of all sentient beings.

The Gaia hypothesis, proposed by James Lovelock, infuses our philosophical contemplation with additional depth. It portrays Earth as a sentient superorganism with interconnected systems. This model encourages us to perceive health not as a static state, but as a dynamic equilibrium within the grand ballet of terrestrial phenomena. The whispers of Gaia urge us to transition from atomistic analyses toward a comprehensive understanding of health dynamics (Lovelock & Margulis, 1974; Gribbin & Gribbin, 2009; Lovelock, 1983).

As we grapple with the epistemological barriers in defining health within a network of interrelationships, the limitations of reductionist methodologies become evident. One Health calls for an enriched lexicon that encompasses concepts of resilience, adaptability, and harmony within interconnected systems. This necessitates a reevaluation of traditional health indicators and the adoption of a more integrative framework for assessing well-being. The ethical principle of equity intersects with One Health, highlighting the rights, responsibilities, and mutualism that bind

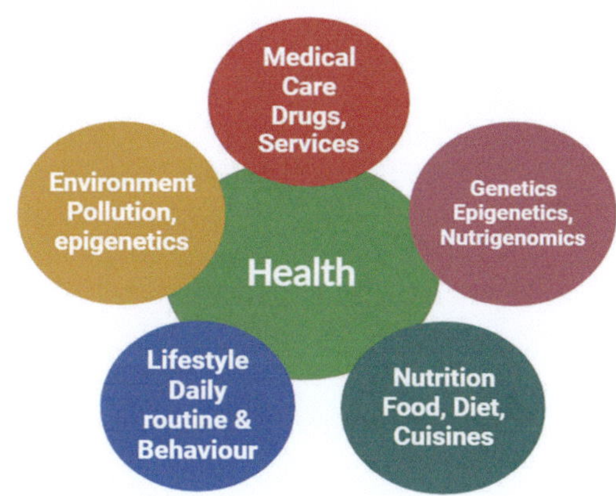

Fig. 1 Key factors influencing health include nutrition, lifestyle, environment, and genetics, which serve as the four fundamental pillars of well-being. When any of these elements are compromised, health can be jeopardized, necessitating medical care as a supportive measure

our existence. Drawing from a mosaic of ethical philosophies, we are urged to extend our moral compass beyond anthropocentric views, recognizing the intrinsic value of all life forms within the tapestry of life (Rousham et al., 1876; Zinsstag et al., 2011; Kahn, 2021).

In the epoch of the Anthropocene, the narrative of One Health intertwines with the overarching challenges of climate change, zoonotic disease transmission, and biodiversity loss. We find ourselves at a crossroads, contemplating profound questions: Is health a privilege or a fundamental right? Can we transcend speciesism and acknowledge our shared destiny within the global bio community? (Fig. 1)

The Swine-Human-Environment Triad

As we investigate the swine-human-environment triad, we delve into its intricacies, utilizing a combination of ecological modeling, socio-economic analysis, and ethical philosophy to decipher the complex interdependence embedded within. At the forefront of our investigation are the environmentally advanced constructs that encapsulate the non-linear, dynamic interactions within the triad (Moraes et al., 2021; Mesquita, 2021). These models challenge simplistic cause-and-effect paradigms, opting instead to embrace the nuanced interplay of feedback loops, threshold phenomena, and temporal lags. They guide us through the theories of resilience and panarchy, shedding light on the adaptive cycles that govern the triad's capacity for both stability and transformation. Focusing on the human element, we dissect the socio-economic forces that shape and are shaped by the swine's health and the environment's state. We trace the economic currents driving swine production and examine the societal determinants influencing human health. This socio-economic fabric unveils a complex interplay, providing a window into the reciprocal relationship between human activities, societal structures, and the health of both swine populations and human communities. Within the sphere of ethics, we encounter a rich array of moral considerations (Oliveira et al., 2018) (Fig. 2).

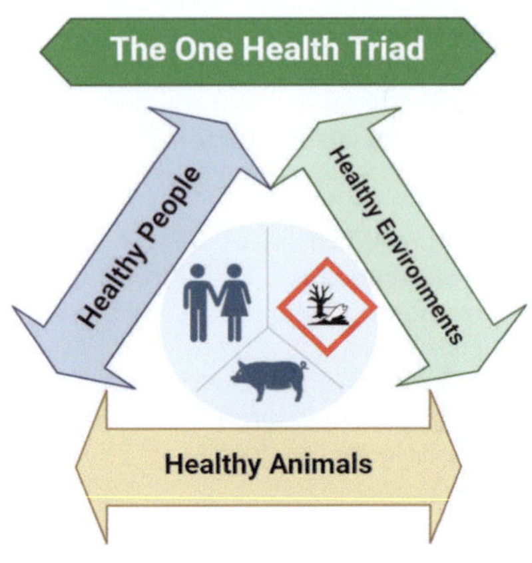

Fig. 2 Schematic representation of the one health triad

Swine as Sentinels: Epidemiological Surveillance and Predictive Modeling

In the landscape of One Health, swine is not merely an agricultural asset but key epidemiological sentinels.

1. *Multilayered Predictive Analytics:* To harness the sentinel capabilities of swine effectively, advanced statistical models and algorithmic approaches are employed. Through the utilization of innovative multilayered neural networks and deep learning algorithms, predictive analytics systematically analyze vast datasets derived from veterinary health records, environmental monitoring initiatives, and human disease surveillance systems. This systematic analysis allows for the identification of subtle patterns and correlations within complex, high-dimensional datasets, enabling the early detection of potential zoonotic spillover events. By proactively identifying emerging trends and forecasting potential disease outbreaks, these advanced analytical methodologies serve as indispensable tools in preemptively mitigating public health risks at the interface of human, animal, and environmental health (Suresh et al., 2021; Arulmozhi et al., 2021; Fernandes et al., 2020; van Klompenburg & Kassahun, 2022).
2. *High-Resolution Risk Mapping:* High-resolution risk mapping represents a pinnacle of technological innovation, harnessing advanced spatial statistics and innovative machine-learning techniques to analyze satellite imagery and environmental data with unprecedented granularity and accuracy. At the heart of high-resolution risk mapping lie algorithms such as support vector machines (SVM) and random forests. These algorithms excel at processing vast volumes of spatial and environmental data, extracting intricate patterns and correlations that may signify potential disease outbreak hotspots. By leveraging the power of machine learning, these algorithms adapt and refine their predictions based on real-time data inputs, ensuring continuous improvement in accuracy and reliability. The process begins with the acquisition of satellite imagery and environmental data, which are then processed and analyzed using advanced computational

techniques. Machine learning algorithms sift through these datasets, identifying spatial patterns and environmental factors that correlate with disease transmission. By applying spatial statistics, the algorithms generate predictive models that can forecast the likelihood of disease outbreaks in different geographic regions. The output of high-resolution risk mapping is a series of detailed maps that highlight areas of elevated disease risk with unprecedented accuracy. These maps serve as invaluable tools for public health officials, enabling them to prioritize surveillance efforts, implement targeted control measures, and allocate resources where they are most needed (Lee et al., 2019; Pittiglio et al., 2018; Alkhamis et al., 2018; Cheng et al., 2023).

3. *Dynamic Network Modeling:* Dynamic network modeling emerges as a tool for understanding the complex interactions within and between swine populations over time. By leveraging principles from graph theory and temporal network analysis, these models provide insights into the evolving contact patterns that underpin disease transmission dynamics. At the core of dynamic network modeling lie intricate algorithms that analyze temporal data to identify key nodes and links within the network. These algorithms consider the dynamic nature of contact patterns, capturing fluctuations in connectivity over time. By applying graph theory concepts such as centrality measures and community detection algorithms, dynamic network models pinpoint critical nodes and links that play pivotal roles in facilitating disease spread. Through the integration of temporal network analysis, dynamic network models offer a nuanced understanding of the temporal dynamics of disease transmission. These models track changes in contact patterns over time, identifying periods of heightened connectivity and potential disease outbreaks. By uncovering temporal patterns in network dynamics, dynamic network modeling provides valuable insights into the underlying mechanisms driving disease transmission dynamics within swine populations (Dorjee et al., 2013; Sartore et al., 2020; Bastard et al., 2020; Hammami et al., 2022; Makau et al., 2021).

Swine as Prognostic Indicators of Zoonotic Threats

1. *Retrospective Analysis of Epidemic Precursors:* In the quest to bolster disease surveillance and response mechanisms, retrospective analyses of past zoonotic events, with swine populations acting as early indicators, offer invaluable insights. These analyses delve into historical datasets, providing a wealth of information for refining surveillance strategies and response protocols. At the forefront of these retrospective analyses are advanced statistical methods, including time-series anomaly detection and cluster analysis. These methodologies meticulously scrutinize temporal data, identifying anomalous patterns and clustering of events that may signify the onset of epidemics. By leveraging these statistical techniques, researchers gain a deeper understanding of epidemic precursors, enabling more proactive and targeted surveillance efforts. Through the retrospective analysis of past zoonotic events involving swine populations,

researchers can identify key factors and indicators associated with disease emergence and transmission. This knowledge serves as a foundation for the development of robust surveillance frameworks and response strategies, enhancing our capacity to detect and mitigate future outbreaks (Nelson & Vincent, 2015; Flanagan et al., 2012; Weiss & Sankaran, 2022; Cardenas et al., 2022; Puspitarani et al., 2023; Lentz et al., 2016).

2. *Real-Time Surveillance and Monitoring Systems:* The integration of real-time surveillance and monitoring systems marks a significant advancement in disease detection and management, particularly within swine populations. This innovative approach harnesses innovative technologies such as the Internet of Things (IoT), remote sensing, and edge computing to create a network of biosensors that continuously stream data for real-time analysis. At the core of these systems lies the Internet of Things, enabling interconnected devices to collect and transmit data seamlessly. Remote sensing technologies, including satellite imagery and drones, provide high-resolution data on environmental conditions and animal behavior. Meanwhile, edge computing facilitates data processing and analysis at the source, minimizing latency and enabling rapid decision-making. By transforming swine populations into a network of biosensors, real-time surveillance systems offer unprecedented insights into disease dynamics and environmental factors that influence health outcomes. Data streams from individual animals, environmental sensors, and other sources are fed into predictive models for real-time analysis. These models utilize advanced algorithms to detect patterns, anomalies, and early indicators of disease outbreaks, enabling timely interventions to mitigate risks and prevent the spread of infectious diseases (Martínez-Avilés et al., 2017; Alba-Casals et al., 2020).
3. *Validation of Predictive Outcomes:* The validation of predictive outcomes stands as a critical aspect within the integration of real-time data streams and complex predictive models for disease outbreak anticipation. Central to this validation process are techniques such as cross-validation and receiver operating characteristic (ROC) curve analysis. Cross-validation involves partitioning the available data into subsets, with each subset utilized for both training and validation purposes. This iterative approach helps assess the generalizability and robustness of predictive models by evaluating their performance across multiple data partitions. Additionally, ROC curve analysis provides a comprehensive evaluation of predictive model performance by plotting the true positive rate against the false positive rate across various threshold values. This graphical representation allows for the determination of optimal model thresholds and facilitates comparisons between different predictive models. By employing these validation techniques, researchers can effectively assess the accuracy and reliability of predictive outcomes derived from real-time data streams and complex models. This ensures that swine populations serve as dependable epidemiological sentinels, capable of providing early warnings for potential disease outbreaks. Furthermore, validated predictive models contribute to the development of proactive surveillance and response strategies, thereby enhancing overall public health prepared-

ness and mitigating the impact of emerging infectious diseases (Maltecca et al., 2019; van Staaveren et al., 2017).

Human Health Dynamics: Sociocultural and Economic Dimensions

Sociocultural Influences on Health

1. *Behavioral Epidemiology:* In examining the epidemiology of diseases, including those transmitted from swine, it is imperative to consider the profound impact of sociocultural factors. Behavioral epidemiology serves as a crucial framework for analyzing how cultural practices and societal behaviors influence disease transmission dynamics. This analysis delves into the cultural determinants of health, exploring how beliefs, traditions, and social structures shape individuals' interactions with their environment and affect their susceptibility to diseases transmitted from swine (Overgaauw et al., 2020). Behavioral epidemiology provides insight into the intricate relationship between cultural norms and disease transmission patterns. By studying case studies and conducting ethnographic research, researchers gain a deeper understanding of how sociocultural factors contribute to disease risk and transmission pathways. These investigations illuminate the contextual factors that influence health behaviors and shape the dynamics of disease outbreaks within human populations. Ethnographic research and case studies play a pivotal role in unraveling the complexities of sociocultural influences on health. Through immersive fieldwork and meticulous analysis, researchers elucidate the cultural contexts in which interactions between humans and swine occur. By capturing the nuances of everyday life and community dynamics, ethnographic research provides valuable insights into the social determinants of health and informs the development of targeted interventions to mitigate disease transmission (Friedler, 2021; Chadborn et al., 2023; Cole et al., 2000; Kerdsin et al., 2022).
2. *Health Beliefs and Practices:*

Cross-Cultural Perspectives

By examining health beliefs and practices through a cross-cultural lens, researchers gain valuable insights into the diverse approaches to disease prevention and management. Cultural determinants such as ethnomedical beliefs, traditional healing practices, and religious rituals profoundly influence individuals' perceptions of health and illness. These cultural nuances significantly shape health-related behaviors, decision-making processes, and community responses to swine-related diseases.

Impact on Preventive Measures

The analysis elucidates how cultural beliefs and practices influence the uptake of preventive measures, including vaccination, sanitation practices, and disease surveillance initiatives. Cultural factors such as perceived susceptibility to illness, beliefs about the efficacy of preventive measures, and trust in healthcare authorities impact individuals' willingness to engage in preventive behaviors. Understanding and addressing these cultural determinants are essential for designing effective public health campaigns and interventions that resonate with diverse cultural contexts.

Access to Healthcare

Health beliefs and practices also exert a profound influence on access to healthcare services, including diagnosis, treatment, and follow-up care for swine-related diseases. Cultural factors such as health-seeking behaviors, attitudes toward modern medicine, and social norms surrounding illness and treatment significantly influence individuals' utilization of healthcare services. Disparities in healthcare access stemming from cultural barriers can exacerbate the burden of swine-related diseases within marginalized communities, underscoring the need for culturally sensitive healthcare delivery models.

Implications for Public Health Interventions

A comparative analysis of health belief models offers valuable insights into the underlying determinants of health-related behaviors and decision-making processes across diverse cultural contexts. Models such as the Health Belief Model, the Theory of Planned Behavior, and the Socioecological Model provide theoretical frameworks for understanding how cultural factors interact with individual beliefs, attitudes, and social environments to shape health outcomes. Integrating these models into public health interventions enables policymakers to develop culturally tailored strategies that address the unique cultural beliefs and practices of diverse populations affected by swine-related diseases (Trnka & Lorencova, 2022) (Fig. 3).

Economic Impact and Health Outcomes

1. *Health Economics:* An analysis of the economic burden of diseases originating from swine populations provides critical insights into their cost implications for healthcare systems and society at large. This assessment encompasses direct healthcare costs, including medical treatment expenses, hospitalization fees, and pharmaceutical expenditures, as well as indirect costs such as productivity losses, absenteeism, and reduced economic output due to illness. Economic modeling techniques play a pivotal role in quantifying the impact of swine-related diseases on healthcare systems and economies (Calderón Díaz et al., 2020). These models utilize epidemiological data, healthcare utilization statistics, and economic parameters to estimate the direct and indirect costs associated with disease outbreaks. By simulating various scenarios and interventions, economic models inform decision-makers about the potential economic consequences of different policy options and intervention strategies. Efficient resource allocation is essential for effectively preventing and controlling diseases originating from swine populations. This section examines strategies for optimizing

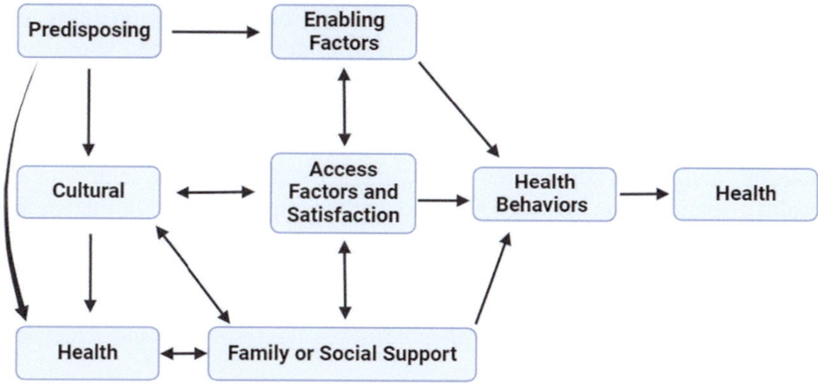

Fig. 3 The Sociocultural Health Behavior Model to investigate the factors influencing health conditions in a target population

resource allocation, considering the economic costs and benefits of different intervention measures. By prioritizing interventions based on their cost-effectiveness and impact on disease burden reduction, policymakers can maximize the efficiency and effectiveness of limited healthcare resources (Mason-D'Croz et al., 2020). Cost-benefit and cost-effectiveness analyses serve as valuable tools for evaluating the economic feasibility and efficiency of disease prevention and control measures. These analyses compare the costs of implementing interventions against their anticipated benefits or outcomes, providing decision-makers with evidence-based insights into the economic viability of different policy options. By weighing the costs and benefits of interventions in monetary terms, policymakers can make informed decisions about resource allocation and policy formulation.

2. *Socioeconomic Status and Health Disparities:* Socioeconomic status encompasses various indicators of an individual's or community's economic and social standing, including income, education, occupation, and access to resources. These factors profoundly shape individuals' living conditions, access to healthcare services, and health-related behaviors, influencing their susceptibility to diseases and health outcomes. Vulnerability to zoonotic diseases is not evenly distributed across populations, with individuals and communities of lower socioeconomic status often bearing a disproportionate burden of disease (Kerdsin et al., 2022). Factors such as limited access to clean water and sanitation, overcrowded living conditions, and occupational exposures increase the risk of zoonotic disease transmission among marginalized populations. Additionally, disparities in healthcare access and utilization further exacerbate health inequities, leading to delayed diagnosis, inadequate treatment, and poorer health outcomes among socioeconomically disadvantaged groups. Access to healthcare services is a fundamental determinant of health outcomes, yet socioeconomic disparities persist in access to quality healthcare. Individuals of lower socioeconomic status face barriers such as financial constraints, lack of health insurance,

geographic remoteness, and limited availability of healthcare facilities, which impede their ability to seek timely and appropriate medical care. These disparities in healthcare access contribute to inequities in disease prevention, diagnosis, and treatment, perpetuating health inequalities among different population groups. The social determinants of health, including education, employment, housing, and social support networks, interact with economic factors to shape health disparities. Socioeconomic disadvantage often results in limited access to education and employment opportunities, unstable housing conditions, and social isolation, all of which contribute to poorer health outcomes. Moreover, economic shocks, such as recessions or economic downturns, can exacerbate existing health inequities by further constraining resources and exacerbating social disparities.

Integrating Sociocultural and Economic Factors in One Health

1. *Interdisciplinary Approaches:* Recognizing that human health is intricately linked to the health of animals and the environment, interdisciplinary approaches are essential for addressing the multifaceted determinants of health outcomes. Sociocultural and economic factors significantly influence disease transmission dynamics, healthcare access, and community resilience to health threats. By integrating perspectives from diverse disciplines, One Health strategies can more effectively identify root causes, develop targeted interventions, and promote sustainable solutions that address the complex nature of health challenges. Effective collaboration among anthropologists, sociologists, economists, and public health experts is crucial for leveraging the complementary expertise of each discipline (Baudoin et al., 2021). Anthropologists provide insights into cultural beliefs, practices, and community dynamics that influence health behaviors and disease transmission patterns. Sociologists offer perspectives on social networks, power dynamics, and structural inequalities that shape health disparities and access to healthcare. Economists contribute expertise in resource allocation, cost-benefit analysis, and policy evaluation to inform evidence-based decision-making in health interventions. Public health experts bring together knowledge from various disciplines to design and implement integrated strategies for disease prevention, surveillance, and response. Methodologies for interdisciplinary research include qualitative and quantitative approaches that bridge disciplinary boundaries and generate comprehensive insights into complex health issues. Qualitative methods such as ethnography, interviews, and focus groups enable researchers to explore sociocultural contexts, perceptions, and experiences related to health and illness. Quantitative methods such as statistical analysis, economic modeling, and spatial mapping provide empirical evidence and quantitative assessments of health outcomes, resource distribution, and intervention effectiveness. The mixed methods approach combines qualitative and quantitative data to triangulate findings and generate a more nuanced understanding of health phenomena (Brown et al., 2021).

2. *Policy Implications:* Effective policies in the realm of One Health must be inherently sensitive to the sociocultural and economic contexts in which they are implemented. Sociocultural factors, including cultural beliefs, practices, and social norms, profoundly influence health behaviors, disease transmission dynamics, and community resilience. Similarly, economic factors such as income inequality, access to healthcare, and resource distribution shape individuals' and communities' vulnerability to health threats. Policies that fail to account for these contextual nuances risk overlooking the root causes of health disparities and may inadvertently exacerbate existing inequalities. Policy formulation in One Health should prioritize integrated approaches that recognize the interconnectedness of human, animal, and environmental health. This entails fostering collaboration among stakeholders from diverse sectors, including healthcare, agriculture, environmental protection, and community development. By promoting interdisciplinary research, data sharing, and knowledge exchange, policymakers can develop comprehensive strategies that address the complex determinants of health outcomes and promote synergies across sectors. Integrated policies that consider the health implications of agricultural practices, land use decisions, and urban planning can lead to more sustainable and resilient communities. Implementing policies that address sociocultural and economic dynamics poses both challenges and opportunities at various levels of governance. Challenges may include navigating political interests, securing funding, and overcoming institutional barriers to collaboration. Additionally, addressing deeply entrenched social inequalities and cultural barriers requires sustained commitment and investment in community engagement and capacity building. However, there are also opportunities to leverage existing policy frameworks, international collaborations, and technological innovations to drive positive change. Empowering local communities, fostering cross-sectoral partnerships, and promoting evidence-based decision-making can enhance the effectiveness and sustainability of One Health policies.

The Environmental Matrix: Ecosystem Services and Biodiversity

Ecosystem Services: Sustaining Health Across Species

1. *Provisioning Services:* Swine production relies heavily on ecosystem services for its sustenance and productivity. Provisioning services, including the supply of food, water, and raw materials, are indispensable for meeting the nutritional needs of swine populations, supporting their growth, and maintaining their health. Agricultural landscapes provide vital resources such as grains, vegetables, and forage crops that constitute the primary feed for swine (Leroy et al., 2024). Additionally, access to clean, freshwater sources is essential for hydration, sanitation, and overall well-being. While provisioning services support swine production, their utilization can also exert significant pressure on ecosys-

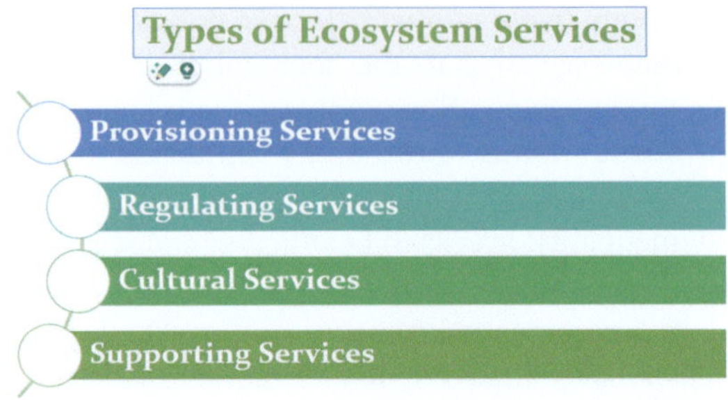

Fig. 4 The Millennium Ecosystem Assessment (MA), a significant UN-sponsored initiative identified four major categories of ecosystem services

tem health and resilience. Intensive agricultural practices, such as monoculture farming, chemical inputs, and land conversion, may lead to habitat destruction, soil degradation, and water pollution (Adla et al., 2022). These environmental impacts can disrupt ecosystem functions, diminish biodiversity, and compromise the long-term availability of provisioning services. Thus, the sustainability of swine production is intricately linked to the health and integrity of the ecosystems from which it derives its resources. Achieving a balance between the utilization of provisioning services and their sustainability is paramount for ensuring the long-term viability of swine production systems. Sustainable agricultural practices, such as agroecology, organic farming, and integrated pest management, prioritize ecosystem health and resilience while meeting the nutritional needs of swine populations. By adopting regenerative practices that enhance soil fertility, conserve water resources, and promote biodiversity, farmers can minimize their ecological footprint and safeguard the provision of essential services for future generations (Bergez et al., 2022; Luty et al., 2021) (Fig. 4).

2. *Regulating Services:*

Disease Regulation

Swine populations can significantly impact disease regulation within ecosystems. The section explores the role of swine as potential reservoirs for zoonotic pathogens, including viruses, bacteria, and parasites, which can pose risks to both animal and human health. Intensive swine production systems, characterized by high stocking densities and limited biosecurity measures, may facilitate the transmission of infectious diseases, leading to outbreaks with far-reaching consequences. Understanding the dynamics of disease transmission between swine and other species is crucial for implementing effective disease control measures and mitigating public health risks.

Climate Regulation

Swine production systems can also influence climate regulation through their emissions of greenhouse gases (GHGs) and their impact on land use and vegetation cover. The section examines the contribution of swine operations to GHG emissions, particularly methane and nitrous oxide, which are potent drivers of climate change. Additionally, deforestation and land conversion for swine farming can lead to the loss of carbon sinks and biodiversity, further exacerbating climate-related challenges. Implementing sustainable practices, such as carbon sequestration, agroforestry, and waste management, can mitigate the environmental footprint of swine production and enhance climate resilience (Hörtenhuber et al., 2020).

Water Purification

Swine populations can affect water purification processes through their waste production and management practices. The section discusses the potential contamination of water bodies by nutrients, pathogens, and pharmaceutical residues from swine operations, which can compromise water quality and ecosystem health. Pollution of freshwater sources poses risks to human health, including the transmission of waterborne diseases and the accumulation of harmful pollutants in food chains. Implementing stringent regulations, improving waste treatment technologies, and promoting sustainable manure management practices are essential for safeguarding water resources and protecting public health.

Implications for Human Health

The section concludes by highlighting the implications of swine populations' impact on regulating services for human health. Uncontrolled disease transmission, climate change-induced hazards, and waterborne contamination pose significant health risks to individuals and communities, particularly those living near swine production facilities. Addressing these challenges requires a holistic approach that integrates environmental stewardship, public health interventions, and policy measures to promote sustainable swine farming practices and safeguard human well-being.

3. *Cultural Services:*

Recreational Benefits

Ecosystems offer a myriad of recreational opportunities that nurture physical and mental well-being, fostering a deep connection between individuals and nature. Parks, forests, and natural landscapes provide spaces for outdoor activities such as hiking, camping, and wildlife observation, offering respite from urban life and promoting physical fitness. Engaging in recreational activities in natural settings has been shown to reduce stress, alleviate symptoms of anxiety and depression, and enhance overall quality of life. By providing opportunities for relaxation, rejuvenation, and leisure, cultural ecosystem services contribute to the holistic health and well-being of individuals and communities.

Spiritual Enrichment

Ecosystems hold profound spiritual significance for many cultures and communities, serving as sacred sites, pilgrimage destinations, and places of reflection and contemplation. Natural landscapes evoke feelings of awe, wonder, and reverence, inspiring spiritual connections, and deepening individuals' sense of belonging to the natural world. Spiritual experiences in nature can foster a sense of inner peace, harmony, and interconnectedness, providing solace during times of adversity and uncertainty. Recognizing and preserving the spiritual values inherent in ecosystems is essential for nurturing cultural identity, promoting social cohesion, and supporting mental and emotional resilience.

Educational Opportunities

Ecosystems serve as living laboratories for experiential learning, offering valuable educational opportunities for individuals of all ages. Natural environments provide platforms for environmental education, ecological research, and direct learning experiences that foster ecological literacy, critical thinking, and stewardship ethics. Schools, nature centers, and environmental organizations utilize ecosystems as outdoor classrooms, facilitating immersive learning experiences that deepen students' understanding of ecological processes, biodiversity conservation, and sustainable living practices. By integrating environmental education into formal and informal learning settings, cultural ecosystem services promote environmental awareness, empower future generations, and inspire informed action for the protection of nature and human health.

4. *Biodiversity: A Cornerstone of One Health.*
   - *Biodiversity and Disease:* Biodiversity loss, driven by factors such as habitat destruction, species extinction, and ecosystem degradation, disrupts the ecological balance and creates conditions conducive to the proliferation of pathogens. Reduced biodiversity may lead to the proliferation of reservoir hosts and vectors, amplifying disease transmission pathways and increasing the likelihood of spillover events between wildlife, domestic animals, and humans. The ramifications of biodiversity loss extend to heightened disease transmission pathways and increased risks of spillover events between wildlife, domestic animals, and humans. As biodiversity dwindles, the proliferation of reservoir hosts and vectors escalates, amplifying the transmission of pathogens across ecosystems (Baines et al., 2024). This amplification effect intensifies the likelihood of diseases jumping species barriers, leading to outbreaks with significant implications for public health and ecosystem stability. The consequences of biodiversity loss reverberate through swine and human populations, elevating the risk of infectious disease emergence and spread. Reduced biodiversity alters ecosystem dynamics, facilitating the encroachment of wildlife into human-dominated landscapes and enhancing opportunities for pathogen transmission. Moreover, weakened natural disease regulation mechanisms exacerbate disease transmission pathways, posing substantial threats to both swine and human health. Understanding the intricate relationship between biodiversity and disease dynamics is paramount for devising effective disease surveillance, prevention, and control strategies. By recognizing the role of biodiversity in shaping disease transmission pathways, stakeholders can implement targeted interventions to mitigate risks and safeguard the health of swine, humans, and the broader ecosystem (Hörtenhuber et al., 2020; Wilcox & Steele, 2021; Ogunseitan, 2022).

- *Genetic Diversity in Swine Populations:* Genetic variability, manifested through diverse gene pools, fosters a robust immune response repertoire, critical for combating pathogenic onslaughts. Specifically, a broad genetic base confers resilience against infectious agents by ensuring a diverse array of immune-related genes, thereby enhancing the capacity to recognize and mount effective defenses against a spectrum of pathogens (Wu et al., 2020). However, industrial farming practices, characterized by intensive selection pressures and narrow breeding objectives, pose formidable challenges to preserving genetic diversity. Selective breeding programs, aimed at maximizing traits like growth rate and meat quality, often prioritize a handful of superior genotypes, inadvertently eroding genetic variability across swine populations. Consequently, this homogenization renders herds increasingly vulnerable to disease susceptibility, as the loss of genetic diversity compromises the collective ability to withstand novel pathogen threats. Recognizing the intricate interplay between genetic diversity and disease resilience is imperative for informing sustainable breeding strategies within swine populations. By integrating genomic selection methodologies, breed conservation initiatives, and biosecurity protocols, stakeholders can mitigate the erosion of genetic diversity and fortify swine populations against the ever-evolving landscape of infectious diseases and environmental stressors (Scherrer et al., 2020; Wang et al., 2020; Jiang et al., 2020).
- *Conservation Strategies:* Conservation methodologies are multifaceted, encompassing a suite of interventions grounded in ecological principles and informed by robust scientific research. Habitat preservation strategies leverage ecological modeling techniques to identify priority areas for conservation, considering factors such as habitat quality, species richness, and landscape connectivity (Van Ba et al., 2020). These models employ spatial analysis tools, such as Geographic Information Systems (GIS) and remote sensing technologies, to delineate habitat corridors and designate protected areas essential for maintaining biodiversity hotspots and facilitating species movement. Restoration initiatives employ ecological restoration frameworks rooted in ecological succession theory, aiming to re-establish native vegetation communities, enhance ecosystem functions, and promote habitat heterogeneity. Techniques such as native species reintroduction, soil stabilization, and hydrological restoration are employed to accelerate ecosystem recovery and promote resilience to environmental stressors. Species reintroduction programs integrate genetic analyses, population modeling, and habitat suitability assessments to inform captive breeding protocols and release strategies, ensuring the genetic diversity and demographic viability of reintroduced populations. Furthermore, sustainable resource management practices integrate ecological principles with socio-economic considerations, employing techniques such as ecosystem-based fisheries management, forest certification schemes, and integrated watershed management approaches to balance conservation objectives with human needs. The effectiveness of conservation strategies is evaluated through rigorous monitoring and evaluation frame-

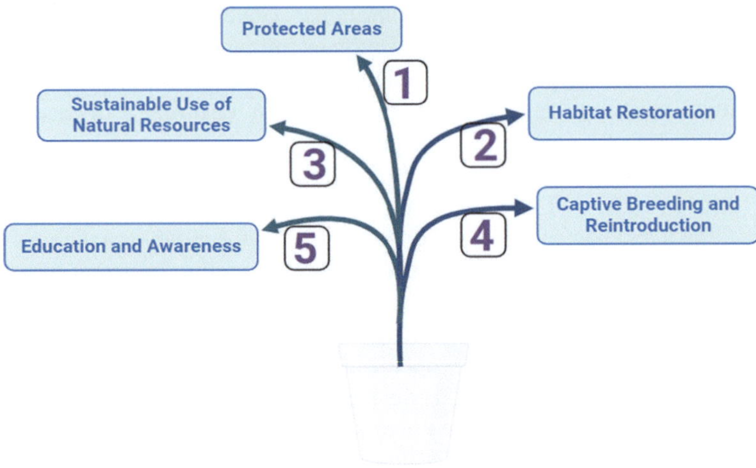

Fig. 5 Biodiversity Conservation through the Lens of Natural Selection

works, incorporating ecological indicators, species population trends, and socio-economic metrics to assess conservation outcomes and inform adaptive management strategies (Fig. 5).

Ethical Considerations and Moral Imperatives

Navigating Ethical Dilemmas

At the heart of One Health lie ethical quandaries that demand thoughtful consideration and nuanced discourse. As stakeholders traverse the interconnected realms of animal welfare, human well-being, and environmental integrity, they encounter ethical crossroads fraught with moral ambiguity. Questions surrounding the equitable distribution of resources, the intrinsic value of non-human life, and the ethical implications of human interventions in natural systems loom large, challenging conventional ethical frameworks and compelling stakeholders to grapple with the ethical complexities of One Health practice (Hernandez et al., 2022; Boudreau LeBlanc et al., 2022).

Philosophical Underpinnings

Embedded within One Health are profound philosophical underpinnings that shape perceptions of morality and ethical conduct. Philosophical traditions spanning utilitarianism, deontology, virtue ethics, and eco-centrism intersect within the One Health framework, offering divergent perspectives on the ethical obligations owed to animals, humans, and the broader biosphere. At the heart of these debates lies the tension between anthropocentric perspectives that prioritize human interests and eco-centric paradigms that advocate for the intrinsic value of all living beings and ecosystems (Hickman et al., 2021; Osterhaus et al., 2020).

Rights, Responsibilities, and Reciprocity

Central to the ethical discourse within One Health are considerations of rights, responsibilities, and reciprocity among diverse stakeholders. As humans wield unprecedented power to shape the fate of ecosystems and species, questions of moral agency, accountability, and intergenerational equity come to the fore. The ethical imperative to uphold the rights of animals, respect the autonomy of ecosystems, and promote justice and fairness across species boundaries underscores the moral imperative inherent in One Health practice.

The Future of One Health

In this visionary exploration, we peer into the horizon of One Health, navigating through scenarios and projections that illuminate the trajectory of this paradigm in a world undergoing rapid transformation. With scenario planning as our compass and innovation as our guiding star, we embark on a journey of foresight and imagination, charting the course of One Health in an era defined by complexity and uncertainty. As we navigate the uncertain waters of the future, scenario planning emerges as a potent tool for charting alternative pathways and anticipating potential challenges and opportunities on the horizon. Drawing upon insights from diverse disciplines and stakeholders, we construct plausible narratives of future worlds—worlds shaped by demographic shifts, technological advances, environmental changes, and socio-economic dynamics. These scenarios serve as windows into futures, inviting us to explore the implications of different trajectories for the practice of One Health and the well-being of humanity and the planet.

At the heart of our vision for the future lies the transformative power of innovation and technology in shaping the landscape of One Health. From breakthroughs in genomics and biotechnology to advancements in artificial intelligence and digital health, technological frontiers offer unprecedented opportunities to revolutionize disease surveillance, diagnosis, and treatment, enhance ecosystem monitoring and management, and empower communities to actively participate in their health and well-being. By harnessing the potential of innovation, we can catalyze a paradigm shift in One Health practice, enabling more proactive, predictive, and participatory approaches to planetary health.

References

Adla, K., Dejan, K., Neira, D., & Dragana, Š. (2022). Degradation of ecosystems and loss of ecosystem services. In *One Health* (pp. 281–327). Elsevier. https://doi.org/10.1016/B978-0-12-822794-7.00008-3

Alba-Casals, A., Allue, E., Tarancon, V., Baliellas, J., Novell, E., Napp, S., & Fraile, L. (2020). Near real-time monitoring of clinical events detected in swine herds in northeastern Spain. *Frontiers in Veterinary Science, 7*. https://doi.org/10.3389/fvets.2020.00068

Alkhamis, M. A., Arruda, A. G., Vilalta, C., Morrison, R. B., & Perez, A. M. (2018). Surveillance of porcine reproductive and respiratory syndrome virus in the United States using risk mapping and species distribution modeling. *Preventive Veterinary Medicine, 150*, 135–142. https://doi.org/10.1016/j.prevetmed.2017.11.011

Arulmozhi, E., Basak, J. K., Sihalath, T., Park, J., Kim, H. T., & Moon, B. E. (2021). Machine learning-based microclimate model for indoor air temperature and relative humidity prediction in a swine building. *Animals, 11*(1), 222. https://doi.org/10.3390/ani11010222

Baines, A. E., Errecaborde, K., Ames, T. R., Goldsmith, T. J., Kinzer, H., Mahero, M., Molitor, T., Molgaard, L., Pelican, K., Ponder, J. B., Travis, D. A., Willette, M., Wolf, T. M., Zou, X., & Wells, S. J. (2024). One Health as a core component of veterinary medicine: defining day-1 public Health competencies for the veterinary workforce. *Journal of Veterinary Medical Education, 51*(2), 176–184. https://doi.org/10.3138/jvme-2023-0016

Bastard, J., Andraud, M., Chauvin, C., Glaser, P., Opatowski, L., & Temime, L. (2020). Dynamics of livestock-associated methicillin resistant staphylococcus aureus in pig movement networks: Insight from mathematical modeling and French data. *Epidemics, 31*, 100389. https://doi.org/10.1016/j.epidem.2020.100389

Baudoin, F., Hogeveen, H., & Wauters, E. (2021). Reducing antimicrobial use and dependence in livestock production systems: A social and economic sciences perspective on an interdisciplinary approach. *Frontiers in Veterinary Science, 8*. https://doi.org/10.3389/fvets.2021.584593

Bergez, J.-E., Béthinger, A., Bockstaller, C., Cederberg, C., Ceschia, E., Guilpart, N., Lange, S., Müller, F., Reidsma, P., Riviere, C., Schader, C., Therond, O., & van der Werf, H. M. G. (2022). Integrating agri-environmental indicators, ecosystem services assessment, life cycle assessment and yield gap analysis to assess the environmental sustainability of agriculture. *Ecological Indicators, 141*, 109107. https://doi.org/10.1016/j.ecolind.2022.109107

Boudreau LeBlanc, A., Williams-Jones, B., & Aenishaenslin, C. (2022). Bio-ethics and One Health: A case study approach to building reflexive governance. *Front Public Health, 10*. https://doi.org/10.3389/fpubh.2022.648593

Brown, V. R., Miller, R. S., McKee, S. C., Ernst, K. H., Didero, N. M., Maison, R. M., Grady, M. J., & Shwiff, S. A. (2021). Risks of introduction and economic consequences associated with African swine fever, classical swine fever and foot-and-mouth disease: A review of the literature. *Transboundary and Emerging Diseases, 68*(4), 1910–1965. https://doi.org/10.1111/tbed.13919

Calderón Díaz, J. A., Fitzgerald, R. M., Shalloo, L., Rodrigues da Costa, M., Niemi, J., Leonard, F. C., Kyriazakis, I., & García Manzanilla, E. (2020). Financial analysis of herd status and vaccination practices for porcine reproductive and respiratory syndrome virus, swine influenza virus, and mycoplasma hyopneumoniae in farrow-to-finish pig farms using a bio-economic simulation model. *Frontiers in Veterinary Science, 7*. https://doi.org/10.3389/fvets.2020.556674

Cardenas, N. C., Sykes, A. L., Lopes, F. P. N., & Machado, G. (2022). Multiple species animal movements: Network properties, disease dynamics and the impact of targeted control actions. *Veterinary Research, 53*(1), 14. https://doi.org/10.1186/s13567-022-01031-2

Chadborn, T., Williams, S., Jorgensen, T., Price, C., Buckel, A., & Altieri, E. (2023). An approach for embedding behavioural science in antimicrobial resistance One Health research. *Journal of Infection and Public Health, 16*, 134–140. https://doi.org/10.1016/j.jiph.2023.11.001

Cheng, M., Liu, X., Sheng, H., & Yuan, Z. (2023). MAPS: A new model using data fusion to enhance the accuracy of high-resolution mapping for livestock production systems. *One Earth, 6*(9), 1190–1201. https://doi.org/10.1016/j.oneear.2023.08.012

Cole, D., Todd, L., & Wing, S. (2000). Concentrated swine feeding operations and public health: A review of occupational and community health effects. *Environmental Health Perspectives, 108*(8), 685–699. https://doi.org/10.1289/ehp.00108685

Cunningham, A. A., Daszak, P., & Wood, J. L. N. (2017). One Health, emerging infectious diseases and wildlife: Two decades of Progress? *Philosophical Transactions of the Royal Society B: Biological Sciences, 372*(1725), 20160167. https://doi.org/10.1098/rstb.2016.0167

Dorjee, S., Revie, C. W., Poljak, Z., McNab, W. B., & Sanchez, J. (2013). Network analysis of swine shipments in Ontario, Canada, to support disease spread modelling and risk-based disease management. *Preventive Veterinary Medicine, 112*(1–2), 118–127. https://doi.org/10.1016/j.prevetmed.2013.06.008

Fernandes, A. F. A., Dórea, J. R. R., Valente, B. D., Fitzgerald, R., Herring, W., & Rosa, G. J. M. (2020). Comparison of data analytics strategies in computer vision systems to predict pig body composition traits from 3D images. *Journal of Animal Science, 98*(8). https://doi.org/10.1093/jas/skaa250

Flanagan, M. L., Parrish, C. R., Cobey, S., Glass, G. E., Bush, R. M., & Leighton, T. J. (2012). Anticipating the species jump: Surveillance for emerging viral threats. *Zoonoses and Public Health, 59*(3), 155–163. https://doi.org/10.1111/j.1863-2378.2011.01439.x

Friedler, A. (2021). Sociocultural, behavioural and political factors shaping the COVID-19 pandemic: The need for a biocultural approach to understanding pandemics and (re)emerging pathogens. *Global Public Health, 16*(1), 17–35. https://doi.org/10.1080/17441692.2020.1828982

Gebreyes, W. A., Dupouy-Camet, J., Newport, M. J., Oliveira, C. J. B., Schlesinger, L. S., Saif, Y. M., Kariuki, S., Saif, L. J., Saville, W., Wittum, T., Hoet, A., Quessy, S., Kazwala, R., Tekola, B., Shryock, T., Bisesi, M., Patchanee, P., Boonmar, S., & King, L. J. (2014). The global One Health paradigm: Challenges and opportunities for tackling infectious diseases at the human, animal, and environment interface in low-resource settings. *PLoS Neglected Tropical Diseases, 8*(11), e3257. https://doi.org/10.1371/journal.pntd.0003257

Gribbin, J., & Gribbin, M. (2009). James Lovelock. Princeton University Press. https://doi.org/10.1515/9781400832859

Hammami, P., Widgren, S., Grosbois, V., Apolloni, A., Rose, N., & Andraud, M. (2022). Complex network analysis to understand trading partnership in French swine production. *PLoS One, 17*(4), e0266457. https://doi.org/10.1371/journal.pone.0266457

Hernandez, E., Llonch, P., & Turner, P. V. (2022). Applied animal ethics in industrial food animal production: Exploring the role of the veterinarian. *Animals, 12*(6), 678. https://doi.org/10.3390/ani12060678

Hickman, R. A., Leangapichart, T., Lunha, K., Jiwakanon, J., Angkititrakul, S., Magnusson, U., Sunde, M., & Järhult, J. D. (2021). Exploring the antibiotic resistance burden in livestock, livestock handlers and their non-livestock handling contacts: A One Health perspective. *Frontiers in Microbiology, 12*. https://doi.org/10.3389/fmicb.2021.651461

Hörtenhuber, S. J., Schauberger, G., Mikovits, C., Schönhart, M., Baumgartner, J., Niebuhr, K., Piringer, M., Anders, I., Andre, K., Hennig-Pauka, I., & Zollitsch, W. (2020). The effect of climate change-induced temperature increase on performance and environmental impact of intensive pig production systems. *Sustainability, 12*(22), 9442. https://doi.org/10.3390/su12229442

Jiang, Y., Li, G., Yu, L., Li, L., Zhang, Y., Zhou, Y., Tong, W., Liu, C., Gao, F., & Tong, G. (2020). Genetic diversity of porcine reproductive and respiratory syndrome virus (PRRSV) from 1996 to 2017 in China. *Frontiers in Microbiology*, 11. https://doi.org/10.3389/fmicb.2020.00618

Kahn, L. H. (2021). Developing a One Health approach by using a multi-dimensional matrix. *One Health, 13*, 100289. https://doi.org/10.1016/j.onehlt.2021.100289

Kerdsin, A., Segura, M., Fittipaldi, N., & Gottschalk, M. (2022). Sociocultural factors influencing human streptococcus suis disease in Southeast Asia. *Foods, 11*(9), 1190. https://doi.org/10.3390/foods11091190

Lee, P., Quintanilla, J. G., Alfonso-Almazán, J. M., Galán-Arriola, C., Yan, P., Sánchez-González, J., Pérez-Castellano, N., Pérez-Villacastín, J., Ibañez, B., Loew, L. M., & Filgueiras-Rama, D. (2019). In vivo ratiometric optical mapping enables high-resolution cardiac electrophysiology in pig models. *Cardiovascular Research, 115*(11), 1659–1671. https://doi.org/10.1093/cvr/cvz039

Lentz, H. H. K., Koher, A., Hövel, P., Gethmann, J., Sauter-Louis, C., Selhorst, T., & Conraths, F. J. (2016). Disease spread through animal movements: A static and temporal network analysis of pig trade in Germany. *PLoS One, 11*(5), e0155196. https://doi.org/10.1371/journal.pone.0155196

Leroy, G., Boettcher, P., Joly, F., Looft, C., & Baumung, R. (2024). Multifunctionality and provision of ecosystem services by livestock species and breeds at global level. *animal, 18*(1), 101048. https://doi.org/10.1016/j.animal.2023.101048

Lovelock, J. E. (1983). Gaia as seen through the atmosphere. In *Biomineralization and biological metal accumulation* (pp. 15–25). Springer. https://doi.org/10.1007/978-94-009-7944-4_2

Lovelock, J. E., & Margulis, L. (1974). Atmospheric homeostasis by and for the biosphere: The gaia hypothesis. *Tellus A: Dynamic Meteorology and Oceanography, 26*(1–2), 2. https://doi.org/10.3402/tellusa.v26i1-2.9731

Luty, L., Musiał, K., & Zioło, M. (2021). The role of selected ecosystem services in different farming systems in Poland regarding the differentiation of agricultural land structure. *Sustainability, 13*(12), 6673. https://doi.org/10.3390/su13126673

Mackenzie, J. S., Jeggo, M., Daszak, P., & Richt, J. A. (Eds.). (2013). *One Health: The human-animal-environment interfaces in emerging infectious diseases* (Current topics in microbiology and immunology) (Vol. 366). Springer. https://doi.org/10.1007/978-3-642-35846-3

Makau, D. N., Paploski, I. A. D., & VanderWaal, K. (2021). Temporal stability of swine movement networks in the U.S. *Preventive Veterinary Medicine, 191*, 105369. https://doi.org/10.1016/j.prevetmed.2021.105369

Maltecca, C., Lu, D., Schillebeeckx, C., McNulty, N. P., Schwab, C., Shull, C., & Tiezzi, F. (2019). Predicting growth and carcass traits in swine using microbiome data and machine learning algorithms. *Scientific Reports, 9*(1), 6574. https://doi.org/10.1038/s41598-019-43031-x

Martínez-Avilés, M., Fernández-Carrión, E., López García-Baones, J. M., & Sánchez-Vizcaíno, J. M. (2017). Early detection of infection in pigs through an online monitoring system. *Transboundary and Emerging Diseases, 64*(2), 364–373. https://doi.org/10.1111/tbed.12372

Mason-D'Croz, D., Bogard, J. R., Herrero, M., Robinson, S., Sulser, T. B., Wiebe, K., Willenbockel, D., & Godfray, H. C. J. (2020). Modelling the global economic consequences of a major African swine fever outbreak in China. *Nature Food, 1*(4), 221–228. https://doi.org/10.1038/s43016-020-0057-2

Mesquita, J. R. (2021). *Emerging and re-emerging diseases—Novel challenges in today's world.* MDPI. https://doi.org/10.3390/books978-3-0365-1896-1

Moraes, D. F. d. S. D., Mesquita, J. R., Dutra, V., & Nascimento, M. S. J. (2021). Systematic review of hepatitis E virus in Brazil: A one-Health approach of the human-animal-environment triad. *Animals, 11*(8), 2290. https://doi.org/10.3390/ani11082290

Nelson, M. I., & Vincent, A. L. (2015). Reverse zoonosis of influenza to swine: new perspectives on the human–animal interface. *Trends in Microbiology, 23*(3), 142–153. https://doi.org/10.1016/j.tim.2014.12.002

Ogunseitan, O. A. (2022). One Health and the environment: From conceptual framework to implementation science. *Environment: Science and Policy for Sustainable Development, 64*(2), 11–21. https://doi.org/10.1080/00139157.2022.2021792

Oliveira, A. R. S., Cohnstaedt, L. W., & Cernicchiaro, N. (2018). Japanese encephalitis virus: Placing disease vectors in the epidemiologic triad. *Annals of the Entomological Society of America*. https://doi.org/10.1093/aesa/say025

Osterhaus, A. D. M. E., Vanlangendonck, C., Barbeschi, M., Bruschke, C. J. M., Christensen, R., Daszak, P., de Groot, F., Doherty, P., Drury, P., Gmacz, S., Hamilton, K., Hart, J., Katz, R., Longuet, C., McLeay, J., Morelli, G., Schlundt, J., Smith, T., Suri, S., Umali, K., van Aken, J., & Wagenaar, J. A. (2020). Make science evolve into a one Health approach to improve HEALTH and security: A white paper. *One Health Outlook, 2*(1), 6. https://doi.org/10.1186/s42522-019-0009-7

Overgaauw, P. A. M., Vinke, C. M., van Hagen, M. A. E., & Lipman, L. J. A. (2020). A One Health perspective on the human–companion animal relationship with emphasis on zoonotic aspects. *International Journal of Environmental Research and Public Health, 17*(11), 3789. https://doi.org/10.3390/ijerph17113789

Pittiglio, C., Khomenko, S., & Beltran-Alcrudo, D. (2018). Wild boar mapping using population-density statistics: From polygons to high resolution raster maps. *PLoS One, 13*(5), e0193295. https://doi.org/10.1371/journal.pone.0193295

Puspitarani, G. A., Fuchs, R., Fuchs, K., Ladinig, A., & Desvars-Larrive, A. (2023). Network analysis of pig movement data as an epidemiological tool: An Austrian case study. *Scientific Reports, 13*(1), 9623. https://doi.org/10.1038/s41598-023-36596-1

Rousham, E. K., Unicomb, L., & Islam, M. A. (1876). Human, animal and environmental contributors to antibiotic resistance in low-resource settings: Integrating behavioural, epidemiological, and One Health approaches. *Proceedings of the Royal Society B: Biological Sciences, 2018*(285), 20180332. https://doi.org/10.1098/rspb.2018.0332

Sartore, L., Wei, Y., Abayomi, E., Riggins, S., Corral, G., Bejleri, V., & Spiegelman, C. (2020). Modeling swine population dynamics at a finer temporal resolution. *Applied Stochastic Models in Business and Industry, 36*(6), 1060–1079. https://doi.org/10.1002/asmb.2597

Scherrer, S., Rosato, G., Spoerry Serrano, N., Stevens, M. J. A., Rademacher, F., Schrenzel, J., Gottschalk, M., Stephan, R., & Peterhans, S. (2020). Population structure, genetic diversity and pathotypes of streptococcus suis isolated during the last 13 years from diseased pigs in Switzerland. *Veterinary Research, 51*(1), 85. https://doi.org/10.1186/s13567-020-00813-w

Suresh, T., Sivarajasekar, N., & Balasubramani, K. (2021). Enhanced ultrasonic assisted biodiesel production from meat industry waste (pig tallow) using green copper oxide nanocatalyst: Comparison of response surface and neural network modelling. *Renewable Energy, 164*, 897–907. https://doi.org/10.1016/j.renene.2020.09.112

Trnka, R., & Lorencova, R. (2022). Indigenous concepts of consciousness, soul, and spirit: A cross-cultural perspective. *Journal of Consciousness Studies, 29*(1), 113–140. https://doi.org/10.53765/20512201.29.1.113

Van Ba, N., Nam, L. Q., Do, D. N., Van Hau, N., & Pham, L. D. (2020). An assessment of genetic diversity and population structures of fifteen Vietnamese indigenous pig breeds for supporting the decision making on conservation strategies. *Tropical Animal Health and Production, 52*(3), 1033–1041. https://doi.org/10.1007/s11250-019-02090-y

van Klompenburg, T., & Kassahun, A. (2022). Data-driven decision making in pig farming: A review of the literature. *Livestock Science, 261*, 104961. https://doi.org/10.1016/j.livsci.2022.104961

van Staaveren, N., Doyle, B., Manzanilla, E. G., Calderón Díaz, J. A., Hanlon, A., & Boyle, L. A. (2017). Validation of carcass lesions as indicators for on-farm Health and welfare of pigs. *Journal of Animal Science, 95*(4), 1528–1536. https://doi.org/10.2527/jas.2016.1180

Wang, Y., Noll, L., Lu, N., Porter, E., Stoy, C., Zheng, W., Liu, X., Peddireddi, L., Niederwerder, M., & Bai, J. (2020). Genetic diversity and prevalence of porcine circovirus type 3 (PCV3) and type 2 (PCV2) in the Midwest of the USA during 2016–2018. *Transboundary and Emerging Diseases, 67*(3), 1284–1294. https://doi.org/10.1111/tbed.13467

Weiss, R. A., & Sankaran, N. (2022). Emergence of epidemic diseases: Zoonoses and other origins. *Faculty Reviews, 11*. https://doi.org/10.12703/r/11-2

Wilcox, B. A., & Steele, J. A. (2021). One Health and emerging zoonotic diseases. In *Handbook of global health* (pp. 1–49). Springer. https://doi.org/10.1007/978-3-030-05325-3_88-2

Wu, F., Sun, H., Lu, S., Gou, X., Yan, D., Xu, Z., Zhang, Z., Qadri, Q. R., Zhang, Z., Wang, Z., Chen, Q., Li, M., Wang, X., Dong, X., Wang, Q., & Pan, Y. (2020). Genetic diversity and selection signatures within Diannan small-ear pigs revealed by next-generation sequencing. *Frontiers in Genetics, 11*. https://doi.org/10.3389/fgene.2020.00733

Zinsstag, J., Schelling, E., Waltner-Toews, D., & Tanner, M. (2011). From "One Medicine" to "One Health" and systemic approaches to health and well-being. *Preventive Veterinary Medicine, 101*(3–4), 148–156. https://doi.org/10.1016/j.prevetmed.2010.07.003

Zoonotic Disease Surveillance and Monitoring in Swine Populations

Sanjay Vaghela and Pranav Anjaria

Abstract

This book chapter provides a comprehensive exploration of zoonotic disease surveillance and monitoring in swine populations, emphasizing the critical intersection of human and animal health. It delves into the common zoonotic diseases prevalent in swine, their transmission patterns, clinical signs, and prevention strategies. It covers various surveillance methods, tools, challenges, and emphasizes the adoption of a One Health approach. It highlights the complexities and intricacies of establishing effective surveillance systems, emphasizing the need for data integration, implementation strategies, and institutional capacity building. The One Health approach is presented as a collaborative framework to enhance zoonotic disease surveillance, involving joint efforts across human, animal, and environmental health domains. It also addresses the challenges in monitoring and controlling zoonotic diseases in swine, proposing potential solutions aligned with the evolving landscape of infectious disease management. It emphasizes the need for sustained investment, coordinated efforts, and innovative approaches to establish and maintain effective zoonotic disease surveillance systems, ultimately safeguarding both animal and human health.

Keywords

Zoonotic diseases · Swine populations · Surveillance · Monitoring · One Health approach

S. Vaghela · P. Anjaria (✉)
Kamdhenu University, Anand, Gujarat, India

R. Deb et al. (eds.), *Emerging Zoonotic Threats from Swine*,
https://doi.org/10.1007/978-981-96-7407-7_3

Introduction

The intersection of human and animal health is a dynamic and critical domain that requires vigilant attention and strategic approaches to mitigate potential threats. Zoonotic diseases—those that can transfer between animals and humans—pose significant public health concerns, with the potential to trigger large-scale outbreaks and pandemics (Cella et al., 2023). Among the various animal populations implicated in zoonotic disease transmission, swine stand out as a crucial reservoir due to their close proximity to humans and the propensity for certain pathogens to traverse species boundaries (Fagre et al., 2022).

Swine, or domestic pigs, play a vital role in the global food supply chain, making their health and well-being of paramount importance. At the same time, the interconnectedness of swine farming with human communities creates an environment conducive to the transmission of pathogens between species. Understanding the dynamics of zoonotic diseases in swine is crucial for devising effective strategies for detection, monitoring, and control, thereby safeguarding both animal and human health (Sharan et al., 2023).

This chapter delves into zoonotic diseases affecting swine, examining pathogens that present risks to human populations (Lin et al., 2023). It then discusses diverse surveillance strategies employed for monitoring zoonotic agents in swine populations. From conventional passive surveillance to advanced diagnostic tools, the chapter provides a comprehensive overview of available methods for disease detection. The importance of epidemiological monitoring frameworks is highlighted as a cornerstone for predicting and preventing outbreaks through the analysis of disease patterns and identification of risk factors (VanderWaal & Deen, 2018). The One Health approach, emphasizing interdisciplinary collaboration, is explored as a comprehensive framework for addressing zoonotic diseases. This approach underscores the interconnected nature of human, animal, and environmental health and advocates for unified action against these complex threats (Brown et al., 2018).

Effective zoonotic disease surveillance in swine populations is riddled with challenges (EMRO, 2020). From the emergence of antimicrobial resistance to the global nature of trade and travel, addressing these hurdles requires innovative solutions like dissecting the challenges faced in monitoring and controlling zoonotic diseases in swine and propose potential solutions that align with the evolving landscape of infectious disease management (Rodríguez-Prieto et al., 2015; Bird & Mazet, 2018). To provide a practical perspective, a series of case studies illustrate successful approaches to zoonotic disease surveillance and monitoring in swine populations. These cases highlight the diverse contexts in which challenges were met and overcome, offering valuable insights for practitioners. Future directions in zoonotic disease surveillance within swine populations must account for advancements in technology, changes in agricultural practices, and the constant evolution of infectious agents. These dynamic factors highlight the growing need for adaptive and anticipatory strategies to effectively monitor, prevent and respond toemerging health threats (Tizzani et al., 2021).

Zoonotic Diseases in Swine

Zoonotic diseases in swine represent a critical intersection between animal and human health, posing significant public health concerns worldwide. Swine are susceptible hosts for a variety of pathogens capable of crossing species barriers and infecting humans, leading to zoonotic transmission (Davies, 2012). Diseases such as influenza A viruses, including the notorious H1N1 strain, and hepatitis E virus are prominent examples of zoonoses associated with swine populations. Additionally, bacteria like Salmonella and Campylobacter species can be transmitted through direct contact with swine or consumption of contaminated pork products, emphasizing the need for robust surveillance strategies to reduce risks (Van Reeth, 2007; Meng, 2012).

Common Zoonotic Disease

A prevalent zoonotic disease in swine is caused by roundworms, particularly *Ascaris suum*. This parasitic infection is primarily spread through the ingestion of eggs found in the environment (Symeonidou et al., 2020). Pigs can contract the infection from contaminated plants, feed, water, or even through contact with infected feces on fomites. The clinical signs of *Ascaris suum* infection typically manifest within a relatively short incubation period of 1–10 days (Nejsum et al., 2012). In young pigs, gastrointestinal symptoms such as a pendulous abdomen may be observed, along with respiratory symptoms like expiratory dyspnea, commonly known as "thumps," and a chronic paroxysmal cough. Additionally, reproductive issues such as delayed estrus and poor conception rates can occur in infected sows (Agustina et al., 2023).

Preventing the spread of *Ascaris suum* infection involves implementing rigorous hygiene measures and management strategies. Regular cleaning and disinfection of pig housing facilities are crucial, along with the prompt removal of manure to minimize environmental contamination. Deworming pigs at appropriate intervals is also essential in controlling the parasite's population within the herd (Nejsum et al., 2012). In addition, adopting effective biosecurity measures, such as thoroughly washing sows before placing them in farrowing crates and early weaning of piglets at 2–4 weeks, can help minimize the risk of transmission. Management strategies like all-in, all-out production systems, and rotational pasture grazing can further assist in controlling the spread of *Ascaris suum* and other zoonotic diseases in swine populations (Symeonidou et al., 2020).

Another major zoonotic disease common in swine populations is brucellosis, caused by *Brucella suis* (Olsen & Tatum, 2016). This bacterial infection can be spread through direct contact with reproductive tissues or fluids, as well as by ingesting contaminated feed or water. Moreover, fomites can act as a source of transmission for the disease. Brucellosis presents with varying incubation periods. Clinical signs often manifest in the reproductive system, leading to issues such as abortion, stillbirths, retained placenta, placentitis, orchitis, and epididymitis (Franco-Paredes et al., 2017). Musculoskeletal symptoms such as arthritis, lameness, and spondylitis, as well as cutaneous manifestations like abscesses, may also occur. Preventive strategies for brucellosis include rigorous cleaning and disinfection practices, along with measures to prevent exposure to wild and feral swine. It's crucial to source animals from Brucella-free suppliers and implement screening protocols to detect infected individuals (Leiser et al., 2013). Infected animals should be promptly isolated or culled, and a separate birthing area should be established to minimize transmission risk. Proper disposal of aborted fetuses and placentas is also essential in preventing the spread of brucellosis within swine herds (Gong et al., 2021).

In addition to roundworms and brucellosis, another common zoonotic disease found in swine populations is erysipelas, caused by the bacterium *Erysipelothrix rhusiopathiae* (Wang et al., 2010). This disease can spread through direct contact with infected animals or their bodily fluids, as well as by ingesting contaminated soil, feed, or water. Cannibalism, especially seen in poultry, may also play a role in transmission, along with mechanical vectors like biting insects (Brooke & Riley, 1999; Habte et al., 2021). Erysipelas has varying incubation periods, typically ranging from 1 to 7 days. The clinical signs vary depending on the stage of infection. Pigs with acute infections may show symptoms such as fever, weakness, red-purple spots on the ears and skin, difficulty breathing, and, in severe cases, death. Subacute cases are characterized by red-purple diamond-shaped skin lesions, while chronically infected pigs may experience joint swelling, lameness, dyspnea, and ultimately death (Opriessnig & Coutinho, 2019).

Preventive strategies for erysipelas encompass a multifaceted approach. It includes maintaining cleanliness and implementing rigorous disinfection protocols to minimize environmental contamination. Controlling rodent populations, which can serve as reservoirs for the bacterium, is also crucial. Vaccination of both pigs and turkeys against erysipelas is recommended to prevent disease outbreaks (Opriessnig et al., 2020). Symptomatic pigs should be promptly culled to prevent further spread of the infection, and infected carcasses should be appropriately disposed of to mitigate the risk of transmission. These thorough prevention measures are crucial for effectively controlling erysipelas and minimizing its impact on both swine health and public health (Habte et al., 2021). Table 1 summarizes different zoonotic diseases prevalent in swine populations, their respective etiologies, transmission patterns, clinical signs, and prevention strategies.

Surveillance Methods

Establishing effective surveillance systems is vital for protecting both swine health and public health. Zoonotic diseases present significant risks to both animal and human populations, whether through direct transmission or foodborne pathways. Given the close interactions between humans and swine in agricultural environments and the potential for zoonotic diseases to spread quickly within swine populations, robust surveillance strategies are essential for early detection, swift response, and disease control (Turlewicz-Podbielska et al., 2020). Surveillance efforts focus

Table 1 Common zoonotic disease in swine (Laber et al., 2002; Rivera-Benitez et al., 2014)

Zoonotic disease (Etiology)	Transmission	Clinical sign	Prevention
Campylobacteriosis (*Campylobacter jejuni, C. coli*)	The disease can be transmitted through the ingestion of feces, reproductive tissues, and contaminated soil or water, direct contact with infected animals, and through fomites	The disease usually presents with an incubation period of 3–25 days, accompanied by gastrointestinal symptoms like enteritis and diarrhea	To curb disease spread, ensure regular cleaning and disinfection, manage manure removal, prevent overcrowding, vaccinate animals (though carriers may persist), isolate aborting individuals, and promptly dispose of aborted fetuses and placentas
Cryptosporidiosis (*Cryptosporidium* spp.)	The disease can be transmitted through the consumption of food, water, and soil contaminated with oocysts, as well as through fomites	After an incubation period of 3–5 days, clinical signs appear, including gastrointestinal symptoms such as watery diarrhea, straining, loss of appetite, and weight loss	Preventive measures include thorough cleaning and disinfection (as the organism is resistant), regular removal of manure, avoiding overcrowding, ensuring colostrum provision, isolating sick animals, and preventing or treating concurrent infections
Cysticercosis/ Taeniasis (*Taenia* spp.)	The disease can be transmitted through ingestion of gravid proglottids found in pastures, as well as through contaminated food, water, or soil	The disease has an extended incubation period ranging from months to years, characterized by gastrointestinal symptoms like unthriftiness, poor appetite, and diarrhea	Preventive measures involve routine cleaning and disinfection, manure removal, deworming of farm dogs and cats, proper disposal of dead animals, avoiding the use of river water for livestock, and keeping animals away from human feces

(continued)

Table 1 (continued)

Zoonotic disease (Etiology)	Transmission	Clinical sign	Prevention
Japanese encephalitis (Flavivirus)	The disease can be transmitted via vectors such as Culex mosquitoes, with potential transmission through semen and transplacental routes	Reproductive symptoms are more common in naïve pigs, resulting in stillborn or mummified fetuses, abortions, orchitis, and infertility	Preventive measures entail thorough cleaning and disinfection, vector control, vaccination particularly in endemic regions like Asia and the Western Pacific, housing animals in screened facilities with well-maintained screens, and minimizing exposure to wild birds
Swine influenza (Influenza virus A Most common: H1N1, H3N2 variant H1N2)	The disease can be transmitted through direct contact with nasal discharge, via fomites, and through the inhalation of droplets and aerosols released during coughing or sneezing	Clinical signs include respiratory symptoms such as fever, loss of appetite, dry cough, difficulty breathing, nasal discharge, and conjunctivitis, as well as possible reproductive problems like abortion	Preventive measures encompass cleaning and disinfection, implementing robust biosecurity protocols, ensuring adequate ventilation, minimizing stress, avoiding exposure to wild birds, and vaccinating pigs
Vesicular stomatitis (Vesiculo virus)	The disease is transmitted through direct contact with skin lesions and vesicles, as well as through contact with saliva and nasal secretions	After an incubation period of 3–7 days, clinical signs of the disease appear, including fever and the presence of papules and vesicles in areas such as the oral cavity, udder, teats, prepuce, interdigital space, and coronary band, along with inflammation, swelling, and pain	Preventive measures include thorough cleaning and disinfection, particularly of milking equipment, milking animals with lesions last, minimizing stress, controlling vectors, quarantining new animals, isolating infected individuals, avoiding hard and abrasive feeds to prevent mucosal injury, and conducting tests to exclude foot-and-mouth disease

on tracking disease prevalence, identifying emerging threats, and guiding evidence-based interventions to reduce the risks linked to zoonotic diseases. By implementing comprehensive surveillance protocols, stakeholders can proactively monitor the health status of swine populations, assess the potential risks to human health, and implement targeted control measures to prevent disease transmission and outbreaks (Burke et al., 2012). The following two surveillance methods for swine zoonotic diseases are active and passive surveillance, which are explained in detail below (Gervasi et al., 2019).

Active Surveillance Method

Periodic Sampling

Health authorities routinely collect samples such as blood, nasal swabs, or feces from swine populations at predetermined intervals. This method serves the purpose of early detection, allowing authorities to identify zoonotic pathogens before they spread widely (Gervasi et al., 2019). Moreover, periodic sampling enables the monitoring of disease prevalence trends over time. It finds application in routine testing of swine herds and targeted sampling during high-risk periods, such as migration seasons for birds that may carry diseases (Hu et al., 2021).

Sentinel Animals

Another active surveillance method involves using specific animals, known as sentinels, to monitor disease prevalence. These sentinels serve as an early warning system, signaling the presence of diseases in a particular area (Corzo et al., 2013). They are particularly useful in high-risk regions where zoonotic threats are known. Sentinel pigs are placed strategically to monitor health and observe clinical signs, though other species like birds or rodents can also serve as sentinels (Gervasi et al., 2019).

Longitudinal Sampling of Vector Populations

This method involves monitoring vectors such as ticks and mosquitoes that transmit diseases among swine. The goal is to identify reservoirs of zoonotic pathogens and evaluate the risk of disease transmission (Gervasi et al., 2019). Longitudinal sampling of vector populations entails studying vector populations in swine environments and collecting samples from vectors to test for pathogens (Alba et al., 2017).

Passive Surveillance Method

Passive surveillance methods are essential components of zoonotic disease monitoring systems, complementing active surveillance approaches. They leverage existing infrastructure and processes to gather data on disease occurrences in swine populations (Gervasi et al., 2019). By relying on reporting systems and abattoir surveillance, authorities can efficiently monitor disease trends, identify emerging threats, and implement appropriate control measures. Collaboration between veterinarians, farmers, laboratories, and regulatory agencies is crucial for the success of passive surveillance efforts, as timely and accurate reporting of disease cases is essential for effective disease management (Corzo et al., 2013).

Reporting Systems

This method involves veterinarians, farmers, and laboratories reporting disease cases as they arise. The aim is to capture naturally occurring cases in swine populations. By maintaining databases of swine disease reports, data can be collected and analyzed to identify trends and patterns in disease (Tsai et al., 2010).

Abattoir Surveillance

During abattoir surveillance, swine carcasses are examined for signs of disease during the slaughter process. This method serves the purpose of detecting diseases that may have been missed during live animal inspections. Routine inspections at abattoirs offer valuable insights into the prevalence of zoonotic diseases in swine populations and play a crucial role in overall disease monitoring efforts (Hoinville et al., 2013).

Tools and Methodologies Supporting Surveillance

Molecular Diagnostics

Utilizing advanced techniques such as PCR (Polymerase Chain Reaction) and ELISA (Enzyme-Linked Immunosorbent Assay) enables the accurate detection of specific pathogens (Tayebeh et al., 2016). Molecular diagnostics offer high sensitivity and yield rapid results, making them invaluable in testing swine samples for zoonotic agents and screening for emerging zoonoses (Sue et al., 2014).

Geographic Information Systems (GIS)

GIS allows the creation of maps to visualize disease occurrences and associated risk factors (Johnson & Johnson, 2001). By conducting spatial analysis, authorities can identify disease hotspots and effectively allocate surveillance efforts. GIS finds application in overlaying disease data with environmental factors, aiding in the planning of targeted interventions based on geographical insights (Dragomir et al., 2014).

Major Obstacles in Implementing Effective Surveillance Systems

Creating a strong surveillance system is inherently intricate, requiring thorough evaluation of various options, efficient distribution of resources, and management of limitations. The complexities in both structure and operation, compounded by regulatory hurdles, present substantial obstacles that may disrupt the smooth operation of these vital networks. Particularly in settings with limited resources, we examined some of these challenges. Below, we propose potential steps to move forward in addressing them.

Improving Data Integration

In resource-limited countries, compiling data on disease outbreaks, surveillance, and mortality/morbidity trends remains a significant challenge. The disconnect between vital registration systems and healthcare networks leads to considerable gaps in understanding disease dynamics and their real-world implications. Administrative and societal constraints further contribute to underreporting of deaths, even in medical facilities, making it difficult to establish clear associations between morbidity and mortality, particularly for infectious diseases.

Additionally, data related to animal trade is often fragmented and unreliable, lacking crucial information on species, trade volume, movement routes, and long-term trends in both legal and illegal trade—domestically and internationally—of livestock and wildlife. Inadequate monitoring and surveillance of wildlife trade heightens the risk of zoonotic disease emergence. A notable instance of this occurred when the monkeypox virus was transmitted from Ghana to Texas through the pet trade, specifically via pouched rats (Sharan et al., 2023).

To mitigate the risk of zoonotic disease transmission and enhance disease surveillance, it is crucial to integrate data systems more effectively. This necessitates strengthening reporting mechanisms and reinforcing monitoring efforts across domestic and wildlife trade sectors. Achieving this goal requires coordinated collaboration at both national and international levels (Bernstein et al., 2022).

Implementation Hurdles

A significant challenge in disease surveillance is the fragmentation of data systems, which separates healthcare utilization records from disease outbreak reporting mechanisms. This disjointed structure has led to inconsistencies in outbreak investigations and reporting, creating gaps that undermine the effectiveness of surveillance efforts (Suthar et al., 2018). To address these challenges, initiatives such as WHO-supported influenza surveillance and the CDC's programs for acute encephalitis syndrome and acute febrile illnesses have been introduced. However, due to resource limitations and varying levels of governmental commitment, these programs have largely remained research-focused pilot initiatives. This highlights the critical need for sustained investment and stronger political commitment to enhance disease surveillance, ensuring a more effective response to emerging public health threats (Hay & McCauley, 2018).

Surveillance Functions Within Distinct Program and Institutional Silos

Programs such as GLEWS and GOARN have played a crucial role in controlling disease transmission, increasing public awareness of zoonotic diseases like COVID-19, rabies, and monkeypox, improving treatment accessibility, and reducing mortality rates. These successes underscore the value of targeted surveillance in managing zoonotic threats. However, despite these advancements, challenges persist in the current disease surveillance framework. A major issue is the fragmentation of surveillance data across separate programs. While these initiatives have made significant progress individually, their data often remains siloed, lacking integration into a comprehensive surveillance system. This disconnect hinders efficient data sharing and utilization. Even when different programs collect overlapping data, mechanisms for coordination and exchange are often absent, leading to inefficiencies and missed opportunities for collaboration. Additionally, existing data systems are underutilized for addressing policy and programmatic questions. The gap between program implementation and research organizations further limits the ability to leverage surveillance data for broader insights and improvements. Without better coordination and information sharing, efforts to strengthen zoonotic disease surveillance remain constrained (Asokan & Mohammed, 2021).

Limited Engagement of the Private Sector

The private healthcare sector encompasses a wide range of providers, from unregistered practitioners to large hospitals, operating on both for-profit and not-for-profit models. Despite its extensive reach, its involvement in disease surveillance has remained limited. Integrating private healthcare into public health surveillance requires addressing several key challenges, including identifying diseases most relevant to private providers, defining appropriate roles for primary care clinics and specialized institutions, ensuring data quality and standardization, and exploring the potential use of private health insurance data for surveillance purposes (Bennett et al., 2017). A citizen-centered approach that merges public and private sector data can enhance real-time disease tracking and provide more comprehensive population coverage. However, effective collaboration with the private sector necessitates strategic planning, clear guidelines, and coordinated efforts to maintain data accuracy, consistency, and relevance for public health decision-making (Gebreyes et al., 2014).

Personnel Challenges

In many countries, the decentralized recruitment of surveillance personnel at state and district levels results in varying responses to human resource shortages in public health surveillance. While disease monitoring is a national priority, health management largely falls under state jurisdiction. However, persistent vacancies and limited capacity pose significant challenges in several regions. A study by Bernstein et al. (2022) highlighted stark disparities in veterinarian availability, ranging from two per 100,000 people in Africa to two per 1000 people in countries such as Spain, Uruguay, and the Falkland Islands. The shortage of well-trained veterinarians, particularly in spillover hotspots, is a serious concern given their crucial role in preventing disease transmission from wildlife and livestock to humans. Understanding and addressing the limited emphasis on public health surveillance by state governments is essential. Factors such as competing priorities, resource constraints, and differing perceptions of surveillance importance may contribute to these gaps. Strengthening public health surveillance requires proactive engagement with state authorities, strategic resource allocation, and enhanced national and international collaboration to bridge workforce shortages and improve disease monitoring capabilities (Jayatilleke, 2020).

Enhancing Institutional Capacity for Training in Core Public Health Competencies

Strengthening institutional capacity through practical, interdisciplinary training programs is essential for effectively monitoring emerging zoonotic disease threats. While many training initiatives focus on public health professionals, some stand out for their impact. For instance, the U.S. Centers for Disease Control and Prevention (CDC) manages the Epidemic Intelligence Service (EIS), a rigorous two-year public health program designed to develop skilled epidemiologists specializing in disease surveillance. Similarly, Canada's Public Health Agency offers the Field Epidemiology Training Program, which plays a crucial role in enhancing public health preparedness for crisis response. Despite these efforts, many countries continue to experience a shortage of trained public health professionals, underscoring the need for sustained investment and collaboration to address gaps in public health capacity building (Doble et al., 2023).

Strengthening Financing for Disease Surveillance to Bolster Global Health Security

Funding for disease surveillance, whether in developed or developing countries, often relies on development aid to address not only financial and material constraints but also workforce-related challenges. Recent assessments indicate that low- and middle-income countries (LMICs) allocate a modest median budget of approximately USD 0.04 per capita annually for surveillance of vaccine-preventable diseases (Himmler et al., 2020). In contrast, studies within the European Union (EU) report an average annual expenditure of EUR 264 per person on surveillance, accounting for about 5% of the total healthcare budget. These figures highlight disparities in disease surveillance funding across regions and raise concerns about the adequacy of available resources. Financial obstacles to sustaining disease surveillance programs can also emerge within organizations responsible for implementing national prevention plans. Challenges often arise when these organizations question the effectiveness of such initiatives or perceive limited direct benefits. Additionally, a lack of collaboration among key stakeholders—such as breeders, livestock brokers, and veterinarians—can further hinder disease control efforts (Hossain et al., 2018). In some cases, professionals in these fields may be reluctant to fully support surveillance programs, believing that health authorities offer insufficient incentives for preventive action. Addressing these human-related barriers, alongside financial and material challenges, is crucial for ensuring the long-term success and sustainability of global disease surveillance initiatives (De Vries et al., 2021).

A One Health Approach to Monitoring Swine Zoonotic Diseases

The One Health approach for monitoring swine zoonotic diseases is based on the collaboration of expertise from various sectors, such as human health, veterinary medicine, and environmental science (EFSA et al., 2023). This integrated approach acknowledges the interconnectedness of health across humans, animals, and ecosystems, emphasizing the need to address health issues at the intersection of these domains. Key to this concept is the understanding that many zoonotic diseases, which affect both animals and humans, originate in animals and may spread to human populations (Heymann & Dixon, 2013). This highlights the importance of taking a comprehensive approach to disease surveillance, with a focus on early detection and response to potential zoonotic risks. By recognizing the intricate relationships between animal, human, and environmental health, the One Health approach offers a framework for proactive and integrated surveillance to protect both animal and human populations from the dangers of swine zoonotic diseases (Shaheen, 2022).

Strengthening Surveillance Systems

The One Health approach aims to strengthen surveillance systems by fostering collaboration among relevant sectors and enhancing the capacity for data sharing and analysis. By promoting strong partnerships between human health, veterinary, and environmental agencies, the surveillance infrastructure can be bolstered to effectively monitor and respond to zoonotic diseases affecting swine populations (Bordier et al., 2020). This collective effort entails creating systems for sharing surveillance data and information among all involved parties, enabling a more thorough understanding of disease dynamics and trends (Stärk et al., 2015). Additionally, investments in diagnostic laboratory systems enable the accurate and timely identification of zoonotic pathogens, further enhancing surveillance capabilities. Furthermore, the establishment of a network for early detection and response to outbreaks ensures swift action in the event of emerging zoonotic threats, mitigating their spread and impact on both animal and human health (Rabozzi et al., 2012).

Key Components of One Health Surveillance

The application of One Health surveillance for swine zoonotic diseases encompasses several essential elements within human, animal, and environmental health sectors. In the human health aspect, healthcare institutions like hospitals, clinics, and public health agencies are crucial for reporting zoonotic cases and carrying out epidemiological investigations to track outbreaks and determine risk factors (Falzon et al., 2019). Similarly, the animal health component involves monitoring swine health at veterinary clinics and livestock farms, with regular sampling of swine populations for early detection of zoonotic pathogens. Swine also serve as sentinel animals, providing early warning signs of potential zoonotic threats circulating in the environment. In the environmental health component, wildlife and vector surveillance are conducted to monitor wild animals and disease-carrying vectors for zoonotic pathogens (Calistri et al., 2013). Additionally, environmental sampling from swine habitats, including water sources and soil, helps identify environmental reservoirs of zoonotic diseases. By combining these elements within the One Health framework, surveillance efforts can be enhanced to efficiently detect, monitor, and reduce the risks posed by swine zoonotic diseases to both animal and human populations (Kaneene et al., 2014).

Conclusions

Monitoring and surveillance of zoonotic diseases in swine populations are essential for protecting both animal and human health. This includes examining various aspects of zoonotic disease surveillance, such as common diseases in swine, surveillance techniques, tools, challenges, and the significance of implementing a One Health approach. Effective surveillance relies on a combination of active and passive methods, supported by tools such as molecular diagnostics and geographic information systems. However, several challenges persist, including limited data integration, implementation hurdles, institutional capacity constraints, and financing issues. Despite these obstacles, the One Health approach, which highlights the interdependence of human, animal, and environmental health, offers a promising framework for improving zoonotic disease surveillance. By encouraging collaboration among diverse stakeholders, such as healthcare providers, veterinarians, policymakers, and researchers, we can enhance our capacity to detect, monitor, and respond to zoonotic disease threats in swine populations. Moving forward, sustained investment, coordinated efforts, and innovative approaches will be essential for establishing and maintaining effective zoonotic disease surveillance systems. By prioritizing proactive surveillance measures and embracing a holistic approach, better protect public health and mitigate the risks posed by zoonotic diseases originating from swine.

References

Agustina, K. K., Wirawan, I. M. A., Sudarmaja, I. M., Subrata, I. M., & Dharmawan, N. S. (2023). Ascaris suum–a zoonosis in Bali, Indonesia. *Tropical Parasitology, 13*(2), 100–106.

Alba, A., Morrison, R. E., Cheeran, A., Rovira, A., Alvarez, J., & Perez, A. M. (2017). OptisampleTM: Open web-based application to optimize sampling strategies for active surveillance activities at the herd level illustrated using porcine respiratory reproductive syndrome (PRRS). *PLoS One, 12*(7), e0176863.

Asokan, G. V., & Mohammed, M. Y. (2021). Harnessing big data to strengthen evidence-informed precise public health response. In *Big data in psychiatry# x0026; neurology* (pp. 325–337). Academic Press.

Bennett, A., Avanceña, A. L., Wegbreit, J., Cotter, C., Roberts, K., & Gosling, R. (2017). Engaging the private sector in malaria surveillance: A review of strategies and recommendations for elimination settings. *Malaria Journal, 16*, 1–19.

Bernstein, A. S., Ando, A. W., Loch-Temzelides, T., Vale, M. M., Li, B. V., Li, H., & Dobson, A. P. (2022). The costs and benefits of primary prevention of zoonotic pandemics. *Science Advances, 8*(5), eabl4183.

Bird, B. H., & Mazet, J. A. (2018). Detection of emerging zoonotic pathogens: An integrated one health approach. *Annual Review of Animal Biosciences, 6*, 121–139.

Bordier, M., Uea-Anuwong, T., Binot, A., Hendrikx, P., & Goutard, F. L. (2020). Characteristics of one health surveillance systems: A systematic literature review. *Preventive Veterinary Medicine, 181*, 104560.

Brooke, C. J., & Riley, T. V. (1999). Erysipelothrix rhusiopathiae: Bacteriology, epidemiology and clinical manifestations of an occupational pathogen. *Journal of Medical Microbiology, 48*(9), 789–799.

Brown, V. R., Bowen, R. A., & Bosco-Lauth, A. M. (2018). Zoonotic pathogens from feral swine that pose a significant threat to public health. *Transboundary and Emerging Diseases, 65*(3), 649–659.

Burke, R. L., Kronmann, K. C., Daniels, C. C., Meyers, M., Byarugaba, D. K., Dueger, E., & Vest, K. G. (2012). A review of zoonotic disease surveillance supported by the armed forces health surveillance center. *Zoonoses and Public Health, 59*(3), 164–175.

Calistri, P., Iannetti, S., Danzetta, L., et al. (2013). The components of 'one world–one health' approach. *Transboundary and Emerging Diseases, 60*, 4–13.

Cella, E., Giovanetti, M., Benedetti, F., Scarpa, F., Johnston, C., Borsetti, A., & Ciccozzi, M. (2023). Joining forces against antibiotic resistance: The one health solution. *Pathogens, 12*(9), 1074.

Corzo, C. A., Culhane, M., Juleen, K., Stigger-Rosser, E., Ducatez, M. F., Webby, R. J., & Lowe, J. F. (2013). Active surveillance for influenza A virus among swine, midwestern United States, 2009–2011. *Emerging Infectious Diseases, 19*(6), 954.

Davies, P. R. (2012). One world, one health: The threat of emerging swine diseases. A North American perspective. *Transboundary and Emerging Diseases, 59*, 18–26.

De Vries, L., Koopmans, M., Morton, A., & van Baal, P. (2021). The economics of improving global infectious disease surveillance. *BMJ Global Health, 6*(9), e006597.

Doble, A., Sheridan, Z., Razavi, A., Wilson, A., & Okereke, E. (2023). The role of international support programmes in global health security capacity building: A scoping review. *PLOS Global Public Health, 3*(4), e0001763.

Dragomir, L., Barliba, C., Barliba, L. L., Calinovici, I., & Eles, G. (2014). GIS-A tool for monitoring and management of epidemics. In *14th international multidisciplinary scientific GeoConference SGEM 2014* (pp. 635–642).

EMRO, W. (2020). Zoonotic disease: Emerging public health threats in the Region. *Regional Committee. Sixty-first session*, pp. 1–4

European Food Safety Authority (EFSA), et al. (2023). Prioritisation of zoonotic diseases for coordinated surveillance systems under the one health approach for cross-border pathogens that threaten the union. *EFSA Journal, 21*(3), e07853.

Fagre, A. C., Cohen, L. E., Eskew, E. A., Farrell, M., Glennon, E., Joseph, M. B., & Albery, G. F. (2022). Assessing the risk of human-to-wildlife pathogen transmission for conservation and public health. *Ecology Letters, 25*(6), 1534–1549.

Falzon, L. C., Alumasa, L., Amanya, F., Kang'Ethe, E., Kariuki, S., Momanyi, K., & Fèvre, E. M. (2019). One health in action: Operational aspects of an integrated surveillance system for zoonoses in western Kenya. *Frontiers in Veterinary Science, 6*, 252.

Franco-Paredes, C., Chastain, D., Taylor, P., Stocking, S., & Sellers, B. (2017). Boar hunting and brucellosis caused by Brucella suis. *Travel Medicine and Infectious Disease, 16*, 18–22.

Gebreyes, W. A., Dupouy-Camet, J., Newport, M. J., Oliveira, C. J., Schlesinger, L. S., Saif, Y. M., & King, L. J. (2014). The global one health paradigm: Challenges and opportunities for tackling infectious diseases at the human, animal, and environment interface in low-resource settings. *PLoS Neglected Tropical Diseases, 8*(11), e3257.

Gervasi, V., Marcon, A., Bellini, S., & Guberti, V. (2019). Evaluation of the efficiency of active and passive surveillance in the detection of African swine fever in wild boar. *Veterinary Sciences, 7*(1), 5.

Gong, Q. L., Sun, Y. H., Yang, Y., Zhao, B., Wang, Q., Li, J. M., & Du, R. (2021). Global comprehensive literature review and meta-analysis of Brucella spp. in swine based on publications from 2000 to 2020. *Frontiers in Veterinary Science, 8*, 630960.

Habte, D., Tamir, D., & Tilahun, T. (2021). Swine erysipelas; it's epidemiology, diagnosis, treatment and control and preventive measures, comprehensive review. *Journal of Clinical Epidemiology & Toxicology, 2*(2), 1–7.

Hay, A. J., & McCauley, J. W. (2018). The WHO global influenza surveillance and response system (GISRS) – A future perspective. *Influenza and Other Respiratory Viruses, 12*(5), 551–557.

Heymann, D. L., & Dixon, M. (2013). The value of the one health approach: Shifting from emergency response to prevention of zoonotic disease threats at their source. *Microbiology Spectrum, 1*(1), 10–1128.

Himmler, S., van Exel, J., Perry-Duxbury, M., & Brouwer, W. (2020). Willingness to pay for an early warning system for infectious diseases. *The European Journal of Health Economics, 21*(5), 763–773.

Hoinville, L., et al. (2013). Systematic literature review of surveillance systems and methods for early detection of exotic, new and re-emerging diseases. *Epidemiology & Infection, 143*(10), 2018–2042.

Hossain, A., Politi, C., Mandalia, N., & Cohen, A. L. (2018). Expenditures on vaccine-preventable disease surveillance: Analysis and evaluation of comprehensive multi-year plans (cMYPs) for immunization. *Vaccine, 36*(45), 6850–6857.

Hu, D., Cheng, T. Y., Morris, P., Zimmerman, J., & Wang, C. (2021). Active regional surveillance for early detection of exotic/emerging pathogens of swine: A comparison of statistical methods for farm selection. *Preventive Veterinary Medicine, 187*, 105233.

Jayatilleke, K. (2020). Challenges in implementing surveillance tools of high-income countries (HICs) in low middle income countries (LMICs). *Current Treatment Options in Infectious Diseases, 12*, 191–201.

Johnson, C. P., & Johnson, J. (2001). GIS: A tool for monitoring and management of epidemics. *Proceedings of Map India*, 1–6.

Kaneene, J. B., Miller, R., Kaplan, B., Steele, J. H., & Thoen, C. O. (2014). Preventing and controlling zoonotic tuberculosis: A one health approach. *Veterinaria Italiana, 50*(1), 7–22. https://doi.org/10.12834/VetIt.1302.08

Laber, K. E., Whary, M. T., Bingel, S. A., Goodrich, J. A., Smith, A. C., & Swindle, M. M. (2002). Biology and diseases of swine. In *Laboratory Animal Medicine* (p. 615). Academic.

Leiser, O. P., Corn, J. L., Schmit, B. S., Keim, P. S., & Foster, J. T. (2013). Feral swine brucellosis in the United States and prospective genomic techniques for disease epidemiology. *Veterinary Microbiology, 166*(1–2), 1–10.

Lin, C. N., Okabayashi, T., Tummaruk, P., & Ooi, P. T. (2023). Zoonotic diseases among pigs. *Frontiers in Veterinary Science, 9*, 1122679.

Meng, X. J. (2012). Emerging and re-emerging swine viruses. *Transboundary and Emerging Diseases, 59*, 85–102.

Nejsum, P., Betson, M., Bendall, R. P., Thamsborg, S. M., & Stothard, J. R. (2012). Assessing the zoonotic potential of Ascaris suum and Trichuris suis: Looking to the future from an analysis of the past. *Journal of Helminthology, 86*(2), 148–155.

Olsen, S. C., & Tatum, F. M. (2016). Swine brucellosis: Current perspectives. *Veterinary Medicine: Research and Reports*, 1–12.

Opriessnig, T., & Coutinho, T. A. (2019). Erysipelas. In *Diseases of swine* (pp. 835–843).

Opriessnig, T., Forde, T., & Shimoji, Y. (2020). Erysipelothrix spp.: Past, present, and future directions in vaccine research. *Frontiers in Veterinary Science, 7*, 174.

Rabozzi, G., Bonizzi, L., Crespi, E., Somaruga, C., Sokooti, M., Tabibi, R., & Colosio, C. (2012). Emerging zoonoses: The "one health approach". *Safety and Health at Work, 3*(1), 77–83.

Rivera-Benitez, J. F., Rosas-Estrada, K., Pulido-Camarillo, E., de la Peña-Moctezuma, A., Castillo-Juárez, H., & Ramírez-Mendoza, H. (2014). Serological survey of veterinarians to assess the zoonotic potential of three emerging swine diseases in Mexico. *Zoonoses and Public Health, 61*(2), 131–137.

Rodríguez-Prieto, V., Vicente-Rubiano, M., Sánchez-Matamoros, A., Rubio-Guerri, C., Melero, M., Martínez-López, B., & Sánchez-Vizcaíno, J. M. (2015). Systematic review of surveillance systems and methods for early detection of exotic, new and re-emerging diseases in animal populations. *Epidemiology & Infection, 143*(10), 2018–2042.

Shaheen, M. N. (2022). The concept of one health applied to the problem of zoonotic diseases. *Reviews in Medical Virology, 32*(4), e2326.

Sharan, M., Vijay, D., Yadav, J. P., Bedi, J. S., & Dhaka, P. (2023). Surveillance and response strategies for zoonotic diseases: A comprehensive review. *Science in One Health*, 100050.

Stärk, K. D., Kuribreña, M. A., Dauphin, G., Vokaty, S., Ward, M. P., Wieland, B., & Lindberg, A. (2015). One health surveillance–more than a buzz word? *Preventive Veterinary Medicine, 120*(1), 124–130.

Sue, M. J., Yeap, S. K., Omar, A. R., & Tan, S. W. (2014). Application of PCR-ELISA in molecular diagnosis. *BioMed Research International, 2014*.

Suthar, A. B., Allen, L. G., Cifuentes, S., Dye, C., & Nagata, J. M. (2018). Lessons learnt from implementation of the international health regulations: A systematic review. *Bulletin of the World Health Organization, 96*(2), 110.

Symeonidou, I., Tassis, P., Gelasakis, A. I., Tzika, E. D., & Papadopoulos, E. (2020). Prevalence and risk factors of intestinal parasite infections in Greek swine farrow-to-finish farms. *Pathogens, 9*(7), 556.

Tayebeh, F., Amani, J., Nazarian, S., Moradyar, M., & Mirhosseini, S. A. (2016). Molecular diagnosis of clinically isolated Klebsiella pneumoniae strains by PCR-ELISA. *Journal Of Applied Biotechnology Reports, 3*(4), 501–505.

Tizzani, M., Muñoz-Gómez, V., De Nardi, M., Paolotti, D., Muñoz, O., Ceschi, P., & Capua, I. (2021). Integrating digital and field surveillance as complementary efforts to manage epidemic diseases of livestock: African swine fever as a case study. *PLoS One, 16*(12), e0252972.

Tsai, P., Scott, K. A., González, M. C., Pappaioanou, M., & Keusch, G. T. (2010). *Sustaining global surveillance and response to emerging zoonotic diseases*. National Academies Press.

Turlewicz-Podbielska, H., Włodarek, J., & Pomorska-Mól, M. (2020). Noninvasive strategies for surveillance of swine viral diseases: A review. *Journal of Veterinary Diagnostic Investigation, 32*(4), 503–512.

Van Reeth, K. (2007). Avian and swine influenza viruses: Our current understanding of the zoonotic risk. *Veterinary Research, 38*(2), 243–260.

VanderWaal, K., & Deen, J. (2018). Global trends in infectious diseases of swine. *Proceedings of the National Academy of Sciences, 115*(45), 11495–11500.

Wang, Q., Chang, B. J., & Riley, T. V. (2010). Erysipelothrix rhusiopathiae. *Veterinary Microbiology, 140*(3–4), 405–417.

Swine Influenza: A Constant Threat to Public Health

Santanu Pal, Bavadharani Mani, Tejpal, and Reddi Lokeswari

Abstract

Acute respiratory disease in pigs caused by influenza A virus results in major economic losses for pig production globally. Various subtypes of influenza A virus of swine (IAV-S) including H1N1, H3N2, and H1N2 were found to co-circulate globally in recent years, yet genetic background, origin, and antigenic properties vary greatly from region to region. Pigs act as either intermediate hosts or a "mixing vessel" thereby viruses of different origins may reassert themselves leading to the production of novel progeny viruses that are capable of replicating and spreading among humans. The receptor for the influenza virus is the same for both pigs and humans which results in inter-species transmission. These potential factors necessitate the control of influenza A viruses in pigs as a public health concern. A key tool in the control of IAV-S is the vaccination. Targeting the major antigenic protein, hemagglutinin (HA), whole inactivated virus (WIV) with adjuvant is available which have been traditionally used. In the absence of maternal antibodies, WIV vaccines are safe and efficient against antigenically identical strains, however reduced efficacy is observed against heterologous strains or in the presence of MDAs. Therefore, a vaccine that is easy to administer and provides a greater immune response against heterologous or even hetero-subtypic strains is needed.

Keywords

Swine · Influenza A virus · Inter-species transmission · Hemagglutinin (HA) · Vaccination

S. Pal (✉) · Tejpal · R. Lokeswari
ICAR-Indian Veterinary Research Institute (ICAR-IVRI), Bareilly, Uttar Pradesh, India

B. Mani
ICAR-Indian Veterinary Research Institute (ICAR-IVRI), Bengaluru, Karnataka, India

R. Deb et al. (eds.), *Emerging Zoonotic Threats from Swine*,
https://doi.org/10.1007/978-981-96-7407-7_4

Introduction

Swine influenza (SI) is a respiratory illness in pigs caused by influenza A viruses. Common symptoms include coughing, difficulty breathing, sneezing, and fever (Kothalwala et al., 2006). Pigs infected with swine influenza may exhibit pneumonia-related lesions when inspected at slaughter (Kothalwala et al., 2006). Subclinical infection is frequently seen particularly in herds with antibodies against closely related strains of swine influenza virus (SIV) (Rose et al., 2013). Influenza A viruses are part of the Orthomyxoviridae family and are enveloped viruses that contain eight segments of single-stranded RNA. The different subtypes of influenza A viruses are classified based on the antigenic and genetic characteristics of two key viral envelope proteins hemagglutinin (HA) and neuraminidase (NA). Swine influenza virus (SIV) consists of eight segments of RNA that encode the proteins, hemagglutinin (HA), neuraminidase (NA), polymerase acidic (PA), polymerase basic 1 (PB1), polymerase basic 2 (PB2), nucleoprotein (NP), matrix (M), and non-structural proteins (NS) (Rose et al., 2013). The ability of the virus to infect is primarily influenced by two proteins HA and NA. HA enables the virus to bind to receptors on the host cell's surface, facilitating entry into the host cell. Meanwhile, NA plays a crucial role in cleaving sialic acid molecules, which helps release newly produced virus particles from the infected cell. Host-adapted influenza A viruses (IAVs) are responsible for one of the most significant viral respiratory diseases affecting both animals and humans. The frequent outbreaks and swiftly followed by dissemination of genetically and antigenically diverse IAVs pose a major challenge to swine production. Influenza A virus (IAV) exemplifies an infectious disease challenge impacting both human and animal health. Addressing swine IAV necessitates One Health strategies to effectively manage zoonotic infections of swine IAV in humans (referred to as "variant" IAV) to create pandemic prevention plans and to reduce the occurrence of reverse zoonoses where human seasonal IAV is transmitted to swine (Rose et al., 2013). H1N1, H1N2, and H3N2 influenza virus subtypes are widespread in swine globally. Despite having only three subtypes in circulation the hemagglutinin (HA) and neuraminidase (NA) genes exhibit significant diversity. A significant portion of the observed diversity in IAV stems from bidirectional transmission between swine and humans (Hemmink et al., 2016; Van Reeth et al., 2012; Kasowski et al., 2011; Ma et al., 2009a, b) and subsequent antigenic drift and shift within swine populations along with viral spread through transportation and trade of live animals. These processes have led to the creation of numerous genetically and antigenically diverse lineages that circulate simultaneously in swine populations globally. Despite the species barriers between humans and swine, influenza A viruses (IAV) swine-adapted H1 and H3 IAV retain receptor binding site (RBS) profiles that prefer binding to α2, 6 sialic acids. This is different from IAV found in waterfowl and domestic poultry which prefer binding to α2,3 sialic acids. However, when human seasonal H3N2 and pre-2009 H1N1 viruses crossed into swine populations they tended to experience substantial adaptations. These adaptations involve losing one or more glycosylation sites on the HA protein, undergoing multiple amino acid substitutions throughout their genome and frequently reassorting with endemic swine IAV which led to the acquisition of various NA and internal gene segment lineages. The remarkable genetic and antigenic diversity of H1 and H3 swine IAV presents perhaps the biggest obstacle to controlling these infections and creating broadly effective vaccines. Similarly, the antigenic variability of swine viruses is a potential threat to humans if human population immunity fails to recognize the resulting swine lineages. This diversity along with the interaction between humans and swine is crucial in the context of variant IAV infections in humans. The likelihood of variant infections depends on animal production systems, animal-human interactions (like live animal markets and exhibitions), the virus's ecology, and other less obvious factors (Hemmink et al., 2016).

Pigs can be infected by both avian and human influenza viruses and they are believed to play a significant role in the ecology of human influenza. Indeed, genetic reassortment between human, avian, and swine influenza viruses can occur. This potential to create new influenza viruses has led to swine being referred to as "mixing vessels". The "mixing vessel" hypothesis is supported by three key facts: (1) swine can be infected by avian and human viruses, (2) reassortment among swine, avian, and human viruses occur in pigs, and (3) pigs can transmit reassorting influenza viruses to humans (Rose et al., 2013). However, when pigs are infected with the virus they may acquire adaptations that allow them to either sustain infection within pig populations thereby creating an additional reservoir for human infection, or develop mutations that enable transmission among humans potentially establishing the virus within the human population (Hemmink et al., 2016).

Historical Evolution of Swine Influenza

A phylogenetically based naming system for swine H1 viruses was established to classify the three main co-circulating lineages as 1A, 1B, and 1C (Kothalwala et al., 2006). The 1A lineage of swine influenza viruses originated from the Spanish influenza pandemic in 1918 (Kothalwala et al., 2006). These viruses constitute the classical swine H1N1 (cH1N1) lineage which spread worldwide. The 1A lineage comprises the H1 hemagglutinin (HA) from the H1N1 pdm09 virus incorporating NA and M genes from the Eurasian avian H1N1 swine lineage as well as genes from the TRIG and classical swine lineages. After the H1N1pdm09 virus spread quickly among humans, it was reintroduced into swine populations worldwide multiple times. A significant factor in these reintroductions was the reassortment of its internal genes with pre-existing endemic H1 and H3 swine viruses. The 1A hemagglutinin (HA) clades are typically associated with an N1 neuraminidase (NA) gene either from the classical swine lineage or the H1N1pdm09 lineage.

In the 1990s a virus identified in the United Kingdom designated as H1N2 possessed the HA gene from a human seasonal H1N1 virus now categorized as 1B.1

while the remaining genes came from the predominant circulating H3N2 swine influenza A virus (IAV). Similarly, human seasonal H1 influenza A viruses also entered US swine populations in the early 2000s and acquired TRIG genes similar to those found in contemporary triple-reassortant viruses (Kothalwala et al., 2006). During the 1970s a lineage originating from an avian H1N1 virus was identified in Europe later spreading to Asia where it is known as the Eurasian avian (EA) 1C lineage. This 1C H1N1 lineage continued to be a dominant lineage in Eurasia and elements of its internal gene makeup played a significant role in shaping the contemporary ecology of influenza A viruses (IAV). Swine H3N2 viruses are primarily categorized based on the time when the putative ancestral human seasonal virus circulates. This classification involves assigning them to specific decades of introduction and defining contemporary strains with numerical clade designations.

Apart from viruses originating from humans, swine are also susceptible to occasional infections from avian influenza viruses. A significant event occurred in 1979 when epidemics of an avian H1N1 influenza virus lineage were observed in Belgian swine. This led to the emergence of the H1N1 virus lineage in Europe which exhibited characteristics similar to avian influenza viruses (Fig. 1). The Eurasian avian-like 1C lineage has persisted in swine populations up to the present time and has been spread to different regions through the international transportation of swine (Rose et al., 2013).

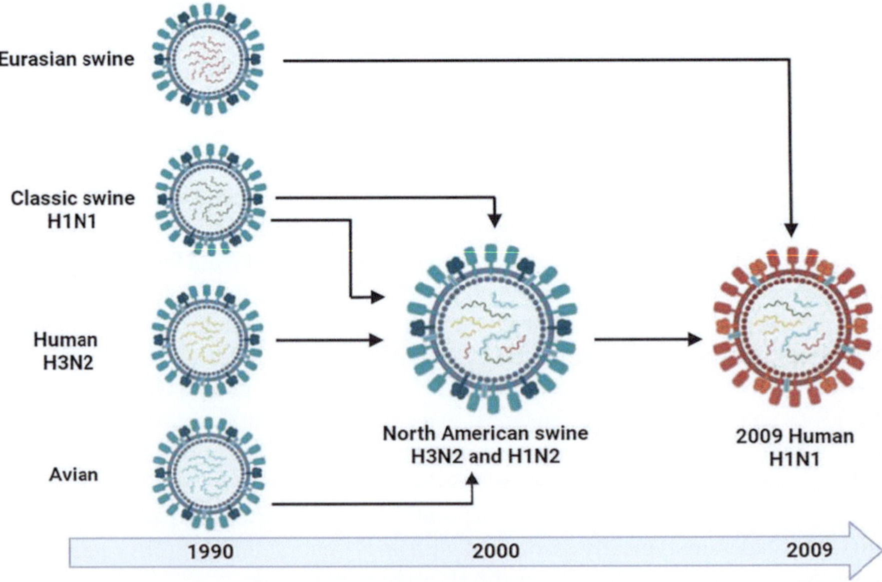

Fig. 1 The evolution of the 2009 influenza A (H1N1) virus involves a series of reassortment events. (Created by the Biorender app)

Geographical Spread and Epidemiology of Swine Influenza

Swine influenza was initially identified in 1918 in the United States, Hungary, and China and today it is one of the most ubiquitous diseases circulating in the global pig population (Brown, 2000). Corzo et al. (2013) found that 4.6% of individual pigs in the United States were infected. In comparison, participating farms showed a herd prevalence of 90.6% throughout 12–24 months using real-time reverse transcription polymerase chain reaction (real-time RT-PCR). In Europe, swine influenza is also prevalent. A study in Belgium, France, Italy, and Spain monitored 80 farrow-to-finish farms from 2006 to 2008. The findings showed that 90% of the farms tested positive for swine influenza virus (SIV) with 62% of individual pigs showing seroprevalence. Among the infected farms, 49% were affected by one subtype of SIV, 38% by two subtypes, and 3.9% by three subtypes (Kyriakis et al., 2013). Swine influenza is endemic in the pig population in China with multiple subtypes currently circulating on farms. Serological studies have shown the presence of H1, H3, H4, H5, H7, and H9 influenza viruses among pig populations in the country (Ding et al., 2021). Swine influenza is also widespread in pig populations across other countries in Southeast Asia. In Vietnam, swine influenza subtypes H1N1, H1N2, and H3N2 are concurrently circulating among the pig population. There have been instances where human-origin influenza viruses have crossed over to infect pigs. Importantly, certain reassortant strains of swine influenza viruses have also infected humans (Baudon et al., 2020). Likewise, these three subtypes are widespread among pigs in Thailand with A(H1N1) pdm09 and its reassortants being the predominant strains observed in the field (Nasamran et al., 2020).

Swine influenza has a presence in numerous countries across North and South America, Europe, Asia, and Africa. Infections on pig farms occur consistently throughout the year with higher numbers typically observed during the spring and winter seasons. Commercial pig farms are generally considered to face a greater risk of infection compared to backyard farms particularly concerning the introduction of new reassortant strains of swine influenza virus (SIV).

Transmission of Swine Influenza Between Pigs

The primary mode of virus transmission between pigs is direct contact between infected and susceptible pigs. Aerosol transmission where the virus spreads through the air is also a common method of indirect transmission of swine influenza virus (SIV). A pig farm can be infected if carrier pigs are introduced or if the virus is brought in by infected visitors, vehicles, or other contaminated objects (fomites). In infected pigs, the swine influenza virus (SIV) is typically found in oral and nasal secretions but not in feces (Botner & Belsham, 2012). Pigs can begin shedding the virus as early as 2 days after infection. While shedding typically lasts for 8–10 days instances of shedding continuing for more than 30 days have been documented. The extended duration of shedding has been suggested to be associated with immune suppression in infected pigs (Choi et al., 2004). SIV can spread quickly among individual pigs within a herd.

Inter-Species Transmission of Swine Influenza

HA subtypes ranging from H1 to H16 circulate among birds, pigs, and humans with specific subtypes predominating in each species (Fig. 2). Wild waterfowl serve as the primary reservoir for H1 to H16 subtypes, while domestic chickens are typically affected by H5, H7, and H9 subtypes. In humans, H1, H2, and H3 subtypes are commonly found while pigs are mainly affected by H1 and H3 subtypes (Short et al., 2015). Pigs can acquire influenza A viruses from various sources, particularly from infected humans and birds (Nelson et al., 2015). Avian influenza viruses have been found in pigs in several countries and regions. For instance, in Canada, H4N6 was isolated from pigs with pneumonia on a commercial swine farm. Similarly, in the United States in 2015 an avian-origin H4N6 virus was isolated from pigs that showed clinical respiratory symptoms. In Nigeria, a study found that 22 out of 129 samples taken from seemingly healthy pigs tested positive for H5N1 influenza virus. Concurrently, there was an outbreak of highly pathogenic avian influenza (HPAI) H5N1 in local poultry (Meseko et al., 2018).

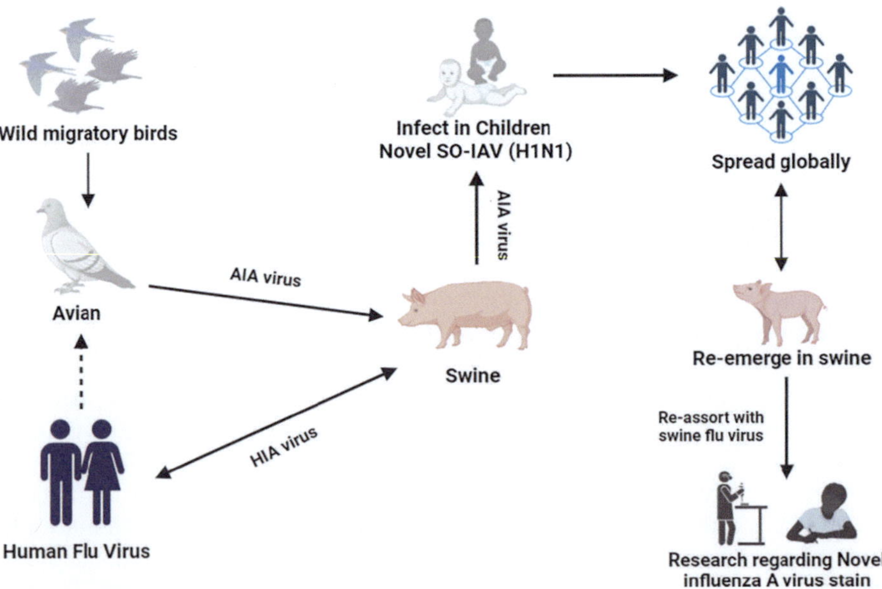

Fig. 2 Dynamic spread and effects of the 2009 H1N1 pandemic influenza with swine as a potential source for reassortment and mixing of influenza A viruses

Zoonotic Potential of Swine Influenza Virus

Human infection with swine influenza A virus (swIAV) typically occurs through close contact with pigs, especially in settings like pig farms or slaughterhouses. Interestingly, pig-to-human transmission of influenza A virus (IAV) has been regularly reported though the number of human infections is lower compared to avian influenza virus (AIV). Although some experts believe that the Spanish influenza pandemic of 1918 was caused by a reassortment of swine H1N1 virus this is controversial with no direct supporting evidence and others contend that it is of avian origin. From 1959 to 2014, only 396 confirmed cases of human infections with swine influenza A virus (swIAV) were reported worldwide (Freidyl et al., 2014). Although human infections with zoonotic influenza viruses are less common than those with seasonal influenza viruses there is a global concern that these zoonotic viruses could mutate in animals or humans potentially enhancing their ability to transmit efficiently from animals to humans or sustain human-to-human transmission. The initial zoonotic influenza pandemic of the twenty-first century the 2009 H1N1 swine flu pandemic emerged in Mexico and was fortunately not highly virulent. Nonetheless, it exposed weaknesses in global pandemic preparedness offering critical insights for improving responses to future major outbreaks. In the wake of the 2009 pandemic a recent review of emerging influenza A infections in humans identified three reassortants that are primarily zoonotic swine influenza variants. In late 2009 a novel A(H1N2) virus was identified in India, comprising a reassortant of the co-circulating A(H1N1) pdm09 and A(H3N2) viruses. In the United States, several human infections with swine H3N2v viruses were reported in the fall of 2011.

The Pig Is a Reservoir Host for Swine Influenza

Pigs are considered "mixing vessels" because they can be infected by avian, swine, and human influenza A viruses. This ability implies that pigs can generate new influenza A virus strains with the potential to cause pandemics (Tchilian & Holzer, 2017). The 2009 pandemic virus emerged from a triple-reassortant event combining six gene segments from at least three different parent viruses with two distinct segments from the H1N1 swine virus lineage to form the novel influenza A virus. The 2009 pandemic H1N1 strain clearly illustrates the significant role pigs play in the emergence of future outbreaks (Sun et al., 2020). In 2020, a new reassortant influenza A virus (IAV) of Eurasian avian-like H1N1 origin known as the G4 genotype was identified during surveillance of pigs in China. This virus contained genes derived from the 2009 pandemic strain and triple-reassortant strains. The G4 influenza A virus (IAV) was antigenically different from human IAVs currently circulating. It exhibited all the necessary traits of a pandemic virus including a preference for binding to α2–6 sialylated glycans. This binding preference is crucial for infecting human cells and is notably similar to the binding site used by the 2009 pandemic

H1N1 IAV strain. Genetic mixing in pigs enables the creation of new influenza virus strains highlighting their role as intermediate hosts in the transmission of influenza viruses.

Pathogenesis of Swine Influenza

Despite the genetic diversity of influenza viruses in swine the replication strategy, clinical disease, and lesions caused by classic H1N1 swine influenza virus, avian-like H1N1 viruses that have adapted to swine, and various reassortants such as H1N1, H1N2, H3N2, and H2N3 (including the 2009 human pandemic H1N1 and subsequent reassortants) are fundamentally similar (Fig. 3). In swine influenza, the virus primarily infects the epithelial cells that line the respiratory tract, ranging from the nasal mucosa to the alveoli. However, the virus has also been detected in glandular epithelial cells associated with larger airways. A characteristic microscopic finding is necrotizing bronchitis and bronchiolitis. Within the first 24 hours post-infection (PI) neutrophils start to accumulate in the blood vessels near bronchioles and there are early signs of lymphocytic infiltration around the airways sometimes appearing before damage to the epithelial cells becomes evident. Between 24 and 48 h PI necrosis and shedding of airway epithelial cells occur along with neutrophils migrating into the airway lumens. By 48 h post-infection (PI) the airways that are affected show a lining of flattened epithelial layers and the neutrophils in the luminal debris are either replaced or are accompanied by macrophages. There is a noticeable increase in lymphocytes accumulating around the airways and nearby blood vessels. As the repair process progresses the epithelial cells lining the airways begin to proliferate. These cells mature into tightly packed tall columnar cells leading to an irregular hyperplastic appearance often observed by 72 h PI. Severely damaged airways may lead to the proliferation of fibroblasts from the exposed subepithelial lamina propria. This can result in the formation of endobronchial polyps or incomplete healing known as bronchiolitis obliterans.

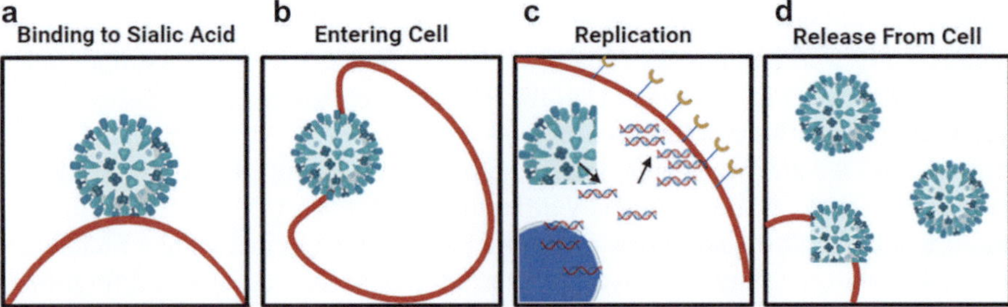

Fig. 3 General mechanism of replication followed by infection with influenza virus

Virulence of Swine Influenza

When discussing how influenza viruses cause disease a common question is whether these viruses differ in their natural ability to cause severe illness. The clinical symptoms linked to natural influenza virus infections in both swine and humans can vary significantly ranging from mild respiratory symptoms to severe difficulty in breathing that can lead to death shortly thereafter. Secondary bacterial infections can exacerbate pneumonia and increase mortality rates in both swine and humans. Epidemics that rapidly spread sometimes with higher mortality rates typically occur when a new virus strain is introduced for which the population has limited immune protection (Table 1). However, there are instances of influenza viral infections without bacterial involvement and outbreaks with unusually high morbidity and mortality rates suggesting that certain viruses may possess inherent capabilities for increased virulence. In swine, occasional influenza outbreaks have been observed with high

Table 1 Genetic subtypes, molecular markers, and their roles in enhancing viral functions and pathogenesis

Genes	Subtypes	Molecular markers and functions
HA	H5	K83, P128, K197, K496 work in two or more combinations to increase binding to α2–6 glycans
	H7	N104K increases affinity to both α2,3- and α2,6-linked SA
	H5	H110Y increases thermostability and pH stability, adaptive mutation for airborne transmission
	H5	S121N enables H5N1 virus binding to both a2–3 and α2–6 glycans
PB2	H5N1	D9N enhances viral polymerase activity, inhibits MAVS to suppress IFN-I production
	H1N1	T271A enhances polymerase activity in human cells
	H7N9, H5N1, H3N2	K526R cooperates with E627K to synergistically increase viral polymerase activity
PB1	H5N1	D3V enhances viral polymerase activity
	H1N1, H5N1, H7N9	K612 SUMOylation is critical for the viral RNA binding activity of PB1, essential for viral pathogenesis and transmission
PA	H7N9	S37A increases polymerase activity in human cells
PA	H7N7	V63I increases viral polymerase activity, viral replication, and virulence in mammalian cells
	H1N1	T552S increases avian virus polymerase activity in mammalian cells
NP	H7N9, H9N2	V41 enhances viral polymerase activity
	H7N9, H9N2	E210D enhances viral polymerase activity
	H7N7	N319K is a mouse-adapted mutation, that improves the binding of NP to importin protein in mammalian cells
M1	H5N1	N30D-T215A increases viral replication and viral virulence in mice
	H9N1	T37A abolishes the phosphorylation site to stabilize the M1 protein and increases viral replication in mammalian species
NS1	H5N1	P42S increases viral virulence in mice by preventing the dsRNA-mediated activation of the NF-κB and IRF – 3 pathways
	H7N9	I106M increases viral virulence in mice by enhanced CPSF30 binding

(Liang, 2023)

mortality rates seemingly caused by the virus alone. In humans, viruses responsible for pandemics typically lead to higher morbidity rates, often indicating greater transmissibility and/or more severe clinical symptoms suggesting higher rates of virus replication compared to seasonal influenza viruses. However, the overall mortality rates may vary and are not necessarily higher during pandemics. Depending on the specific pandemic certain age groups within the population may experience higher rates of infection.

Diagnosis of Swine Influenza

The diagnosis of swine influenza involves a range of diagnostic techniques to ensure accurate detection and identification of the virus (Table 2). The traditional methods, such as virus culture and isolation, remain a gold standard for their specificity but are time-consuming. Serological methods, including immunofluorescence tests, complement fixation, double immunodiffusion, single radial-immunodiffusion, enzyme-linked immunosorbent assay (ELISA), and hemagglutination inhibition tests, are widely used for detecting antibodies and assessing immune responses. Advanced and quick methods, such as rapid influenza detection tests, PCR-based techniques, and non-PCR RNA-specific detection methods, offer high sensitivity and specificity, enabling timely diagnosis. Additionally, biosensors like optical, potentiometric, impedimetric, amperometric, piezoelectric, magnetic, and thermometric biosensors represent cutting-edge diagnostic tools that provide rapid, accurate, and portable solutions for detecting swine influenza, making them invaluable in both clinical and field settings.

1. *Influenza virus antigen detection*: Immunohistochemistry (IHC) and immunofluorescence (IFA) techniques are employed to identify influenza virus antigens in tissues that have been either frozen or fixed with formalin utilizing various antibodies (Hussaini et al., 2022). The nucleoprotein (NP) is highly conserved across influenza A viruses, making anti-NP antibodies useful for detecting all

Table 2 Diagnostic techniques for viral detection and their types

Diagnostic techniques	Types
Traditional method	Virus culture and isolation
Serological method	Immunofluorescence test, complement fixation, double immunodiffusion test, single radial-immunodiffusion test, enzyme-linked immunosorbent assay, Hemagglutination inhibition test
Advanced and quick methods	Rapid influenza detection tests, PCR-based detection methods, non-PCR-based RNA-specific detection methods
Biosensors	Optical biosensors, potentiometric biosensors, Impediametric biosensors, Amperometric biosensor, piezoelectric biosensor, magnetic biosensor, thermometric biosensor

Ravina et al. (2020)

influenza A subtypes. In contrast, the hemagglutinin (HA) protein is specific to subtypes and is used to identify particular influenza virus subtypes. NP antigens are found in both the nucleus and cytoplasm of infected cells. Meanwhile, the hemagglutinin (HA) protein is situated in the cytoplasm and on the cell surface. Direct immunostaining techniques employ antibodies that are tagged with biotin, fluorophores, enzymes, or colloidal gold (Buchwalow and Böcker, 2010).

2. *Virus isolation*: Swine influenza virus (SIV) is routinely isolated using embryonated chicken eggs (ECEs) as well as various cell lines such as Madin-Darby canine kidney (MDCK) cells and the CACO-2 cell line (Chiapponi et al., 2010). The effectiveness of different methods for isolating SIV depends on the specific strains of the virus present. Virus isolation is often challenging, costly, and time-consuming. However, it is essential when a live virus is needed for further research such as assessing the pathogenicity of new SIV strains and screening potential vaccine candidates (Detmer et al., 2013).
3. *Serological methods*: Serological tests for swine influenza virus (SIV) primarily detect host antibodies against the virus. The most commonly used tests are the hemagglutination inhibition (HI) test and enzyme-linked immunosorbent assay (ELISA). Numerous commercial ELISA kits have been developed to detect antibodies to the influenza A nucleoprotein (NP) due to its high conservation across influenza A viruses (Goodell et al., 2016). Several studies have indicated that an NP-blocking ELISA kit originally designed for detecting antibodies in birds is also effective for identifying NP antibodies in pigs. Overall, HI tests are easier to perform, less expensive, and faster compared to ELISAs. However, selecting the appropriate antigen is challenging due to the variety of SIV strains. Moreover, the sensitivity of HI tests may be limited when used exclusively for SIV surveillance in the presence of heterologous viruses; however, they do offer the advantage of being useful for virus subtyping. Serological tests have several advantages: they are generally cost-effective, simpler to conduct than polymerase chain reaction (PCR) tests or virus isolation (VI), and more sensitive in detecting pig exposure to the influenza A virus. This increased sensitivity is due to the longevity of antibodies, which can persist for at least 1.5 months post-infection, making serological tests less dependent on the timing of sample collection. However, serological tests have their limitations. They only offer information on past exposure to SIV and do not provide genetic data or live viruses, which are crucial for assessing the pandemic potential of strains. Additionally, cross-reactions can occur between different lineages within the same subtype or among different subtypes, and maternally derived antibodies can affect the accuracy of the test (Allerson et al., 2013).
4. *Hemagglutination inhibition (HI)*: The agglutination of red blood cells (RBCs) naturally happens when the HA protein is on the virus's surface. Influenza antibodies can specifically inhibit this process, and this inhibition can be measured using a hemagglutination inhibition (HI) assay. For swine influenza viruses (SIVs) optimal HA and HI reactions are achieved with turkey or chicken RBCs which are utilized in standardized testing procedures (OIE, 2008). In the hemagglutination inhibition (HI) test serial two-fold dilutions of the test serum (starting

from 1:10 and ending at 1:640 or 1:1280) are made in 96-well microtiter plates. To each well containing the serum dilutions 4–8 HA units of a specific subtype of influenza virus are added. After incubating for an hour at room temperature, a 0.5% RBC suspension is added to each well. If specific antibodies are absent the virus binds to the RBCs causing hemagglutination. However, if anti-hemagglutinin antibodies are present in the serum from prior exposure or vaccination, they will bind to the hemagglutinin protein on the virus surface preventing hemagglutination. The HI titer of the serum is defined as the reciprocal of the highest serum dilution that inhibits hemagglutination. HI titers equal to or greater than 1:40 are typically regarded as indicative of protective levels (Hancock et al., 2009). The HI test is widely used for detecting antibodies against SIV but it is somewhat subjective and results can vary due to operator differences and test repetition. Additionally, cross-reactivity exists among a, b, and c clusters of the H1 subtype of SIVs, so a positive HI titer may suggest exposure to a related virus without definitive identification. However, HI titers are typically stronger when the virus matches the one of exposure. This test is favored for its standardized, cost-effective, and straightforward nature providing results comparable to more complex tests like serum neutralization.

5. *Serum neutralization (SN) or virus neutralization (VN)*: The serum neutralization (SN) test identifies virus-specific neutralizing antibodies in a serum sample. In this assay, the serum is diluted in two-fold increments along with a known quantity of SIV followed by pre-incubation. The mixture is then added to MDCK cells to ascertain the highest dilution of serum capable of neutralizing virus infection and preventing cytopathic effects (CPE) production. Neutralizing antibodies in serum prevent virus infection in cell cultures stopping cytopathic effects (CPE) production. Without antibodies, the virus infects cells and causes CPE. The SN titer is determined by the highest serum dilution that neutralizes virus infection. Known as micro neutralization for its use of small serum volumes in 96-well microtiter plates this test shows the biological activity of antibodies. Unlike HI and ELISA SN directly measures antibody ability to neutralize virus. Challenges include needing specialized equipment and supplies for virus cultures, longer result times (up to 72 h), and potential SN titer variation upon retesting.
6. *Molecular methods*: Molecular tests on nasal swabs, nasal wipes, or oral fluids are primarily utilized in surveillance to detect SIV RNA and generate amplicons for further sequencing. Standard molecular assays for influenza A viruses focus on a conserved amplicon of the M-gene. For subtyping specific primers must be designed to target different gene segments, primarily HA and NA (Henritzi et al., 2020). The development of real-time RT-PCR assays for detecting SIVs began in 2004. Compared to conventional RT-PCR, real-time RT-PCR can be completed in a few hours and can differentiate between SIV subtypes. Additionally, it is often less expensive than virus isolation (VI) and traditional RT-PCR assays. Most importantly real-time RT-PCR eliminates the need for post-PCR sample handling, thereby minimizing the risk of cross-contamination (Richt et al.,

2004). Multiplex RT-qPCR assays can distinguish between H1, H3, N1, and N2 subtypes of SIV. These multiplex RT-qPCR assays are also able to detect various lineages within the H1 subtype, including 1C "av" (European avian-derived), 1B "hu" (European human-derived), and 1A "pdm" (H1N1pdm09).

Limitations of Diagnostic Assays

In the past decade, influenza A viruses in North American swine have undergone rapid genetic and antigenic changes affecting cross-reactivity in serologic assays. It's crucial to consider these variations when interpreting test results. While some antigenic cross-reactivity exists among the classical and reassorted clusters (a, b, and c) of the swine H1 subtype there is minimal to no cross-reactivity between these clusters and the human-like d cluster. The differences in antigenic cross-reactivity were shown in the 2009 pandemic H1N1 virus among both North American and European swine H1 subtypes using sera from pigs that were experimentally infected or vaccinated (Kyriakis et al., 2010). Within swine H3 viruses there is minimal or no cross-reactivity observed between groups I and IV. Similarly, there is limited to no cross-reactivity between different swine subtypes. This necessitates testing multiple viruses from each subtype to identify the specific virus subtype that induced the antibodies. To address these challenges and expand influenza surveillance samples may first undergo screening using the MultiS-Screen ELISA. Subsequently, more targeted tests like SN and HI assays can be employed to determine the specific virus subtype responsible for the exposure.

Swine Influenza Is a Major Threat to the Pig Industry

Swine influenza is highly contagious with nearly all exposed pigs becoming infected though the mortality rate is typically very low. Even in a previously unexposed pig population, clinical symptoms may only appear in a minority of pigs. However, significant illness and death which lead to economic losses can occur when swine influenza virus infects pigs simultaneously with other swine diseases or when infection happens in pregnant sows during the later stages of pregnancy (Fablet et al., 2012). In Wesley's study in 2004 stillbirths were observed in naturally infected gilts after being exposed to live H3N2 SIV between 80 and 82 days of gestation. The average percentage of stillbirths per litter was 22%, whereas control gilts that were naturally infected but not exposed to live H3N2 SIV had no stillbirths. Additionally, abortions can occur in sows when they are infected with newly emerging strains of swine influenza virus (Wesley, 2004; Gumbert et al., 2020). Swine influenza virus (SIV) infections result in reduced feed conversion efficiency (FCE) and slower growth rates in pigs contributing to productivity losses.

Swine Influenza Is a Public Health Concern

SIVs play a significant role in the potential emergence of pandemic influenza strains in humans contributing to the emergence of 19 reassortant influenza A virus strains in humans since 1918. Out of these three were primarily zoonotic variants of swine influenza A virus (Bui et al., 2017). Numerous instances of swine-to-human transmission have been documented in China and various other countries. In 1999 a case was reported in Hong Kong where a child was infected with swine influenza H3N2 virus (Gregory et al., 2001). Zu et al. (2013) documented a human infection with a European avian-like swine H1N1 influenza virus in Jiangsu province. The virus isolated from the patient's pigs on their smallholding was identical to the one that infected the patient. Killian et al. (2013) studied an H1N1 outbreak at a county fair in Ohio USA in 2007. They identified a triple-reassortant swine H1N1 influenza virus that had infected both humans and pigs (Killian et al., 2013). SIV strains that adapt to humans can lead to global pandemic outbreaks. For example, the H1N1pdm09 strain affected 10–20% of the global population and emerged as a new strain capable of infecting both swine and humans. In Mexico, during the period from 2007 to 2008, 12.9% of pig farm workers tested positive for antibodies against H3N2 SIV while 3.2% tested positive for antibodies against H1N1 SIV. According to Ma et al. (2015) in China 17.3% of workers employed in piggeries and 7.0% of workers in other occupations tested positive for antibodies against swine H3N2 virus. However, the interpretation of results can be complicated by cross-reactivity between antibodies against human seasonal H3N2 influenza virus and swine H3N2 virus. These studies did not exclude this potential issue. In another study, researchers found that individuals who tested positive for antibodies against seasonal H3N2 virus were more likely to also test positive for antibodies against swine H3N2 virus.

Control Measures and Challenges with Swine Influenza

Vaccination against swine influenza (SI) is often administered to sows because it is believed to protect piglets through maternal immunity against closely related influenza A virus strains (Chamba et al., 2019). Allerson et al. (2013) showed that vaccinating sows could effectively decrease the transmission of swine influenza virus (SIV) among piglets. However, there are several challenges associated with SIV vaccination. Primarily the effectiveness of vaccination in the field depends on the presence of antibodies that match the circulating strains. Therefore, it is crucial to vaccinate using strains that are currently circulating to achieve optimal efficacy. Since various strains are prevalent in herds globally the potential ineffectiveness of vaccination due to the absence of local circulating strains in the vaccine formulation cannot be overlooked. Secondly, maternal-derived antibodies (MDA) might interfere with the development of immunity against infection with closely related SIV strains in piglets. One study indicated that piglets with MDA could experience prolonged shedding of the virus if subsequently infected with a homologous SIV strain. Thirdly, there have been reports of vaccine-associated enhanced respiratory disease observed in field conditions which could potentially negate the benefits of using swine influenza virus (SIV) vaccines (Mancera Gracia et al., 2020).

Swine populations worldwide harbor a wide variety of swine influenza viruses which are highly diverse. Novel genotypes and subtypes of these viruses could emerge in pigs at any time due to infections from avian and human influenza viruses. The global movement of live pigs through increasing international trade has sped up virus evolution and made the swine influenza situation more complex worldwide. This has led to the introduction of new swine influenza viruses into previously unexposed swine herds. Examples include the North American triple reassortant and Eurasian avian-like H1N1 swine influenza viruses, which have been introduced into China from North American and European countries (Zhu et al., 2013). This is a major challenge to produce effective vaccines and control swine influenza for the swine industry.

Despite the widespread use of vaccines, swine influenza remains difficult to control, similar to human seasonal influenza. One critical concern is the potential emergence of a novel virus in pigs capable of infecting humans and potentially causing epidemics or pandemics akin to the 2009 pH1N1 virus. It's worth noting that the 2009 pH1N1 virus likely originated in North America particularly Mexico rather than in Southeast Asian "wet markets" which are often associated with pandemic influenza viruses (Shortridge, 1992). This highlights that pandemic-capable viruses can emerge from various locations emphasizing the need for vigilant surveillance of pigs in different regions. Additionally, existing swine viruses like the North American triple reassortant H3N2 virus in the United States and the Eurasian avian-like H1N1 virus in China have gained enhanced infectivity in humans through reassortment with other viruses. This has led to the emergence of H3N2 variant viruses in the United States and reassortant Eurasian H1N1-like viruses in China both of which have caused infections in humans. Hence there is a critical need for enhanced global surveillance of influenza A viruses (IAVs) in pigs to improve our understanding of their ecology. Additionally, it is essential to develop more effective vaccines for swine to safeguard both animal and public health.

Preventive Measure for Swine Influenza in Pigs

Preventing swine influenza in pigs primarily depends on three main approaches: facility management, herd management, and vaccination. Facility management includes practices like disinfection and maintaining controlled temperatures to reduce viral spread in the environment. Herd management involves measures such as preventing overcrowding and isolating pigs showing signs of influenza from those that are not exposed. Vaccination is also critical in preventing swine influenza. Relying solely on vaccinations may not sufficiently prevent swine influenza spillover events without additional prevention and mitigation measures in place.

Preventive Measures to Stop Swine to Human Viral Transmission

Preventing the transmission of H1N1 from swine to humans is critical to reducing the risk of human outbreaks. It's essential not only to lower influenza rates in swine populations but also to focus on preventing transmission from swine to humans. Swine are susceptible to both avian and human strains of H1N1 influenza making them potential "mixing vessels." In these animals, viral reassortment can happen which can lead to the development of new strains of swine influenza through antigenic shifts (Ma et al., 2009). Transmission of the influenza virus from swine to humans typically occurs among individuals closely involved with pigs such as farmers, pork handlers, and veterinarians. It is highly recommended that these individuals wear face masks while interacting with infected animals to prevent transmission through respiratory droplets, as face masks have proven effective in preventing influenza spread.

Preventive Measures to Reduce Human-to-Human Transmission

The primary routes through which zoonotic swine influenza viruses spread among humans are likely through inhalation of respiratory droplets or aerosols, direct mucosal contact, and exposure to contaminated surfaces (fomites). For instance, if a susceptible individual touches a contaminated surface and then contacts their mucous membranes in the nose, mouth, or eyes transmission can occur (Zhang & Li, 2018). It is crucial to address these potential points of transmission during the influenza infectious period. Effective strategies documented to prevent virus spread include regular handwashing with soap and water or alcohol-based hand sanitizers as well as disinfecting household, hospital, and public environments using a diluted bleach solution. In 2009 during the H1N1 influenza pandemic, a vaccine approved by the Food and Drug Administration (FDA) in the United States was found effective by the National Institutes of Health (NIH). Their studies showed that a single dose administered within 10 days of illness was capable of generating protective antibodies against the virus.

Treatment for patients infected with H1N1 influenza varies based on the severity of symptoms. Mild-to-moderate cases typically resolve on their own with rest and oral fluids at home. Symptomatic management may involve medications like paracetamol/acetaminophen for fever, antihistamines for congestion, and pain relievers such as non-steroidal anti-inflammatories or paracetaminophen for headaches, muscle aches, and joint pain. Patients with progressive or severe symptoms should be hospitalized for close monitoring especially if they show signs of respiratory failure, sepsis, or multiple organ dysfunction. Treatment in such cases may include IV fluids to maintain hydration, correction of electrolyte imbalances, and antibiotics if bacterial infections are present. For acute respiratory distress syndrome (ARDS) caused by influenza, patients may require mechanical ventilation either non-invasive or invasive. In severe cases, extracorporeal membrane oxygenation (ECMO) may be necessary (Sukhal et al., 2017).

Conclusion

More than 60% of human infectious diseases are caused by pathogens that can spread from animals to humans. While various zoonotic viruses such as the current SARS-CoV-2 have caused significant human casualties influenza viruses have led to at least four confirmed pandemics within less than a century. Swine influenza A virus (swIAV) imposes a significant disease burden on pigs leading to notable economic impacts and posing a significant threat to human health. The 2009 H1N1 "Swine Flu" pandemic serves as a stark reminder of the severe consequences that could arise for pork production and global food security if another strain were to emerge from pigs similar to the 1918 pandemic. The simultaneous presence of various swine influenza virus (SIV) strains on pig farms can facilitate genetic reassortment among strains leading to the emergence of new strains within pig populations and strains with pandemic potential. Certain farming practices and inadequate biosecurity measures on pig farms increase the risk of SIV infections. Despite the availability of reliable diagnostic tests and ongoing studies monitoring the genetic evolution of swine influenza viruses controlling the disease in pig farms remains challenging. Close interaction between pigs and farm workers provides opportunities for the zoonotic transmission of swine influenza viruses. Effective control of swine influenza in pig farms is crucial to prevent the development of influenza pandemics originating from pigs. As industrial farming practices expand and multi-site systems increase pig movements the chances of viral reassortment rise potentially facilitating the emergence of new and virulent influenza A virus strains. The relevance of each strategy will vary depending on regional factors and the predominant farming systems in place with local infrastructure playing a crucial role in their implementation. Effective control measures aimed at reducing the spread of swine influenza A virus (swIAV) within pig populations and its transmission to humans can enhance economic outcomes in pig production promote the health of farmers and pigs and prevent pigs from becoming a reservoir for new strains of influenza A virus. Monitoring swine for influenza viruses remains critical for both animal and public health, particularly in regions where swine influenza A virus diversity is high and viruses evolve quickly. It is essential to focus on areas where farming practices facilitate viral transmission and movement and where human-pig interactions are frequent enhancing the potential for zoonotic transmission. Due to the rapid evolution of the swine influenza virus (SIV), it is crucial to consistently develop and approve new inactivated SIV vaccines. Current killed influenza vaccines for swine have uncertain effectiveness underscoring the need to select new vaccine strains from current circulating SIVs based on surveillance data. Adopting a vaccine strain selection process akin to that used by the WHO for human influenza vaccines may be necessary to ensure the efficacy of national and regional swine vaccines.

References

Allerson, M., Deen, J., Detmer, S. E., Gramer, M. R., Joo, H. S., Romagosa, A., & Torremorell, M. (2013). The impact of maternally derived immunity on influenza a virus transmission in neonatal pig populations. *Vaccine, 31*(3), 500–505.

Baudon, E., Peyre, M., Tung, D. D., Thi Nga, P., Khong, N. V., Cowling, B. J., & Peiris, M. (2020). Surveillance of swine influenza viruses in sentinel familial farms in hung yen province in northern Vietnam in 2013–2014. *Zoonoses and Public Health, 67*(3), 213–221.

Bøtner, A., & Belsham, G. J. (2012). Virus survival in slurry: Analysis of the stability of foot-and-mouth disease, classical swine fever, bovine viral diarrhoea and swine influenza viruses. *Veterinary Microbiology, 157*(1–2), 41–49.

Brown, I. H. (2000). The epidemiology and evolution of influenza viruses in pigs. *Veterinary Microbiology, 74*(1–2), 29–46.

Buchwalow, I. B., & Böcker, W. (2010). *Immunohistochemistry: Basics and methods*. Springer Science & Business Media.

Bui, C. M., Chughtai, A. A., Adam, D. C., & MacIntyre, C. R. (2017). An overview of the epidemiology and emergence of influenza A infection in humans over time. *Archives of Public Health, 75*, 1–7.

Chamba Pardo, F. O., Wayne, S., Culhane, M. R., Perez, A., Allerson, M., & Torremorell, M. (2019). Effect of strain-specific maternally-derived antibodies on influenza A virus infection dynamics in nursery pigs. *PLoS One, 14*(1), e0210700.

Chiapponi, C., Zanni, I., Garbarino, C., Barigazzi, G., & Foni, E. (2010). Comparison of the usefulness of the CACO-2 cell line with standard substrates for isolation of swine influenza A viruses. *Journal of Virological Methods, 163*(1), 162–165.

Choi, Y. K., Goyal, S. M., & Joo, H. S. (2004). Evaluation of transmission of swine influenza type A subtype H1N2 virus in seropositive pigs. *American Journal of Veterinary Research, 65*(3), 303–306.

Corzo, C. A., Culhane, M., Juleen, K., Stigger-Rosser, E., Ducatez, M. F., Webby, R. J., & Lowe, J. F. (2013). Active surveillance for influenza A virus among swine, midwestern United States, 2009–2011. *Emerging Infectious Diseases, 19*(6), 954.

Detmer, S., Gramer, M., Goyal, S., Torremorell, M., & Torrison, J. (2013). Diagnostics and surveillance for swine influenza. In *Swine influenza* (pp. 85–112).

Ding, F., Li, Y., Huang, B., Edwards, J., Cai, C., Zhang, G., et al. (2021). Infection and risk factors of human and avian influenza in pigs in South China. *Preventive Veterinary Medicine, 190*, 105317.

Fablet, C., Marois-Créhan, C., Simon, G., Grasland, B., Jestin, A., Kobisch, M., et al. (2012). Infectious agents associated with respiratory diseases in 125 farrow-to-finish pig herds: A cross-sectional study. *Veterinary Microbiology, 157*(1–2), 152–163.

Freidl, G. S., et al. (2014). Influenza at the animal–human interface: A review of the literature for virological evidence of human infection with swine or avian influenza viruses other than a (H5N1). *Eurosurveillance, 19*(18), 20793.

Goodell, C. K., Prickett, J., Kittawornrat, A., Johnson, J., Zhang, J., Wang, C., & Zimmerman, J. J. (2016). Evaluation of screening assays for the detection of influenza A virus serum antibodies in swine. *Transboundary and Emerging Diseases, 63*(1), 24–35.

Gregory, V., Lim, W., Cameron, K., Bennett, M., Marozin, S., Klimov, A., et al. (2001). Infection of a child in Hong Kong by an influenza A H3N2 virus closely related to viruses circulating in European pigs. *Journal of General Virology, 82*(6), 1397–1406.

Gumbert, S., Froehlich, S., Rieger, A., Stadler, J., Ritzmann, M., & Zoels, S. (2020). Reproductive performance of pandemic influenza A virus infected sow herds before and after implementation of a vaccine against the influenza A (H1N1) pdm09 virus. *Porcine Health Management, 6*, 1–9.

Hancock, K., Veguilla, V., Lu, X., Zhong, W., Butler, E. N., Sun, H., et al. (2009). Cross-reactive antibody responses to the 2009 pandemic H1N1 influenza virus. *New England Journal of Medicine, 361*(20), 1945–1952.

Hemmink, J. D., Morgan, S. B., Aramouni, M., Everett, H., Salguero, F. J., Canini, L., & Tchilian, E. (2016). Distinct immune responses and virus shedding in pigs following aerosol, intranasal and contact infection with pandemic swine influenza A virus, A (H1N1) 09. *Veterinary Research, 47*, 1–15.

Henritzi, D., Petric, P. P., Lewis, N. S., Graaf, A., Pessia, A., Starick, E., et al. (2020). Surveillance of European domestic pig populations identifies an emerging reservoir of potentially zoonotic swine influenza A viruses. *Cell Host & Microbe, 28*(4), 614–627.

Hussaini, H. M., Seo, B. & Rich, A.M. (2022). Immunohistochemistry and immunofluorescence. In Oral biology: molecular techniques and applications (pp. 439–450). New York, NY: Springer US.

Kasowski, E. J., Garten, R. J., & Bridges, C. B. (2011). Influenza pandemic epidemiologic and virologic diversity: Reminding ourselves of the possibilities. *Clinical Infectious Diseases, 52*(suppl_1), S44–S49.

Killian, M. L., Swenson, S. L., Vincent, A. L., Landgraf, J. G., Shu, B., Lindstrom, S., et al. (2013). Simultaneous infection of pigs and people with triple-reassortant swine influenza virus H1N1 at a US county fair. *Zoonoses and Public Health, 60*(3), 196–201.

Kothalawala, H., Toussaint, M. J. M., & Gruys, E. (2006). An overview of swine influenza. *Veterinary Quarterly, 28*(2), 45–53.

Kyriakis, C. S., Olsen, C. W., Carman, S., Brown, I. H., Brookes, S. M., Van Doorsselaere, J., & Van Reeth, K. (2010). Serologic cross-reactivity with pandemic (H1N1) 2009 virus in pigs, Europe. *Emerging Infectious Diseases, 16*(1), 96.

Kyriakis, C. S., Rose, N., Foni, E., Maldonado, J., Loeffen, W. L. A., Madec, F., et al. (2013). Influenza a virus infection dynamics in swine farms in Belgium, France, Italy and Spain, 2006–2008. *Veterinary Microbiology, 162*(2–4), 543–550.

Liang, Y. (2023). Pathogenicity and virulence of influenza. *Virulence, 14*(1), p.2223057.

Ma, W., Lager, K. M., Vincent, A. L., Janke, B. H., Gramer, M. R., & Richt, J. A. (2009). The role of swine in the generation of novel influenza viruses. *Zoonoses and public health, 56*(6–7), 326–337.

Ma, W., Lager, K. M., Vincent, A. L., Janke, B. H., Gramer, M. R., & Richt, J. A. (2009a). The role of swine in the generation of novel influenza viruses. *Zoonoses and Public Health, 56*(6–7), 326–337.

Ma, W., Kahn, R. E., & Richt, J. A. (2009b). The pig as a mixing vessel for influenza viruses: Human and veterinary implications. *Journal of Molecular and Genetic Medicine, 3*(1), 158.

Ma, M., Anderson, B. D., Wang, T., Chen, Y., Zhang, D., Gray, G. C., & Lu, J. (2015). Serological evidence and risk factors for swine influenza infections among Chinese swine workers in Guangdong Province. *PLoS One, 10*(5), e0128479.

Mancera Gracia, J. C., Pearce, D. S., Masic, A., & Balasch, M. (2020). Influenza A virus in swine: Epidemiology, challenges and vaccination strategies. *Frontiers in Veterinary Science, 7*, 647.

Meseko, C., Globig, A., Ijomanta, J., Joannis, T., Nwosuh, C., Shamaki, D., et al. (2018). Evidence of exposure of domestic pigs to highly pathogenic avian influenza H5N1 in Nigeria. *Scientific Reports, 8*(1), 5900.

Nasamran, C., Janetanakit, T., Chiyawong, S., Boonyapisitsopa, S., Bunpapong, N., Prakairungnamthip, D., et al. (2020). Persistence of pdm2009-H1N1 internal genes of swine influenza in pigs, Thailand. *Scientific Reports, 10*(1), 19847.

Nelson, M. I., Stratton, J., Killian, M. L., Janas-Martindale, A., & Vincent, A. L. (2015). Continual reintroduction of human pandemic H1N1 influenza a viruses into swine in the United States, 2009 to 2014. *Journal of Virology, 89*(12), 6218–6226.

OIE [World Organization for Animal Health] (2008) Manual of diagnostic tests and vaccines for terrestrial animals. Chapter 2.8.8: Swine Influenza.

Ravina, Dalal, A., Mohan, H., Prasad, M. & Pundir, C.S. (2020). Detection methods for influenza A H1N1 virus with special reference to biosensors: a review. *Bioscience reports, 40*(2), p.BSR20193852.

Richt, J. A., Lager, K. M., Clouser, D. F., Spackman, E., Suarez, D. L., & Yoon, K. J. (2004). Real–time reverse transcription–polymerase chain reaction assays for the detection and differentiation of north American swine influenza viruses. *Journal of Veterinary Diagnostic Investigation, 16*(5), 367–373.

Rose, N., Hervé, S., Eveno, E., Barbier, N., Eono, F., Dorenlor, V., & Simon, G. (2013). Dynamics of influenza a virus infections in permanently infected pig farms: Evidence of recurrent infections, circulation of several swine influenza viruses and reassortment events. *Veterinary Research, 44*, 1–14.

Short, K. R., Richard, M., Verhagen, J. H., van Riel, D., Schrauwen, E. J., van den Brand, J. M., et al. (2015). One health, multiple challenges: The inter-species transmission of influenza A virus. *One Health, 1*, 1–13.

Shortridge, K. F. (1992). Pandemic influenza: a zoonosis? *Seminars in Respiratory Infections, 7*(1), 11–25.

Sukhal, S., Sethi, J., Ganesh, M., Villablanca, P. A., Malhotra, A. K., & Ramakrishna, H. (2017). Extracorporeal membrane oxygenation in severe influenza infection with respiratory failure: A systematic review and meta-analysis. *Annals of Cardiac Anaesthesia, 20*(1), 14–21.

Sun, H., Xiao, Y., Liu, J., Wang, D., Li, F., Wang, C., et al. (2020). Prevalent Eurasian avian-like H1N1 swine influenza virus with 2009 pandemic viral genes facilitating human infection. *Proceedings of the National Academy of Sciences, 117*(29), 17204–17210.

Tchilian, E., & Holzer, B. (2017). Harnessing local immunity for an effective universal swine influenza vaccine. *Viruses, 9*(5), 98.

Van Reeth, K., Brown, I. H., & Olsen, C. W. (2012). Influenza virus. In *Diseases of swine* (Vol. 10, pp. 557–571).

Wesley, R. D. (2004). Exposure of sero-positive gilts to swine influenza virus may cause a few stillbirths per litter. *Canadian Journal of Veterinary Research, 68*(3), 215.

Zhang, N., & Li, Y. (2018). Transmission of influenza A in a student office based on realistic person-to-person contact and surface touch behaviour. *International Journal of Environmental Research and Public Health, 15*(8), 1699.

Zhu, H., Webby, R., Lam, T. T., Smith, D. K., Peiris, J. S., & Guan, Y. (2013). History of swine influenza viruses in Asia. In *Swine influenza* (pp. 57–68).

Zu, R., Dong, L., Qi, X., Wang, D., Zou, S., Bai, T., et al. (2013). Virological and serological study of human infection with swine influenza A H1N1 virus in China. *Virology, 446*(1–2), 49–55.

The Silent Threat: Understanding Nipah Virus and Its Implications

Varun Asediya, Pranav Anjaria, Gyanendra Singh Sengar, Seema Rani Pegu, and Rajib Deb

Abstract

This review aims to unravel the enigma of the Nipah virus, a zoonotic pathogen with a high mortality rate. We systematically analyze the current understanding of the virus's epidemiology, pathogenesis, diagnostic methods, and control measures. Our objective is to identify gaps in the existing body of knowledge and suggest potential areas for future research. This review serves as a valuable resource for researchers in the field, providing a consolidated overview of the current landscape of Nipah virus research and offering insights into the next steps for this important area of study.

Keywords

Nipah virus · Zoonotic pathogen · Epidemiology · Pathogenesis · Viral transmission · Immune response · Vaccine development · Public health impact

Introduction

In the shadow of the global pandemic, a silent specter lurks. The Nipah virus, a zoonotic pathogen with a chilling mortality rate between 40% and 75% (Conroy, 2023), is a ticking time bomb. The most recent outbreak in Kerala, India, has

V. Asediya
M.B. Veterinary College, Dungarpur, Rajasthan, India

P. Anjaria
College of Veterinary Science & Animal Husbandry, Kamdhenu University, Anand, Gujarat, India

G. S. Sengar · S. R. Pegu · R. Deb (✉)
National Research Centre on Pig, Indian Council of Agricultural Research, Guwahati, Assam, India

R. Deb et al. (eds.), *Emerging Zoonotic Threats from Swine*,
https://doi.org/10.1007/978-981-96-7407-7_5

infected six people, two of whom have tragically lost their lives. This is the fourth outbreak to hit Kerala in 5 years, a grim reminder of the virus's persistent threat (Conroy, 2023).

Imagine, for a moment, a world where Nipah becomes the next pandemic. With no approved vaccines or treatments, our healthcare systems would be pushed to the brink, echoing the harrowing scenes from the COVID-19 crisis. The virus, carried mainly by fruit bats but also capable of infecting domestic animals such as pigs (Halpin & Rota, 2023), could spread unchecked, its reach extending far beyond the current hotspots.

This review aims to shed light on the various facets of the Nipah virus. We delve into its epidemiology, exploring the patterns of its outbreaks and its modes of transmission. We examine its pathogenesis, seeking to understand how it infects cells and causes disease. We also review the current diagnostic methods and discuss their strengths and limitations.

Moreover, we evaluate the existing measures for preventing and controlling Nipah virus outbreaks. By identifying gaps in these areas, we hope to provide a roadmap for future research efforts. As we navigate through the complexities of the Nipah virus, we invite readers to join us on this journey of discovery. Together, we can work toward a future where the threat of the Nipah virus is effectively managed.

Methods

This review adheres to a rigorous and systematic approach to ensure the comprehensiveness and reliability of the information collated. The methodology is divided into four key stages:

- Database Search: A meticulous search of the literature was conducted across several databases, including PubMed, Scopus, Web of Science, and Google Scholar. The search parameters were confined to studies published in English. A combination of keywords was employed to yield the most relevant studies. These included: "Nipah virus", "epidemiology", "pathogenesis", "control measures", "outbreaks", and "public health response".
- Inclusion and Exclusion Criteria: The search results were subjected to a thorough screening process to identify peer-reviewed articles that offered a focused examination of the Nipah virus and provided comprehensive details on the methodologies employed and the results obtained. Studies that failed to meet these criteria were excluded. Additionally, the reference lists of the selected studies and pertinent reviews were scrutinized for potential inclusion of other relevant studies.
- Data Extraction: A standardized data extraction form was utilized to collate data from each study. This form included fields for authors, year of publication, title, objectives, methods, results, conclusions, and limitations. This ensured uniformity in the data extraction process and facilitated subsequent analysis.
- Data Synthesis: The selected studies were categorized based on their primary focus areas: epidemiology of Nipah virus; pathogenesis of Nipah virus; public

health response to Nipah virus outbreaks; and control measures for Nipah virus. A narrative synthesis was conducted for each category, summarizing the main features, applications, advantages, disadvantages, and challenges pertinent to understanding and controlling the Nipah virus.

This systematic approach guarantees a comprehensive review that encapsulates the most relevant and recent studies on the Nipah virus. It also facilitates a critical assessment of the current state of knowledge on the subject, thereby identifying gaps in the existing literature and suggesting potential avenues for future research. This methodology ensures that our review is not only thorough but also unique, providing a fresh perspective on the current understanding of the Nipah virus.

Epidemiology of Nipah Virus

Nipah virus (NiV) is a single-stranded, negative-sense, enveloped RNA virus of the genus Henipavirus within the family Paramyxoviridae (Hauser et al., 2021). NiV is a zoonotic virus that can be transmitted to humans from animals (such as bats or pigs), or contaminated foods and can also be transmitted directly from human to human (Whitmer et al., 2021). The known geographic distribution of NiV correlates with the range of its reservoir species—flying foxes of the genus Pteropus-including Australia and Southeast Asia to India and the Eastern African islands (Soman Pillai et al., 2020). The RNA genome of NiV encodes six structural proteins: nucleocapsid (N), phosphoprotein (P), matrix (M), fusion glycoprotein (F), attachment glycoprotein (G), and large polymerase (L). The F and G proteins mediate cellular attachment and entry into the host cell by inducing membrane fusion4. NiV infection can cause severe respiratory and neurological disease in humans, with a case fatality rate ranging from 40% to 75% depending on the strain and outbreak location (Thakur et al., 2022). NiV is classified as a biosafety level 4 (BSL-4) pathogen and a potential bioterrorism agent. There are no approved vaccines or specific antiviral treatments for NiV infection, but several candidates are under investigation (Widerspick et al., 2022).

The emergence and re-emergence of NiV outbreaks in different regions of the world pose a significant threat to public health and animal welfare (Kojom & Singh, 2021; Biswas et al., 2023; Uwishema et al., 2022). The factors that influence the spillover of NiV from bats to humans are not fully understood, but anthropogenic activities and climate change are likely to play a role (Lawrence & Escudero-Pérez, 2022; Islam et al., 2023a; Latinne & Morand, 2022; Epstein et al., 2020; Shaheen, 2022). The genetic diversity and evolution of NiV strains also have implications for the pathogenesis, transmission, and diagnosis of NiV infection (Hauser et al., 2021). The current understanding of the Nipah virus is limited by the lack of comprehensive surveillance, laboratory capacity, and research funding in the endemic areas (Raut et al., 2023; Qiu et al., 2023). Therefore, there is a need for a multidisciplinary and collaborative approach to address the challenges and knowledge gaps in the prevention and control of NiV outbreaks (Ferri & Lloyd-Evans, 2021; Plowright et al., 2019; Gwenzi et al., 2022; Granerod et al., 2023).

Transmission Patterns

NiV is a zoonotic virus that can be transmitted to humans through various routes of exposure to infected animals or their secretions (Sayed et al., 2019). The main reservoir hosts of NiV are fruit bats of the genus Pteropus, which can shed the virus in their saliva, urine, and feces without showing any signs of illness (Mougari et al., 2022; Gokhale et al., 2022; Olival et al., 2020). Humans can acquire NiV infection by direct contact with these bats or their excretions, such as by drinking palm sap or eating fruits that have been contaminated by bat saliva (Nahar et al., 2020; Nazmunnahar et al., 2023; Chimire et al., 2022). NiV can also infect pigs and other domestic animals, which can transmit the virus to humans through direct contact or aerosols (Sayed et al., 2019). Human-to-human transmission of NiV has been documented in several outbreaks, especially in hospital settings, where close contact with patients or their body fluids (such as respiratory droplets, urine, or blood) can facilitate the spread of the virus (Chaiyes et al., 2022; Alam et al., 2022). NiV transmission patterns involve multiple pathways and require strict infection control measures to prevent further outbreaks (Chaiyes et al., 2022).

The transmission dynamics of NiV are influenced by several factors, such as the ecology and behavior of the bat reservoirs, the susceptibility and density of the intermediate and amplifying hosts, the environmental and climatic conditions, and the human activities and practices that increase the risk of exposure (Yahya et al., 2021). The spillover of NiV from bats to humans is likely to occur when the bats are stressed, immunocompromised, or undergoing seasonal changes in their reproductive or migratory cycles, which may affect their viral shedding and distribution (Epstein et al., 2020). The spillover events may also be triggered by the loss or fragmentation of the bat habitats due to deforestation, urbanization, or agricultural expansion, which may force the bats to seek alternative food sources or roosting sites near human settlements. The transmission of NiV from pigs to humans is dependent on the pig population size, density, and movement, as well as the level of biosecurity and hygiene practices in the pig farms (Islam et al., 2023a). The transmission of NiV from humans to humans is influenced by the viral load and duration of shedding of the infected individuals, the type and frequency of contact with the patients or their body fluids, and the availability and use of personal protective equipment and isolation facilities in the health care settings (Chaiyes et al., 2022).

The transmission patterns of NiV may also vary depending on the genetic diversity and evolution of the virus strains (Rahman et al., 2021). NiV strains can be classified into two main lineages: NiV-Malaysia and NiV-Bangladesh, based on their geographic origin and phylogenetic analysis (Sayed et al., 2019). NiV-Malaysia was first identified in the 1998–1999 outbreak in Malaysia and Singapore, where it caused severe respiratory disease in pigs and humans, with a case fatality rate of 40% in humans (Singh et al., 2019a). NiV-Bangladesh was first identified in the 2001 outbreak in Bangladesh, where it caused severe encephalitis in humans, with a case fatality rate of 75% in humans (Rahman et al., 2021). NiV-Bangladesh has been responsible for most of the subsequent outbreaks in Bangladesh and India, where it has also shown evidence of human-to-human transmission and possible airborne transmission (Nazmunnahar et al., 2023). NiV strains can also undergo genetic recombination, mutation, and adaptation, which may affect their virulence, tropism, and antigenicity (Olatunji et al., 2023). The genetic diversity and evolution of NiV strains have implications for the development of diagnostic tools, vaccines, and therapeutics, as well as the assessment of the risk of emergence and spread of new NiV variants (Rahman et al., 2021).

Clinical Symptoms of NiV Infection

The incubation period for Nipah virus (NiV) in humans can vary from 2 weeks to 2 months (Uwishema et al., 2022). The severe form of NiV encephalitis is often characterized by high fever, headache, nausea, vomiting, abnormal eye reflexes, vasomotor abnormalities, seizures, and myoclonic jerks, all of which suggest dysfunction in the brainstem (Alam, 2022). Patients typically exhibit neurological symptoms such as aseptic meningitis, extensive encephalitis, and localized brainstem involvement, often accompanied by cerebellar symptoms (Kenmoe et al., 2019). Some patients may also exhibit psychological symptoms such as depression, personality disorders, and difficulties in focusing and speaking (Bruno et al., 2022). In some cases, NiV patients may experience relapses and late-onset encephalitis that can persist for months or even years after the initial acute illness (Tan et al., 2002; Ng et al., 2004). For example, a small percentage of patients who survived the 1998–1999 Malaysia-Singapore outbreak experienced relapses following their recovery from acute encephalitis, while others developed late-onset encephalitis. Segmental myoclonus, characterized by rhythmic involuntary contractions of muscle groups supplied by contiguous segments of the brainstem or spine, was more common in Malaysia than in outbreaks that occurred in Bangladesh and India. A significant number of NiV survivors (about one-third) have shown neurological and cognitive issues. Among them, more than half displayed behavioral and neuropsychiatric alterations like those observed in Malaysia and Singapore, and nearly all experienced chronic fatigue syndrome (Mishra et al., 2023).

Knowledge Gaps

The Nipah virus (NiV), with significant mortality rates, has been the subject of extensive virological and epidemiological research. Despite these efforts, our understanding of NiV and its pathogenesis is hindered by several unresolved research gaps (Gurley et al., 2020).

1. Strain Diversity in NiV Research

Current NiV research is primarily based on studies involving two primary strains, NiV-Malaysia, and NiV-Bangladesh (Rahman et al., 2021). This limited strain diversity restricts our ability to extrapolate findings across different NiV strains, particularly in relation to pathogenicity, viral shedding, transmission dynamics, and countermeasure efficacy (McKee et al., 2022). Future research should incorporate a wider range of NiV strains to provide a more holistic understanding of the virus.

2. Zoonotic Transmission Dynamics

The mechanisms of NiV infection within its primary reservoir, Pteropus spp. fruit bat populations, remain largely elusive (Alam et al., 2022; Rees et al., 2021). Key factors influencing these dynamics, including viral shedding and spillover event frequency, are yet to be fully elucidated. Additionally, the role of intermediate hosts in facilitating spillover events and the potential for human-to-animal transmission warrant further investigation (Sayed et al., 2019).

3. Human Infection and Pathogenesis

Our understanding of NiV pathogenesis in humans is rudimentary. The rapid progression of the disease and the lack of rapid diagnostic tools often result in late diagnoses (Liew et al., 2022; Pelissier et al., 2019). Furthermore, cultural and religious considerations often prevent the performance of diagnostic autopsies, limiting opportunities for biological sample collection (Gurley et al., 2020).

4. Treatment and Countermeasures

Encephalitis and acute respiratory distress, common clinical manifestations of NiV infection, pose significant treatment challenges. The absence of best practice guidelines for supportive care complicates patient management. While the Coalition for Epidemic Preparedness Innovations (CEPI) is funding clinical trials of vaccine candidates, similar efforts for NiV therapeutics are lacking (Gouglas et al., 2019; Gómez Román et al., 2020; Monath et al., 2022; Pischel et al., 2021; Kitikiti et al., 2022) (Table 1).

Progress in Diagnostic Techniques

Molecular Diagnostic Techniques for NiV

Current state-of-the-art diagnostic technologies for Nipah virus (NiV) are often slow and require laboratory infrastructure that may not be accessible in all endemic regions (Mazzola & Kelly-Cirino, 2019). To overcome these limitations, several innovative techniques have been developed:

- Reverse Transcription Recombinase-Based Isothermal Amplification with Lateral Flow Detection: These assays feature a simple, rapid one-step sample processing method that inactivates the BSL-4 pathogen, eliminating the need for multi-step RNA purification and ensuring safer testing (Pollak et al., 2023).

Table 1 Animal models for studying NiV pathology

Animal model	Route of infection	Dose	Outcome	References
Golden hamster	IP or IN	Lethal	Death in 6–10 dpi, virus in urine, increased viral proliferation, pathology, and mortality with NiVM	Guillaume et al. (2009)
Ferret	Oral	5000 to 50,000 TCID50	Respiratory and neurological symptoms, systemic vasculitis, rhinitis, tonsillitis, nasopharyngitis, non-suppurative meningitis, viral antigens in brain and meninges	Bossart et al. (2009)
African green monkey	Intratracheal	2×10^4 pfu	Fatal infection and disease, virus dissemination to multiple organs, vasculitis, endothelial syncytia, acute respiratory and neurological disease	Geisbert et al. (2010)
Guinea pig	IP	6×10^4 PFU	Severe clinical illness, death in 4–8 dpi, virus excretion in urine, placenta, and fetal fluids, high viral load in various tissues, extensive damage in uterus and urinary bladder	Geisbert et al. (2012)
Pig	Subcutaneous or oral	50,000 TCID50	Fever, sickness, lack of coordination, mucosal nasal discharge, chronic cough, reduced pathogenesis, brief rise in body temperature, momentary respiratory symptoms, slight depressive symptoms, slumped posture	Middleton et al. (2002), Berhane et al. (2008), Chua (2003), Gao et al. (2022)
Cat	Oronasal	50,000 TCID50	Severe meningitis, early febrile reaction, mild behavioral changes, severe respiratory illness, tiny hemorrhagic nodules in lungs	Mungall et al. (2006)
Mouse (Balb/c and C57BL/6)	IP or IN	Not specified	No symptoms, seropositive between 2 and 15 days after injection, infectious virus detectable mainly in lungs	Gao et al. (2022)

Abbreviations: *IP* intraperitoneal, *IN* intranasal, *dpi* days post-infection, *NiVM* Nipah virus Malaysia strain, *NiVB* Nipah virus Bangladesh strain, *TCID50* 50% tissue culture infectious dose, *pfu* plaque-forming unit

Designed to detect the nucleocapsid protein (N) gene, these tests demonstrate an analytical sensitivity of 1000 copies/μL for synthetic NiV RNA while avoiding cross-reactivity with flaviviruses or Chikungunya virus, which present with similar febrile symptoms (Pollak et al., 2023). Two specific tests identified 50,000–100,000 $TCID_{50}$/mL (100–200 RNA copies/reaction) of both NiV

Bangladesh (NiV B) and NiV Malaysia (NiV M) strains, delivering results within 30 minutes. Their simplicity, speed, and minimal equipment requirements make them well-suited for use in resource-limited settings (Pollak et al., 2023).

- Advancements in Serological and Nucleic Acid Amplification Techniques: Several in-house assays using serological and nucleic acid amplification techniques have been developed to diagnose NiV. Some early multiplex panels have also been designed to differentiate NiV infection from other febrile illnesses (Mazzola & Kelly-Cirino, 2019).
- Enzyme-Linked Immunosorbent Assays (ELISA) and Polymerase Chain Reaction (PCR): Various ELISA-based tests and molecular methods using PCR have been developed for NiV diagnosis, offering reliable detection capabilities (Singh et al., 2019a).
- Isothermal Reverse Transcription-Loop-Mediated Isothermal Amplification (RT-LAMP): A rapid RT-LAMP assay was developed to detect NiV by targeting the nucleocapsid protein (N) gene. This method, which operates at 65 °C, has been evaluated against conventional RT-PCR, demonstrating its potential for efficient NiV detection (Ma et al., 2019).

These advancements mark significant progress toward the development of near-patient NiV diagnostics that offer high sensitivity for initial screening, robustness across diverse settings, and the capability to be performed safely outside high-containment laboratories (Pollak et al., 2023).

Recent Advances in Understanding the Virus

Recent advancements in our understanding of the Nipah virus (NiV) have been significant. The molecular architecture of the Nipah virus (NiV) is crucial for its entry and replication in host cells. Recent cryo-electron microscopy studies have revealed the three-dimensional structures of two key components of the NiV envelope: the G glycoprotein tetramer and the nucleocapsid protein (N) (Talukdar et al., 2023; Ker et al., 2021). The G glycoprotein tetramer is responsible for binding to the cellular receptors ephrin-B2 and ephrin-B3 and mediates the fusion of the viral and cellular membranes (Talukdar et al., 2023; Wang et al., 2022a). The nucleocapsid protein forms a helical assembly that encapsulates the viral RNA genome and interacts with the viral polymerase and phosphoprotein (Ker et al., 2021). These structural insights provide a basis for understanding the molecular mechanisms of NiV infection and for developing novel therapeutics and vaccines against this emerging pathogen.

Moreover, a mathematical test provides (Agarwal & Singh, 2020) a comprehensive depiction of NiV's transmission dynamics within a specific population. This model employs a differential operator with the Mittag-Leffler function, offering a more accurate portrayal of the virus's spread by considering factors such as waiting distribution and memory effects. This approach underscores the importance of innovative mathematical models in understanding and predicting the behavior of infectious diseases like NiV.

Another study (Samreen et al., 2023) has a mathematical model to investigate the dynamics and control interventions of the Nipah virus. The model, governed by a nonlinear fractional-order system of differential equations, considers two transmission modes: Food-borne and human-to-human. It identifies three equilibrium states and performs a thorough theoretical analysis. Sensitivity analysis is performed to obtain effective time-dependent controls, and the most effective strategy for disease eradication is determined through numerical simulations.

Moreover, another study (Diekmann et al., 2010) has a comprehensive understanding of the basic reproduction number (R0), a crucial quantity in infectious disease epidemiology. The authors present a detailed recipe for constructing the Next-Generation Matrix (NGM) from basic ingredients derived directly from the specifications of the model. They define two related matrices, the NGM with large domain and the NGM with small domain. These matrices, along with the NGM, reflect the range of possibilities encountered in the literature for the characterization of R0. The authors establish that these matrices have the same non-zero eigenvalues, the largest of which is the basic reproduction number R0. This work provides valuable insights into the construction of next-generation matrices for compartmental epidemic models.

Treatment Strategies, Prevention, and Control Measures

The current treatment strategies for Nipah virus infection are limited to supportive care, including rest, hydration, and treatment of symptoms as they occur (Islam et al., 2023b). There are no specific antiviral treatments available for the Nipah virus till now (Johnson et al., 2021).

However, there are promising treatments under trial. One promising treatment is Remdesivir, an experimental antiviral drug that has shown complete effectiveness against Nipah virus infection in monkeys (Lo et al., 2019). Additionally, India is importing monoclonal antibodies from Australia to treat Nipah virus infection in Kerala (Sahay et al., 2020). These treatments are still under investigation and are not yet approved for use.

There is no specific antiviral treatment or vaccine available for NiV infection in humans or animals (Singh et al., 2019b). The current management of NiV infection is mainly supportive and symptomatic, such as hydration, oxygen therapy, anticonvulsants, and antibiotics for secondary infections. The use of ribavirin (Rababi & Nag, 2023), a broad-spectrum antiviral drug, has been reported to have some efficacy in reducing the mortality of NiV infection in vitro and in animal models, but its clinical benefit in humans is unclear and controversial. Recently, a human monoclonal antibody m102.4 (Tit-oon et al., 2020; Banerjee et al., 2019) that targets the NiV G protein has been developed and tested in animal models and has shown promising results in preventing and treating NiV infection (Doyle et al., 2021; Dsouza & Selvaa Kumar, 2023; Wang et al., 2022b). However, the safety and efficacy of this antibody in humans have not been established yet, and its availability and accessibility are limited.

Therefore, the prevention and control of NiV infection relies heavily on the implementation of effective and comprehensive measures at the individual, community, and national/international levels. These measures include:

Individual level: People should practice good personal hygiene and avoid contact with sick or dead animals, especially bats and pigs, and their products (Zumla et al., 2016). People should also avoid consuming raw or partially cooked date palm sap, fruits, or other food items that could be contaminated by bat saliva or urine. People who have contact with suspected or confirmed cases of NiV infection should wear appropriate personal protective equipment (PPE) and follow standard infection control practices to prevent nosocomial transmission. People who develop symptoms of NiV infection, such as fever, headache, cough, sore throat, vomiting, or altered mental status, should seek medical attention as soon as possible and inform the healthcare workers about their exposure history ((Satter et al., 2022).

Community level: Public health education and awareness campaigns should be conducted to inform the population about the signs, symptoms, and risk factors of NiV infection, and to promote safe and hygienic practices (Singh et al., 2019b). Community engagement and participation are essential to ensure the acceptance and compliance of the prevention and control measures, and to reduce stigma and discrimination against affected individuals and groups. Surveillance and reporting systems should be established and strengthened to detect and monitor NiV outbreaks and to facilitate timely and effective response. Rapid diagnostic tests and laboratory confirmation should be available and accessible to confirm suspected cases and to guide clinical management and contact tracing (Kitikiti et al., 2022). Isolation and quarantine facilities should be prepared and equipped to provide adequate and appropriate care for the patients and to prevent further spread of the infection. Contact tracing and follow-up should be conducted to identify and monitor the contacts of confirmed cases and to provide them with prophylaxis or treatment if needed. Outbreak investigation and research should be conducted to understand the epidemiology, ecology, and transmission dynamics of NiV and to identify potential reservoirs and sources of infection (Epstein et al., 2020).

National and international level: Policies and regulations should be developed and implemented to prevent and control the introduction and spread of NiV and other emerging infectious diseases. These include strengthening animal health and veterinary services, implementing biosecurity and biosafety measures, regulating the trade and movement of animals and animal products, and enhancing the collaboration and coordination among different sectors and stakeholders (Ambat et al., 2019). Regional and global networks and platforms should be established and maintained to share information, resources, and expertise, and to provide technical and financial support for the prevention and control of NiV and other zoonotic diseases. Research and development should be prioritized and funded to develop new and improved tools and strategies for the diagnosis, treatment, and prevention of NiV infection, such as vaccines and antivirals (Irving et al., 2021).

Future Directions

The Nipah virus is a zoonotic pathogen that poses a serious threat to human and animal health. Despite the efforts of researchers and public health authorities, there are still many gaps in the current knowledge and understanding of the virus, its transmission, its epidemiology, and its prevention and control. Therefore, it is imperative to conduct more research and surveillance to address these challenges and to prepare for potential future outbreaks. Some of the areas for future research include:

The molecular and evolutionary mechanisms of the virus, especially the factors that influence its virulence, host range, and transmissibility. Understanding the genetic diversity and evolution of the virus can help to identify potential targets for vaccines and therapeutics, as well as to monitor the emergence of new strains or variants (Talukdar et al., 2023). Moreover, elucidating the molecular pathogenesis of the virus, such as the role of the fusion (F) and attachment (G) proteins in cellular interactions and the role of the polymerase (L) protein in viral replication, can help to reveal the molecular determinants of the disease severity and the immune response (Sen et al., 2019).

The ecology and behavior of the natural reservoirs of the virus, mainly the fruit bats of the genus Pteropus. Studying the distribution, migration, and feeding habits of these bats can help to elucidate the spillover events and the environmental drivers of the virus transmission (Shariff et al., 2023; Cable et al., 2022; Gómez Román et al., 2022; Rzymski et al., 2023). Furthermore, investigating the dynamics of the virus infection and shedding in bats, as well as the factors that modulate the viral load and the immune response in bats, can help to understand the persistence and the transmission of the virus in the natural host (Irving et al., 2021; Subudhi et al., 2019; Gurley et al., 2017; Gupta et al., 2021).

The risk factors and modes of transmission of the virus among humans and animals, particularly the role of person-to-person transmission and the role of intermediate hosts such as pigs. Investigating the epidemiological and social determinants of the virus spread can help to design effective interventions and to reduce the exposure and contact with infected animals or people (Halpin & Rota, 2023). Additionally, exploring the mechanisms of cross-species transmission and adaptation of the virus, as well as the genetic and immunological factors that influence the susceptibility and the outcome of the infection in different hosts, can help to assess the risk and the impact of the virus emergence (Conroy, 2023).

The development and evaluation of vaccines and therapeutics for the prevention and treatment of the Nipah virus infection (Shariff et al., 2023). Currently, there are no approved vaccines or drugs for the virus, and the management of the infection relies on supportive care and infection control measures. Developing safe and effective vaccines and therapeutics can improve the clinical outcomes and the survival rates of the infected individuals, as well as to prevent or contain the outbreaks. Some of the promising candidates include mRNA-based vaccines that can induce robust and durable immune responses, monoclonal antibodies that can neutralize the virus and protect against disease, and antiviral drugs that can inhibit the viral entry or replication.

The importance of continued surveillance and research on the Nipah virus cannot be overstated. The virus has a high mortality rate, a wide host range, and a potential for adaptation and emergence (Lin, 2023). Moreover, the virus is influenced by environmental and anthropogenic changes, such as land use conversion, climate change, and human-animal interactions, that can increase the risk and the frequency of outbreaks. Therefore, it is essential to monitor the virus activity and the disease occurrence, to enhance the laboratory and diagnostic capacities, to strengthen the collaboration and communication among the stakeholders, and to raise the awareness and the preparedness of the public and the health workers (Anjaria et al., 2023). By doing so, we can improve our knowledge and our response to the Nipah virus, and ultimately, protect the health and the well-being of humans and animals.

In the realm of infectious disease management, Artificial Intelligence (AI) emerges as a powerful ally in the battle against the Nipah virus. This insidious pathogen, capable of causing devastating outbreaks, demands innovative approaches for prediction, understanding, and containment. This content explores seven key facets where AI plays a pivotal role:

1. *Predictive Modeling*: AI can help in creating predictive models to forecast potential outbreaks by analyzing various factors such as climate change, deforestation, and urbanization (Rolnick et al., 2023). These models can be based on machine learning algorithms that learn from past data to predict future outcomes (Asediya & Anjaria, 2023).
2. *Virus Evolution Study*: Machine learning algorithms can be used to understand the genetic diversity and evolution of the virus (Kannan & Priya, 2023; Varma et al., 2014; Randhawa et al., 2020). This involves analyzing the genetic sequences of the virus to understand its mutation patterns and evolutionary history (Deka & Morshed, 2018; Ghosh et al., 2022).
3. *Host Identification:* AI has been used to identify bat species with the potential to host the Nipah virus (Li et al., 2020). This involves using machine learning algorithms to analyze the traits of different bat species and predict their potential to host the virus.
4. *Epidemiological Research*: AI can assist in studying the epidemiological and social determinants of the virus transmission among humans and animals. This involves analyzing large datasets of epidemiological data to understand patterns and trends in virus transmission (Anjaria et al., 2023).
5. *Drug Discovery*: AI can speed up drug discovery by identifying potential compounds that can inhibit the virus. This involves using machine learning algorithms to analyze the structures of different compounds and predict their potential to inhibit the virus (Pathania et al., 2020; Abduljalil et al., 2023).
6. *Understanding Strain Diversity*: AI can help in understanding the diversity of Nipah virus strains in endemic countries. This involves sequencing the virus from different individuals and using machine learning algorithms to analyze the sequences and understand strain diversity (Li et al., 2020).

7. *Public Health Response*: AI can also assist in the public health response to Nipah virus outbreaks. For example, machine learning algorithms can be used to analyze data from social media and other sources to track the spread of the virus and inform public health interventions (Kannan & Priya, 2023; Deka & Morshed, 2018).

Conclusion

The review has meticulously dissected the mystery surrounding the Nipah virus, a formidable zoonotic adversary with alarming mortality rates. It has navigated through the labyrinth of the virus's epidemiology, pathogenesis, diagnostic techniques, and counteractive strategies. The review has illuminated the shadowy corners of our current understanding and pinpointed the unexplored territories awaiting scientific exploration. Serving as a beacon for researchers, this review offers a unified panorama of the Nipah virus research terrain. The insights gleaned from this review are anticipated to chart the course for future investigations, steering us toward the ultimate destination—the mitigation of this lethal viral threat.

Bibliography

Abduljalil, J. M., Elfiky, A. A., Sayed, E.-S. T. A., & AlKhazindar, M. M. (2023). *In silico* structural elucidation of Nipah virus L protein and targeting RNA-dependent RNA polymerase domain by nucleoside analogs. *Journal of Biomolecular Structure & Dynamics, 41*, 8215–8229.

Agarwal, P., & Singh, R. (2020). Modelling of transmission dynamics of Nipah virus (Niv): A fractional order approach. *Physica A: Statistical Mechanics and its Applications, 547*, 124243.

Alam, A. M. (2022). Nipah virus, an emerging zoonotic disease causing fatal encephalitis. *Clinical Medicine, 22*, 348–352.

Alam, M. G. S., Billah, M. M., Sharif, A. R., Sultana, S., Shano, S., Rahman, M. K., Islam, A., Alamgir, A. S. M., Shirin, T., & Flora, M. S. (2022). Secondary human-to-human transmission of Nipah virus in an ambulance, northwestern Bangladesh, February 2019. *Outbreak, Surveillance, Investigation & Response (OSIR) Journal, 15*.

Ambat, A. S., Zubair, S. M., Prasad, N., Pundir, P., Rajwar, E., Patil, D. S., & Mangad, P. (2019). Nipah virus: A review on epidemiological characteristics and outbreaks to inform public health decision making. *Journal of Infection and Public Health, 12*, 634–639.

Anjaria, P., Asediya, V., Bhavsar, P., Pathak, A., Desai, D., & Patil, V. (2023). Artificial intelligence in public health: Revolutionizing epidemiological surveillance for pandemic preparedness and equitable vaccine access. *Vaccines (Basel), 11*, 1154.

Asediya, V., & Anjaria, P. (2023). Quantum leap: Is the conflux of artificial intelligence, personalized medicine, nutrigenetics and nutrigenomics the path to optimal health? *Epigenomics, 15*, 397–400.

Banerjee, S., Niyas, V. K. M., Soneja, M., Shibeesh, A. P., Basheer, M., Sadanandan, R., Wig, N., & Biswas, A. (2019). First experience of ribavirin postexposure prophylaxis for Nipah virus, tried during the 2018 outbreak in Kerala, India. *Journal of Infection, 78*, 491–503.

Berhane, Y., Weingartl, H. M., Lopez, J., Neufeld, J., Czub, S., Embury-Hyatt, C., Goolia, M., Copps, J., & Czub, M. (2008). Bacterial infections in pigs experimentally infected with Nipah virus. *Transboundary and Emerging Diseases, 55*, 165–174.

Biswas, J. K., Mukherjee, P., Vithanage, M., & Prasad, M. N. V. (2023). Emergence and re-emergence of emerging infectious diseases (EIDs). In *One health* (pp. 19–37). Wiley.

Bossart, K. N., Zhu, Z., Middleton, D., Klippel, J., Crameri, G., Bingham, J., McEachern, J. A., Green, D., Hancock, T. J., Chan, Y.-P., Hickey, A. C., Dimitrov, D. S., Wang, L.-F., & Broder, C. C. (2009). A neutralizing human monoclonal antibody protects against lethal disease in a new ferret model of acute Nipah virus infection. *PLoS Pathogens, 5*, e1000642.

Bruno, L., Nappo, M. A., Ferrari, L., Di Lecce, R., Guarnieri, C., Cantoni, A. M., & Corradi, A. (2022). Nipah virus disease: Epidemiological, clinical, diagnostic and legislative aspects of this unpredictable emerging zoonosis. *Animals, 13*, 159.

Cable, J., Fauci, A., Dowling, W. E., Günther, S., Bente, D. A., Yadav, P. D., Madoff, L. C., Wang, L., Arora, R. K., Van Kerkhove, M., Chu, M. C., Jaenisch, T., Epstein, J. H., Frost, S. D. W., Bausch, D. G., Hensley, L. E., Bergeron, É., Sitaras, I., Gunn, M. D., Geisbert, T. W., Muñoz-Fontela, C., Krammer, F., de Wit, E., Nordenfelt, P., Saphire, E. O., Gilbert, S. C., Corbett, K. S., Branco, L. M., Baize, S., van Doremalen, N., Krieger, M. A., Clemens, S. A. C., Hesselink, R., & Hartman, D. (2022). Lessons from the pandemic: Responding to emerging zoonotic viral diseases – A keystone symposia report. *Annals of the New York Academy of Sciences, 1518*, 209–225.

Chaiyes, A., Duengkae, P., Suksavate, W., Pongpattananurak, N., Wacharapluesadee, S., Olival, K. J., Srikulnath, K., Pattanakiat, S., & Hemachudha, T. (2022). Mapping risk of Nipah virus transmission from bats to humans in Thailand. *EcoHealth, 19*, 175–189.

Chimire, K., Kasarla, R. R., Adhikari, S. R., & Pathak, L. (2022). An emerging zoonosis of public health concern: A comprehensive review on Nipah virus infection. *Journal of Universal College of Medical Sciences, 10*, 71–76.

Chua, K. B. (2003). Nipah virus outbreak in Malaysia. *Journal of Clinical Virology, 26*, 265–275.

Conroy, G. (2023). Nipah virus outbreak: What scientists know so far. *Nature*. https://doi.org/10.1038/d41586-023-02967-x

Deka, M., & Morshed, N. (2018). Mapping disease transmission risk of Nipah virus in south and Southeast Asia. *Tropical Medicine and Infectious Disease, 3*, 57.

Diekmann, O., Heesterbeek, J. A. P., & Roberts, M. G. (2010). The construction of next-generation matrices for compartmental epidemic models. *Journal of the Royal Society Interface, 7*, 873–885.

Doyle, M. P., Kose, N., Borisevich, V., Binshtein, E., Amaya, M., Nagel, M., Annand, E. J., Armstrong, E., Bombardi, R., Dong, J., Schey, K. L., Broder, C. C., Zeitlin, L., Kuang, E. A., Bornholdt, Z. A., West, B. R., Geisbert, T. W., Cross, R. W., & Crowe, J. E. (2021). Cooperativity mediated by rationally selected combinations of human monoclonal antibodies targeting the henipavirus receptor binding protein. *Cell Reports, 36*, 109628.

Dsouza, N., & Selvaa Kumar, C. (2023). Predicting the changes in neutralizing antibody interaction with G protein derived from Bangladesh isolates of Nipah virus: Molecular dynamics based approach. *Journal of Biomolecular Structure & Dynamics, 42*, 1–11.

Epstein, J. H., Anthony, S. J., Islam, A., Kilpatrick, A. M., Ali Khan, S., Balkey, M. D., Ross, N., Smith, I., Zambrana-Torrelio, C., Tao, Y., Islam, A., Quan, P. L., Olival, K. J., Khan, M. S. U., Gurley, E. S., Hossein, M. J., Field, H. E., Fielder, M. D., Briese, T., Rahman, M., Broder, C. C., Crameri, G., Wang, L.-F., Luby, S. P., Lipkin, W. I., & Daszak, P. (2020). Nipah virus dynamics in bats and implications for spillover to humans. *Proceedings of the National Academy of Sciences, 117*, 29190–29201.

Ferri, M., & Lloyd-Evans, M. (2021). The contribution of veterinary public health to the management of the COVID-19 pandemic from a one health perspective. *One Health, 12*, 100230.

Gao, Z., Li, T., Han, J., Feng, S., Li, L., Jiang, Y., Xu, Z., Hao, P., Chen, J., Hao, J., Xu, P., Tian, M., Jin, N., Huang, W., & Li, C. (2022). Assessment of the immunogenicity and protection of a Nipah virus soluble G vaccine candidate in mice and pigs. *Frontiers in Microbiology, 13*.

Geisbert, T. W., Daddario-DiCaprio, K. M., Hickey, A. C., Smith, M. A., Chan, Y.-P., Wang, L.-F., Mattapallil, J. J., Geisbert, J. B., Bossart, K. N., & Broder, C. C. (2010). Development of an acute and highly pathogenic nonhuman primate model of Nipah virus infection. *PLoS One, 5*, e10690.

Geisbert, T. W., Feldmann, H., & Broder, C. C. (2012). Animal challenge models of henipavirus infection and pathogenesis. In *Henipavirus: Ecology, molecular virology, and pathogenesis* (pp. 153–177).

Ghosh, D., Chakraborty, S., Kodamana, H., & Chakraborty, S. (2022). Application of machine learning in understanding plant virus pathogenesis: Trends and perspectives on emergence, diagnosis, host-virus interplay and management. *Virology Journal, 19*, 42.

Gokhale, M., Sudeep, A. B., Mathapati, B., Balasubramanian, R., Ullas, P. T., Mohandas, S., Patil, D. R., Shete, A. M., Gopale, S., Sawant, P., Jain, R., Holeppanavar, M., Suryawanshi, A. T., Chopade, G., Dhaigude, S., Patil, D. Y., Mourya, D. T., & Yadav, P. D. (2022). Serosurvey for Nipah virus in bat population of southern part of India. *Comparative Immunology, Microbiology and Infectious Diseases, 85*, 101800.

Gómez Román, R., Wang, L.-F., Lee, B., Halpin, K., de Wit, E., Broder, C. C., Rahman, M., Kristiansen, P., & Saville, M. (2020). Nipah@20: Lessons learned from another virus with pandemic potential. *mSphere, 5*.

Gómez Román, R., Tornieporth, N., Cherian, N. G., Shurtleff, A. C., L'Azou Jackson, M., Yeskey, D., Hacker, A., Mungai, E., & Le, T. T. (2022). Medical countermeasures against henipaviruses: A review and public health perspective. *The Lancet Infectious Diseases, 22*, e13–e27.

Gouglas, D., Christodoulou, M., Plotkin, S. A., & Hatchett, R. (2019). CEPI: Driving progress toward epidemic preparedness and response. *Epidemiologic Reviews, 41*, 28–33.

Granerod, J., Huang, Y., Davies, N. W. S., Sequeira, P. C., Mwapasa, V., Rupali, P., Michael, B. D., Solomon, T., & Easton, A. (2023). Global landscape of encephalitis: Key priorities to reduce future disease burden. *Clinical Infectious Diseases, 77*, 1552. https://doi.org/10.1093/cid/ciad417

Guillaume, V., Wong, K. T., Looi, R. Y., Georges-Courbot, M.-C., Barrot, L., Buckland, R., Wild, T. F., & Horvat, B. (2009). Acute Hendra virus infection: Analysis of the pathogenesis and passive antibody protection in the hamster model. *Virology, 387*, 459–465.

Gupta, P., Singh, M. P., Goyal, K., Tripti, P., Ansari, M. I., Obli Rajendran, V., Dhama, K., & Malik, Y. S. (2021). Bats and viruses: A death-defying friendship. *Virus, 32*, 467–479.

Gurley, E. S., Hegde, S. T., Hossain, K., Sazzad, H. M. S., Hossain, M. J., Rahman, M., Sharker, M. A. Y., Salje, H., Islam, M. S., Epstein, J. H., Khan, S. U., Kilpatrick, A. M., Daszak, P., & Luby, S. P. (2017). Convergence of humans, bats, trees, and culture in Nipah virus transmission, Bangladesh. *Emerging Infectious Diseases, 23*, 1446–1453.

Gurley, E. S., Spiropoulou, C. F., & de Wit, E. (2020). Twenty years of Nipah virus research: Where do we go from here? *The Journal of Infectious Diseases, 221*, S359–S362.

Gwenzi, W., Skirmuntt, E. C., Musvuugwa, T., Teta, C., Halabowski, D., & Rzymski, P. (2022). Grappling with (re)-emerging infectious zoonoses: Risk assessment, mitigation framework, and future directions. *International Journal of Disaster Risk Reduction, 82*, 103350.

Halpin, K., & Rota, P. A. (2023). A review of Hendra virus and Nipah virus infections in man and other animals. In *Zoonoses: Infections affecting humans and animals* (pp. 1–17). Springer International Publishing.

Hauser, N., Gushiken, A. C., Narayanan, S., Kottilil, S., & Chua, J. V. (2021). Evolution of Nipah virus infection: Past, present, and future considerations. *Tropical Medicine and Infectious Disease, 6*, 24.

Irving, A. T., Ahn, M., Goh, G., Anderson, D. E., & Wang, L.-F. (2021). Lessons from the host defences of bats, a unique viral reservoir. *Nature, 589*, 363–370.

Islam, A., Cannon, D. L., Rahman, M. Z., Khan, S. U., Epstein, J. H., Daszak, P., Luby, S. P., Montgomery, J. M., Klena, J. D., & Gurley, E. S. (2023a). Nipah virus exposure in domestic and peridomestic animals living in human outbreak sites, Bangladesh, 2013–2015. *Emerging Infectious Diseases, 29*, 393–396.

Islam, M. R., Dhar, P. S., & Rahman, M. M. (2023b). Newly outbreak of Nipah virus: Epidemiology, symptoms, transmission, diagnostic testing, treatment, and global health concern. *International Journal of Surgery, 109*, 507–508.

Johnson, K., Vu, M., & Freiberg, A. N. (2021). Recent advances in combating Nipah virus. *Faculty Reviews, 10*, 74.

Kannan, M., & Priya, C. (2023). A research on prediction of bat-borne disease infection through segmentation using diffusion-weighted MR imaging in deep-machine learning approach. *Materials Today Proceedings, 81*, 994–999.

Kenmoe, S., Demanou, M., Bigna, J. J., Nde Kengne, C., Fatawou Modiyinji, A., Simo, F. B. N., Eyangoh, S., Sadeuh-Mba, S. A., & Njouom, R. (2019). Case fatality rate and risk factors for Nipah virus encephalitis: A systematic review and meta-analysis. *Journal of Clinical Virology, 117*, 19–26.

Ker, D.-S., Jenkins, H. T., Greive, S. J., & Antson, A. A. (2021). CryoEM structure of the Nipah virus nucleocapsid assembly. *PLoS Pathogens, 17*, e1009740.

Kitikiti, N. S., Soumyanarayanan, U., Vogel, S., & Lim, J. C. W. (2022). Science, innovation, and Society in the age of pandemics: Reflections from the inaugural sir Alasdair Breckenridge lecture. *Clinical Pharmacology and Therapeutics, 111*, 548–550.

Kojom, L. P., & Singh, V. (2021). A review on emerging infectious diseases prioritized under the 2018 WHO Research and Development blueprint: Lessons from the Indian context. *Vector-Borne and Zoonotic Diseases, 21*, 149–159.

Latinne, A., & Morand, S. (2022). Climate anomalies and spillover of bat-borne viral diseases in the Asia–Pacific region and the Arabian peninsula. *Viruses, 14*, 1100.

Lawrence, P., & Escudero-Pérez, B. (2022). Henipavirus immune evasion and pathogenesis mechanisms: Lessons learnt from natural infection and animal models. *Viruses, 14*, 936.

Li, K., Yan, S., Wang, N., He, W., Guan, H., He, C., Wang, Z., Lu, M., He, W., Ye, R., Veit, M., & Su, S. (2020). Emergence and adaptive evolution of Nipah virus. *Transboundary and Emerging Diseases, 67*, 121–132.

Liew, Y. J. M., Ibrahim, P. A. S., Ong, H. M., Chong, C. N., Tan, C. T., Schee, J. P., Gómez Román, R., Cherian, N. G., Wong, W. F., & Chang, L.-Y. (2022). The Immunobiology of Nipah virus. *Microorganisms, 10*, 1162.

Lin, H. (2023). Nipah virus: A zoonotic virus transmitted from bats and pigs, causing an epidemic in Southeast Asia. *Advances in Infectious Disease, 13*, 283–290.

Lo, M. K., Feldmann, F., Gary, J. M., Jordan, R., Bannister, R., Cronin, J., Patel, N. R., Klena, J. D., Nichol, S. T., Cihlar, T., Zaki, S. R., Feldmann, H., Spiropoulou, C. F., & de Wit, E. (2019). Remdesivir (GS-5734) protects African green monkeys from Nipah virus challenge. *Science Translational Medicine, 11*.

Ma, L., Chen, Z., Guan, W., Chen, Q., & Liu, D. (2019). Rapid and specific detection of all known Nipah virus strains' sequences with reverse transcription-loop-mediated isothermal amplification. *Frontiers in Microbiology, 10*, 10.

Mazzola, L. T., & Kelly-Cirino, C. (2019). Diagnostics for Nipah virus: A zoonotic pathogen endemic to Southeast Asia. *BMJ Global Health, 4*, e001118.

McKee, C. D., Islam, A., Rahman, M. Z., Khan, S. U., Rahman, M., Satter, S. M., Islam, A., Yinda, C. K., Epstein, J. H., Daszak, P., Munster, V. J., Hudson, P. J., Plowright, R. K., Luby, S. P., & Gurley, E. S. (2022). Nipah virus detection at bat roosts after spillover events, Bangladesh, 2012–2019. *Emerging Infectious Diseases, 28*, 1384–1392.

Middleton, D. J., Westbury, H. A., Morrissy, C. J., van der Heide, B. M., Russell, G. M., Braun, M. A., & Hyatt, A. D. (2002). Experimental Nipah virus infection in pigs and cats. *Journal of Comparative Pathology, 126*, 124–136.

Mishra, G., Prajapat, V., & Nayak, D. (2023). Advancements in Nipah virus treatment: Analysis of current progress in vaccines, antivirals, and therapeutics. *Immunology*. https://doi.org/10.1111/imm.13695

Monath, T. P., Nichols, R., Tussey, L., Scappaticci, K., Pullano, T. G., Whiteman, M. D., Vasilakis, N., Rossi, S. L., Campos, R. K., Azar, S. R., Spratt, H. M., Seaton, B. L., Archambault, W. T., Costecalde, Y. V., Moore, E. H., Hawks, R. J., & Fusco, J. (2022). Recombinant vesicular stomatitis vaccine against Nipah virus has a favorable safety profile: Model for assessment of live vaccines with neurotropic potential. *PLoS Pathogens, 18*, e1010658.

Mougari, S., Gonzalez, C., Reynard, O., & Horvat, B. (2022). Fruit bats as natural reservoir of highly pathogenic henipaviruses: Balance between antiviral defense and viral tolerance. *Current Opinion in Virology, 54*, 101228.

Mungall, B. A., Middleton, D., Crameri, G., Bingham, J., Halpin, K., Russell, G., Green, D., McEachern, J., Pritchard, L. I., Eaton, B. T., Wang, L.-F., Bossart, K. N., & Broder, C. C. (2006). Feline model of acute Nipah virus infection and protection with a soluble glycoprotein-based subunit vaccine. *Journal of Virology, 80*, 12293–12302.

Nahar, N., Asaduzzaman, M., Mandal, U. K., Rimi, N. A., Gurley, E. S., Rahman, M., Garcia, F., Zimicki, S., Sultana, R., & Luby, S. P. (2020). Hunting bats for human consumption in Bangladesh. *EcoHealth, 17*, 139–151.

Nazmunnahar, A. I., Roknuzzaman, A. S. M., & Islam, M. R. (2023). The recent Nipah virus outbreak in Bangladesh could be a threat for global public health: A brief report. *Health Science Reports, 6*, e1423.

Ng, B.-Y., Lim, C. C. T., Yeoh, A., & Lee, W. L. (2004). Neuropsychiatric sequelae of Nipah virus encephalitis. *The Journal of Neuropsychiatry and Clinical Neurosciences, 16*, 500–504.

Olatunji, G., Kokori, E., Abdulrahmon, M. A., & Aderinto, N. (2023). Addressing the recurrent Nipah virus outbreaks: A call for vigilance, collaboration, and preparedness. *New Microbes New Infections, 54*, 101184.

Olival, K. J., Latinne, A., Islam, A., Epstein, J. H., Hersch, R., Engstrand, R. C., Gurley, E. S., Amato, G., Luby, S. P., & Daszak, P. (2020). Population genetics of fruit bat reservoir informs the dynamics, distribution and diversity of Nipah virus. *Molecular Ecology, 29*, 970–985.

Pathania, S., Randhawa, V., & Kumar, M. (2020). Identifying potential entry inhibitors for emerging Nipah virus by molecular docking and chemical-protein interaction network. *Journal of Biomolecular Structure & Dynamics, 38*, 5108–5125.

Pelissier, R., Iampietro, M., & Horvat, B. (2019). Recent advances in the understanding of Nipah virus immunopathogenesis and anti-viral approaches. *F1000Res, 8*, 1763.

Pischel, L., Yildirim, I., & Omer, S. B. (2021). Fast development of high-quality vaccines in a pandemic. *Chest, 160*, e1–e3.

Plowright, R. K., Becker, D. J., Crowley, D. E., Washburne, A. D., Huang, T., Nameer, P. O., Gurley, E. S., & Han, B. A. (2019). Prioritizing surveillance of Nipah virus in India. *PLoS Neglected Tropical Diseases, 13*, e0007393.

Pollak, N. M., Olsson, M., Marsh, G. A., Macdonald, J., & McMillan, D. (2023). Evaluation of three rapid low-resource molecular tests for Nipah virus. *Frontiers in Microbiology, 13*.

Qiu, Y., Guitian, J., Webster, J. P., Musallam, I., Haider, N., Drewe, J. A., & Song, J. (2023). Global prioritization of endemic zoonotic diseases for conducting surveillance in domestic animals to protect public health. *Philosophical Transactions of the Royal Society B: Biological Sciences, 378*.

Rababi, D., & Nag, A. (2023). Evaluation of therapeutic potentials of selected phytochemicals against Nipah virus, a multi-dimensional in silico study. *3 Biotech, 13*, 174.

Rahman, M. Z., Islam, M. M., Hossain, M. E., Rahman, M. M., Islam, A., Siddika, A., Hossain, M. S. S., Sultana, S., Islam, A., Rahman, M., Rahman, M., Klena, J. D., Flora, M. S., Daszak, P., Epstein, J. H., Luby, S. P., & Gurley, E. S. (2021). Genetic diversity of Nipah virus in Bangladesh. *International Journal of Infectious Diseases, 102*, 144–151.

Randhawa, G. S., Soltysiak, M. P. M., El Roz, H., de Souza, C. P. E., Hill, K. A., & Kari, L. (2020). Machine learning using intrinsic genomic signatures for rapid classification of novel pathogens: COVID-19 case study. *PLoS One, 15*, e0232391.

Raut, J., Joshi, A., Mudey, A., & Mehendale, A. M. (2023). The past, present, and future of one health in India: A narrative review. *Cureus, 15*, e44992. https://doi.org/10.7759/cureus.44992

Rees, E. M., Minter, A., Edmunds, W. J., Lau, C. L., Kucharski, A. J., & Lowe, R. (2021). Transmission modelling of environmentally persistent zoonotic diseases: A systematic review. *Lancet Planet Health, 5*, e466–e478.

Rolnick, D., Donti, P. L., Kaack, L. H., Kochanski, K., Lacoste, A., Sankaran, K., Ross, A. S., Milojevic-Dupont, N., Jaques, N., Waldman-Brown, A., Luccioni, A. S., Maharaj, T., Sherwin, E. D., Mukkavilli, S. K., Kording, K. P., Gomes, C. P., Ng, A. Y., Hassabis, D., Platt, J. C., Creutzig, F., Chayes, J., & Bengio, Y. (2023). Tackling climate change with machine learning. *ACM Computing Surveys, 55*, 1–96.

Rzymski, P., Szuster-Ciesielska, A., Dzieciątkowski, T., Gwenzi, W., & Fal, A. (2023). mRNA vaccines: The future of prevention of viral infections? *Journal of Medical Virology, 95.*

Sahay, R. R., Yadav, P. D., Gupta, N., Shete, A. M., Radhakrishnan, C., Mohan, G., Menon, N., Bhatnagar, T., Suma, K., Kadam, A. V., Ullas, P. T., Anu Kumar, B., Sugunan, A. P., Sreekala, V. K., Khobragade, R., Gangakhedkar, R. R., & Mourya, D. T. (2020). Experiential learnings from the Nipah virus outbreaks in Kerala towards containment of infectious public health emergencies in India. *Epidemiology and Infection, 148*, e90.

Samreen, U. S., Nawaz, R., AlQahtani, S. A., Li, S., & Hassan, A. M. (2023). A mathematical study unfolding the transmission and control of deadly Nipah virus infection under optimized preventive measures: New insights using fractional calculus. *Results in Physics, 51*, 106629.

Satter, S. M., Nazneen, A., Aquib, W. R., Sultana, S., Rahman, M. Z., Klena, J. D., Montgomery, J. M., & Shirin, T. (2022). Vertical transfer of humoral immunity against Nipah virus: A novel evidence from Bangladesh. *Tropical Medicine and Infectious Disease, 8*, 16.

Sayed, A., Bottu, A., Qaisar, M., Mane, M. P., & Acharya, Y. (2019). Nipah virus: A narrative review of viral characteristics and epidemiological determinants. *Public Health, 173*, 97–104.

Sen, N., Kanitkar, T. R., Roy, A. A., Soni, N., Amritkar, K., Supekar, S., Nair, S., Singh, G., & Madhusudhan, M. S. (2019). Predicting and designing therapeutics against the Nipah virus. *PLoS Neglected Tropical Diseases, 13*, e0007419.

Shaheen, M. N. F. (2022). The concept of one health applied to the problem of zoonotic diseases. *Reviews in Medical Virology, 32*, e2326.

Shariff, S., Siddiq, A., Itani, R., Nazir, A., & Uwishema, O. (2023). The role of surveillance and early detection in controlling Nipah virus outbreaks in Bangladesh. *International Journal of Surgery: Globalization and Health, 6.*

Singh, R. K., Dhama, K., Chakraborty, S., Tiwari, R., Natesan, S., Khandia, R., Munjal, A., Vora, K. S., Latheef, S. K., Karthik, K., Singh Malik, Y., Singh, R., Chaicumpa, W., & Mourya, D. T. (2019a). Nipah virus: Epidemiology, pathology, immunobiology and advances in diagnosis, vaccine designing and control strategies – A comprehensive review. *The Veterinary Quarterly, 39*, 26–55.

Singh, R. K., Dhama, K., Chakraborty, S., Tiwari, R., Natesan, S., Khandia, R., Munjal, A., Vora, K. S., Latheef, S. K., Karthik, K., Singh Malik, Y., Singh, R., Chaicumpa, W., & Mourya, D. T. (2019b). Nipah virus: Epidemiology, pathology, immunobiology and advances in diagnosis, vaccine designing and control strategies – A comprehensive review. *Veterinary Quarterly, 39*, 26–55.

Soman Pillai, V., Krishna, G., & Valiya, V. M. (2020). Nipah virus: Past outbreaks and future containment. *Viruses, 12*, 465.

Subudhi, S., Rapin, N., & Misra, V. (2019). Immune system modulation and viral persistence in bats: Understanding viral spillover. *Viruses, 11*, 192.

Talukdar, P., Dutta, D., Ghosh, E., Bose, I., & Bhattacharjee, S. (2023). Molecular pathogenesis of Nipah virus. *Applied Biochemistry and Biotechnology, 195*, 2451–2462.

Tan, C. T., Goh, K. J., Wong, K. T., Sarji, S. A., Chua, K. B., Chew, N. K., Murugasu, P., Loh, Y. L., Chong, H. T., Tan, K. S., Thayaparan, T., Kumar, S., & Jusoh, M. R. (2002). Relapsed and late-onset Nipah encephalitis. *Annals of Neurology, 51*, 703–708.

Thakur, V., Thakur, P., & Ratho, R. K. (2022). Nipah outbreak: Is it the beginning of another pandemic in the era of COVID-19 and Zika. *Brain, Behavior, and Immunity, 99*, 25–26.

Tit-oon, P., Tharakaraman, K., Artpradit, C., Godavarthi, A., Sungkeeree, P., Sasisekharan, V., Kerdwong, J., Miller, N. L., Mahajan, B., Khongmanee, A., Ruchirawat, M., Sasisekharan, R., & Fuangthong, M. (2020). Prediction of the binding interface between monoclonal antibody m102.4 and Nipah attachment glycoprotein using structure-guided alanine scanning and computational docking. *Scientific Reports, 10*, 18256.

Uwishema, O., Wellington, J., Berjaoui, C., Muoka, K. O., Onyeaka, C. V. P., & Onyeaka, H. (2022). A short communication of Nipah virus outbreak in India: An urgent rising concern. *Annals of Medicine & Surgery, 82.*

Varma, S., Botlani, M., & Leighty, R. E. (2014). Discerning intersecting fusion-activation pathways in the Nipah virus using machine learning. Proteins: Structure. *Function, and Bioinformatics, 82*, 3241–3254.

Wang, Z., Amaya, M., Addetia, A., Dang, H. V., Reggiano, G., Yan, L., Hickey, A. C., DiMaio, F., Broder, C. C., & Veesler, D. (2022a). Architecture and antigenicity of the Nipah virus attachment glycoprotein. *Science, 1979*(375), 1373–1378.

Wang, Z., Dang, H. V., Amaya, M., Xu, Y., Yin, R., Yan, L., Hickey, A. C., Annand, E. J., Horsburgh, B. A., Reid, P. A., Smith, I., Eden, J.-S., Xu, K., Broder, C. C., & Veesler, D. (2022b). Potent monoclonal antibody–mediated neutralization of a divergent Hendra virus variant. *Proceedings of the National Academy of Sciences, 119*, 119.

Whitmer, S. L. M., Lo, M. K., Sazzad, H. M. S., Zufan, S., Gurley, E. S., Sultana, S., Amman, B., Ladner, J. T., Rahman, M. Z., Doan, S., Satter, S. M., Flora, M. S., Montgomery, J. M., Nichol, S. T., Spiropoulou, C. F., & Klena, J. D. (2021). Inference of Nipah virus evolution, 1999–2015. *Virus Evolution, 7*.

Widerspick, L., Vázquez, C. A., Niemetz, L., Heung, M., Olal, C., Bencsik, A., Henkel, C., Pfister, A., Brunetti, J. E., Kucinskaite-Kodze, I., Lawrence, P., Muñoz Fontela, C., Diederich, S., & Escudero-Pérez, B. (2022). Inactivation methods for experimental Nipah virus infection. *Viruses, 14*, 1052.

Yahya, E. B., et al. (2021). Asian nipah virus and the potential of new pandemic. *Pakistan Journal of Biotechnology, 18*, 17–22.

Zumla, A., Dar, O., Kock, R., Muturi, M., Ntoumi, F., Kaleebu, P., Eusebio, M., Mfinanga, S., Bates, M., Mwaba, P., Ansumana, R., Khan, M., Alagaili, A. N., Cotten, M., Azhar, E. I., Maeurer, M., Ippolito, G., & Petersen, E. (2016). Taking forward a 'one health' approach for turning the tide against the Middle East respiratory syndrome coronavirus and other zoonotic pathogens with epidemic potential. *International Journal of Infectious Diseases, 47*, 5–9.

Streptococcus suis: An Emerging Zoonotic Pathogen from Swine

Santanu Pal, Dumala Naveen, Reddi Lokeswari, Bavadharani Mani, Priyanshi Yadav, and Shivali Khandelwal

Abstract

Streptococcus suis ranks among the key bacterial pathogens with high prevalence causing significant economic impacts in the swine sector, as the global trend shifts away from prophylactic antimicrobial use. Moreover, it poses a major emerging zoonotic threat, impacting individuals in direct proximity to infected pigs or pork products. Besides certain Asian countries, *S. suis* is recognized as a significant public health concern globally affecting both livestock and human populations. The pathogen's ability to spread through respiratory droplets, direct contact, or contaminated food products poses a risk to individuals involved in the swine industry and pork consumption. Moreover, the emergence of antibiotic-resistant strains complicates treatment and control measures. While previously viewed as sporadic incidences, human infections caused by this pathogen have been reported over the past four and a half decades, with two prominent outbreaks recorded in China in 1998 and 2005. These infections cause a range of complications, such as purulent meningitis, septic shock, endocarditis, pneumonic syndromes, uveitis-endophthalmitis, and arthritis in both pigs and human beings. Over the past few decades, ongoing efforts have led to significant advancements in our understanding of this zoonotic infectious organism, contributing to unveiling the molecular mechanisms that underlie its high pathogenicity. This chapter will offer background information on the biology and

S. Pal (✉) · D. Naveen · R. Lokeswari · P. Yadav · S. Khandelwal
ICAR-Indian Veterinary Research Institute (ICAR-IVRI), Izatnagar, Bareilly, Uttar Pradesh, India

B. Mani
ICAR-Indian Veterinary Research Institute (ICAR-IVRI), Hebbal, Bengaluru, Karnataka, India

R. Deb et al. (eds.), *Emerging Zoonotic Threats from Swine*,
https://doi.org/10.1007/978-981-96-7407-7_6

molecular characteristics of this Gram-positive bacterium, along with detailing the clinical signs, pathology, epidemiology, diagnosis, treatment, and prevention of the occurrence of the disease in both animals and humans.

Keywords

Streptococcus suis · Pigs · Zoonosis · Pathogenesis · Virulence factors · Epidemiology

Introduction

The prevalence of *Streptococcus suis*-related diseases presents considerable economic challenges and raises concerns regarding animal well-being within swine farming. Moreover, the pathogen poses a significant public health risk given its considerable potential for zoonotic transmission. The early human case of *S. suis* was reported in Denmark in 1968 (Perch et al., 1968). Since then, human infection with *S. suis* has evolved into a significant zoonosis and roughly 1600 cases of *S. suis* infections have been reported in humans across over 30 countries or regions globally with intensive swine production. In many Western countries, *Streptococcus suis* is commonly viewed as an occupational hazard primarily affecting individuals employed in the swine or pork sectors. However, in Southeast Asian regions, the major population faces exposure primarily through close interaction with animals or the consumption of uncooked pork products. Before 2005, over 200 cases had been reported globally, mostly from European and Asian countries and regions (Geffner Sclarsky et al., 2001). In July 2005, a significant outbreak of human *S. suis* infection occurred in Sichuan province, China, accompanied by several isolated cases in other provinces (Wang et al., 2005). This marked the third reported outbreak of human *S. suis* infections in China, following earlier outbreaks in Jiangsu province in 1998 and 1999 (Du et al., 2020). These recurrent and intensive outbreaks of human *S. suis* infection have sparked considerable global public concern regarding this pathogen as an emerging zoonotic agent. *Streptococcus suis* poses a significant threat to pig populations globally, particularly in regions where intensive pig farming is common. Additionally, it's increasingly being found in various mammalian species, birds, and the environment. In humans, *S. suis* is recognized as an emerging zoonotic pathogen, causing systemic infections such as meningitis, which can lead to hearing loss or balance problems. Other clinical manifestations include endocarditis, cellulitis, peritonitis, muscle breakdown, joint inflammation, spinal disc infections, pneumonia, eye inflammation, and severe eye infections. Human infections primarily occur as an occupational hazard, affecting individuals who have contact with contaminated animal blood, secretions, or pork-based products. There are currently 33 identified capsular serotypes of the bacterium. Among these, Serotype 2 stands out as the most aggressive, causing severe infections in both pigs and humans on a global scale.

To reduce the threat to humans, food safety, health education, and hygiene should be promoted (Kerdsin et al., 2020). One of the biggest threats to world health is antibiotic resistance. If preventive measures (such as effective immunizations) are not taken, *S. suis* could become more resistant to antibiotics and spread its resistance genes to bacteria that are not part of their host animal species. High levels of resistance to tetracyclines (exceeding 90%) and macrolides (over 70%) have been observed in *S.* suis isolates from pigs worldwide. This resistance trend was noted as early as the 1980s, as indicated by a retrospective analysis of historical pig samples in Denmark. Similarly, resistance to tetracyclines and macrolides in human strains was documented in the latter half of the 2000s, although retrospective studies revealed that it had already become prevalent in the preceding decades. The dual nature of *Streptococcus suis*, functioning both as a harmless colonizer and a highly aggressive pathogen, has led to uncertainties regarding diagnostic interpretation and the definition of virulence. Consequently, a significant research hurdle lies in pinpointing specific markers of virulence that can distinguish between strains that are merely commensal and those that are truly pathogenic. This task is made challenging by the considerable variability in both physical traits and genetic makeup observed in *S. suis*, exemplified by the existence of at least 33 capsular serotypes. The nasopharynx serves as a reservoir for *S. suis* and various other potentially harmful microorganisms and harmless inhabitants. Among these inhabitants, some are considered innocent bystanders, naturally colonizing the respiratory mucosa without causing harm, while others, known as pathobionts, can become opportunistic pathogens under certain conditions, contributing to clinical disease. When pathogens exert significant influence over changes in the microbiota and manipulate the host response, they are termed keystone pathogens, capable of intensifying the virulence of pathobionts and leading to dysbiosis and inflammatory conditions. In the case of *S. suis*, collaborative interactions with other bacterial agents like Pasteurella multocida or Mycoplasma hyopneumoniae, as well as respiratory viruses such as porcine reproductive and respiratory syndrome virus (PRRSV), porcine circovirus type 2, and swine influenza virus (SIV), can heighten the risk of invasive infections.

Biological Features

S. suis is a Gram-positive facultative anaerobe, typically appearing as coccoid or ovoid cells occurring singly, in pairs, or in short chains. Initially, when the first classification of *S. suis* was proposed, the Lancefield test facilitated the categorization of strains into the R, S, and T groups of Streptococci. However, this classification method is influenced by how bacterial extracts are prepared. Especially, since *S. suis* is an encapsulated bacterium (a characteristic discovered later), early classification attempts relied on preparations of capsular antigens rather than antigens located in the bacterial wall. Based on the carbohydrate composition of bacterial cell wall antigens, Lancefield grouping has been used to classify streptococci since the 1930s. De Moor divided *Streptococcus* strains from septicemic infections in pigs into Lancefield groups with the designations R, S, RS, and T at the beginning of the

1960s. Nevertheless, Moor's R and S groups were identified as subgroups of Lancefield group D by Elliott in 1966, which resulted in the identification of these strains as a novel species, "*Streptococcus suis*." Subsequent research revealed that, instead of the components of their cell walls, the main antigens of Moor's R and S groups originated from their capsular polysaccharides (CPSs). Later, Moor's streptococci (S, R, and RS) were reclassified as serotypes 1, 2, and 1/2 of *S. suis*, respectively. Six additional serotypes (serotypes 3–8) were identified by Perch et al. in 1983. Later, between 1989 and 1995, 26 more serotypes (serotypes 9–34) were identified. It was reported in 2013 that many *S. suis* serotype 21/29 strains were isolated from healthy pigs. Furthermore, Pan et al. discovered the new serotype Chz in *S. suis* isolates from pigs with meningitis in 2015 (Okura et al., 2016). *S. suis* falls under groups R and S in the Lancefield classification (Okura et al., 2016). There are 35 known serotypes of *S. suis*, which are categorized serologically according to the unique antigenicity of their capsular polysaccharides (CPSs). A novel serotype called Chz was proposed (Pan et al., 2015). In sick pigs, *S. suis* isolates from specific serotypes—like serotypes 2, 3, 7, and 9—were often found. Serotype 2 is the most common in *S. suis* infections in pigs and humans, while serotypes 4, 5, 9, 14, 16, 21, 24, and 31 are all related to human infections (Dutkiewicz et al., 2017).

As of present, genetic analysis has led to the reclassification of *S. suis* into 29 serotypes (Okura et al., 2016). Previously, *S. suis* was known to include 35 serotypes (serotypes 1/2 and 1–34). However, serotypes 20, 22, 26, 32, 33, and 34 have been re-identified as belonging to other species and are now referred to as *S. suis*-like bacteria (Higgins et al., 1995; Nishibori et al., 2013). Understanding information about serotypes is crucial as not all are linked to zoonotic potential or disease severity. Certain serotypes, like serotypes 2 and 14, are correlated with zoonotic infections. Notably, serotype 2 stands out as the most prevalent serotype in both human and swine populations worldwide. Among these serotypes, type 2 is most commonly associated with diseases in both pigs and humans and is the most frequently reported worldwide. While there have been isolated human *S. suis* infection cases attributed to types 1 and 14, the vast majority of human infections are caused by type 2.

Diversity of *Streptococcus suis*

S. suis displays significant genetic and phenotypic diversity as a bacterial species. Strains belonging to distinct capsular serotypes, or even those within the same serotype, exhibit genetic variations from one another. Multilocus sequence typing (MLST) serves as a method for genetic characterization, offering detailed insights into the epidemiology, strain relationships, and virulence properties of pathogens. King et al. (2002) developed an MLST model specific to *Streptococcus suis*, utilizing seven distinct housekeeping genes (cpn60, dpr, recA, aroA, thrA, gki, and mutS). Each gene contains multiple alleles, and the combination of these alleles within an isolate defines its sequence type (ST). Isolates sharing the same ST are considered to belong to the same clone. Interestingly, instances may occur where isolates with the same ST possess different serotypes, and conversely, isolates with the same serotype may belong to different STs. In various regions worldwide, specific sequence types (STs) of *Streptococcus suis* have been consistently linked to clinical cases in both pigs and humans. For instance, ST1 is frequently associated with clinical infections in Europe, Asia, and Argentina. Conversely, ST7 has been identified as the culprit behind significant outbreaks in China during 1998 and 2005 and appears to be endemic in China and Hong Kong. In North America, the predominant STs among serotype 2 strains isolated from both pigs and humans are ST25 and ST28. ST28 has also been detected in Japan and other countries. Additionally, ST101 to ST104 is endemic in Thailand, while ST20 has been exclusively found in human cases in Europe, particularly in the Netherlands and France.

Epidemiology

Streptococcus suis is widely distributed as a pathobiont and is increasingly recognized as a zoonotic pathogen. Its primary reservoir hosts are domestic pigs and wild boars. Subclinically infected pigs, which show no outward signs of illness, play a crucial role in the spread of *S. suis*, serving as the main source of infection for both pigs and humans. In the respiratory tract, *S. suis* exhibits two distinct phases or "faces": firstly, as a harmless colonization commensal bacterium, and secondly, as an invasive pathogen capable of breaching various defense barriers. The transition between these phases is influenced by several factors, including bacterial, host, and environmental elements. Susceptible pigs, particularly weaning piglets, can suffer from a range of serious infections including meningitis, septicemia, pneumonia, endocarditis, or polyarthritis. The primary mode of transmission is horizontal, occurring through nose-to-nose contact. However, vertical transmission from infected sows to piglets during farrowing is also possible. The *S. suis* infection primarily manifests as sporadic. But outbreaks are also documented. A large-scale *S. suis* outbreak in humans happened in China in 2005; out of 204 infected individuals, 38 died (Lun et al., 2007). A recent epidemic of *S. suis* infections in Thailand's Nakhon Ratchasima region in March 2021 resulted in 19 cases of meningitis and septicemia as well as two fatalities. Through epidemiological inquiry and whole genome sequencing (WGS), the source of the epidemic was identified as an offering of raw pork that was served during a Buddhist ritual that 241 people attended. Furthermore, the strain showed resistance to several antibiotics, such as linezolid, erythromycin, clindamycin, tetracycline, and chloramphenicol. The acquisition of a transposon from the IS1216 family containing optrA and ermA, as well as an integrative and conjugative element (ICE) carrying the tetO and ermB resistance genes, was suggested to be the cause of this resistance. This study emphasizes the emergence of *S. suis* zoonotic lineages resistant to many drugs, highlighting the persistent threat posed by these strains to human health (Brizuela et al., 2023).

The regional distribution of *S. suis* serotypes predominance varies from region to region (Fig. 1). For example, serotypes 2 and 3 are more prevalent in the United States and Canada, while serotype 9 is more common in other European nations

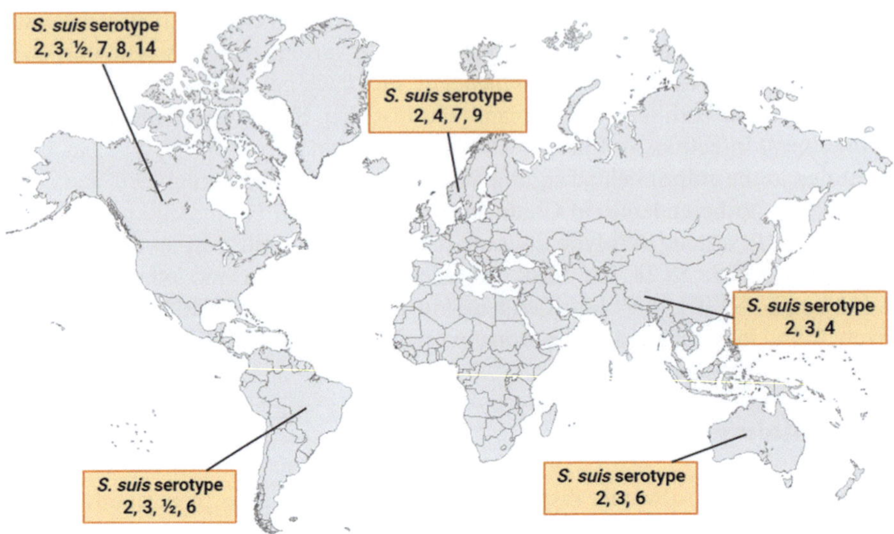

Fig. 1 The distribution of infectious *S. suis* serotypes in different continents worldwide

(Goyette et al., 2014). The strains of *S. suis* typically isolated from infected pigs predominantly fall within serotypes 1 to 8, with serotype 2 being the most commonly encountered (Goyette-Desjardins et al., 2014). Serotype 2 strains are widely recognized as the most virulent, although not all strains of this serotype exhibit high virulence. The three serotypes most commonly isolated from clinical cases of *S. suis* infection in pigs globally are serotype 2 (28% prevalence), serotype 9 (19.4%), and serotype 3 (15.9%). The distribution of serotypes isolated from infected pigs varies across geographical regions. In North America, dominant serotypes include serotype 2 (24.3%), serotype 3 (21%), and serotype 1/2 (13%). Brazil predominantly reports serotypes 2 (57.6%), 1/2 (9.6%), and 14 (8.8%). In Asia, serotype 2 is the most prevalent (44.2%), followed by serotypes 3 (12.4%) and 4 (5.6%). Notably, serotype 9 is frequently isolated from swine infections in Europe (61%), while serotypes 2 (18.4%) and 7 (6.7%) are also encountered (Goyette-Desjardins et al., 2014). As of now, a total of 1642 cases of human infections have been reported, with 74.7% attributed to serotype 2 strains.

Swine as a Reservoir of *S. suis*

In the recent outbreak, all instances of human disease were epidemiologically linked to contact with pigs. Although most cases involved broken skin, the exact mode of transmission remained unspecified. Additional sporadic cases of zoonotic *S. suis* infections have been associated with accidental injuries caused by lacerations or inhalation of infected aerosols from carcasses of infected animals. It is worth noting that *S. suis* can also be present in the feces and on surfaces (fomites) of infected pigs. Besides transmission through direct contact with infected pigs or exposure to airborne pathogens, the recent outbreak might have been partly influenced by the consumption of contaminated pork, suggesting a potential avenue for foodborne transmission. *S.* suis commonly establishes early colonization in the upper respiratory tract of pigs. Indeed, finding pigs free of *S. suis* under natural circumstances is challenging, indicating the pathogen's adeptness at adapting to its porcine host reservoir. However, *S. suis* also possesses the capability to induce severe, potentially fatal illnesses. Earlier research indicated that a significant proportion, ranging from 40% to 80%, of healthy pig's harbor *S. suis* in various anatomical sites such as the nasal cavities, tonsils, vagina, and digestive tract (Goyette-Desjardins et al., 2015). Colonization of pigs by *S. suis* can occur through vertical transmission during birth or through horizontal transmission via aerosols. Comparing the levels of *Streptococcus suis* in saliva samples across different growth stages indicated that the saliva of sows was the most likely reservoir and primary source of infection for pigs.

Transmission Dynamics

Animals can become contaminated through vertical transmission, where piglets contract microorganisms from their mother's bacterial flora, or through horizontal transmission via contact with other members of the herd. The aerosolization of *S. suis* has also been identified as a mode of transmission. Virulent and viable strains of *S. suis* have been isolated from aerosols present inside pig sties (Bonifait et al., 2014). Pigs in a healthy state often harbor *S. suis*, primarily in their tonsils and upper respiratory tracts, which can lead to several conditions such as meningitis, endocarditis, arthritis, sepsis, and pneumonia. It has been confirmed that *S. suis* is a novel zoonotic disease that can infect human beings through direct contact with diseased pigs, eating raw pork products, being around pigs at work butchering, processing, and slaughtering ill or deceased pigs, alcohol consumption, male sex, and skin aberrations are the risk factors (Rayanakorn et al., 2018). Animals such as cattle, sheep, goats, boars, cats, dogs, horses, and birds can also occasionally acquire *S. suis* infection, in addition to humans and pigs (Fig. 2).

Zoonotic Potential of *S. suis*

The majority of newly emerging infectious diseases are zoonoses, many of which fall under the category of "neglected" diseases. Zoonoses, being infections that affect both humans and animals, present a dual burden (Bari et al., 2022). In humans *S. suis* infection presents as meningitis. Patients with meningitis can develop permanent hearing loss. In humans one common clinical sign of an infection with *S. suis* is meningitis. Furthermore, endocarditis, septicemia, arthritis, and hearing loss are a frequent side effect that may be significant, bilateral, or irreversible (Kim et al., 2023). Since its first reported case of meningitis in Denmark in 1968 by Perch,

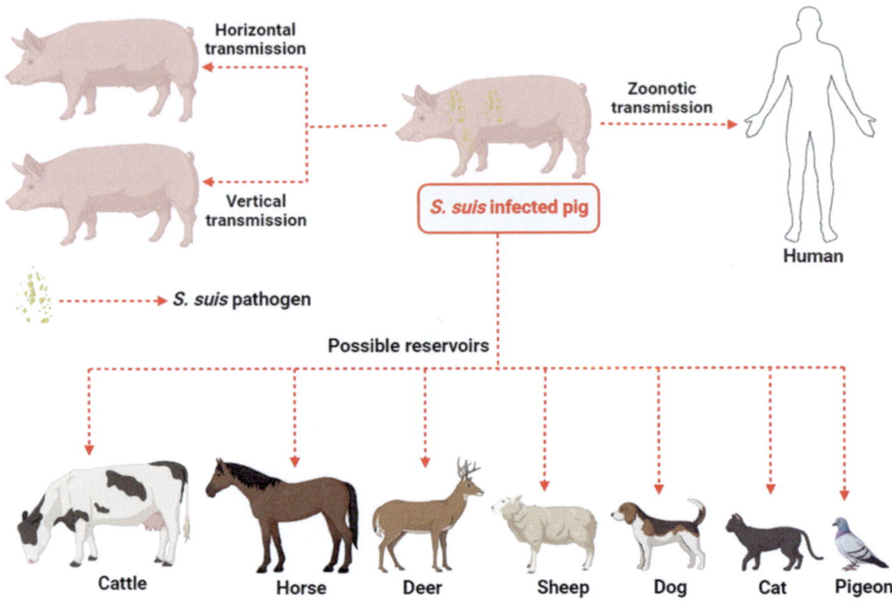

Fig. 2 Transmission dynamics of *S. suis*, detailing how the bacteria spreads through various pathways to infect hosts

Streptococcus suis has been recognized as a zoonotic agent. Subsequently, sporadic human infections have been documented in various European countries such as those reported by Watkins et al. (2001), Pedroli et al. (2003), and Manzin et al. (2008). Similarly, cases have been reported in Asian countries including Thailand (Pootong, 1993; BOE, 2005; Rusmeechan and Sribusara, 2008), Hong Kong (Hui et al., 2005), China (Ye et al., 2006), and Vietnam (Mai et al., 2008). While human infections with *Streptococcus suis* have been sporadically documented in North America, the first reported case in the United States didn't occur until 2006, as noted by Willenburg et al. (2006). In Greece, the initial case of *S. suis* septicemia and meningitis was reported in 2005 by Mazokopakis et al. (2005). This case involved septicemia caused by S22, complicated by meningitis and subsequent deafness in an elderly woman with a history of prior contact with unprocessed pork meat. The causative agent was isolated from both blood cultures and cerebrospinal fluid. Individuals in regular contact with pigs, such as pig farmers, abattoir workers, pork transporters, meat inspectors, and butchers, typically contract the infection through the skin, often via cuts, wounds, or abrasions, as documented by Robertson and Blackmore (1989) and Tarradas et al. (2001). The majority of human infections occur among pork handlers, particularly those working in slaughterhouses, and are often the result of minor injuries or skin abrasions contaminated by raw pork or pig viscera, as highlighted by Clifton-Hadley et al. (1984) and Breton et al. (1986).

Pathogenesis and Virulence Factors

Pathogenesis of *S. suis* is complex in that it involves several niche environments and upper respiratory tract of pigs being the common colonization site. It was found that throughout all stages of the pathogenic process, *S. suis* interacts with various types of immunocompetent host cells, including polymorphonuclear leukocytes, mononuclear macrophages, lymphocytes, dendritic cells, and microglia with over 100 different virulence factors to evade the host's innate and adaptive immune defenses and to overcome environmental stress (Fig. 3). The first barrier at odds with *S. suis* infection is the respiratory epithelial cells. Though the mechanisms by which the strains of *S. suis* breach the mucosal barrier are not clearly understood, the main pathway for invasive infection is through dissemination from the nasopharynx. Human infection occurs through eating contaminated pork but can also occur as occupational exposure to the people who are in contact with infected animals like butchers and abattoir workers. Nasopharyngeal colonization of *S. suis* has been disclosed as a major cause of disease in humans. A theoretical framework was proposed to account for the systemic infection of piglets with *S. suis* and this model led to the finding of *S. suis* in the tonsillar lymphoid tissue and also a high concentration of CD169+ macrophages (Segura et al., 2020). According to this model, virulent strains of *S. suis* may multiply in the tonsils due to physical and environmental stressors that lessen the microbiota's competition. This leads to an increase in *S. suis* in the tonsils, which can then enter the bloodstream through the numerous tiny

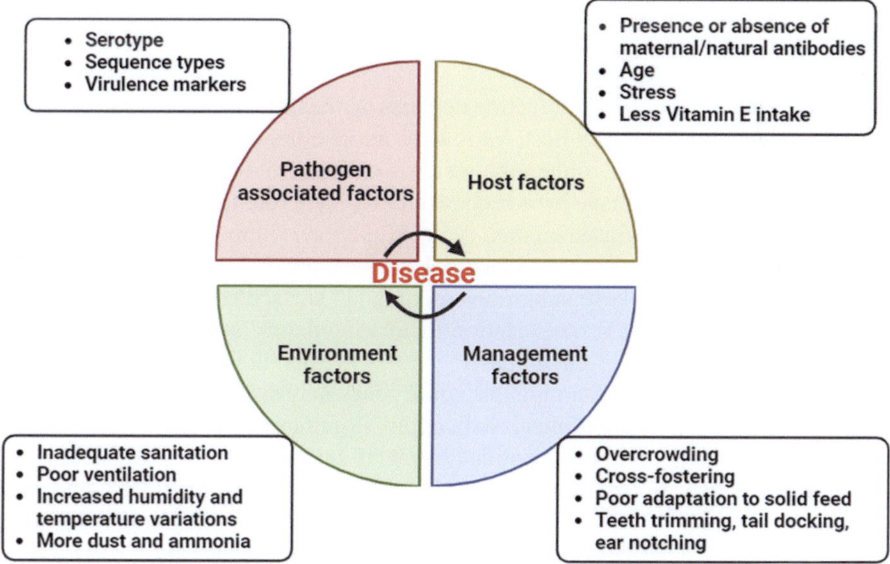

Fig. 3 The figure highlighting the key factors that contribute to the transmission of *S. suis* infection

blood vessels that permeate the lymphoid tissue. CD169+ macrophages may serve as reservoirs for this replication. A scenario like this would also make sense given the observation that invasive infection is more frequently linked to serotype 2 strains that engage with the CD169 Siglec 1 receptor through their sialylated CPS. Co-infection with viruses like Porcine Reproductive and Respiratory Syndrome Virus or Swine Influenza Virus can subvert the innate functions of CD169+ macrophages, which could aid in *S. suis* survival and bloodstream dissemination (Segura et al., 2020). In this regard, nothing is known about the possible methods that *S. suis* serotypes lacking sialic acid in their CPSs may employ. It is also possible that the ability of the organism to survive and/or replicate in this specific fraction of macrophages is specific to strains that cause infection. The major virulence factor associated with *S. suis* infection is the capsular polysaccharide (CPS) and the cps gene locus is exchanged between different serotypes. The increase in the zoonotic potential of *S. suis* may be ascribed mainly to the CPS switch whereas loss or acquisition of other genes may also lead to disparity in virulence potential (Matajira et al., 2019). Various other potential virulence factors are found associated with the infection including extracellular protein factor, suilysin, muramidase-released protein, hyaluronate lyase, several adhesins, and surface antigen 1. In animal infection models except capsular polysaccharides, no other virulence factors were found to be important for virulence. Among human isolates, there was diverse response for the presence of muramidase-released protein and extracellular protein factor. Suilysin (SLY) is a member of the cholesterol-dependent pore-forming toxin family and is the major toxin of *S. suis* in a mouse model (Seitz et al., 2016).

Molecular Processes Involved in *S. suis* Infection

The clinical outcome of *S. suis* infection depends on the intricate interaction between this zoonotic pathogen and its host. Various bacterial components and host cell factors collectively contribute to the pathogenesis of *S. suis* infection. To date, nearly 60 bacterial components have been recognized to play a role in the infection and/or pathogenicity of *S. suis*. Based on their typical functions within bacterial life cycles, these bacterial virulence-associated factors have been provisionally categorized into three main subgroups. These subgroups include (1) surface/secreted elements, (2) enzymes/proteases, and (3) transcription factors/regulatory systems. Additionally, there is a fourth subgroup encompassing other factors such as transporters and secretion systems. It's worth noting that some genes may exhibit characteristics that could place them within multiple classifications simultaneously.

In addition to the previously identified elements such as capsular polysaccharides (CPS), extracellular protein factor (EF), fibronectin binding factor (FBP), muramidase-released protein (MRP), a 38 kDa surface-localized protein, and thio-activated hemolysin, several additional members have been identified (Feng et al., 2014). These include SspA, a surface-associated subtilisin-like serine protease, HtpS, a newly discovered immunogenic protein exposed on the cell surface, and Sat surface protein. Similar to FBP, the gene SSU05_1311, with an unknown function, has been recognized as another surface-anchored fibronectin-binding protein. Notably, this surface protein has been shown to play a crucial role in vivo by aiding in the traversal of mucosal epithelia, indicating its significance as a novel virulence factor.

Clinical Manifestations

The outbreak of *S. suis* most recurrently occurs in pigs that are 2–6 weeks old upon weaning, when there is an acute drop in maternal antibody levels. The maternal antibody levels will not increase till they reach 8 weeks old and this explains the lower incidence of disease in grower and finisher pigs (Corsaut et al., 2021). Sudden death due to septicemia in pigs and streptococcal toxic shock-like syndrome in humans are the common features of the infection (Segura et al., 2020). The common clinical manifestations in humans include meningitis and sepsis (Brizuela et al., 2023). Septic shock is ascribed as the most common cause of death and animals showed disseminated intravascular coagulopathy. Other common clinical signs include anorexia, fever, reddening of skin, depression, lameness, paralysis, shaking, and convulsions (Kim et al., 2023) (Fig. 4).

Diagnostic Techniques

Identification of *S. suis* traditionally involves labor-intensive processes such as bacterial isolation, culture, and subsequent biochemical assays, which are both time-consuming and prone to inaccuracies. To address these drawbacks, more precise detection methods have been adopted, including immunological and nucleic acid-based approaches, along with immunosensor technologies (Table 1). Immunological

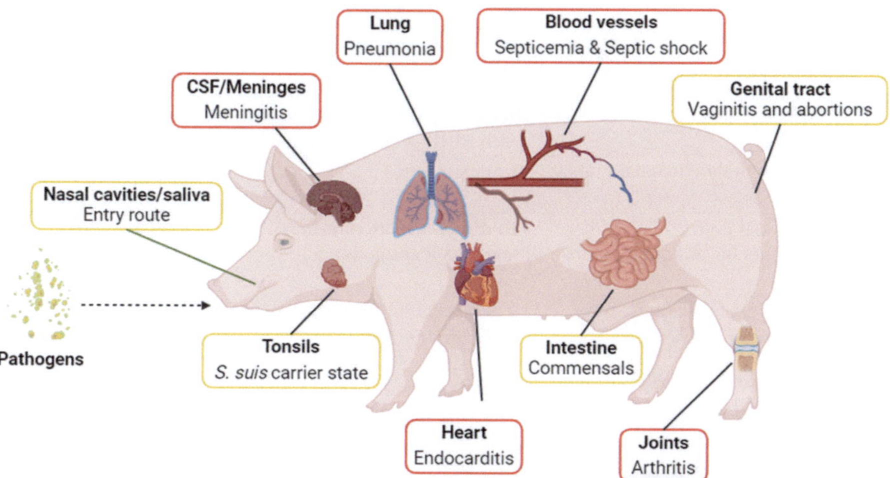

Fig. 4 A schematic representation of the pathogenic process involved in *S. suis* infections

Table 1 Various methods for detecting, identifying, and characterizing different strains of *S. suis*

Sl. no.	Diagnostic methods	Description	References
1.	*Microbiological methods*		
2.	Selective medium-based culture	A modified Todd-Hewitt Broth agar containing 5% defibrinated sheep blood and crystal violet	Kataoka et al. (1991)
3.	*Molecular tests*		
4.	Conventional PCR	Only glutamate dehydrogenase (gdh) as a target gene	Okwumabua et al. (2003)
5.	Swabs PCR	Only extracellular protein factor (epf) as a target gene	Swildens et al. (2005)
6.	Nested PCR	To differentiate *S. suis* from other bacteria like *Hemophilus parasuis*	Kang et al. (2012)
7.	Single-tube LAMP assay	Loop-mediated isothermal amplification (LAMP) with 100 to 1000 times higher sensitivity than the conventional PCR assay	Zhang et al. (2013)
8.	Real-time PCR	cps2J, glutamate dehydrogenase (gdh)	Yang et al. (2010)
9.	RFLP	Used for ribotyping	Okwumabua et al. (1995)
10.	ISR-RFLP	PCR amplification of 16S-23S rDNA intergenic spacer region (ISR) that was followed by restriction fragment length polymorphism (RFLP) analysis (ISR-RFLP)	Marois et al. (2006)
11.	*Immunological assays*		
12.	An enzyme-based in-situ hybridization method	16S rRNA as a target gene	Madsen et al. (2001)
13.	MRP/EF-based ELISA	Muramidase-released protein (MRP)/ extracellular protein factor (EF) protein as capture antigen	Vecht et al. (1993)
14.	CPS-based indirect ELISA	Capsular polysaccharide (CPS) as capture antigen	Kataoka et al. (1996)
15.	SERS	Surface-enhanced Raman scattering with MRP protein as capture antigen	Chen et al. (2012)
16.	ICS (immunochromatographic strip)	To detect anti-CPS antibody	Yang et al. (2007)
17.	Colloidal gold immunochromatographic strips	To direct detection of the *S. suis* serotype 2 antigens	Ju et al. (2010)
18..	Electrochemiluminescence (ECL) immunosensor	It is based on l-cysteine combined with mimicking bi-enzyme synergetic catalysis	Wang et al. (2013)

methods such as enzyme-linked immunosorbent assay (ELISA), dot-immunobinding, and colloidal gold-based immunochromatographic assays (GICA) have emerged as convenient and reliable alternatives. GICA, in particular, integrates various technologies including colloidal gold labeling, immunoassay, chromatography, monoclonal antibody technology, and other novel material techniques, offering definitive results without the need for specialized equipment or complex procedures. These advancements mark a significant stride in clinical and quarantine diagnostics (Ju et al., 2010; Nakayama et al., 2014). Nucleic acid-based techniques such as polymerase chain reaction (PCR), loop-mediated isothermal amplification (LAMP), DNA microarray, and typing-oriented analyses like pulsed-field gel electrophoresis (PFGE) and restriction fragment length polymorphism (RFLP) provide insights into genomic variations among different strains and serotypes of *S. suis*. Multi-locus sequence typing (MLST) directly identifies nucleotide sequence variations for typing purposes (Feng et al., 2014). These methods collectively offer valuable insights into *S. suis* diversity and evolution. Immunosensors, leveraging antigen-antibody interactions and nanomaterial signal amplification, exhibit high sensitivity and selectivity (Xia et al., 2018). They are compact, user-friendly, and open to automation, expanding their utility across diverse applications in *S. suis* detection. Frequently, routine microbiological testing is insufficient to detect neuroinvasive infections. As *S. suis* meningitis has a relatively low clinical incidence (3%) it is frequently misdiagnosed, particularly when combined with Listeria monocytogenes meningitis (36%) and pneumococcal meningitis (20%) (Koopmans et al., 2013). A promising and all-encompassing technique for detecting pathogens that offer "unbiased" results is metagenomic next-generation sequencing (mNGS). Consequently, it applies to the clinical diagnosis of diverse infections, including some that are rare (Gu et al., 2019). Despite the array of available methods, each approach has its limitations. Therefore, a comprehensive diagnostic strategy should integrate multiple techniques, emphasizing the development of standardized diagnostic protocols. This intensive effort is crucial for advancing rapid diagnosis, prevention, and control measures against swine streptococcal disease.

Antimicrobial Resistance

Since the 1980s, when *Streptococcus suis* was first shown to have antimicrobial resistance (AMR), the rate of AMR has steadily increased. The widespread occurrence and fatality associated with *S. suis* infections, coupled with the absence of an effective and universally applicable vaccine to deter, or reduce their occurrence, have resulted in the extensive utilization of antibiotics. Additionally, *S. suis* is exposed to antibiotics due to its commensal nature, which is beneficial for promoting growth, preventing infections, and treating other infectious conditions. The development of antibiotic-resistant *S. suis* isolates is mostly attributable to the convergence of these factors (Uruén et al., 2022).

The most commonly used antibiotics in the swine industry are beta-lactams, tetracyclines, and macrolides. Resistance to aminoglycosides, fluoroquinolones, amphenicols, and glycopeptides has previously been documented globally, with significant rates of resistance to macrolides and tetracyclines. To counteract the effects of antibiotic action, *S. suis* has developed a variety of resistance mechanisms, the most common of which include target site mutations, the manufacture enzymes of target-protective and antibiotic-modifying or degrading, as well as antibiotic exporters (Uruén et al., 2022). Antibiotic resistance genes encode the majority of resistance mechanisms, and a significant portion are carried by mobile genetic elements (MGEs) that can spread horizontally by gene transfer (Tempier et al., 2021). Compared to other *Streptococcus* species, *S. suis* revealed greater levels of MGEs, as determined by the study of streptococcal genomes. Because of this, *S. suis* is thought to be an AMR gene reservoir with the ability to quickly gather and spread MGEs (Huang et al., 2016).

The pattern of antibiotic usage, which varies among countries, regions, and even farms, has a substantial impact on the AMR profile of *S. suis*. *S. suis* has been shown by numerous researchers to be 100% resistant to various antimicrobial treatments. It was reported that 87% of the isolates were resistant to at least four antibiotics, while 6% were resistant to at least six antimicrobials (Devi et al., 2017). Hoa et al. report that multidrug resistance to erythromycin, tetracycline, and chloramphenicol was present in *S. suis*-infected individuals and that this resistance grew dramatically from 6% in 1999 to 23% in 2006 and 2007. Furthermore, it is also reported that tetracyclines, macrolides, and lacosamide have high AMR rates (> 80%) of all over the world (Uruén et al., 2022). It is evident from these results that *S. suis* is a global-spreading bacterial superbug. In certain regions, resistance to β-lactams, quinolones, and amphenicols is still negligible. Their resistance mechanism or the fact that fewer people are using these antibiotics could be the cause of this.

Treatment options for *Streptococcus suis* are limited as the bacteria develop resistance to numerous medicines. This implies that more research needs to be done on stronger or other antibiotics, which could result in increased healthcare costs. Treatment failures in swine herds have a detrimental effect on farmer revenue and can compromise the safety and availability of food. Concerns related to the zoonotic transfer of animal-to-human resistance strains are also raised by this situation, as it puts public health at risk by reducing the efficacy of antibiotics in treating individual patients as well as managing outbreaks and preventing infections in communities. The resistant forms of the bacterium could be hard to control and completely eradicate, leading to long-lasting or recurrent outbreaks that harm both animal and human populations.

Genetic Underpinnings of Antibiotic Resistance in *S. suis*

To evade the effects of antibiotics, *S. suis* has evolved diverse resistance mechanisms, typically categorized into four groups: (i) target mutation, which hampers antibiotic binding to its target, (ii) enzymatic modification of targets, (iii) alteration of antibiotics, involving degradation or modification to prevent target binding, and (iv) expulsion of antibiotics from the cell through enhanced production of efflux pumps.

The primary mechanisms of resistance to β-lactam antibiotics include (i) limited access to penicillin-binding proteins (PBPs), (ii) decreased binding affinity of PBPs, and (iii) degradation of the antibiotic by β-lactamases. The main cause of resistance to β-lactams in streptococci stems from mutations occurring within the pbp2x and pbp2b genes (Yu et al., 2023). While the cpoA and murM genes exist in *S. suis* genomes, any mutations within these genes that could potentially contribute to β-lactam resistance have not yet been documented. Resistance to macrolide, lincosamide, and streptogramin (MLS) antibiotics arises from multiple mechanisms, with one of the most prevalent being the methylation of the ribosome at the macrolide-binding site.

Extensive metagenomic analysis of resistant isolates has revealed that the majority of corresponding antimicrobial resistance (AMR) genes are located within mobile genetic elements (MGEs) such as integrative and conjugative elements (ICEs), integrative and mobilizable elements (IMEs), and their derivatives. These elements possess genes enabling autonomous conjugation and integration of the MGE into the bacterial chromosome. Conjugation appears to be a highly efficient method for gene dissemination in *S. suis*, as evidenced by the widespread presence of MGEs in *S. suis* genomes across various genetic lineages. Comparative genomic studies of streptococcal species indicate a higher abundance of these elements in *S. suis* compared to other pathogenic *Streptococcus* species. Consequently, *S. suis* is recognized as an AMR gene reservoir capable of accumulating and transmitting MGEs at a high frequency.

Streptococcus suis has the potential to transfer pbp resistance alleles via horizontal gene transfer (HGT). However, since these alleles are not situated within mobile genetic elements (MGEs), the gene transfer process must be facilitated by natural transformation or other mechanisms besides conjugation and transduction. Natural transformation is an inducible process activated by the quorum-sensing system, various environmental factors, and potentially unidentified host factors.

Preventive Measures Against *S. suis* Infection

The infected pigs are the primary sources of disease transmission to humans. Therefore, preventing transmission to humans relies heavily on controlling diseased animals. There are several preventive measures available to be adopted, including vaccination of healthy individuals, enhancing pig-raising conditions, disinfecting, or fumigating animal houses, and quickly isolating sick animals during disease outbreaks. In the treatment of *Streptococcus suis* meningitis in pigs, it is advised to include adjunctive therapy with an anti-inflammatory agent. However, animals with advanced septicemia, meningitis, and arthritis often show poor response to treatment, necessitating re-evaluation of all cases 3 days after treatment initiation. Additionally, pigs housed in the same pen as affected animals should receive treatment administered through feed or water. Preventative measures for controlling the disease in piglets may involve isolating farrowing sows and fumigating the housing between animals. Administering long-acting penicillin injections to piglets at birth could potentially prevent the onset of the disease. Employing all-in, all-out husbandry methods can help minimize the spread of infection. Additionally, meditated early weaning has been successful in eradicating the disease from a herd, although the most reliable method remains slaughter, disinfection, and repopulation, as noted by Higgins and Gottschalk (1999). Commercial or autogenous bacterin vaccines have been utilized thus far, though their effectiveness is currently under scrutiny, as indicated by research studies conducted by Wisselink et al. (2000) and Baums et al. (2009).

To minimize antimicrobial usage, prevention efforts for *S. suis* disease should primarily focus on managing predisposing factors and, notably, vaccination. Despite extensive research efforts resulting in various vaccine candidate antigens, there has yet to be a universally effective commercial *S. suis* vaccine (Table 2). The pursuit of a universal cross-protective vaccine is particularly challenging due to the extensive genomic diversity observed in *S. suis*. Currently, no vaccine is available for human beings to prevent *S. suis* infection. Therefore, during severe outbreaks, implementing stringent controls on animal trading and slaughtering is imperative to mitigate transmission from pigs to humans. Additionally, raising awareness of the disease

Table 2 Comprehensive list of protective antigens and potential vaccine candidates for the development of effective vaccines against *S. suis*

Sl. no.	Candidate vaccine Ag	Properties	Animal model	References
1.	EF	Extracellular factor	Pigs	Wisselink et al. (2001)
2.	38 kDa	A protein of 38 kDa localized on the bacterial surface and/or cell wall	Pigs	Okwumabua and Chinnapapakkagari (2005)
3.	MRP	Muramidase-released protein	Pigs, CD1 mice	Huang et al. (2012)
4.	SLY	Suilysin	Mice	Du et al. (2013)
5.	Enolase	A surface-localized enzyme of central metabolism, catalyzing the dehydration of 2-phospho-D-glycerate to phosphoenolpyruvate	Mice	Zhang et al. 2009)
6.	SsPepO	A secretary immunogenic protein discovered by immuno-proteomic techniques	Mice/pigs	Li et al. (2011a)
7.	IBP	Immunoglobulin G (IgG)-binding protein	Mice	Liu et al. (2009)
8.	ESA	Epidermal surface antigen	Mice	Liu et al. (2009)
9.	RfeA	RTX family exoprotein A	Mice	Liu et al. (2009)
10.	Sat (HP0272)	Immunogenic surface protein sat	Mice	Chen et al. (2010)
11.	HP0197	An immunogenic protein	Mice/piglets	Zhang et al. 2009)
12.	HP0245	In vivo-induced protein located on the cell surface	Mice	Li et al. (2011)
13..	6PGD	6-Phosphogluconate dehydrogenase (6PGD) localized on cell surface	Piglets	Tan et al. (2009)

among populations at high risk is crucial to prevent human infection. The important safety measures include protecting the skin from pig bites or injuries caused by sharp tools for those occupationally exposed to pigs and pig products, immediately disinfecting and dressing wounds and abrasions sustained at work, wearing appropriate masks or respirators to protect the respiratory tract, seeking medical advice in case of fever after exposure to pigs or pork meat, and avoiding occupations linked with pig and pork exposure for immunocompromised individuals. Education efforts should extend to individuals involved in the preparation and cooking of pork, including those in domestic settings. Adequate cooking is also vital in preventing *S. suis* infection. The World Health Organization (WHO) advises that pork should be cooked thoroughly, reaching an internal temperature of 70 °C, or until the juices run clear rather than pink.

One Health Approach

To improve health outcomes, One Health is a collaborative approach that focuses on developing and implementing laws, policies, and programs. Among the relevant issues include zoonoses, antibiotic resistance, environmental degradation, and food safety and security (Osei et al., 2022). Owing to its comprehensive methodology and awareness of the intricate relationships that exist among animals, humans, and the environment, the One Health perspective is crucial for understanding and treating *Streptococcus suis* infections. This point of view emphasizes interdisciplinary teamwork in tackling health challenges while accounting for factors such as immunization regimens, biosecurity policies, animal husbandry practices, and monitoring systems. AMR is an issue for One Health since it affects not only the human-livestock interaction but also environmental reservoirs such as soil, water bodies, and animal waste (Young et al., 2019; Checcucci et al., 2020). One Health actively combats *Streptococcus suis*'s resistance to antibiotics by promoting sensible antibiotic use in both human and veterinary medicine. To combat *Streptococcus suis* infection, the veterinary, medical, and environmental sectors collaborate and use a variety of strategies targeted at disease prevention, control, and treatment. Systems of coordinated monitoring are put in place to track the incidence and spatial distribution of infections caused by *Streptococcus suis* in both human and animal populations. Scientists are working together to better understand the virulence mechanisms, risk factors, and dynamics of *Streptococcus suis*. This research contributes significantly to our understanding of the disease's epidemiology and guides the creation of efficient preventative measures. Together, veterinarians, doctors, and environmental specialists launch public education campaigns aimed at farmers, healthcare providers, and the general public to encourage infection-prevention activities like good hygiene and biosecurity protocols.

Future Perspectives and Research Directions

Further investigation into alternative therapeutic methods including antibiotic peptides, immunomodulators, and bacteriophage therapy is necessary. Numerous plant essential oils (EOs) have demonstrated their ability to eradicate pathogenic strains of *S. suis* in vitro. It is advised that more studies be done to evaluate the efficacy and safety of EOs in vivo and investigate any potential positive interactions with antibiotics (Peterfalvi et al., 2019). To develop vaccines and immunotherapeutic approaches, it is essential to look into the host immunological responses to *S. suis* infection. Finding genetic markers related to pathogenicity and antibiotic resistance can also be aided by whole-genome sequencing and comparative genomics studies. To manage and early identification of epidemics, we must adopt a One Health approach that incorporates monitoring the health of humans and animals (Purushothaman et al., 2022).

Concluding Remarks

The diversity of *S. suis* strains poses a significant obstacle to advancing the development of effective control measures and epidemiological monitoring. Moreover, the rise of antibiotic-resistant strains of *S. suis*, to commonly used antibiotics along with concerns about antibiotic use in the swine industry, has escalated the challenge of controlling *S. suis* infections. Establishing molecular tools capable of distinguishing virulent strains is crucial. As a potential solution to combat *S. suis* infection, utilization of bacteriophage derivatives or individual phages has been explored. Initial evaluations have indicated promising benefits, particularly in terms of biofilm destruction when combined with antibiotics. Numerous non-virulent strains of *S. suis*, isolated from healthy pigs, have shown the capability to produce active bacteriocins against virulent serotypes. Consequently, these bacteriocins could also be considered for use alongside antibiotics. Significant progress in understanding the virulence factors of *S. suis* and their potential for vaccination holds great promise for the development of a universal vaccine against this pathogen.

Author Contributions Conceptualization: S.P. and D.N.; Literature review: S.P., D.N., R.L., and B.M.; Writing original draft of the manuscript: S.P., D.N., R.L., and B.M.; Preparation of tables and figures: S.P., and B.M.; Review and revision of the manuscript: P.Y., and S.K.; Compilation and preparation of final version: S.P.

References

Bonifait, L., Veillette, M., Létourneau, V., Grenier, D., & Duchaine, C. (2014). Detection of *Streptococcus* suis in bioaerosols of swine confinement buildings. *Applied and Environmental Microbiology, 80*(11), 3296–3304.

Brizuela, J., Kajeekul, R., Roodsant, T. J., Riwload, A., Boueroy, P., Pattanapongpaibool, A., et al. (2023). *Streptococcus suis* outbreak caused by an emerging zoonotic strain with acquired multi-drug resistance in Thailand. *Microbial Genomics, 9*(2), mgen000952.

Checcucci, A., Trevisi, P., Luise, D., Modesto, M., Blasioli, S., Braschi, I., & Mattarelli, P. (2020). Exploring the animal waste resistome: The spread of antimicrobial resistance genes through the use of livestock manure. *Frontiers in Microbiology, 11*, 1416.

Chen, B., Zhang, A., Li, R., Mu, X., He, H., Chen, H., & Jin, M. (2010). Evaluation of the protective efficacy of a newly identified immunogenic protein, HP0272, of *Streptococcus* suis. *FEMS Microbiology Letters, 307*(1), 12–18.

Chen, K., Han, H., & Luo, Z. (2012). *Streptococcus* suis II immunoassay based on thorny gold nanoparticles and surface enhanced Raman scattering. *Analyst, 137*(5), 1259–1264.

Corsaut, L., Martelet, L., Goyette-Desjardins, G., Beauchamp, G., Denicourt, M., Gottschalk, M., & Segura, M. (2021). Immunogenicity study of a *Streptococcus suis* autogenous vaccine in preparturient sows and evaluation of passive maternal immunity in piglets. *BMC Veterinary Research, 17*(1), 1–15.

Devi, M., Dutta, J. B., Rajkhowa, S., Kalita, D., Saikia, G. K., Das, B. C., Hazarika, R. A., & Mahato, G. (2017). Prevalence of multiple drug resistant *Streptococcus suis* in and around Guwahati, India. *Veterinary World, 10*(5), 556.

Du, H., Huang, W., Xie, H., Ye, C., Jing, H., Ren, Z., & Xu, J. (2013). The genetically modified suilysin, rSLYP353L, provides a candidate vaccine that suppresses proinflammatory response and reduces fatality following infection with *Streptococcus* suis. *Vaccine, 31*(38), 4209–4215.

Dutkiewicz, J., Sroka, J., Zajac, V., Wasinski, B., Cisak, E., Sawczyn, A., Kloc, A., & Wojcik-Fatla, A. (2017). *Streptococcus* suis: A re-emerging pathogen associated with occupational exposure to pigs or pork products. Part I–Epidemiology. *Annals of Agricultural and Environmental Medicine, 24*, 683–695.

Feng, Y., Zhang, H., Wu, Z., Wang, S., Cao, M., Hu, D., & Wang, C. (2014). *Streptococcus suis* infection: An emerging/reemerging challenge of bacterial infectious diseases? *Virulence, 5*(4), 477–497.

Geffner Sclarsky, D. E., Moreno Muñoz, R., Campillo Alpera, M. S., Pardo Serrano, F. J., Gómez Gómez, A., & Martínez-Lozano, M. D. (2001, June). *Streptococcus suis* meningitis. *Anales de Medicina Interna (Madrid, Spain: 1984), 18*(6), 317–318.

Goyette-Desjardins, G., Auger, J. P., Xu, J., Segura, M., & Gottschalk, M. (2014). Streptococcus suis, an important pig pathogen and emerging zoonotic agent—An update on the worldwide distribution based on serotyping and sequence typing. *Emerging Microbes & Infections, 3*(1), 1–20.

Gu, W., Miller, S., & Chiu, C. Y. (2019). Clinical metagenomic next-generation sequencing for pathogen detection. *Annual Review of Pathology, 14*, 319–338.

Higgins, R., Gottschalk, M., Boudreau, M., Lebrun, A., & Henrichsen, J. (1995). Description of six new capsular types (29–34) of *Streptococcus suis*. *Journal of Veterinary Diagnostic Investigation, 7*(3), 405–406.

Huang, D., Zhu, H., Lin, H., Xu, J., & Lu, C. (2012). First insights into the protective effects of a recombinant swinepox virus expressing truncated MRP of *Streptococcus* suis type 2 in mice. *Berliner und Munchener Tierarztliche Wochenschrift, 125*(3–4), 144–152.

Huang, J., Ma, J., Shang, K., Hu, X., Liang, Y., Li, D., Wu, Z., Dai, L., Chen, L., & Wang, L. (2016, October 7). Evolution and diversity of the antimicrobial resistance associated mobilome in *Streptococcus* suis: A probable mobile genetic elements reservoir for other streptococci. *Frontiers in Cellular and Infection Microbiology, 6*, 118. https://doi.org/10.3389/fcimb.2016.00118. PMID: 27774436; PMCID: PMC5053989.

Ju, Y., Hao, H. J., Xiong, G. H., Geng, H. R., Zheng, Y. L., Wang, J., Cao, Y., Yang, Y. H., Cai, X. H., & Jiang, Y. Q. (2010). Development of colloidal gold-based immunochromatographic assay for rapid detection of *Streptococcus suis* serotype 2. *Veterinary Immunology and Immunopathology, 133*(2–4), 207–211.

Kang, I., Kim, D., Han, K., Seo, H. W., Oh, Y., Park, C., et al. (2012). Optimized protocol for multiplex nested polymerase chain reaction to detect and differentiate Haemophilus parasuis, *Streptococcus* suis, and mycoplasma hyorhinis in formalin-fixed, paraffin-embedded tissues from pigs with polyserositis. *Canadian Journal of Veterinary Research, 76*(3), 195–200.

Kataoka, Y., Sugimoto, C., Nakazawa, M., & Kashiwazaki, M. (1991). Detection of *Streptococcus* suis type 2 in tonsils of slaughtered pigs using improved selective and differential media. *Veterinary Microbiology, 28*(4), 335–342.

Kataoka, Y., Yamashita, T., Sunaga, S., Imada, Y., Ishikawa, H., Kishima, M., & Nakazawa, M. (1996). An enzyme-linked immunosorbent assay (ELISA) for the detection of antibody against *Streptococcus* suis type 2 in infected pigs. *Journal of Veterinary Medical Science, 58*(4), 369–372.

Kerdsin, A., Takeuchi, D., Nuangmek, A., Akeda, Y., Gottschalk, M., & Oishi, K. (2020). Genotypic comparison between *Streptococcus suis* isolated from pigs and humans in Thailand. *Pathogens, 9*, 50.

Kim, J. G., Seong, G. M., Kim, Y. R., Heo, S. T., & Yoo, J. R. (2023). *Streptococcus suis* causes bacterial meningitis with hearing loss in patients without direct exposure to pigs in a regional pork industry territory. *Journal of Medicine and Life Science, 20*(1), 43–47.

Koopmans, M. M., Brouwer, M. C., Bijlsma, M. W., Bovenkerk, S., Keijzers, W., & van der Ende, A. (2013). Listeria monocytogenes sequence type 6 and increased rate of unfavorable outcome in meningitis: Epidemiologic cohort study. *Clinical Infectious Diseases, 57*(2), 247–253.

Li, J., Xia, J., Tan, C., Zhou, Y., Wang, Y., Zheng, C., et al. (2011a). Evaluation of the immunogenicity and the protective efficacy of a novel identified immunogenic protein, SsPepO, of *Streptococcus* suis serotype 2. *Vaccine, 29*(38), 6514–6519.

Li, W., Hu, X., Liu, L., Chen, H., & Zhou, R. (2011b). Induction of protective immune response against *Streptococcus* suis serotype 2 infection by the surface antigen HP0245. *FEMS Microbiology Letters, 316*(2), 115–122.

Liu, L., Cheng, G., Wang, C., Pan, X., Cong, Y., Pan, Q., et al. (2009). Identification and experimental verification of protective antigens against *Streptococcus* suis serotype 2 based on genome sequence analysis. *Current Microbiology, 58*, 11–17.

Madsen, L. W., Boye, M., & Jensen, H. E. (2001). An enzyme-based in situ hybridisation method for the identification of *Streptococcus* suis note: Brief report. *APMIS, 109*(10), 665–669.

Mai, N. T. H., Hoa, N. T., Nga, T. V. T., Linh, L. D., Chau, T. T. H., Sinh, D. X., Phu, N. H., Chuong, L. V., Diep, T. S., Campbell, J., Nghia, H. D. T., Minh, T. N. H., Chau, N. V. V., de Jong, M. D., Chinh, N. T., Hien, T. T., Farrar, J., & Schultsz, C. (2008). *Streptococcus suis* meningitis in adults in Vietnam. *Clinical Infectious Diseases, 46*, 659–667.

Marois, C., Le Devendec, L., Gottschalk, M., & Kobisch, M. (2006). Molecular characterization of *Streptococcus* suis strains by 16S–23S intergenic spacer polymerase chain reaction and restriction fragment length polymorphism analysis. *Canadian Journal of Veterinary Research, 70*(2), 94.

Matajira, C. E. C., Moreno, L. Z., Poor, A. P., Gomes, V. T. M., Dalmutt, A. C., Parra, B. M., de Oliveira, C. H., et al. (2019). *Streptococcus suis* in Brazil: Genotypic, virulence, and resistance profiling of strains isolated from pigs between 2001 and 2016. *Pathogens, 9*(1), 31.

Nakayama, T., Zhao, J., Takeuchi, D., Kerdsin, A., Chiranairadul, P., Areeratana, P., Loetthong, P., Pienpringam, A., Akeda, Y., & Oishi, K. (2014). Colloidal gold-based immunochromatographic strip test compromising optimized combinations of anti-*S. suis* capsular polysaccharide polyclonal antibodies for detection of *Streptococcus* suis. *Biosensors and Bioelectronics, 60*, 175–179.

Nishibori, T., Nishitani, Y., Nomoto, R., & Osawa, R. (2013). Reappraisal of the taxonomy of *Streptococcus suis* serotypes 20, 22, 26, and 33 based on DNA–DNA homology and sodA and recN phylogenies. *Veterinary Microbiology, 162*(2–4), 842–849.

Okura, M., Osaki, M., Nomoto, R., Arai, S., Osawa, R., Sekizaki, T., & Takamatsu, D. (2016). Current taxonomical situation of *Streptococcus suis*. *Pathogens, 5*(3), 45.

Okwumabua, O., & Chinnapapakkagari, S. (2005). Identification of the gene encoding a 38-kilodalton immunogenic and protective antigen of *Streptococcus* suis. *Clinical and Vaccine Immunology, 12*(4), 484–490.

Okwumabua, O. G. I., Staats, J., & Chengappa, M. M. (1995). Detection of genomic heterogeneity in *Streptococcus* suis isolates by DNA restriction fragment length polymorphisms of rRNA genes (ribotyping). *Journal of Clinical Microbiology, 33*(4), 968–972.

Okwumabua, O., O'Connor, M., & Shull, E. (2003). A polymerase chain reaction (PCR) assay specific for *Streptococcus* suis based on the gene encoding the glutamate dehydrogenase. *FEMS Microbiology Letters, 218*(1), 79–84.

Osei, E. K., Mahony, J., & Kenny, J. G. (2022). From farm to fork: *Streptococcus suis* as a model for the development of novel phage-based biocontrol agents. *Viruses, 14*(9), 1996.

Pan, Z., Ma, J., Dong, W., Song, W., Wang, K., Lu, C., & Yao, H. (2015). Novel variant serotype of *Streptococcus suis* isolated from piglets with meningitis. *Applied and Environmental Microbiology, 81*, 976–985.

Perch, B., Kristjansen, P., & Skadhauge, K. N. (1968). Group R streptococci pathogenic for man. Two cases of meningitis and one fatal case of sepsis. *Acta Pathologica et Microbiologica Scandinavica, 74*(1), 69–76.

Peterfalvi, A., Miko, E., Nagy, T., Reger, B., Simon, D., Miseta, A., et al. (2019). Much more than a pleasant scent: A review on essential oils supporting the immune system. *Molecules, 24*(24), 4530.

Purushothaman, S., Meola, M., & Egli, A. (2022). Combination of whole genome sequencing and metagenomics for microbiological diagnostics. *International Journal of Molecular Sciences, 23*(17), 9834.

Rayanakorn, A., Goh, B. H., Lee, L. H., Khan, T. M., & Saokaew, S. (2018). Risk factors for *Streptococcus suis* infection: A systematic review and meta-analysis. *Scientific Reports, 8*(1), 13358.

Segura, M., Aragon, V., Brockmeier, S. L., Gebhart, C., Greeff, A. D., Kerdsin, A., et al. (2020). Update on *Streptococcus suis* research and prevention in the era of antimicrobial restriction: 4th international workshop on *S. suis*. *Pathogens, 9*(5), 374.

Seitz, M., Valentin-Weigand, P., & Willenborg, J. (2016). Use of antibiotics and antimicrobial resistance in veterinary medicine as exemplified by the swine pathogen *Streptococcus* suis. In *How to overcome the antibiotic crisis: Facts, challenges, technologies, and future perspectives* (pp. 103–121). Springer.

Swildens, B., Wisselink, H. J., Engel, B., Smith, H. E., Nielen, M., Verheijden, J. H., & Stegeman, J. A. (2005). Detection of extracellular factor-positive *Streptococcus* suis serotype 2 strains in tonsillar swabs of live sows by PCR. *Veterinary Microbiology, 109*(3–4), 223–228.

Tan, C., Liu, M., Liu, J., Yuan, F., Fu, S., Liu, Y., et al. (2009). Vaccination with *Streptococcus* suis serotype 2 recombinant 6PGD protein provides protection against S. suis infection in swine. *FEMS Microbiology Letters, 296*(1), 78–83.

Uruén, C., García, C., Fraile, L., Tommassen, J., & Arenas, J. (2022). How *Streptococcus suis* escapes antibiotic treatments. *Veterinary Research, 53*(1), 1–33.

Vecht, U., Wisselink, H. J., Anakotta, J., & Smith, H. E. (1993). Discrimination between virulent and nonvirulent *Streptococcus* suis type 2 strains by enzyme-linked immunosorbent assay. *Veterinary Microbiology, 34*(1), 71–82.

Wang, H., Dong, D., & Xie, Q. (2005). Analysis of infectious syndrome caused by *Streptococcus suis* II. *Jiangsu Medical Journal, 31*(6), 419.

Wang, H., Yuan, R., Chai, Y., Cao, Y., Gan, X., Chen, Y., & Wang, Y. (2013). An ultrasensitive peroxydisulfate electrochemiluminescence immunosensor for *Streptococcus* suis serotype 2 based on l-cysteine combined with mimicking bi-enzyme synergetic catalysis to in situ generate coreactant. *Biosensors and Bioelectronics, 43*, 63–68.

Wisselink, H. J., Vecht, U., Smith, H. E., & Stockhofe-Zurwieden, N. (2001). Protection of pigs against challenge with virulent *Streptococcus* suis serotype 2 strains by a muramidase-released protein and extracellular factor vaccine. *Veterinary Record, 148*(15), 473–477.

Xia, X., Wang, X., Wei, X., Jiang, J., & Hu, J. (2018). Methods for the detection and characterization of *Streptococcus suis*: From conventional bacterial culture methods to immunosensors. *Antonie Van Leeuwenhoek, 111*(12), 2233–2247.

Yang, J., Jin, M., Chen, J., Yang, Y., Zheng, P., Zhang, A., et al. (2007). Development and evaluation of an immunochromatographic strip for detection of *Streptococcus* suis type 2 antibody. *Journal of Veterinary Diagnostic Investigation, 19*(4), 355–361.

Yang, W., Cai, X., Hao, Y., Liu, Y., Wang, S., Xing, R., et al. (2010). Characterization of *Streptococcus* suis serotype 2 blood infections using RT-qPCR to quantify glutamate dehydrogenase copy numbers. *Journal of Microbiological Methods, 83*(3), 326–329.

Young, C., Kharmacharya, D., Bista, M., Sharma, A., Goldstein, T., Anthony, S. J., Smith, W., Mazet, J., & Johnson, C. (2019). Sharing of antimicrobial resistance genes among animals, humans, and the environment in Nepal: A one health case study. *International Journal of Infectious Diseases, 79*, 20.

Yu, D., Guo, D., Zheng, Y., & Yang, Y. (2023). A review of penicillin binding protein and group A streptococcus with reduced-β-lactam susceptibility. *Frontiers in Cellular and Infection Microbiology, 13*, 1117160.

Zhang, A., Chen, B., Mu, X., Li, R., Zheng, P., Zhao, Y., et al. (2009). Identification and characterization of a novel protective antigen, Enolase of *Streptococcus* suis serotype 2. *Vaccine, 27*(9), 1348–1353.

Zhang, J., Zhu, J., Ren, H., Zhu, S., Zhao, P., Zhang, F., et al. (2013). Rapid visual detection of highly pathogenic *Streptococcus* suis serotype 2 isolates by use of loop-mediated isothermal amplification. *Journal of Clinical Microbiology, 51*(10), 3250–3256.

Swine-Associated Methicillin-Resistant *Staphylococcus aureus* (MRSA)

Abhilash Surakaram, Tapan Kumar Dutta, E. N. P. Sneha, and Belore Balaji Manoher

Abstract

Staphylococcus aureus is a concerning pathogen in both veterinary and public health due to its ability to cause a wide variety of infections. *Staphylococcus aureus*, which is resistant to methicillin, or known as methicillin-resistant *Staphylococcus aureus* (MRSA), has resistance to the majority of β-lactam antibiotics. Pigs are the reservoir hosts for MRSA, which poses risks to both animal and human health. The frequency of MRSA in pigs varies both systemically and regionally. Direct contact, contaminated environments, and human-to-animal transmission are the three ways that MRSA can infect pigs. Additionally, swine-associated MRSA strains may spread to humans through occupational exposure, food-borne transmission, and community interaction. According to genetic analysis, MRSA strains isolated from pigs are often linked to livestock-associated lineages, which are identified by specific genetic markers such as the absence of staphylococcal enterotoxins (SE) or Panton-Valentine Leukocidin (PVL) genes and the staphylococcal cassette chromosome mec (SCCmec) type IV or V. On the other hand, the possibility of genetic exchange between human-adapted

A. Surakaram (✉) · E. N. P. Sneha
Department of Veterinary Microbiology, ICAR-Indian Veterinary Research Institute (ICAR-IVRI), Bareilly, Uttar Pradesh, India

T. K. Dutta
Department of Veterinary Microbiology, CVSc&AH, Central Agricultural University, Aizawl, Mizoram, India

B. B. Manoher
Department of Veterinary Microbiology, ICAR-Indian Veterinary Research Institute (ICAR-IVRI), Bareilly, Uttar Pradesh, India

Animal Science Department, University Of Connecticut, Connecticut, USA

R. Deb et al. (eds.), *Emerging Zoonotic Threats from Swine*,
https://doi.org/10.1007/978-981-96-7407-7_7

MRSA strains and swine-associated bacteria highlights the significance of ongoing molecular characterization and surveillance programs.

Keywords

Staphylococcus aureus · Swine-associated MRSA · livestock-associated MRSA · β-lactam · Staphylococcal enterotoxins (SE) · Panton-Valentine Leukocidin (PVL) · Molecular characterization

Introduction

The effective prevention and treatment of infectious diseases is threatened by the impending public health crisis of antibiotic resistance. The abuse and misuse of antibiotics in veterinary and human medicine, animal husbandry, and agricultural contexts accelerates the development of antimicrobial resistance (Landers et al., 2012). Staphylococci are a persistent and ubiquitous pathogen in the environment because they can withstand a broad range of temperatures, from 7 to 40 °C, and they may even thrive in adverse environments like dryness and dehydration (Gnanamani et al., 2017). Methicillin-resistant *Staphylococcus aureus* (MRSA) is a strain of *Staphylococcus aureus* that possesses genes encoding *mecA* and *mecC,* which confer resistance against drugs known to be β-lactam (Decline et al., 2020). There are three main categories of MRSA, which can be differentiated by epidemiological and molecular typing: hospital-associated MRSA (HA-MRSA), community-associated MRSA (CA-MRSA), and livestock-associated MRSA (LA-MRSA). Hospital-related MRSA (HA-MRSA), which was initially discovered in humans in the late 1980s, is one example of the first kind. The second one is community-acquired (CA)-MRSA, which was first identified in people in the mid-1990s; the third is livestock-associated MRSA (LA-MRSA), which was first identified in humans in 2005 (Khairullah et al., 2023). The antimicrobial susceptibility of *S. aureus* isolates in animals has historically been less consistently reported than in humans. When MRSA was discovered in dairy cows (Devriese et al., 1972) and canines (Decline et al., 2020) in 1972, the occurrence of MRSA in animals was first documented. However, a human strain of MRSA was the cause of this initial occasional incident. After being initially detected, the sequence type ST398 known as LA-MRSA was eventually discovered in food products as well as animals originating from ongoing transmission and reservoirs (Khairullah et al., 2020). The sequence type (ST) 398 of clonal complex (CC) 398 is the most prevalent LA-MRSA in the world. Pigs are the primary reservoir for this clone, despite the fact that LA-MRSA ST398 has been isolated from a variety of other animals, including horses, poultry, and veal calves (Crombe et al., 2013).

LA-MRSA Emergence

Alexander Fleming discovered penicillin G, the first beta-lactam antibiotic, in 1928, and it was first used as a chemotherapeutic treatment on humans in 1941 (Fletcher, 1984). Ten years later, penicillin resistance was already present in more than half of the isolates in large hospitals (Shlaes & Projan, 2009). The discovery of methicillin and other antimicrobials was prompted by the need to design antibiotics that could withstand the action of β-lactamases produced by staphylococci. But not long after this antibiotic was introduced, methicillin-resistant *S. aureus* (MRSA) was discovered (Stapleton & Taylor, 2002). Methicillin resistance is caused by the synthesis of a novel penicillin-binding protein (PBP), called PBP2a, which has a low affinity for methicillin and other β-lactam antibiotics. This PBP2a stops the antibiotic from entering its target site, resulting in resistance (Fishovitz et al., 2014). The primary gene in charge of methicillin resistance is the mecA gene. This gene is located on the staphylococcal cassette chromosome mec (SCCmec) genetic locus (Shore et al., 2011). Despite being the most prevalent PBP2a-encoding gene (mecA), the discovery of a new mec gene has been reported lately. This gene is called mecC. MecC, a member of SCCmec type XI, has been found in both *S. aureus*, environmental and CONS animal samples (MacFadyen et al., 2018; Porrero et al., 2014). Two less common mec genes have been identified, mecB and mecD, they were both detected in *Macrococcus caseolyticus*, while the mecB gene has also been recently found in *S. aureus* (Lakhundi & Zhang, 2018; Becker et al., 2018).

Importance of LA-MRSA from Pigs

Pigs play a significant role in the transmission of livestock-associated methicillin-resistant *Staphylococcus aureus* (LA-MRSA) CC398 to humans. Pigs can serve as reservoirs for MRSA CC398, carrying the bacteria asymptomatically, shedding the bacteria into the environment, and potentially transmitting it to humans. Pig farmers, veterinarians, and slaughterhouse workers have frequent and close contact with pigs which further increases the likelihood of transmission of MRSA between pigs and humans (Wang et al., 2017).

Swine-Associated MRSA

ST398 seems to be primarily related to pigs, sheep, and cows, but is characterized by colonization abilities of several host species, including poultry, and may cause severe human infections (Rasigade et al., 2010). Although farmers of pigs and poultry are easily colonized by ST398, the transmission of farmers to their families is not frequent, and decolonization occurs quickly after the removal of the infection reservoir (Graveland et al., 2011). However, human ST398 infection occurs without obvious contact with livestock or livestock workers, so some ST398 isolates may be stored in reserves outside pig farms (Mee-Marquet et al., 2011). Recent microarray studies have examined the genetic content of ST398 strains from pigs and human sources (Hallin et al., 2011). Although Hallin and his colleagues found no significant gene differences between isolates from different hosts, McCarthy and colleagues discovered a b-converting prophage in ST398 human isolates, suggesting that some strains were adapted to human host. Therefore, one or more ST398 subtypes are circulating in human populations. There is considerable genetic diversity among ST398 isolates, as shown by a large number of identified staphlococcal protein A (spa) genes (Argudin et al., 2010). A recent important study by Price and his colleagues using a whole genome sequence approach to study the evolution of ST398 strains revealed the ancestors of LA-MRSA strains. Furthermore, this study has demonstrated multiple independent SCCmec acquisition events, suggesting that antibiotic selective pressure exists in the livestock industry, and has promoted the development of antibiotic resistance among ST398 strains (Price et al., 2012). In general, ST398 strains have resistance to tetracycline, macrolides, lincosamide, and aminoglycosides (Kadlec et al., 2009). Furthermore, some strains were recently identified as having resistance to phenolic acid and apramycin genes in ST398 isolates. Historically, resistance to methicillin in *S. aureus* from cattle has rarely been observed, but the recent emergence of ST398 LA-MRSA clones and the identification of new mecA alleles in cloned human and bovine isolates are major concerns.

Microbiology and General Biochemical Characteristics

Staphylococcus is a gram-positive, non-motile, and non-spore-forming bacteria (Silva et al., 2020; Gnanamani et al., 2017). More than 50 species of *Staphylococcus* are listed in the List of Prokaryotic Names with Standing in Nomenclature database, despite *S. aureus* being the most common bacterium in its genus (Rossi et al., 2020). In nutrient agar media, *S. aureus* forms large yellow or white colonies. The yellow colour of the colonies is due to carotenoids, which are produced by the organism. The term aureus is a Latin word, which means the colour of gold (Liu et al., 2005). The organism often produces four types of hemolysins (alpha, beta, gamma, and delta) and shows hemolytic properties in blood agar (Blair, 1958; Dinges et al., 2000). The majority of isolates produce the virulence factor coagulase enzyme, which aids in the identification of the organism. The organism is catalase-positive and oxidase-negative. Because of its salt tolerance, the organism can thrive in mannitol salt agar media with 7.5% NaCl (Brown et al., 2005).

Epidemiology

Since its first discovery in 2005 in pigs in the Netherlands, LA-MRSA has spread to pigs in several other nations. Numerous research and surveys conducted in various countries have illustrated its prevalence rate and spread in pigs (Hoefer et al., 2022). In pig breeding and production farms in different European countries, the average positive rate of LA-MRSA is 14% and 26.9%, respectively (Abreu et al., 2019).

Comparing the molecular typing results of LA-MRSA isolates in pigs revealed regional variations in the distribution of genetic variants. The main LA-MRSA strain found in pig production farms in Europe, the United States, and Canada was CC398. Non-CC398 LA-MRSA strains that are commonly found include CC1, CC9, CC30, and CC97. The most common spa types found in Europe within the CC398 lineage were t011, t034, and t108, primarily found in pig breeding and production farms (Abreu et al., 2019). Pig farms in China, Thailand, Pakistan, and Vietnam are the primary locations for LA-MRSA CC9 strains. The most spa types found in Asia within the CC9 lineage were t899 and t337. In contrast to the CC398 strains, the CC9 strains possess enterotoxin and TST-1 genes encoding the toxic shock syndrome toxin (Khairullah et al., 2023).

Transmission of LA-MRSA

Transmission from Pigs to Pigs

Since pigs have been recognized as a significant LA-MRSA reservoir, research has been done to identify the pathways of transmission both within and across herds. LA-MRSA can be transmitted among pigs by direct and indirect contact. The most common method of LA-MRSA transmission between pigs is most likely direct contact (Khairullah et al., 2023).

Transmission from Pigs to Humans

People who live or work on pig farms, such as farmers and their families, veterinarians, and abattoir employees, are more likely to contract LA-MRSA, according to several studies (Crombe et al., 2013). The transmission of *S. aureus* between hosts is mediated primarily by physical contacts. The dust in MRSA-coated pig stables is highly contaminated (Schulz et al., 2012). It is therefore likely that the colonization of human workers in these areas may be caused by inhalation of MRSA-contaminated dust (Bos et al., 2014). 77%–86% of people working in MRSA-positive stables had nasal colonization (Cuny et al., 2009). The expansion of the colony seems to depend on the duration of exposure and the intensity of contact with animals (Graveland et al., 2011).

Pathogenesis

The pathogenesis of *S. aureus* infections involves five stages. They are (1) colonization, (2) local infection, (3) systemic dissemination and/or sepsis, (4) metastatic infections, and (5) toxinosis (Gnanamani et al., 2017). The first crucial stage in colonizing a new host is adhesion to host cells or matrix elements. *S. aureus* possesses a variety of adhesion factors and processes that facilitate binding and the establishment of a permanent colonization. Moreover, *S. aureus* has the potential to possess several additional virulence factors, which enable it to cause infections. The LA-MRSA CC398 harbours genes encoding the significant hemolytic toxins alpha- and beta-toxins (hla and hlb), which can be released into the environment under specific growth circumstances.

Virulence Factors

The virulence components of LA-MRSA are encoded either in the core genome or onMGEs, including phages, transposons, chromosomal cassettes, and pathogenicity islands. The virulence properties of LA-MRSA CC398 differ from those of the conventional human-adapted CA- and HA-MRSA clonal lineages. DNA microarray analysis shows that genes encoding virulence factors, such as adhesions, accessory gene regulators (agr), capsular polysaccharides (cap), and enzymes, are present in all LA-MRSA isolates, while the genes encoding exotoxins differed amongst them. In LA-MRSA, enterotoxins and toxic shock syndrome toxin 1 (TSST-1) are absent or rarely present. LA-MRSA produces hemolytic toxins which are encoded by the hla and hlb genes. Panton Valentine leukocidin (PVL) toxin genes present in the majority of CA-MRSA are absent in the case of LA-MRSA. The leukocidin genes, like the lukS/F-PV genes, were also not found in LA-MRSA (Table 1) (Ballhausen et al., 2017).

Table 1 Presence and absence of important virulence genes and characteristics in LA-MRSA

Virulence factors which are involved in attachment	**Characteristics**
Microbial surface components recognizing adhesive matrix molecules (MSCRAMM) cna gene	Tissue attachment is facilitated by cell surface proteins that interact with host molecules like collagen, fibronectin, and fibrinogen.
Virulence factors which are involved in evasion of host immune system Panton-valentine leukocidin (PVL) and lukS/F-PV (absent in LA-MRSA)	**Characteristics** Most community-associated MRSA (CA-MRSA) contains PVL. PVL forms porins on the host cell membrane which leads to drainage of cell contents and cell death.
Hemolysin (hla and hlb)	Alpha toxin interacts with ADAM10 receptor which is located on epithelial cells and responsible for its pathogenesis
Virulence factors which are involved toxin production Enterotoxins (absent or rarely found in LA-MRSA) (sep, sek/seq, seb)	**Characteristics** Several enterotoxins are produced by *S. Aureus*, which causes food poisoning due to the intoxication of these toxins.
Toxic shock syndrome toxin-1 (TSST-1) (absent or rarely found in LA-MRSA)	Few enterotoxins and TSST-1 are called as pyrogenic toxin superantigens

Antibiotic Resistance Genes Present in LA-MRSA

LA-MRSA strain genome includes different types of antibiotic resistance genes. LA-MRSA which has mecA gene shows resistance to cefoxitin. CC97 isolates which are showing gentamicin and kanamycin resistance are generally positive for aacA-aphD genes. CC96 isolates which are having erm(C) gene show resistance to erythromycin and clindamycin. CC398 isolates which are resistant to MLS-B are mediated by erm(A) and erm(C). Generally, CC96 and CC97 isolates containing fusB and fusC genes show resistance to fusidic acid. CC97 isolates which are resistant to tetracycline carry tet(K) gene (Boswihi et al., 2020).

Mechanisms of Antibiotic Resistance

Antimicrobials are drugs that inhibit or stop the growth of microbes; as a result, they are frequently used to treat and prevent diseases. They fall into the bacteriostatic or bactericidal categories. While bacteriostatic medications prevent the growth and multiplication of germs, bactericidal medications work by directly killing the bacterium. Aminoglycosides, β-lactams, fluoroquinolones, and glycopeptides are among the primary classes of bactericidal antibiotics; bacteriostatic medications include lincosamides, oxazolidinones, and macrolides. Bacteriological resistance to antibiotics can be intrinsic, based largely on the typical and unique biology of the bacterium, or extrinsic, resulting from horizontal gene transfer, in which new genes are acquired and transferred by integrons, plasmids, transposons, integrons, or bacteriophages (Brown-Jaque et al., 2015). There are a number of ways in which bacterial resistance to antimicrobials can appear, including inhibition of cell wall synthesis, inhibition of cytoplasmic membrane synthesis or damage, inhibition of protein synthesis in ribosomes, modifications to nucleic acid synthesis, and alteration of cellular metabolisms (Tenover, 2006).

Detection Methods

Methicillin resistance can be found using a variety of techniques, such as screening methods using solid culture media containing oxacillin, methods that identify the mecA gene or its protein product, and traditional methods for measuring MICs (disc diffusion, Etest, or broth dilution). The reference technique for identifying methicillin resistance is thought to be the detection of the mecA gene (Velasco et al., 2005). Detection methods involve phenotypic and genotypic methods.

Phenotypic and Genotypic MRSA Detection Methods

Sample (Nasal swabs from swine, swine workers, environmental swabs)

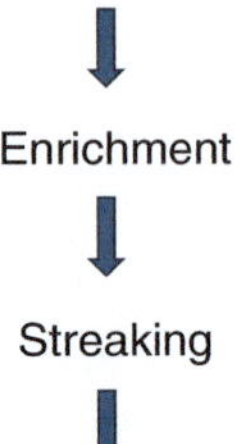

Enrichment

Streaking

Examine plates for typical colonies (sheep blood agar-*S. aureus* shows double zone of hemolysis and produces white or yellow-coloured colonies)

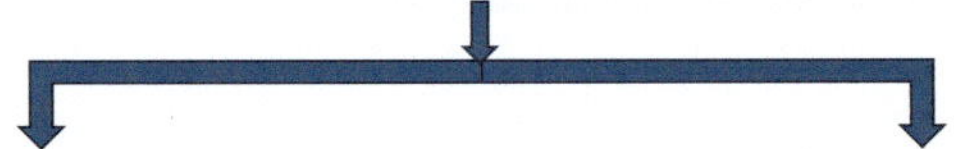

Phenotypic confirmation by Biochemical tests:

- catalase and coagulase - positive
- Gram staining - gram - positive cocci in clusters

Molecular confirmation by screening for species specific gene *nuc* for *S. aureus*

Phenotypic detection of MRSA using MeReSa

Molecular detection of methicillin resistant genes *mecA, mecC*

Phenotypic Detection of antibiotic susceptibility pattern by disk diffusion test and MIC

Molecular Detection of AMR by screening for presence of AMR genes

Molecular typing of the isolates using MLST, spa typing, PFGE, *SCCmec* typing.

Chromogenic medium has emerged as a useful technique in recent years for the quick detection of MRSA in clinical samples (Perry, 2017). Researchers are increasingly using the MLST approach, especially to understand the growth and evolution of MRSA clones and to investigate long-term population relatedness (Robinson & Enright, 2003). The PFGE technique uses restriction endonucleases to break down bacterial DNA. Because there are comparatively few restriction sites, the resulting fragments are smaller but significantly larger than those produced by traditional constant-field agarose gel electrophoresis. In PFGE, the DNA fragments embedded in agarose plugs can be sorted by size because of periodic changes in the electric field's orientation, or "pulsing." Multiple isolates can be analysed and compared more easily because of the restriction pattern of chromosomal DNA provided by PGFE analysis, which is made up of distinct fragments (Tenover et al., 1995). The primary characteristic of PCR is its capacity to generate many copies of the target sequence by replicating a specific DNA sequence. For the genetic investigation of *S. aureus*, AP-PCR, or random amplified polymorphic DNA (RAPD), is one of the PCR-based typing methods (Belkum et al., 1995). The short sequence repeat (SSR) or polymorphic X region of the protein A gene is sequenced as part of the spa typing technique. Unlike MLST, which integrates data from seven loci for *S. aureus* typing, spa typing uses information from a single locus. Spa typing has been compared to PFGE for the purpose of typing well-characterized *S. aureus* strains (Shopsin et al., 1999). Multiplex PCR is used in the SCCmec typing approach to ascertain the existence of the various ccr genes and the structure of the mec complex (Lakhundi & Zhang, 2018). Gene chips have been used by researchers to examine the relatedness of MRSA strains. In this instance, the researchers examined the relatedness of MRSA isolates using an Affymetrix GeneChip that displayed anticipated open reading frames from six genetically distinct *S. aureus* strains as well as new GenBank entries (Dunman et al., 2004). When used to analyse MRSA outbreaks, NGS has proven to be incredibly accurate, quick, and discriminatory. Researchers have also used WGS phylogenetics to find MRSA and MSSA clonal complexes and have shown that this method is better than conventional typing methods (Bowers et al., 2018) Numerous standardized manual and commercial techniques can be used to analyse *S. aureus*'s antimicrobial susceptibility to a wide range of antibiotics.

Zoonotic Potential

Individuals who come into close contact with animals that are MRSA-positive are more likely to contract MRSA themselves. This has been reported for personnel employed in livestock production environments, as well as companion animal and equine clinics (Morgan, 2008). It has been demonstrated that MRSA ST398 may colonize and infect a variety of hosts, indicating that it has minimal host specificity. The processes of host adaptability remain poorly known to this day (Cuny et al., 2010). Nevertheless, MRSA ST398 has been inadvertently shown to generate outbreaks and serious (invasive) infections thus far (Kluytmans, 2010). Hospitals that use humans as vectors pose the danger of introducing MRSA from the animal reservoir. As a result, the "Search and Destroy" strategy in the Netherlands classified farmers of cattle and pigs as risk groups. The rise of LA-MRSA has consequently led to an increase in the yearly number of patients in the Netherlands who are admitted to hospitals with suspected MRSA colonization and need MRSA screening. The healthcare system is heavily burdened by this (van Rijen et al., 2008; Wassenberg & Bonten, 2010). The successful implementation of the "Search and Destroy" policy depends on the identification of risk factors and understanding of the persistence of LA-MRSA in humans. Hospital infection control and antibiotic policies may be significantly impacted by a better knowledge of the processes behind persistence and transmission as well as the part exposure plays in LA-MRSA carriage in humans and animals. Additionally, it offers data for evidence-based recommendations on the creation of fresh strategies and defences against MRSA. Risk factors for the occurrence of ST398 in people and animals were not extensively studied. Pig farming has been linked to a significant risk of ST398 transmission from animals to humans (Lewis et al., 2008; Smith et al., 2009; van den Broek et al., 2009). MRSA carriage in veal calf rearing was found to be directly related to MRSA carriage in people (Graveland et al., 2010). It was shown that the number of MRSA-positive animals on the farm and the intensity of animal contact were highly correlated with LA-MRSA carriage among veal farmers, their family members, and staff. Nonetheless, it is evident that a positive farmer increases the likelihood that family members will carry MRSA. According to Wulf et al. (2008), veterinarians who interact with pigs are likewise more likely to contract MRSA. It has been established in human medicine that the use of antibiotics and the existence of MRSA are causally related (Tacconelli et al., 2008). Animals are thought to exhibit a similar association (de Neeling et al., 2007; Wulf and Voss, 2008). The use of common antimicrobial medications for pigs appears to be a risk factor for MRSA transmission in pig farms (van Duijkeren et al., 2008). It has been demonstrated that in veal farming, calves treated with antibiotics were more likely to be detected as MRSA-positive (Graveland et al., 2010). However, additional quantification is required. MRSA frequency in veal calves seemed to be correlated with improved farm hygiene (Graveland et al., 2010).

Health Impact on Humans

LA-MRSA, a strain of MRSA, causes various infections like skin and respiratory infections, sometimes severe (Foster 2002; Richardson et al., 2018). It's resistant to multiple antibiotics, complicating treatment and leading to longer illnesses and hospital stays (Albur et al., 2012). Severe cases may need hospitalization, with risks of serious complications like sepsis or necrotizing fasciitis. MRSA strains can cause several human infections, including acne, wound healing, food poisoning, urinary tract infections, bacterial pneumonia, endocarditis, neuro-aetiology infections, osteomyelitis, health-related infections, otitis, mastritis, and septicaemia (Boucher & Corey, 2008).

Control Measures

The frequent use of antibiotics in humans and animals led to the development of MDR-MRSA. A health approach to MDR-MRSA infections requires cooperation between public health experts, microbiologists, epidemiologists, veterinarians, and medical doctors. Today, most commercial antibiotics resist MRSA infections. In order to control the problem of antibiotic resistance in animals and humans, antibiotic sensitivity tests (disc distribution methods) are needed to investigate and examine the resistant species (Algammal et al., 2020). There are various ways that MRSA might be introduced onto a farm. The three most significant ones are the transfer of MRSA-colonized animals across farms, direct contact with infected people, and animal contact with contaminated transportation vehicles (van Duijkeren et al., 2008). For this reason, while introducing live animals onto a farm, proper external biosecurity procedures should be followed. Only stock from herds that are MRSA-negative should be used for introduction. Since MRSA has been demonstrated to be airborne and transmitted in this way, they should be confined at a distance of 550 meters from the remainder of the herd for at least 6 weeks (Shiomori et al., 2001). Animals should be tested for MRSA during quarantine and allowed to join the main herd only if it has been proven that they are MRSA-negative. When animals are handled, gloves should be worn, and all human beings working or visiting the farm must wash their hands before entering and washing their hands when they leave the farm. The number of visitors entering the farm must be kept to a minimum, but if necessary, visitors must not have been at another farm in the previous 48 h, because LA-MRSA can still be transported during that period (Angen et al., 2017). In addition, farm visitors should wear masks to reduce transmission to herd (Angen et al., 2019). Meat products must not be allowed on farms because MRSA can survive in them (Pondit et al., 2018). The use of antimicrobials in farms should be minimized. When MRSA enters the farm for the first time, the use of antimicrobials helps to choose MRSA strains, destroying non-resistant strains (Broens et al., 2012). In a model for assessing the effectiveness of interventions in the spread of MRSA in Danish pig farms, it was predicted that reducing the use of antimicrobials, restricting animal movement, and reducing human transmission would be highly effective if introduced in areas with low MRSA prevalence (Schulz et al., 2019). In 2013, Norway launched a national control strategy to eradicate MRSA in pig farms (Grontvedt et al., 2016). This strategy not only covers annual monitoring of all pigs, but also involves a human population surveillance programme in accordance with the one health approach. Hospitals and veterinary authorities must take general precautions to reduce the spread of MRSA in the community, and it is necessary to follow general hygiene practices, infection control systems and environmental disinfection. HACCP guidelines should be implemented in the processing and processing of meat, dairy and milk products in order to minimize MRSA contamination in human food. The MRSA-infected animal must be isolated and treated, and the MRSA-infected wound must be disinfected and covered (Algammal et al., 2020).

Future Perspectives and Research Directions

According to research conducted thus far, MRSA CC398 has a high capacity for transmission and a high likelihood of persisting in the pig population under intensive farming conditions. Furthermore, the pig habitat is an ideal environment for these bacteria, which could serve as an additional source of MRSA contamination. Therefore, it should be anticipated that controlling or eliminating MRSA CC398 from pig herds using intensive farming techniques will be exceedingly challenging.

References

Abreu, R., Rodríguez-Álvarez, C., Lecuona, M., Castro, B., González, J. C., Aguirre-Jaime, A., & Arias, Á. (2019). Increased antimicrobial resistance of MRSA strains isolated from pigs in Spain between 2009 and 2018. *Veterinary Sciences, 6*(2), 38.

Albur, M., Bowker, K., Weir, I., & MacGowan, A. (2012). Factors influencing the clinical outcome of methicillin-resistant Staphylococcus aureus bacteraemia. *European Journal of Clinical Microbiology & Infectious Diseases, 31*, 295–301.

Algammal, A. M., Hetta, H. F., Elkelish, A., Alkhalifah, D. H. H., Hozzein, W. N., Batiha, G. E., El Nahhas, N., & Mabrok, M. A. (2020). Methicillin-resistant Staphylococcus aureus (MRSA): One health perspective approach to the bacterium epidemiology, virulence factors, antibiotic-resistance, and zoonotic impact. *Infection and Drug Resistance, 13*, 3255–3265.

Angen, Ø., Feld, L., Larsen, J., Rostgaard, K., Skov, R., Madsen, A. M., & Larsen, A. R. (2017). Transmission of methicillin-resistant Staphylococcus aureus to human volunteers visiting a swine farm. *Applied and Environmental Microbiology, 83*(23), e01489–e01417.

Angen, Ø., Skade, L., Urth, T. R., Andersson, M., Bækbo, P., & Larsen, A. R. (2019). Controlling transmission of MRSA to humans during short-term visits to swine farms using dust masks. *Frontiers in Microbiology, 9*, 3361.

Argudín, M. A., Fetsch, A., Tenhagen, B. A., Hammerl, J. A., Hertwig, S., Kowall, J., Rodicio, M. R., Käsbohrer, A., Helmuth, R., Schroeter, A., Mendoza, M. C., Bräunig, J., Appel, B., & Guerra, B. (2010). High heterogeneity within methicillin-resistant Staphylococcus aureus ST398 isolates, defined by Cfr9I macrorestriction-pulsed-field gel electrophoresis profiles and spa and SCCmec types. *Applied and Environmental Microbiology, 76*(3), 652–658.

Ballhausen, B., Kriegeskorte, A., van Alen, S., Jung, P., Köck, R., Peters, G., Bischoff, M., & Becker, K. (2017). The pathogenicity and host adaptation of livestock-associated MRSA CC398. *Veterinary Microbiology, 200*, 39–45.

Becker, K., van Alen, S., Idelevich, E. A., Schleimer, N., Seggewiß, J., Mellmann, A., Kaspar, U., & Peters, G. (2018). Plasmid-encoded transferable mecB-mediated methicillin resistance in Staphylococcus aureus. *Emerging Infectious Diseases, 24*(2), 242–248.

Blair, J. E. (1958). Factors determining the pathogenicity of staphylococci. *Annual Review of Microbiology, 12*, 491–506.

Bos, M. E., Verstappen, K. M., van Cleef, B. A., Dohmen, W., Dorado-García, A., Graveland, H., Duim, B., Wagenaar, J. A., Kluytmans, J. A., & Heederik, D. J. (2014). Transmission through air as a possible route of exposure for MRSA. *Journal of Exposure Science & Environmental Epidemiology, 17*, 263.

Boswihi, S. S., Udo, E. E., Mathew, B., Noronha, B., Verghese, T., & Tappa, S. B. (2020). Livestock-associated methicillin-resistant Staphylococcus aureus in patients admitted to Kuwait hospitals in 2016-2017. *Frontiers in Microbiology, 10*, 2912.

Boucher, H. W., & Corey, G. R. (2008). Epidemiology of methicillin-resistant Staphylococcus aureus. *Clinical Infectious Diseases, 46*(Suppl 5), S344–S349.

Bowers, J. R., Driebe, E. M., Albrecht, V., McDougal, L. K., Granade, M., Roe, C. C., Lemmer, D., Rasheed, J. K., Engelthaler, D. M., Keim, P., & Limbago, B. M. (2018). Improved subtyping of Staphylococcus aureus clonal complex 8 strains based on whole-genome phylogenetic analysis. *mSphere, 3*(3), e00464–e00417.

Broens, E. M., Espinosa-Gongora, C., Graat, E. A., Vendrig, N., Van Der Wolf, P. J., Guardabassi, L., Butaye, P., Nielsen, J. P., De Jong, M. C., & Van De Giessen, A. W. (2012). Longitudinal study on transmission of MRSA CC398 within pig herds. *BMC Veterinary Research, 8*, 58.

Brown, D. F., Edwards, D. I., Hawkey, P. M., Morrison, D., Ridgway, G. L., Towner, K. J., Wren, M. W., et al. (2005). Guidelines for the laboratory diagnosis and susceptibility testing of methicillin-resistant Staphylococcus aureus (MRSA). *The Journal of Antimicrobial Chemotherapy, 56*(6), 1000–1018.

Brown-Jaque, M., Calero-Cáceres, W., & Muniesa, M. (2015). Transfer of antibiotic-resistance genes via phage-related mobile elements. *Plasmid, 79*, 1–7.

Crombe, F., Argudín, M. A., Vanderhaeghen, W., Hermans, K., Haesebrouck, F., & Butaye, P. (2013). Transmission dynamics of methicillin-resistant Staphylococcus aureus in pigs. *Frontiers in Microbiology, 4*, 57.

Cuny, C., Nathaus, R., Layer, F., Strommenger, B., Altmann, D., & Witte, W. (2009). Nasal colonization of humans with methicillin-resistant Staphylococcus aureus (MRSA) CC398 with and without exposure to pigs. *PLoS One, 4*(8), e6800.

Cuny, C., Friedrich, A., Kozytska, S., Layer, F., Nübel, U., Ohlsen, K., Strommenger, B., Walther, B., Wieler, L., & Witte, W. (2010). Emergence of methicillin-resistant Staphylococcus aureus (MRSA) in different animal species. *International Journal of Medical Microbiology, 300*(2–3), 109–117.

de Neeling, A. J., van den Broek, M. J., Spalburg, E. C., van Santen-Verheuvel, M. G., Dam-Deisz, W. D., Boshuizen, H. C., van de Giessen, A. W., van Duijkeren, E., & Huijsdens, X. W. (2007). High prevalence of methicillin resistant Staphylococcus aureus in pigs. *Veterinary Microbiology, 122*(3–4), 366–372.

Decline, V., Effendi, M. H., Rahmaniar, R. P., Yanestria, S. M., & Harijani, N. (2020). Profile of antibiotic-resistant and presence of methicillin-resistant Staphylococcus aureus from nasal swab of dogs from several animal clinics in Surabaya, Indonesia. *International Journal of One Health, 6*(1), 90–94.

Devriese, L. A., Van Damme, L. R., & Fameree, L. (1972). Methicillin (cloxacillin)-resistant Staphylococcus aureus strains isolated from bovine mastitis cases. *Zentralblatt für Veterinärmedizin Reihe B, 19*(7), 598–605.

Dinges, M. M., Orwin, P. M., & Schlievert, P. M. (2000). Exotoxins of Staphylococcus aureus. *Clinical Microbiology Reviews, 13*(1), 16–34.

Dunman, P. M., Mounts, W., McAleese, F., Immermann, F., Macapagal, D., Marsilio, E., McDougal, L., Tenover, F. C., Bradford, P. A., Petersen, P. J., Projan, S. J., & Murphy, E. (2004). Uses of Staphylococcus aureus GeneChips in genotyping and genetic composition analysis. *Journal of Clinical Microbiology, 42*(9), 4275–4283.

Fishovitz, J., Hermoso, J. A., Chang, M., & Mobashery, S. (2014). Penicillin-binding protein 2a of methicillin-resistant Staphylococcus aureus. *IUBMB Life, 66*(8), 572–577.

Fletcher, C. (1984). First clinical use of penicillin. *British Medical Journal, 289*(6460), 1721–1723.

Foster, T. J. (2002). Staphylococcus aureus. *Molecular Medical Microbiology*, 839–888.

Gnanamani, A., Hariharan, P., & Paul-Satyaseela, M. (2017). Staphylococcus aureus: Overview of bacteriology, clinical diseases, epidemiology, antibiotic resistance and therapeutic approach. *Frontiers in Staphylococcus Aureus, 4*(28), 10–5772.

Graveland, H., Wagenaar, J. A., Heesterbeek, H., Mevius, D., van Duijkeren, E., & Heederik, D. (2010). Methicillin resistant Staphylococcus aureus ST398 in veal calf farming: Human MRSA carriage related with animal antimicrobial usage and farm hygiene. *PLoS One, 5*(6), e10990.

Graveland, H., Wagenaar, J. A., Bergs, K., Heesterbeek, H., & Heederik, D. (2011). Persistence of livestock associated MRSA CC398 in humans is dependent on intensity of animal contact. *PLoS One, 6*(2), e16830.

Grontvedt, C. A., Elstrøm, P., Stegger, M., Skov, R. L., Skytt Andersen, P., Larssen, K. W., Urdahl, A. M., Angen, Ø., Larsen, J., Åmdal, S., Løtvedt, S. M., Sunde, M., & Bjørnholt, J. V. (2016). Methicillin-resistant Staphylococcus aureus CC398 in humans and pigs in Norway: A "one health" perspective on introduction and transmission. *Clinical Infectious Diseases, 63*(11), 1431–1438.

Hallin, M., De Mendonça, R., Denis, O., Lefort, A., El Garch, F., Butaye, P., Hermans, K., & Struelens, M. J. (2011). Diversity of accessory genome of human and livestock-associated ST398 methicillin resistant Staphylococcus aureus strains. *Infection, Genetics and Evolution, 11*(2), 290–299.

Hoefer, A., Becker, A. A. M. J., Moodley, A., Boyen, F., & Butaye, P. (2022). Presence of methicillin resistant Staphylococcus aureus (MRSA) in feces of the small Indian mongooses (Urva auropunctata) on Saint Kitts and Nevis, West Indies. *Antibiotics (Basel, Switzerland), 11*(8), 990.

Kadlec, K., Ehricht, R., Monecke, S., Steinacker, U., Kaspar, H., Mankertz, J., & Schwarz, S. (2009). Diversity of antimicrobial resistance pheno- and genotypes of methicillin-resistant Staphylococcus aureus ST398 from diseased swine. *The Journal of Antimicrobial Chemotherapy, 64*(6), 1156–1164.

Khairullah, A. R., Ramandinianto, S. C., & Effendi, M. H. (2020). A review of livestock-associated methicillin-resistant Staphylococcus aureus (LA-MRSA) on bovine mastitis. *Systematic Reviews in Pharmacy, 11*(7), 172–183.

Khairullah, A. R., Kurniawan, S. C., Effendi, M. H., Sudjarwo, S. A., Ramandinianto, S. C., Widodo, A., Riwu, K. H. P., Silaen, O. S. M., & Rehman, S. (2023). A review of new emerging livestock-associated methicillin-resistant Staphylococcus aureus from pig farms. *Veterinary World, 16*(1), 46–58.

Kluytmans, J. A. (2010). Methicillin-resistant Staphylococcus aureus in food products: Cause for concern or case for complacency? *Clinical Microbiology and Infection, 16*(1), 11–15.

Lakhundi, S., & Zhang, K. (2018). Methicillin-resistant Staphylococcus aureus: Molecular characterization, evolution, and epidemiology. *Clinical Microbiology Reviews, 31*(4), e00020–e00018.

Landers, T. F., Cohen, B., Wittum, T. E., & Larson, E. L. (2012). A review of antibiotic use in food animals: Perspective, policy, and potential. *Public Health Reports, 127*, 4–22.

Lewis, H. C., Molbak, K., Reese, C., Aarestrup, F. M., Selchau, M., Sorum, M., & Skov, R. L. (2008). Pigs as source of methicillin-resistant Staphylococcus aureus CC398 infections in humans, Denmark. *Emerging Infectious Diseases, 14*(9), 1383–1389.

Liu, G. Y., Essex, A., Buchanan, J. T., Datta, V., Hoffman, H. M., Bastian, J. F., Fierer, J., & Nizet, V. (2005). Staphylococcus aureus golden pigment impairs neutrophil killing and promotes virulence through its antioxidant activity. *The Journal of Experimental Medicine, 202*(2), 209–215.

MacFadyen, A. C., Harrison, E. M., Ellington, M. J., Parkhill, J., Holmes, M. A., & Paterson, G. K. (2018). A highly conserved mecC-encoding SCCmec type XI in a bovine isolate of methicillin-resistant staphylococcus xylosus. *The Journal of Antimicrobial Chemotherapy, 73*(12), 3516–3518.

Morgan, M. (2008). Methicillin-resistant Staphylococcus aureus and animals: Zoonosis or humanosis? *The Journal of Antimicrobial Chemotherapy, 62*(6), 1181–1187.

Perry, J. D. (2017). A decade of development of chromogenic culture media for clinical microbiology in an era of molecular diagnostics. *Clinical Microbiology Reviews, 30*(2), 449–479.

Pondit, A., Haque, Z. F., Sabuj, A. A. M., Khan, M. S. R., & Saha, S. (2018). Characterization of Staphylococcus aureus isolated from chicken and quail eggshell. *Journal of Advanced Veterinary and Animal Research, 5*(4), 466–471.

Porrero, M. C., Harrison, E. M., Fernández-Garayzábal, J. F., Paterson, G. K., Díez-Guerrier, A., Holmes, M. A., & Domínguez, L. (2014). Detection of mecC-methicillin-resistant Staphylococcus aureus isolates in river water: A potential role for water in the environmental dissemination. *Environmental Microbiology Reports, 6*(6), 705–708.

Price, L. B., Stegger, M., Hasman, H., Aziz, M., Larsen, J., Andersen, P. S., Pearson, T., Waters, A. E., Foster, J. T., Schupp, J., Gillece, J., Driebe, E., Liu, C. M., Springer, B., Zdovc, I., Battisti, A., Franco, A., Zmudzki, J., Schwarz, S., Butaye, P., et al. (2012). Staphylococcus aureus CC398: Host adaptation and emergence of methicillin resistance in livestock. *MBio, 3*(1), e00305–e00311.

Rasigade, J. P., Laurent, F., Hubert, P., Vandenesch, F., & Etienne, J. (2010). Lethal necrotizing pneumonia caused by an ST398 Staphylococcus aureus strain. *Emerging Infectious Diseases, 16*(8), 1330.

Richardson, E. J., Bacigalupe, R., Harrison, E. M., Weinert, L. A., Lycett, S., Vrieling, M., et al. (2018). Gene exchange drives the ecological success of a multi-host bacterial pathogen. *Nature Ecology & Evolution, 2*(9), 1468–1478.

Robinson, D. A., & Enright, M. C. (2003). Evolutionary models of the emergence of methicillin-resistant Staphylococcus aureus. *Antimicrobial Agents and Chemotherapy, 47*(12), 3926–3934.

Rossi, C. C., Pereira, M. F., & Giambiagi-deMarval, M. (2020). Underrated staphylococcus species and their role in antimicrobial resistance spreading. *Genetics and Molecular Biology, 43*, e20190065.

Schulz, J., Friese, A., Klees, S., Tenhagen, B. A., Fetsch, A., Rösler, U., & Hartung, J. (2012). Longitudinal study of the contamination of air and of soil surfaces in the vicinity of pig barns by livestock-associated methicillin-resistant Staphylococcus aureus. *Applied and Environmental Microbiology, 78*(16), 5666–5671.

Schulz, J., Boklund, A., Toft, N., & Halasa, T. (2019). Effects of control measures on the spread of LA-MRSA among Danish pig herds between 2006 and 2015–a simulation study. *Scientific Reports, 9*(1), 691.

Shiomori, T., Miyamoto, H., & Makishima, K. (2001). Significance of airborne transmission of methicillin-resistant Staphylococcus aureus in an otolaryngology-head and neck surgery unit. *Archives of Otolaryngology Head and Neck Surgery, 127*(6), 644–648.

Shlaes, D. M., & Projan, S. J. (2009). Antimicrobial resistance versus the discovery and development of new antimicrobials. In D. L. Mayers (Ed.), *BT-antimicrobial drug resistance: Mechanisms of drug resistance* (pp. 43–50). Humana Press.

Shopsin, B., Gomez, M., Montgomery, S. O., Smith, D. H., Waddington, M., Dodge, D. E., Bost, D. A., Riehman, M., Naidich, S., & Kreiswirth, B. N. (1999). Evaluation of protein a gene polymorphic region DNA sequencing for typing of Staphylococcus aureus strains. *Journal of Clinical Microbiology, 37*(11), 3556–3563.

Shore, A. C., Deasy, E. C., Slickers, P., Brennan, G., O'Connell, B., Monecke, S., Ehricht, R., & Coleman, D. C. (2011). Detection of staphylococcal cassette chromosome mec type XI carrying highly divergent mecA, mecI, mecR1, blaZ, and ccr genes in human clinical isolates of clonal complex 130 methicillin-resistant Staphylococcus aureus. *Antimicrobial Agents and Chemotherapy, 55*(8), 3765–3773.

Silva, V., Caniça, M., Capelo, J. L., Igrejas, G., & Poeta, P. (2020). Diversity and genetic lineages of environmental staphylococci: A surface water overview. *FEMS Microbiology Ecology, 96*, fiaa191.

Smith, T. C., Male, M. J., Harper, A. L., Kroeger, J. S., Tinkler, G. P., Moritz, E. D., Capuano, A. W., Herwaldt, L. A., & Diekema, D. J. (2009). Methicillin-resistant Staphylococcus aureus (MRSA) strain ST398 is present in midwestern U.S. swine and swine workers. *PLoS One, 4*(1), e4258.

Stapleton, P. D., & Taylor, P. W. (2002). Methicillin resistance in Staphylococcus aureus: Mechanisms and modulation. *Science Progress, 85*(Pt 1), 57–72.

Tacconelli, E., De Angelis, G., Cataldo, M. A., Pozzi, E., & Cauda, R. (2008). Does antibiotic exposure increase the risk of methicillin-resistant Staphylococcus aureus (MRSA) isolation? A systematic review and meta-analysis. *The Journal of Antimicrobial Chemotherapy, 61*(1), 26–38.

Tenover, F. C. (2006). Mechanisms of antimicrobial resistance in bacteria. *The American Journal of Medicine, 119*(6 Suppl 1), S3–S70.

Tenover, F. C., Arbeit, R. D., Goering, R. V., Mickelsen, P. A., Murray, B. E., Persing, D. H., & Swaminathan, B. (1995). Interpreting chromosomal DNA restriction patterns produced by pulsed-field gel electrophoresis: Criteria for bacterial strain typing. *Journal of Clinical Microbiology, 33*(9), 2233–2239.

van Belkum, A., Kluytmans, J., van Leeuwen, W., Bax, R., Quint, W., Peters, E., Fluit, A., Vandenbroucke-Grauls, C., van den Brule, A., & Koeleman, H. (1995). Multicenter evaluation of arbitrarily primed PCR for typing of Staphylococcus aureus strains. *Journal of Clinical Microbiology, 33*(6), 1537–1547.

Van Den Broek, I. V. F., Van Cleef, B. A. G. L., Haenen, A., Broens, E. M., Van Der Wolf, P. J., Van Den Broek, M. J. M., et al. (2009). Methicillin-resistant Staphylococcus aureus in people living and working in pig farms. *Epidemiology & Infection, 137*(5), 700–708.

van der Mee-Marquet, N., François, P., Domelier-Valentin, A. S., Coulomb, F., et al. (2011). Emergence of unusual bloodstream infections associated with pig-borne-like Staphylococcus aureus ST398 in France. *Clinical Infectious Diseases, 52*(1), 152–153.

van Duijkeren, E., Ikawaty, R., Broekhuizen-Stins, M. J., Jansen, M. D., Spalburg, E. C., de Neeling, A. J., Allaart, J. G., van Nes, A., Wagenaar, J. A., & Fluit, A. C. (2008). Transmission of methicillin-resistant Staphylococcus aureus strains between different kinds of pig farms. *Veterinary Microbiology, 126*(4), 383–389.

van Rijen, M. M., Van Keulen, P. H., & Kluytmans, J. A. (2008). Increase in a Dutch hospital of methicillin-resistant Staphylococcus aureus related to animal farming. *Clinical Infectious Diseases, 46*(2), 261–263.

Velasco, D., del Mar Tomas, M., Cartelle, M., Beceiro, A., Perez, A., Molina, F., Moure, R., Villanueva, R., & Bou, G. (2005). Evaluation of different methods for detecting methicillin (oxacillin) resistance in Staphylococcus aureus. *The Journal of Antimicrobial Chemotherapy, 55*(3), 379–382.

Wang, X. L., Li, L., Li, S. M., Huang, J. Y., Fan, Y. P., Yao, Z. J., et al. (2017). Phenotypic and molecular characteristics of Staphylococcus aureus and methicillin-resistant Staphylococcus aureus in slaughterhouse pig-related workers and control workers in Guangdong Province, China. *Epidemiology & Infection, 145*(9), 1843–1851.

Wassenberg, M. W., & Bonten, M. J. (2010). The Dutch MRSA policy can and should be different. *Nederlands Tijdschrift voor Geneeskunde, 154*(45), A2575.

Wulf, M., & Voss, A. (2008). MRSA in livestock animals-an epidemic waiting to happen? *Clinical Microbiology and Infection, 14*(6), 519–521.

Wulf, M. W., Sørum, M., van Nes, A., Skov, R., Melchers, W. J., Klaassen, C. H., & Voss, A. (2008). Prevalence of methicillin-resistant Staphylococcus aureus among veterinarians: An international study. *Clinical Microbiology and Infection, 14*(1), 29–34.

Brucellosis in Swine and Its Implications for Human Health

Shivali Khandelwal, Santanu Pal, Priyanshi Yadav, Vishal Yadav, and Taruna Bhati

Abstract

Brucella suis, pathogen of swine brucellosis, specifically biovars 1 and 3, is prevalent in various regions worldwide with a significant zoonotic risk in humans. *B. suis* exhibits genomic diversity and its pathogenicity is attributed to mechanisms such as evasion of innate and adaptive immune responses. The bacterium's ability to modulate host immune pathways contributes to its virulence and persistence within host cells. Brucellosis manifests with manifestations like pyrexia, weakness, ortholegia, and softness of tissue and can be transmitted through various routes including ingestion, inhalation, and contact with infected animals or their products. Diagnosis relies primarily on serological testing due to the limitations of bacterial isolation. However, serological assays may yield false-positive results, necessitating confirmation through molecular methods like PCR. Currently, there are no commercially available vaccines for *B. suis* in pigs in India. Control measures primarily focus on herd depopulation, approaches to develop effective vaccines, and therapeutic options for managing swine brucellosis. This chapter will provide an overall understanding of the complex interplay between the bacterium, host immune responses, and diagnostic methods essential for effectively controlling and preventing swine brucellosis and its zoonotic implications.

S. Khandelwal (✉) · S. Pal · P. Yadav
ICAR-Indian Veterinary Research Institute (ICAR-IVRI), Bareilly, Uttar Pradesh, India

V. Yadav
ICAR-National Dairy Research Institute (ICAR-NDRI), Karnal, Haryana, India

T. Bhati
Department of Veterinary Microbiology and Biotechnology, College of Veterinary and Animal Science, Bikaner, Rajasthan, India

R. Deb et al. (eds.), *Emerging Zoonotic Threats from Swine*,
https://doi.org/10.1007/978-981-96-7407-7_8

Keywords

Brucellosis · *Brucella suis* · Pigs · Zoonotic risk · Preventive methods

Introduction

Brucellosis in pigs, an infectious ailment owing its origin to an intracellular bacteria belonging to the genus *Brucella*, is a global health concern (Franco-Paredes et al., 2017). Although the disease is associated with worldwide pig reproductive losses, its primary importance lies in its capacity to transmit to humans through zoonotic infections (Gusi et al., 2019). Due to this, some nations have formulated regulatory initiatives to combat brucellosis in pigs. *Brucella suis* is a species zoonotic importance known to inhabitants of domestic and wild animals worldwide. As man-to-man transmission is rarely reported, infection in humans comes from animal reservoirs. Like other Brucella species, wild or feral pig populations are important reservoir hosts in many regions of the world. For a number of reasons, there is little knowledge about brucellosis in pigs. These include the disease's varied presentation at the individual and herd levels, its complicated epidemiology with many contributing factors, its capacity to infect a broad spectrum of hosts, and issues with the specificity of pig serological testing. Furthermore, the pig industry's brief commercial cycles might be a factor in the paucity of thorough illness data (Ducrotoy et al., 2017). Current diagnostics need the use of herds rather than individual animals due to limits in sensitivity and specificity. At present, India does not own any commercialized licensed vaccines as prophylactic measures of brucellosis in pigs. The most effective regulatory approach to control swine brucellosis is to cull whole herd which is not feasible.

Taxonomy of *Brucella suis*

The etiological bacterium of the genus *Brucella* is a facultative intracellular, Gram-negative cocco-bacilli or short rods that are not spore-forming, non-capsulated, and nonmotile. Predilecting site of Brucella in infected animals is within the phagocytic, reticuloendothelial, and specialized epithelial cells. *Brucella suis* is one of 10 species that are now found in the genus. According to Olsen and Palmer (2014), a number of additional species are being contemplated for inclusion. As confirmed scientifically in 1980 that strains of Brucella might form a genetically single "species," according to genomic techniques (Verger et al., 1985), the epidemiologic and diagnostic benefits of classifying Brucella strains into different "nomenspecies" according to their host preferences and distinctive phenotypic traits are stronger. The discovery that newly identified Brucella species exhibit greater genetic diversity than the six traditional Brucellae species (Verger et al., 2000) and the results of whole-genome sequencing that reveal distinct lineages unique to each species (Foster et al., 2009) provide additional support for the current classification scheme.

However, it should be mentioned that a range of hosts can be spontaneously infected by the most virulent species of Brucella (Oslen et al., 2014).

As per metabolomics, Brucella species are further divided into biovars depending on multiplication in thionin or basic fuschin dyes, and agglutination patterns due to monoclonal antibodies aiming the R, A, or M forms of the lipopolysaccharide (LPS)-O-side-chain (Alton et al., 1988). The *B. suis* isolates consistently express the smooth shape of the LPS O side chain. Before being identified and categorized as a new species within the *Brucellae* genus, it was specified as a unique strain of *Brucella abortus* based on pathogenicity (Huddleson, 1929).

It is impossible to visually differentiate *B. suis* colonies from isolates of other smooth Brucella species. There are currently five distinct biovars of *B. suis*, and pigs can contract brucellosis from biovars 1, 2, and 3. While biovars 1 and 3 are zoonotic, pathogenic, and endemic in America and Asia, causing reproductive issues in pigs and serious infections in humans, biovar 2 is reported to occur in Europe and Egypt and seems an extremely rare etiological factor of infection in humans (Elmonir et al., 2022; Spickler, 2018). Only found in subarctic locations, biovar 4 isolates are considered as zoonotic, mostly infecting wild caribou (*Rangifer tarandus*) and reindeer. Wolves (*Canis lupus*), moose (*Alces alces*), and arctic foxes (*Alopex lagopus*) in subarctic locations have also reported this biovar (Olsen et al., 2014). Additionally, only rodents in the USSR have yielded the isolates in biovar 5 (Alton et al., 1988).

There are four known brucella species that can infect people, i.e., *Brucella suis* (found in pigs and reindeer), *Brucella melitensis* (found in goats), *Brucella abortus* (found in cattle, bison, and elk), and *Brucella canis* (found in dogs). In contrast to *B. abortus*, *B. suis* does not require a high CO_2 environment for multiplication, which is a noteworthy characteristic when produced in laboratory settings. Its colonies have a sleek appearance. Serological agglutination assays employing monospecific anti-sera or anti-smooth Brucella antibodies can be used to identify isolates from pigs as Brucella tentatively. Standard typing techniques, such as the formation of hydrogen sulfide (a trait of biovar 1) and growth in the presence of dyes, are used to discriminate between species and biovariety. Only specific strains of biovar 1 and all strains of biovar 3 grow when basic fuchsin is present, whereas all three biovars grow when thionine is present (Alton, 1990).

Genetic Characteristics of *Brucella suis*

All of the *B. suis* biovars' representative genomes have been sequenced and examined (Paulen et al., 2002; Tae et al., 2011). Except for biovar 3 of *Brucella suis* owing a single chromosome of ~3.1 Mbp, others have two circular chromosomes of ~1.2 and 2.1 Mbp, respectively. The replication origin of the small chromosome is plasmid-like but the large chromosome is typical as of other bacteria. Approximately 3200–3400 open reading frames are encoded by the nearly identical GC content of the two chromosomes, which have an average GC value of 58–59%. *B. suis* branch is thought to contain the highest genetic variability intraspecifically among the six conventional Brucella species, despite the genus's remarkable homogeneity (*B. suis, B. melitensis, B. ovis, B. neotomae, B. abortus, and B. canis*). According to the phylogenetic analysis, the *B. suis* strains seem to have broken apart from the *B. foetus* and *B. melitensis* clades (Foster et al., 2009).

According to comparative bioinformatics, Brucella as a bacteria has evolved from its ancestors in lithosphere and adapted to the eukaryotic cell's intracellular environment by acquiring a secretion system, i.e., the VirB type 4 and a restricted-metal inhabitant (Wattam et al., 2014). This VirB type 4 secretion system more or less similar to that of Brucella was also confirmed on a plasmid having broad host range, isolated from an unknown bacteria in the lucerne rhizosphere, despite Brucella not having any reported natural plasmids that could permit the genetical transfer including antibiotic resistance (Schneiker et al., 2001). A roughly 30% reduction in genome size was also linked to the evolution of the Brucellae, especially in proteins involved in the metabolism, biosynthesis, and utilization of carbohydrates and amino acids (Wattam et al., 2014). According to Tay et al. (2015), to encode factors responsible for pathogenicity Brucella possess genomic islands, which are primarily proteins and enzymes hypothetically and are frequently linked to DNA (acquired horizontally), such as integrases and transposases. To understand the genetic and epidemiologic connections among *B. suis* and the remaining species of this genus, a variety of molecular approaches have been used. Additionally, strain separation and comparisons of genetic strain lineages have been made possible by the finding of multiple-locus variable-number tandem-repeat sequences (Duvnjak et al., 2015).

Immune Evasion Strategies of *Brucella suis*

Avoiding adaptive immunity, decreasing cellular immunity, dodging innate immunity, and developing intracellular parasitism are the primary processes in Brucella's pathogenicity and immune evasion strategy (Elrashedy et al., 2022). Nonetheless, a number of strategies have been employed by Brucella species, including *B. suis*, to avoid immunological detection in vivo (Olsen, 2013). Brucella species are well known for their ability to lessen the stimulation of Toll-like receptors (TLRs) and other pathogen recognition receptors (PRRs), in addition to establishing a replicative niche that decreases host recognition. In the cytoplasm, PRRs detect pathogens' RNA or DNA as well as trigger the type I interferons synthesis and remaining cytokines of inflammatory cause. Furthermore, several of the traditional structures—such as fimbria, pilli, plasmids, and capsules—known to activate PRRs are absent in Brucella (Kagan & Iwasaki, 2012). In addition to being present in the phagosome and having the ability to coordinate innate and adaptive immunity processes, cell membrane-linked PRRs are also engaged in the recognition of microbes that are responsible for the recruitment of antimicrobial activities to phagosomes and phagocytosis. The LPS produced by Brucella has a noncanonical structure, its stimulatory impact on Toll-like 4 receptors is diminished, and its cell membrane is extremely hydrophobic.

LPS-O-side-chain on and the major histocompatibility complex class II molecules can combine to form complexes that stop macrophages from presenting foreign proteins. TLR signaling may be interfered with or disrupted by proteins identified in brucella that are similar to TLR adaptor molecules. Compared to the endotoxin of other Gram-negative bacteria, the lipid A of the LPS of Brucella strains causes a significantly lower inflammatory response in mammalian hosts (Barquero-Calvo et al., 2007). Brucella characterizes reduced dendritic cell activation and maturation as well as a diminished innate immune response in comparison to other Gram-negative bacteria. Infected pigs can develop antibody responses and direct B-cell activation due to the highly immunogenic, T-cell-independent LPS of *B. suis*. Cytotoxic T cells linked to cellular immunity that generate cytokines (interleukin-2, interleukin-12, TNF-α, and interferon) in TH1-type patterns are thought as a basis for protection related to immunological origin. The innate immune system plays a crucial role in inducing cellular immune responses through the cross-presentation pathway, which allows internalized antigens to enter the ER through phagosome-ER-derived vesicles fusion and antigen attached to class I MHC complex for cell surface and molecular presentation. According to Olsen (2013), acquired or adaptive immune responses may also be directed toward a TH-1 pathway by the innate immune system's release of the proper cytokines in response to pathogen interaction.

Intracellular Trafficking by *Brucella suis*

Usually, brucella enters the host via piercing mucosal membranes. From there, they move freely or inside phagocytic cells to neighboring lymph nodes, where they begin to multiply. They then dispersed all over the body. By interacting with lipid rafts areas on the cell surface that contain certain lipids and proteins phagocytic cells can absorb smooth forms of Brucella, such as *B. suis* (Cutler et al., 2005). The bacteria first live inside a membrane-bound space known as a phagosome after they are inside the cell. By turning on a type IV secretion system, changing its pH, and blocking fusion with lysosomes, they control this compartment. According to Olsen and Tatum (2016), this allows Brucella to generate a replicating niche after entering endoplasmic reticulum (ER) called as a Brucella-containing vacuole (BOV), which allows it to elude the immune system. Brucella continues to interact with the ER and facilitates its reproduction by enlisting proteins from the endoplasmic reticulum and secretory vesicles (Fugier et al., 2009). The formation of the BOV enables certain bacteria to survive intracellularly, even if the fusion of phagosomes with lysosomes may kill a sizable percentage of the bacteria. To survive in a nutrient-deficient environment, Brucella uses tactics including nutrient scavenging and stationary-phase physiology (e.g., collecting iron by employing siderophores) inside the host cells (Bellaire et al., 2003).

Free radicals, the primary tool the host immune cells use to combat intracellular infections, can also be detoxified by Brucella species. It appears that the bacterial lipopolysaccharide (LPS) O side chain is essential for invasion and defense against different host defenses. Furthermore, *B. suis* can prevent phagocytic cells from dying through programmed cell death, extending their survival inside the host and shielding them from immunological reactions (Jimenez et al., 2004). The basis for creating and maintaining chronic infections is Brucella's capacity to adapt for long-term survival within cells, despite food restrictions, and avoid immune detection (Gross et al., 2000).

Route of *B. suis* Transmission

Infection often enters a domestic pig population primarily by the introduction of an infected animal, either male or female. Moreover, the virus may be transmitted by direct contact with afflicted wild pigs or by sharing the use of an infected male pig. Unlike *Brucella abortus*, this disease can be transmitted by mating with an infected male pig. The most common way for animals to infect one another is by oral contact with tainted reproductive resources from an infected female pig (Alton, 1990). Humans can contract swine brucellosis by aerosols, such as respiratory tissues and the mouth, or as an opportunistic pathogen through fissures. The disease can be acquired by hunting or other contact with feral pigs, but it is most commonly associated with agricultural laborers, veterinarians, and abattoir workers. Although handling seropositive wild hosts of other Brucella species has long been known to offer a minimal risk of infection for human workers, processing ill pigs in a slaughterhouse setting poses a high risk of infection (Hendricks et al., 1962; Heineman and Dziamski, 1976). According to certain evidence, handling meat from sick pigs may increase the risk of acquiring a zoonotic infection caused by *B. suis* (Deqiu et al., 2002). *B. suis* zoonotic infection through raw milk remains a public health concern because sick cattle can excrete high amounts of bacteria in milk, despite typically being asymptomatic (Beattie & Rice, 1934). According to Jordan et al. (1943), drinking unpasteurized milk from calves infected with *B. suis* used to induce several infections in humans rather than just the occasional one. Humans can contract the disease by eating raw or tainted milk or milk products, coming into intimate contact with diseased animals or animal carcasses, or coming into contact with tainted reproductive materials. Millions of people worldwide are at risk of infection, particularly in the Third World, where sanitary and hygienic conditions are frequently subpar. Infection rates can reach 78 cases per 100,000 persons in the Mediterranean region, the Middle East, southern Europe, and South America. In the United States, hunters, lab technicians, abattoir workers, farmers, ranchers, and veterinarians are the main groups with brucellosis, a zoonotic disease. In humans, the infection is frequently restricted to laboratory workers and those who work with pigs. However, *B. suis* has the capacity to colonize cow udders, which could cause serious human epidemics (Fig. 1).

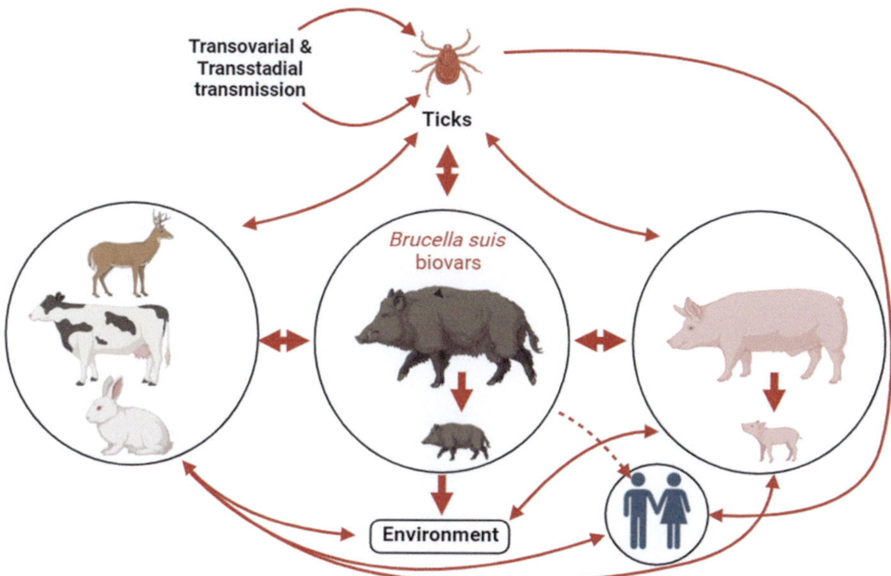

Fig. 1 Schematic diagram showing the transmission of *Brucella suis* biovars through several routes involving wild boars (*Sus scrofa*) and ticks (Dermacentor) as main reservoirs

Pathogenesis and Clinical Signs of *Brucella suis* Infection in Pigs

The pathophysiology of brucellosis in pigs is similar to that of infections in other animals. After an oral or vaginal invasion, the organisms will remain and grow in the targeted lymph node or nodes for a week to 10 days. The bacteremia that follows may last for 34 weeks (Alton, 1990). The incubation period is the amount of time that passes between exposure and the manifestation of clinical symptoms or a positive serological test. Depending on several variables, the incubation period may extend from 2 weeks to many months. The reticular endothelium system contains cells where Brucella nests and multiplies. The spleen, lymph nodes, liver, bone marrow, epididymis, and placenta are therefore thought to be ideal sites for isolating Brucella species. This is due to the fact that these organs, which are referred to as "gold organs," contain a significant number of Brucella organisms (Gonzalez-Espinoza et al., 2021). The increased chance of recovering Brucella organisms from these macrophage-rich reticuloendothelial system tissues is the justification for obtaining tissue specimens for molecular studies, such as bone marrow aspirates, liver biopsy specimens, or lymph nodes (Greenfield et al., 2002) (Fig. 2).

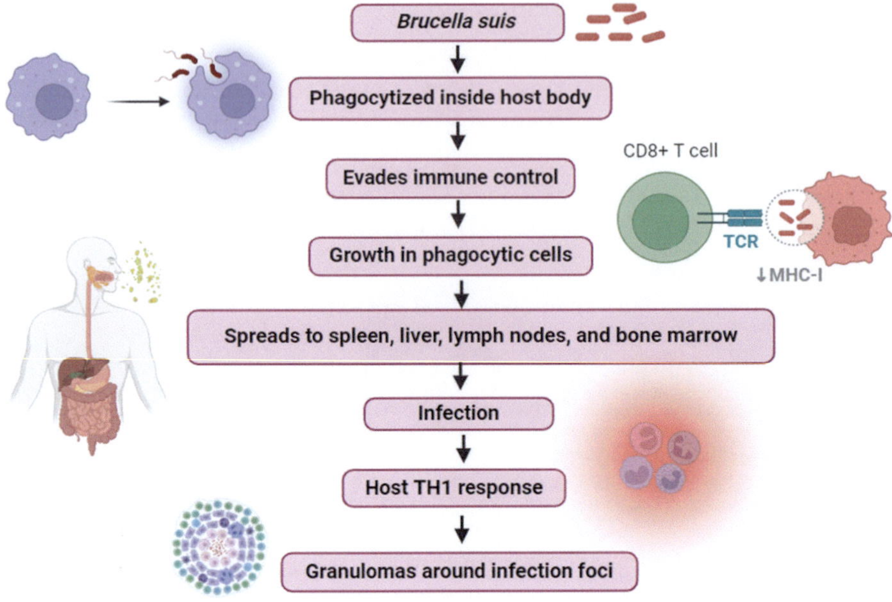

Fig. 2 The steps involved in the pathogenic process of *B. suis* infection

Status of Swine Brucellosis in India

Pigs' clinical symptoms may vary greatly depending on the herd's infection stage and the location of the bacterium's development in each individual animal. The bacteria enter the body through mucosal membranes, coitus, and food. It is possible to isolate brucellae from nearly any tissue following the bacteremic phase, but the lymph nodes are the most common source. It is quite dangerous to handle the animals because of this widespread infection. Although a cellular immune response starts to emerge earlier, antibodies show up 2 weeks after infection (Deyoe, 1967; Kaneene et al., 1978). Pigs with reproductive issues may have infertility, abortion, or stillbirth as symptoms. Infected animals may also exhibit other symptoms of sickness, such as lameness and swelling of the joints. Subclinical infections also exist (Deyoe, 1981).

The characteristics of brucellosis in swine and large or small ruminants (*B. abortus* or *B. melitensis*) differ significantly. These traits include prolonged shedding from mucosal surfaces or in urine, the possibility of disease transmission through coitus, and chronic bacteremia. In contrast to ruminant brucellosis, males and non-pregnant pigs appear to be able to contribute to the spread of the disease. Since transmission necessitates direct or intimate contact, environmental persistence is typically thought to have little epidemiological influence (Blood et al., 1983). To keep *B. suis* in a community, it is thought that ongoing host infection is required. Despite the widespread belief that abortion is a significant clinical symptom linked to *B. suis* in field settings, it typically represents a minor aspect of the presentation of suis infection in pigs. After researching the organ-level evolution of illnesses in populations of gigantic pigs, several authors have given credit to the myth that *B. suis* was initially found from an aborted fetus (Johnson & Huddleson, 1931). Clinical signs are not a reliable indicator of brucellosis, even if *B. suis* is linked to reproductive losses in pigs, because placental and fetal lesions can be difficult to distinguish from other infectious agents (Manthei, 1970). The little fetuses that are expelled in placental tissues as a result of placentitis lesions of varying severity that might form in females who naturally contract the disease are rarely seen by farmers. Between days 21 and 27, these lesions may result in fetal death. A return to estrus 40–45 days after spontaneous breeding may be the earliest indication of an early miscarriage. The results of experimental infections support this, showing that contaminated semen implanted in sows during the early stages of pregnancy caused reproductive losses as early as 22 days after infection and an irregular recovery to estrus 30–45 days later (Manthei, 1970). Additionally, there is experimental evidence that infection after day 40 of pregnancy is the cause of mid-to-late gestational abortions. Field abortions are typically linked to oral exposure between 50 and 100 days of gestation. Sometimes, between 100 and 110 days of gestation, sows will discharge weak or stillborn fetuses. Although uterine infections often disappear 30–40 days after an abortion, they may result in uterine or vaginal shedding that lasts for up to 36 months. In the small percentage of females with chronic uterine infections, this shedding can continue for up to 36 months and is linked to either temporary or permanent infertility (Manthei, 1970). Metritis and placental retention are possible outcomes for infected sows. The severity of the uterine lesions and the length of the sickness are directly related to infertility (Thomseon, 1934). In pigs, the disease is characterized by septicemia and chronic inflammatory lesions (hygromas) in the joints and reproductive organs of both sexes.

There are very few reports of brucellosis in pigs in India. An isolation report of *B. suis* (biovar 2) is available in the literature (Mathur, 1985). Several Indian states, including Tamil Nadu (Kumar & Rao, 1980), Karnataka, Andhra Pradesh, Madhya Pradesh, Punjab (Shome et al., 2016) and Uttar Pradesh, Assam (Nath et al., 2009) have documented seroprevalences of Brucella in pigs. Pigs with a history of abortions had the highest seroprevalence in Assam, the state that borders Meghalaya. Meghalaya has only reported one case of pig brucellosis, with a zero seroprevalence rate (Shome et al., 2016).

In India, there are hardly any reports of brucellosis in pigs. The literature has an isolation report of *B. suis* (biovar 2) (Mathur, 1985). Brucella seroprevalences in pigs have been reported in a number of Indian states, including Tamil Nadu (Kumar & Rao, 1980), Karnataka, Andhra Pradesh, Madhya Pradesh, Punjab (Shome et al., 2016), and Uttar Pradesh, Assam (Nath et al., 2009). Assam, the state that borders Meghalaya, had the greatest seroprevalence of pigs with a history of abortions. Meghalaya has a 0% seroprevalence rate and has only recorded one case of pig brucellosis (Shome et al., 2016).

Potential for Zoonotic Species

According to Sankarasubramanian et al. (2016), the five biovars of *Brucella suis* are known as 1 through 5. Domestic pigs, cattle, sheep, and even people can contract brucellosis from *Brucella suis* biovars 1, 2, and 3. According to Olsen and Tatum (2016), brucellosis in pigs caused by *Brucella suis* is less dangerous than that caused by *Brucella melitensis* and *Brucella abortus*, but it frequently leaves a persistent infection that is difficult to detect. The epidemic's scope and infection range could be increased if it spreads to nearby livestock and other animals (Szulowski et al., 2013). Menshawy et al. (2014) state that *Brucella suis* biovars 1 and 3 are responsible for the bulk of swine-borne illnesses in humans. It is simple for people to interact directly with these biovars, especially among farmers, veterinarians, and abattoir staff (Galinska & Zagórski, 2013; Zheng et al., 2018). In regions where *Brucella melitensis* infection is not prevalent, *Brucella suis* has been identified as the primary cause of human brucellosis. However, as swine brucellosis has become more common, human brucellosis has also become less common due to advancements in swine management. Human brucellosis has been linked to several species of Brucella, including *Brucella melitensis*, *Brucella abortus*, and biovars 1, 2, 3, and 4 of *Brucella suis*. Occasionally, marine animal species such as *Brucella canis* have also been linked to human brucellosis (Lopes et al., 2010).

In people, the disease typically takes 1–3 weeks to incubate, but it might take months. There are two types of illness: mild and self-limiting and severe. It always includes a persistent, sporadic, or irregular fever, which might begin abruptly or gradually. Similar to other feverish illnesses, this one also has a major impact on the musculoskeletal system, as demonstrated by the related widespread aches and pains, exhaustion, disorientation, and despair. The infection and/or sickness may persist permanently if antibiotics are not taken (WHO/OMS, 1998). Treating the disease in the animal host is the most cost-effective method of preventing human brucellosis, and nations with low incidence of human brucellosis are also those that control animal brucellosis. Clinical signs of human brucellosis typically appear weeks to months after the illness first manifests as a chronic, slow-onset illness. The pathophysiology of human brucellosis typically varies from that of reservoir host brucellosis (Fig. 3).

Clinical Signs and Symptoms in Human Being

Human brucellosis is characterized by chills, pyrexia (undulant fever), cephalalgia, malaise, excessive perspiration, weakness, joint and muscle soreness, and exhaustion. A typical core body temperature in the afternoon can be as high as 40 °C. Indications of the infection include headache, arthralgia, constipation, anorexia, sleeplessness, night sweats, sexual dysfunction, and even neurological problems. These symptoms are not pathognomonic in nature. The primary routes of human infection are inhaling aerosolized Brucella particles, consuming raw milk, dairy products, and undercooked meat, and coming into touch with ill animals while

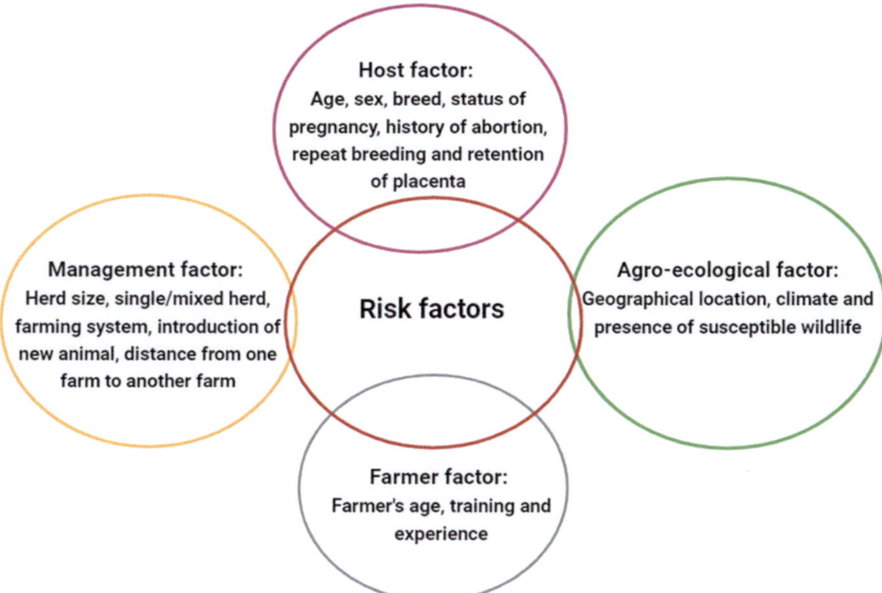

Fig. 3 Factors contributing to the risk of Brucella infection in animals followed by zoonotic transmission to humans are categorized into four groups

at work or during leisure (CDC, 2009). The symptoms of Brucella are clinically linked to inflammatory lesions caused by the bacteria's localization, and it can spread to nearly any tissue or in vivo area. The most frequent negative effect is osteoarticular disease, which may include spondylitis, sacroiliitis, and peripheral arthritis. Human brucellosis frequently has a low death rate, even in cases where therapy is not received. Although relapses of infection are common, they are typically not linked to the emergence of antibiotic-resistant strains of Brucella, partly because the organism lacks naturally occurring plasmids (Pappas et al., 2005).

More recently, human brain tumors have been connected to Brucella infection. They did not, however, allow for accurate distinction to species of *B. suis*, *B. melitensis*, or *B. abortus*. According to Zhang et al. (2011), DNA sequences obtained using PCR amplification from formalin-fixed tissues were associated with 25% of metastatic carcinomas, 60% of glioblastomas, and 25% of medulloblastomas. Despite regional variations in exposure risk, *B. suis* continues to pose a hazard to human zoonotic infection worldwide. Swine populations that are wild or feral continue to be important sources of swine brucellosis transmission to domestic animals and people. Because human brucellosis symptoms and clinical indicators are so vague, doctors may struggle to diagnose it. A conclusive diagnosis requires the proper serology and bacteriology, as well as a history of contact with pigs or pig corpses. The common broad-spectrum antibiotics do not work on Brucella species. To treat, a long-term course of streptomycin or rifampin combined with tetracycline or doxycycline is necessary.

Diagnosis of Swine Brucellosis

The gold standard for diagnosing swine brucellosis is still bacterial isolation (Olsen et al., 2014). However, because of the slow growth of Brucella in vitro, the poor recovery of isolates from chronically infected pigs, the high expense of microbiologic testing, and the biosafety concerns when handling *B. suis* isolates, bacterial isolation is frequently not a practical diagnostic technique. Serologic testing is the accepted method for diagnosing swine brucellosis because of these factors. The smooth LPS of *B. suis* strains may be recognized by monoclonal antibodies against the A and M antigens and common (C) LPS epitopes shared with cross-reacting strains, despite slight strain variations (Tae et al., 2011).

Additionally, based on metabolic traits, a semiautomated metabolic system has been shown to have good specificity in differentiating between Brucella species and biovars (Al Dahouk et al., 2010). Common tests for swine brucellosis include the following: buffered plate antigen, mercaptoethanol, rivanol, complement fixation test (CFT), card test (Rose Bengal test [RBT]), competitive enzyme-linked immunosorbent assay (c-ELISA), and fluorescent polarization assay (FPA) (Lord et al., 1997; Nielsen et al., 1999; Olsen et al., 2012). When compared to an indirect enzyme-linked immunosorbent assay (ELISA), FPA, and RBT for the diagnosis of swine brucellosis, data from two studies demonstrated that the c-ELISA had the highest specificity (mean SPs 99% and 86% but equivalent SP with RBT in one study) and the highest sensitivity (mean estimates of sensitivity 95% and 96%) (Nagalingam et al., 2012).

A bioengineered recombinant glycoprotein polysaccharide antigen of *B. suis* was demonstrated to exhibit high sensitivity (98%) and specificity (100%) when used as the target antigen in an ELISA in pigs infected with biovars 1 and 2 (Cortina et al., 2016). Recent years have seen the development of additional serologic assays for swine brucellosis, which reduce false-positive results, especially when testing for biovar 2 infections in Europe. However, tests that use the LPS O side-chain as an antigen (such as RBT, ELISAs, and FPA) showed lower diagnostic specificity when it came to handling false-positive results (McGiven et al., 2012). However, tests that use Brucella protein extracts without the O-polysaccharide, like indirect ELISAs, gel immunodiffusion, counterimmunoelectrophoresis, and latex agglutination, were found to have high specificity and moderate sensitivity when it came to identifying *B. suis* and distinguishing false-positive results on serologic tests (Dieste-Perez et al., 2015).

The Brucellin skin test, also known as the delayed-type hypersensitivity reaction, uses cytoplasmic proteins that are isolated from rough strain and clear of lipopolysaccharides (LPS). Furthermore, *B. suis* disorders and infections brought on by cross-reacting bacteria, such as *Yersinia enterocolitica* O:9, can be distinguished using *B. melitensis* strain B115104 as a diagnostic tool. The skin test is successful at the herd level since pigs that undergo it do not create cross-reacting antibodies that are reactive in RBT, CFT, or ELISA tests (EFSA, 2009).

Numerous serological tests can be used to identify animals that have brucella. According to Alton et al. (1975), the most widely utilized of these are the Serum

Agglutination Test (SAT), the Rose Bengal Plate Test (RBPT), and the Complement Fixation Test (CFT).

The FPA, the Rose Bengal rapid agglutination test (RBT), the i-ELISA and c-ELISA, and the CFT are the serological tests for swine brucellosis listed in the World Organization for Animal Health Manual of Diagnostic Tests and Vaccines; however, the CFT is not recommended (OIE, 2009). None of the aforementioned tests have optimal sensitivity values, and even fewer have optimal specificity for specific diagnostic purposes due to false-positive results, which are most likely caused by cross-reactions with other bacteria and mostly with *Y. enterocolitica* O:9. Sometimes swine serum contains non-specific antibodies, most frequently IgM, which reduces the specificity of conventional diagnostics, especially serum agglutination assays. Furthermore, pro-complementary activity from guinea-pig and swine complement reduces the sensitivity of the CFT (Febo et al., 2012).

Handling an Infection Caused by *Brucella suis*

As of right now, India lacks a commercially available vaccination to prevent *B. suis* infection in domestic or wild pigs. This may be partly because *B. suis* is receiving less attention than *B. fetus* and *B. melitensis*. Changes to swine production systems that emphasize confinement housing to lower exposure risk, the significantly higher prevalence in a wildlife reservoir compared to the low prevalence in domestic livestock in many countries, and the belief that swine brucellosis was essentially under control in domestic swine populations that emerged 30–40 years ago in developed nations can all contribute to this. Compared to the other two Brucella species, people could believe that *B. suis* presents a lesser danger of brucellosis in humans. In contrast to the development of a vaccination for *B. foetus* and *B. melitensis*, the lack of a standardized, repeatable challenge paradigm that replicates infection and clinical disease in pigs under field conditions further impedes the development of vaccines and therapeutic options. Therefore, further efforts to standardize the experimental challenge approach will be beneficial for the development of effective vaccines against swine brucellosis. Similar to brucellosis vaccines for large and small ungulates, a successful vaccination would be a useful tool, but it is expected that a vaccine by itself will not be enough to eradicate *B. suis*. If the ultimate objective is to eradicate the disease, vaccination will probably need to be employed in combination with other tactics (such as test and kill, selective depopulation, etc.). The currently recommended regulatory strategy to prevent swine brucellosis is complete herd depopulation; however, in many cases, this approach is costly and unfeasible.

Vaccine for Swine Brucellosis

There is currently no approved vaccination to prevent brucellosis that is both safe and effective. Nevertheless, China has approved the *B. suis* strain S2 vaccine. The S2 vaccine, which is currently registered as a multi-species vaccination that protects cattle, small ruminants, and pigs against all three species of Brucella, was created in 1952 at the China Institute of Veterinary Drug Control (IVDC) from a naturally weakened strain found in a swine fetus (Sun et al., 2021). It is frequently used in China to vaccinate male and female cattle, sheep/goats, and pigs against brucellosis.

The S2 immunization provides cattle with 2 years of protection against *B. abortus*, pigs with 1 year of protection against *B. suis*, and sheep and goats with 3 years of protection against *B. melitensis*. Without the need for an adjuvant, it can be administered subcutaneously, intramuscularly, conjunctivally, or orally (in combination with drinking water) (Li et al., 2023). In China, the oral method is approved for all of the previously specified animals, even those that are pregnant. Additionally, subcutaneous and intramuscular procedures are approved for all species except pregnant calves and tiny fat-tailed sheep (Liang et al., 2020) (Fig. 4).

Conclusion

In conclusion, a serious global health issue for both humans and animals is swine brucellosis, which is caused by an infection with *Brucella suis*. This contagious and recently discovered zoonosis is disregarded in most endemic countries, including India. The sickness not only renders pigs incapable of procreating, but it also presents a potential zoonotic risk to humans. The genetic diversity of the *B. suis* species, which includes five biovars, demonstrates the pathogen's complexity and adaptability to a variety of hosts and environments. The main ways that *B. suis* spreads among domestic pig populations are by direct contact with infected animals, sharing use of diseased males, and oral contact with contaminated reproductive materials. Humans can become infected through ingestion of contaminated food products, contact with diseased animals or their tissues, or aerosolization. Unsanitary circumstances raise the risk of contracting *B. suis* zoonotic infections, which can have major negative effects on public health, particularly in regions with high infection rates. Epidemiology shows that *B. suis* biovars 1 and 3 are the primary cause of human swine-related disorders, especially outside of Europe. Swine populations, notably wild and feral pigs, serve as significant disease reservoirs in many parts of the world, prolonging the disease's duration. Pigs can display a variety of brucellosis clinical signs, making diagnosis challenging, especially in light of the limits of existing diagnostic methods in terms of sensitivity and specificity. Although bacterial isolation remains the gold standard, serologic testing is often used due to practical constraints. However, in suspicious instances, molecular techniques must be utilized for validation because false positives and negatives are common. Eating contaminated animal products or having direct contact with infected animals is the major way that

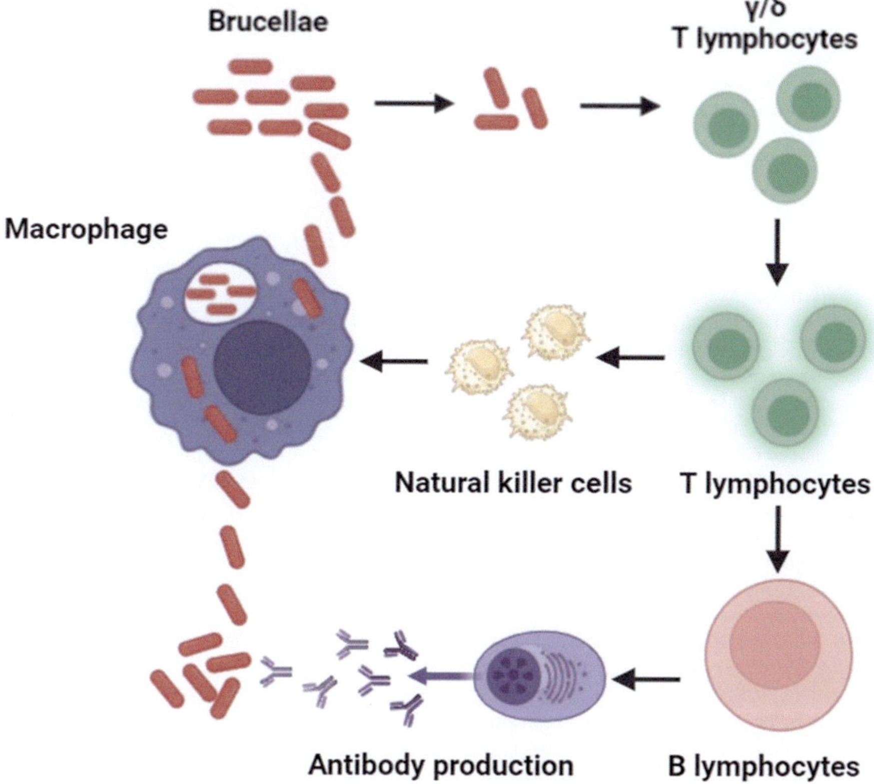

Fig. 4 Host immune response against *B. suis* infection in the natural environment as a basis for vaccine development

human brucellosis, a chronic illness with nebulous symptoms, is disseminated. Neurological problems and potential links to particular cancer types are among the illness's serious health effects. Swine brucellosis is controlled by regulatory programs and biosecurity measures; whole-herd depopulation is the recommended strategy for controlling epidemics. However, this approach is often costly and unfeasible. Pig brucellosis is infrequently reported because diagnostics are not accessible or because bovine brucellosis is the main focus. Effective vaccine development and diagnostic technology advancement are crucial for the effective control and eventual eradication of swine brucellosis, necessitating additional study as well as cross-disciplinary and cross-regional cooperation.

References

Alton, G. G., Maw, J., Rogerson, B. A., & McPherson, G. G. (1975). The serological diagnosis of bovine brucellosis: Eradication of the CFT, SAT and RBPT. *Australian Veterinary Journal, 51*, 57–63.

Alton, G. G., Jones, L. M., Angus, R. D., & Verger, J. M. (1988). *Techniques for the brucellosis laboratory*. INRA Publications.

Alton, G. G., Nielsen, K., & Duncan, J. R. (1990). Brucella suis. *Animal brucellosis*, 412–422.

Barquero-Calvo, E., Chaves-Olarte, E., Weiss, D. S., Guzman-Verri, C., Chacon-Diaz, C., Rucavado, A., et al. (2007). *Brucella abortus* uses a stealthy strategy to avoid activation of the innate immune system during the onset of infection. *PLoS One, 2*(7), e631.

Beattie, C. P., & Rice, R. M. (1934). Undulant fever due to Brucella of the porcine type-*Brucella Suis*: Report of a milk-borne epidemic. *Journal of the American Medical Association, 102*(20), 1670–1674.

Bellaire, B. H., Elzer, P. H., Baldwin, C. L., & Roop, R. M. (2003). Production of the siderophore 2, 3-dihydroxybenzoic acid is required for wild-type growth of Brucella abortus in the presence of erythritol under low-iron conditions in vitro. *Infection and Immunity, 71*(5), 2927–2932.

Centers for Disease Control and Prevention (CDC). (2009). *Brucella suis* infection associated with feral swine hunting-three states, 2007-2008. MMWR. *Morbidity and Mortality Weekly Report, 58*(22).

Cortina, M. E., Balzano, R. E., Rey Serantes, D. A., Caillava, A. J., Elena, S., Ferreira, A. C., et al. (2016). A bacterial glycoengineered antigen for improved serodiagnosis of porcine brucellosis. *Journal of Clinical Microbiology, 54*(6), 1448–1455.

Cutler, S. J., Whatmore, A. M., & Commander, N. J. (2005). Brucellosis–new aspects of an old disease. *Journal of Applied Microbiology, 98*(6), 1270–1281.

Dahouk, A., et al. (2010). Differential phenotyping of Brucella species using a newly developed semi-automated metabolic system. *BMC Microbiology, 10*, 269.

Deqiu, S., Donglou, X., & Jiming, Y. (2002). Epidemiology and control of brucellosis in China. *Veterinary Microbiology, 90*(1–4), 165–182.

Deyoe, B. L. (1967). Pathogenesis of three strains of *B. suis* in swine. *American Journal of Veterinary Research, 28*, 951–957.

Deyoe, B. L. (1981). In A. D. Lehman (Ed.), *Diseases of swine* (5th ed.). Lowa State University Press.

Di Febo, T., Luciani, M., Portanti, O., Bonfini, B., Lelli, R., & Tittarelli, M. (2012). Development and evaluation of diagnostic tests for the serological diagnosis of brucellosis in swine. *Veterinaria Italiana, 48*(2), 133–156.

Dieste-Perez, L., Blasco, J. M., De Miguel, M. J., Moriyon, I., & Munoz, P. M. (2015). Diagnostic performance of serological tests for swine brucellosis in the presence of false positive serological reactions. *Journal of Microbiological Methods, 111*, 57–63.

Ducrotoy, M., Bertu, W. J., Matope, G., Cadmus, S., Conde-Álvarez, R., Gusi, A. M., et al. (2017). Brucellosis in sub-Saharan Africa: Current challenges for management, diagnosis and control. *Acta Tropica, 165*, 179–193.

Duvnjak, S., Račić, I., Špičić, S., Zdelar-Tuk, M., Reil, I., & Cvetnić, Ž. (2015). Characterisation of Brucella suis isolates from Southeast Europe by multi-locus variable-number tandem repeat analysis. *Veterinary Microbiology, 180*(1–2), 146–150.

EFSA (European Food Safety Authority), AHAW Panel (ESA Panel on Animal Health and Welfare). (2009). Porcine brucellosis (*Brucella suis*). *EFSA Journal, 1144*, 1–112.

Elmonir, W., Abdel-Hamid, N. H., Hamdy, M. E., Beleta, E. I., El-Diasty, M., Melzer, F., et al. (2022). Isolation and molecular confirmation of Brucella suis biovar 2 from slaughtered pigs: An unanticipated biovar from domestic pigs in Egypt. *BMC Veterinary Research, 18*(1), 224.

Elrashedy, A., Gaafar, M., Mousa, W., Nayel, M., Salama, A., Zaghawa, A., et al. (2022). Immune response and recent advances in diagnosis and control of brucellosis. *German Journal of Veterinary Research, 2*(1), 10–24.

Foster, J. T., Beckstrom-Sternberg, S. M., Pearson, T., Beckstrom-Sternberg, J. S., Chain, P. S., Roberto, F. F., et al. (2009). Whole-genome-based phylogeny and divergence of the genus Brucella. *Journal of Bacteriology, 191*(8), 2864–2870.

Franco-Paredes, C., Chastain, D., Taylor, P., Stocking, S., & Sellers, B. (2017). Boar hunting and brucellosis caused by *Brucella suis*. *Travel Medicine and Infectious Disease, 16*, 18–22.

Fugier, E., Salcedo, S. P., de Chastellier, C., Pophillat, M., Muller, A., Arce-Gorvel, V., et al. (2009). The glyceraldehyde-3-phosphate dehydrogenase and the small GTPase Rab 2 are crucial for Brucella replication. *PLoS Pathogens, 5*(6), e1000487.

Galinska, E. M., & Zagórski, J. (2013). Brucellosis in humans-etiology, diagnostics, clinical forms. *Annals of Agricultural and Environmental Medicine, 20*(2), 233.

González-Espinoza, G., Arce-Gorvel, V., Mémet, S., & Gorvel, J. P. (2021). Brucella: Reservoirs and niches in animals and humans. *Pathogens, 10*(2), 186.

Greenfield, R. A., Drevets, D. A., Machado, L. J., Voskuhl, G. W., Cornea, P., & Bronze, M. S. (2002). Bacterial pathogens as biological weapons and agents of bioterrorism. *The American Journal of the Medical Sciences, 323*(6), 299–315.

Gross, A., Terraza, A., Ouahrani-Bettache, S., Liautard, J. P., & Dornand, J. (2000). In vitro Brucella suis infection prevents the programmed cell death of human monocytic cells. *Infection and Immunity, 68*(1), 342–351.

Gusi, A. M., Bertu, W. J., Jesús de Miguel, M., Dieste-Pérez, L., Smits, H. L., Ocholi, R. A., et al. (2019). Comparative performance of lateral flow immunochromatography, iELISA and rose Bengal tests for the diagnosis of cattle, sheep, goat and swine brucellosis. *PLoS Neglected Tropical Diseases, 13*(6), e0007509.

Heineman, H. S., & Dziamski, I. M. (1976). *Brucella suis* infection in Philadelphia. A survey of hog fever and asymptomatic brucellosis. *American Journal of Epidemiology, 103*(1), 88–100.

Hendricks, S. L., Borts, I. H., Heeren, R. H., Hausler, W. J., & Held, J. R. (1962). Brucellosis outbreak in an Iowa packing house. *American Journal of Public Health and the Nations Health, 52*(7), 1166–1178.

Huddleson, I. F., & Hallman, E. T. (1929). The pathogenicity of the species of the genus Brucella for monkeys. *The Journal of infectious diseases*, 293–303

Jiménez de Bagüés, M. P., Terraza, A., Gross, A., & Dornand, J. (2004). Different responses of macrophages to smooth and rough Brucella spp.: Relationship to virulence. *Infection and Immunity, 72*(4), 2429–2433.

Johnson, H. W., & Huddleson, I. F. (1931). Natural Brucella infection in swine. *Journal of American Veterinary Medical Association, 78*, 849–862.

Jordan, C. F., Borts, I. H., Harris, D. M., & Jennings, J. R. (1943). Brucellosis: Consideration of its epidemiology, diagnosis and control. *American Journal of Public Health and the Nations Health, 33*(7), 773–779.

Kagan, J. C., & Iwasaki, A. (2012). Phagosome as the organelle linking innate and adaptive immunity. *Traffic, 13*(8), 1053–1061.

Kaneene, J. M., et al. (1978). Cell-mediated immune responses in swine from a herd infected with Brucella suis. *American Journal of Veterinary Research, 39*(10), 1607–1611.

Kumar, R., & Rao, C. V. N. (1980). Porcine brucellosis in Tamil Nadu. *Indian Veterinary Journal, 57*(1), 1–4.

Li, P., Jiang, H., Feng, Y., Zhang, G., Banai, M., & Ding, J. (2023). The advances of the Chinese Brucella suis strain 2 vaccine. *Animal Research and One Health, 1*(1), 115–126.

Liang, P. F., Zhao, Y., Zhao, J. H., Pan, D. F., & Guo, Z. Q. (2020). Human distribution and spatial-temporal clustering analysis of human brucellosis in China from 2012 to 2016. *Infectious diseases of poverty, 9*, 1–9

Lopes, L. B., Nicolino, R., & Haddad, J. P. A. (2010). Brucellosis-risk factors and prevalence: A review. *The Open Veterinary Science Journal, 4*(1), 72.

Lord, V. R., Cherwonogrodzky, J. W., Marcano, M. J., & Melendez, G. (1997). Serological and bacteriological study of swine brucellosis. *Journal of Clinical Microbiology, 35*(1), 295–297.

Manthei, C. A. (1970). Aspectos clínicos y patologicos de la brucelosis suina [Clinical and pathological aspects of brucellosis suis]. *Review of the National Institute of Hygiene, 7*, 105–106.

Mathur, T. N. (1985). The epidemiology of brucellosis. In *Proceedings of the brucellosis symposium and annual conference of the Indian association of pathologists and microbiologists (IAPM)* (Vol. 25, pp. 9–10).

McGiven, J. A., Nicola, A., Commander, N. J., Duncombe, L., Taylor, A. V., Villari, S., et al. (2012). An evaluation of the capability of existing and novel serodiagnostic methods for porcine brucellosis to reduce false positive serological reactions. *Veterinary Microbiology, 160*(3–4), 378–386.

Menshawy, A., Perez-Sancho, M., Garcia-Seco, T., Hosein, H. I., García, N., Martinez, I., et al. (2014). Assessment of genetic diversity of zoonotic Brucella spp. recovered from livestock in Egypt using multiple locus VNTR analysis. *BioMed Research International, 2014*, 1.

Nagalingam, M., Shome, R., Balamurugan, V., Shome, B. R., NarayanaRao, K., Vivekananda, ... & Prabhudas, K. (2012). Molecular typing of Brucella species isolates from livestock and human. *Tropical animal health and production, 44*(1), 5–9.

Nath, A. J., Barman, N. N., Sarma, D. K., Das, S. K., & Bora, D. P. (2009). Seroprevalence of brucella and parvovirus infections in pigs. *Indian Veterinary Journal, 86*(4), 339–341.

Nielsen, K., Gall, D., Smith, P., Vigliocco, A., Perez, B., Samartino, L., et al. (1999). Validation of the fluorescence polarization assay as a serological test for the presumptive diagnosis of porcine brucellosis. *Veterinary Microbiology, 68*(3–4), 245–253.

Olsen, S. C. (2013). Recent developments in livestock and wildlife brucellosis vaccination. *International Office of Epizootics, 32*(1), 207–217.

Olsen, S. C., & Palmer, M. V. (2014). Advancement of knowledge of Brucella over the past 50 years. *Veterinary Pathology, 51*(6), 1076–1089.

Olsen, S. C., & Tatum, F. M. (2016). Swine brucellosis: Current perspectives. *Veterinary Medicine: Research and Reports, Volume 8*, 1–12.

Pappas, G., Akritidis, N., Bosilkovski, M., & Tsianos, E. (2005). Brucellosis. *The New England journal of medicine, 352*(22), 2325–2336. https://doi.org/10.1056/NEJMra050570

Paulsen, I. T., Seshadri, R., Nelson, K. E., Eisen, J. A., Heidelberg, J. F., Read, T. D., et al. (2002). The Brucella suis genome reveals fundamental similarities between animal and plant pathogens and symbionts. *Proceedings of the National Academy of Sciences, 99*(20), 13148–13153.

Sankarasubramanian, J., Vishnu, U. S., Gunasekaran, P., & Rajendhran, J. (2016). A genome-wide SNP-based phylogenetic analysis distinguishes different biovars of *Brucella suis*. *Infection, Genetics and Evolution, 41*, 213–217.

Schneiker, S., Keller, M., Dröge, M., Lanka, E., Pühler, A., & Selbitschka, W. (2001). The genetic organization and evolution of the broad host range mercury resistance plasmid pSB102 isolated from a microbial population residing in the rhizosphere of alfalfa. *Nucleic Acids Research, 29*(24), 5169–5181.

Shome, R., Triveni, K., Shankaranarayana, P. B., Sahay, S., Rao, N., Shome, B. R., et al. (2016). Record of porcine brucellosis in India by indigenously developed indirect ELISA. *Asian Pacific Journal of Tropical Disease, 6*(11), 892–894.

Spickler, A. R. (2018). Brucellosis: Canine Brucellosis. Retrieved from http://www.cfsph.iastate.edu/DiseaseInfo/factsheets

Sun, S., Jiang, H., Li, Q., Liu, Y., Gao, Q., Liu, W., et al. (2021). Safety and transcriptome analysis of live attenuated brucella vaccine strain S2 on non-pregnant cynomolgus monkeys without abortive effect on pregnant cynomolgus monkeys. *Frontiers in Veterinary Science, 8*, 641022.

Szulowski, K., Iwaniak, W., Weiner, M., & Zlotnicka, J. (2013). Brucella suis biovar 2 isolations from cattle in Poland. *Annals of Agricultural and Environmental Medicine, 20*(4), 672.

Tae, H., Shallom, S., Settlage, R., Preston, D., Adams, L. G. and Garner, H. R. (2011). Revised genome sequence of *Brucella suis* 1330.

Tay, B. Y., Ahmad, N., Hashim, R., Mohamed Zahidi, J. A., Thong, K. L., Koh, X. P., & Mohd Noor, A. (2015). Multiple-locus variable-number tandem-repeat analysis (MLVA) genotyping of human Brucella isolates in Malaysia. *BMC Infectious Diseases, 15*, 1–7.

Thomseon, A. (1934). Brucella infection in swine. Studies from an epizootic in Denmark. *Acta Pathologica et Microbiologica Scandinavica, 21*, 115–130.

Verger, J. M., Grimont, F., Grimont, P. A., & Grayon, M. (1985). Brucella, a monospecific genus as shown by deoxyribonucleic acid hybridization. *International Journal of Systematic and Evolutionary Microbiology, 35*(3), 292–295.

Verger, J. M., Grayon, M., Cloeckaert, A., Lefèvre, M., Ageron, E., & Grimont, F. (2000). Classification of Brucella strains isolated from marine mammalsusing DNA–DNA hybridization and ribotyping. *Research in Microbiology, 151*(9), 797–799.

Wattam, A. R., Foster, J. T., Mane, S. P., Beckstrom-Sternberg, S. M., Beckstrom-Sternberg, J. M., Dickerman, A. W., et al. (2014). Comparative phylogenomics and evolution of the Brucellae reveal a path to virulence. *Journal of Bacteriology, 196*(5), 920–930.

World Organisation for Animal Health (Office International des Épizooties: OIE). (2009). Porcine brucellosis. In *Manual of diagnostic tests and vaccines for terrestrial animals* (pp. 1–7). OIE.

Zhang, B., Izadjoo, M., Horkayne-Szakaly, I., Morrison, A., & Wear, D. J. (2011). Medulloblastoma and brucellosis-molecular evidence of Brucella sp in association with central nervous system cancer. *Journal of Cancer, 2*, 136.

Zheng, R., Xie, S., Lu, X., Sun, L., Zhou, Y., Zhang, Y., & Wang, K. (2018). A systematic review and meta-analysis of epidemiology and clinical manifestations of human brucellosis in China. *BioMed Research International, 2018*, 1.

Salmonellosis: A Major Foodborne Zoonotic Disease Linked to Swine

Sanjeev Kumar, Fatema Akter, and Tapan Kumar Dutta

Abstract

Annually, 600 million individuals worldwide acquire foodborne diseases, leading to 420,000 fatalities. Human salmonellosis is regarded as a significant foodborne infection worldwide. Mostly, human salmonellosis has been related to ingestion of *Salmonella*-contaminated animal-derived dietary products. Pork consumption ranks number one globally, followed by poultry, beef, and goat/sheep. Consequently, pork and its derivatives serve as a possible reservoir of *Salmonella* for humans. The *S.* 1,4,[5],12:i:-, *S. typhimurium*, along with *S. derby,* are prevalent *Salmonella* serovars that have been isolated from pork in Europe. *Salmonella* is widely distributed in environment and intestines of many livestock species and poultry. The pervasive presence of *Salmonella* complicates its eradication, yet many mitigating methods can be implemented to decrease *Salmonella* levels in pork production. Cross-contamination at retail shops and homes has also been reported to spread *Salmonella* to humans. The critical investigation of each case of foodborne infection is essential to know the source of *Salmonella* and to adopt appropriate mitigation strategies.

S. Kumar (✉)
Department of Veterinary Microbiology, Institute of Veterinary Science and Animal Husbandry, Siksha 'O' Anusandhan (Deemed to be University), Bhubaneswar, Odisha, India

F. Akter
Department of Veterinary Microbiology, ICAR-Indian Veterinary Research Institute, Hebbal Campus, Bengaluru, Karnataka, India

T. K. Dutta
Department of Veterinary Microbiology, College of Veterinary Sciences and Animal Husbandry, Central Agricultural University, Selesih, Mizoram, India

R. Deb et al. (eds.), *Emerging Zoonotic Threats from Swine*,
https://doi.org/10.1007/978-981-96-7407-7_9

Keywords

Foodborne pathogen · *Salmonella* · Swine · Zoonosis

Introduction

Infections due to *Salmonella* are very common in swine. It is a primary contributor to economic losses within pork industry (Soliani et al., 2023). Furthermore, *Salmonella* is a principal foodborne bacterium responsible for foodborne illnesses in humans, hence representing a considerable danger to worldwide public health (Soliani et al., 2023). In humans, ingestion of contaminated food, especially that of animal origin, regarded as primary source of *Salmonella* infections (Heredia & García, 2018). The UN Food and Agriculture Organization states that pork constitutes most consumed meat globally at 36%, followed by poultry at 33%, beef at 24%, as well as goat/sheep at 5%. Pigs and pork products are possible sources of *Salmonella* that can cause foodborne illness in people. According to estimates from the Centers for Disease Control and Prevention (CDC), *Salmonella* bacteria lead to 1.35 million illnesses, 26,500 hospitalizations, as well as 420 fatalities annually in the United States. In all these illnesses, food is identified as the primary source of *Salmonella*. A survey by the European CDC indicated that human salmonellosis ranked second after campylobacteriosis, with an incidence of 23.4 cases per 100,000 population (Galán-Relaño et al., 2023).

The United States Department of Agriculture Economic Research Service (USDA ERS) has estimated an annual economic burden of $15.5 billion attributed to 15 pathogens (*Clostridium perfringens*, *Cyclospora cayetanensis, Cryptosporidium, Listeria monocytogenes, Salmonella, Shigella*, *Toxoplasma gondii*, *Norovirus,* STEC O157:H7, STEC non-O157:H7, *Vibrio* other non-cholera species, *Vibrio parahaemolyticus*, *Vibrio vulnificus*, and *Yersinia enterocolitica*) accountable for 95% of 9.4 million cases of foodborne illness. Among the 15 pathogens, five—*Salmonella* (24%), *Toxoplasma gondii* (21%), *Listeria monocytogenes* (18%), *Norovirus* (15%), as well as *Campylobacter* (12%)—constitute 90% of the economic burden, with Salmonella incurring the highest cost at $3666.6 million (Hoffmann et al., 2015).

In swine, *Salmonella* causes serious acute septicemia or chronic debilitating intestinal disease. In humans, mild to severe gastroenteritis is the most common manifestation of salmonellosis. Symptoms include fever, stomach pain, diarrhea (sometimes bloody diarrhea), nausea, and vomiting. Most individuals recuperate from salmonellosis within 4–7 days without medical intervention. Systemic infection resulting from host-restricted *Salmonella* (*S. typhi*, *S. paratyphi* A) may arise and can be deadly to the individual if not promptly treated with antibiotics. Individuals under 5 years of age, pregnant women, elderly, and those having compromised immune systems (including individuals with cancer or other debilitating conditions) are at an elevated risk of contracting salmonellosis and are more prone to experiencing severe symptoms (Kuria, 2023).

Salmonella

Salmonella was initially isolated by Theobald Smith in 1885, a research assistant at Bureau of Animal Industry, United States Department of Agriculture, under the guidance of Daniel Elmer Salmon. The *Salmonella* isolated by Smith and Salmon was *Salmonella enterica* subspecies *enterica* serovar Choleraesuis. The genus is named in honor of Daniel Elmer Salmon for his discovery with other scientists. The genus *Salmonella* is a member of family *Enterobacteriaceae* and comprises 2 species: *S. bongori*, *S. enterica*. *Salmonella enterica* comprises 6 subspecies: *Salmonella enterica* subspecies *enterica* (subspecies I), *Salmonella enterica* subspecies *salamae* (subspecies II), *Salmonella enterica* subspecies *arizonae* (subspecies IIIa), *Salmonella enterica* subspecies *diarizonae* (subspecies IIIb), *Salmonella enterica* subspecies *houtenae* (subspecies IV), as well as *Salmonella enterica* subspecies *indica* (subspecies VI). The genus *Salmonella* is categorized into many serotypes according to Kauffmann and White classification system, which relies on surface antigens, including flagellar (H) antigen, somatic (O) antigen, in some cases, capsular (Vi) antigen. This classification was introduced by Philip Bruce White and Fritz Kauffmann in 1934. The genus *Salmonella* contains more than 2600 serotypes. *Salmonella* can be classified broadly into two categories based on the type of clinical infection: typhoidal salmonellae, which causes typhoid fever, and non-typhoidal salmonellae, which causes gastroenteritis and food poisoning.

Salmonella is gram-negative, rod-shaped bacterium that belongs to the family *Enterobacteriaceae*. It's non-lactose fermenting, non-spore-forming, catalase-positive, as well as oxidase-negative facultative anaerobe. Most bacteria belonging to the genus *Salmonella* are motile except *S*. Gallinarum and *S*. Pullorum. The biofilm formation has been seen in *Salmonella*, especially in the serovars that can colonize multiple hosts, giving them an advantage to persist longer in the environment inside the infected host (Harrell et al., 2021). The curlin subunit gene D (*csgD*) expression of *Salmonella* is essential for forming biofilm (Grantcharova et al., 2010). It is well established that the persistence of *Salmonella* for more extended period in the environment is often associated with the formation of biofilm on inanimate as well as on animate surfaces. Whereas biofilm formation within the host is still not fully established. Most isolates of *Salmonella* did not show *csgD* gene (regulate biofilm formation) expression at 37 °C or more (Sokaribo et al., 2020).

Intestinal tract of both warm-blooded as well as cold-blooded animals serves as the primary reservoir for *Salmonella* and functions as a subclinical excretor. *Salmonella* can persist for several months to years in environments such as moist soil, water, fecal matter, as well as animal feed (Shikov et al., 2022).

All strains of salmonellae have a single chromosome. The genome size of *Salmonella* varies from 4.50 to 5.15Mbp, with a mean length of 4.78Mbp. A pan-genome analysis of 341 *S. enterica* isolates obtained from retail meat in Beijing, China, revealed 13,931 genes, with 3635 genes identified in the core genome. A limited number of genes, or occasionally a single gene, exhibit variations in guanine-cytosine concentration inside the core genome, known as "pathogenicity islands." These pathogenicity islands are recognized for augmenting the virulence potential of a species. In addition to chromosomal DNA, *Salmonella* may possess extrachromosomal DNA in the form of plasmids. These plasmids frequently contain virulence genes or antibiotic resistance genes. The *Salmonella* genus is increasingly characterized by complex interactions between pathogenicity islands, bacteriophages, plasmids, and other mobile components that may be the reason for their vast diversity (Lyu et al., 2021).

Salmonellosis in Swine

Salmonellae are categorized into three groups according to host range: host-adapted serovars, host-restricted serovars, as well as host-non-restricted serovars, as seen in Table 1 (Cheng et al., 2019). *S.* Typhisuis is a host-restricted serovar of *Salmonella,* which infects only single species, i.e., pigs. Host-adapted serovars are related to specific host species. However, they can induce sickness in other hosts; for instance, *S.* Cholerasuis, suited to pigs, can infect people. The unrestricted serovars can infect a diverse array of host animals, but commonly induce self-limiting gastroenteritis in several species, including humans, cattle, pigs, mice, as well as poultry. Unrestricted serovars encompass *S.* Typhimurium as well as *S.* Enteritidis (Bonardi, 2017).

The outcome of a disease is influenced by multiple factors. These factors include host factors, i.e., immune cells and their products, and pathogen factors, i.e., adhesins, invasins, capsules, exotoxin, endotoxins, biofilm, etc. The interaction between host factors and pathogen factors decides the final outcome, severity, and prognosis of a disease. Upon ingestion, S. enterica enters the colon and confronts human reactions aimed at eliminating the infection (Ruby et al., 2012). *Salmonella* generates multiple virulence factors, including type1 secretion systems, flagella, fimbriae, flagellin, and virulence plasmids, to counteract the host response. The virulence factors produced by *Salmonella* and their role in the pathogenesis are given in Table 2. Many virulence factors are encoded on *Salmonella* Pathogenicity Islands (SPI) on the chromosome. Most notably, type III secretion system 1 (T3SS1) and type III secretion system 2 (T3SS2) are encoded on SPI1 and SPI2, respectively (Ibarra and Steele-Mortimer, 2009; Lou et al., 2019).

The feco-oral route is considered the main route for spreading salmonellosis among pigs, although the upper respiratory tract and lungs have also been demonstrated to act as routes of entry into the host (Bonardi, 2017). Those bacterial cells survive the gastric juices' bactericidal effect and reach the intestine (Pradhan &

Table 1 Classification of salmonellae infecting pigs based on host range

Group	Serovar	Host
Host restricted serovar	*S.* Typhisuis	Pigs
Host adapted serovar	*S.* Choleraesuis	Pigs and humans
Host unrestricted serovars	*S.* Typhimurium *S.* Enteritidis	Humans, poultry, swine, bovines, and rodents Humans, poultry, swine, bovines, and rodents

Table 2 Virulence factors of *Salmonella* and their function

Virulence factor	Function
Fimbriae	Adhesion and invasion
Flagella	Adhesion and invasion
Virulence plasmids	Destabilizes the cytoskeleton and causes host cell cytotoxicity
Type I secretion systems	Invasion/adhesion
Type 3 secretion systems	Needle-like structure injects the effector proteins directly into the enterocyte
Lipid A part of LPS	Endotoxic shock
Salmonella cytolethal distending toxin	DNA damage in host cells
Superoxide dismutase	Prevent the killing of intracellular pathogens from reactive oxygen species
Iron acquisition system	Help in acquiring the iron in the eukaryotic host

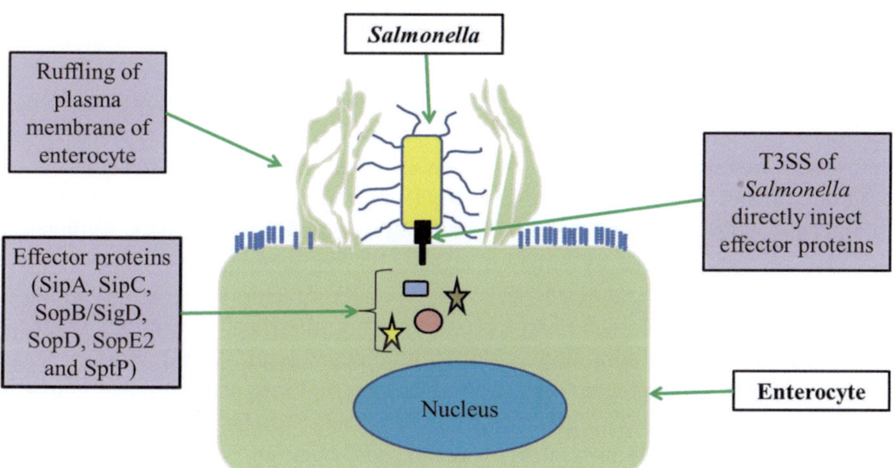

Fig. 1 Ruffling of the plasma membrane of enterocyte by *Salmonella* after injection of effector proteins using T3SS

Negi, 2019). The M-cells (Micro-fold cells) of intestine capture the *Salmonella* and present it to professional phagocytes, i.e., macrophage and dendritic cells, to perform phagocytosis to produce the antibody response against the pathogen. Moreover, *Salmonella* injects effector proteins (SipA, SipC, SopD, SopB/SigD, SopE2, SptP) directly into enterocytes using type III secretion system (T3SS), which results in reorganization of actin protein near the plasma membrane of enterocyte to give the appearance of cytoplasmic process (ruffles formation) as depicted in Fig. 1. The ruffling helps internalize the *Salmonella* into the enterocyte (Eng et al., 2015). Besides M-cell-mediated phagocytosis and T3SS1-mediated invasion, various additional virulence factors, including fimbriae as well as non-fimbrial adhesins upon the surface of *Salmonella*, might facilitate the attachment as well as the internalization of *Salmonella* (Singh, 2015). Following internalization, *Salmonella* endure as well as proliferate within a modified phagosome referred to as *Salmonella*-containing vacuole (SCV) (Diacovich et al., 2017). T3SS-1 and T3SS-2 are essential for the survival of *Salmonella* within enterocytes and phagocytes (Wang et al., 2020).

Salmonella's pathogen-associated molecular patterns (PAMPs), along with innate immune system's pattern recognition receptors (PRRs), combine to produce proinflammatory cytokines (IL-1β, IL-18). Inflammation of small and large intestines is brought on by pro-inflammatory cytokines (IL-1β, IL-18). In addition to causing diarrhea, acute inflammatory reactions may induce mucosal damage as well as ulceration. A systemic disease could result if *Salmonella* enters the bloodstream from the intestine. *Salmonella* species express a variety of PAMPs that PRRs can identify, including T3SS, flagella, fimbriae, LPS (Vi antigen), as well as bacterial DNA (De Jong et al., 2012). Relevant PRRs encompass nucleotide-binding and oligomerization domain (NOD)-like receptors along with Toll-like receptors (TLRs). The onset of invasive salmonellosis is significantly influenced by the toll-like receptor-4 (TLR-4). Mice lacking TLR4 had a higher vulnerability to salmonellosis. Flagellin and LPS are recognized by TLR5 and TLR4, respectively. However, Salmonella's cell surface contains the Vi antigen, which inhibits TLR4 from recognizing LPS (De Jong et al., 2012).

Clinical manifestations of salmonellosis in swine range from gastroenteritis to systemic illness. Host-unrestricted serovars (S. Typhimurium) primarily cause gastroenteritis, while host-adapted (S. Choleraesuis) and host-restricted (S. Typhisuis) serovars primarily cause systemic disease with septicemia. Pigs infected with S. Typhisuis and S. Choleraesuis serovars typically develop swine paratyphoid, a severe systemic illness marked by fever, shivering, diarrhea, respiratory distress, and depression that is sometimes fatal (Lamichhane et al., 2024). Within 36 to 48 hours of infection, infected pigs show clinical symptoms, and within 24 hours of exposure, they excrete S. Cholerasuis in their feces. Globally, S. Choleraesuis, including the variation Kunzendorf, was the most common serovar to be isolated from pigs. The primary symptoms of a *Salmonella* Choleraesuis infection are bluish discolorations of the ears, nose, chest, and abdomen, though they can also affect the feet, ventral area of the neck, and belly. Furthermore, there is either no diarrhea or very mild diarrhea, along with pyrexia, drowsiness, inappetence, moist cough, along with hard breathing (Bonardi, 2017). S. Cholerasuis infection in swine typically results in splenomegaly, gastric mucosa infarction, gastritis, along with erosions, enlarged as well as lung congestion and pneumonia, swollen mesenteric and gastrohepatic lymph nodes, occasional white foci of necrosis in liver, as well as enterocolitis. The presence of scattered foci of coagulative necrosis along with the infiltration of neutrophils along with histiocytes in liver characterize the primary microscopic lesions. Similar lesions have been discovered in spleen as well as lymph nodes. Fibrinoid thrombi are seen in pulmonary arteries, kidneys (affecting glomerular capillaries), stomach mucosa, and cyanotic cutaneous venules. The lungs may exhibit interstitial pneumonia or suppurative bronchopneumonia. Localized necrotizing encephalitis, as well as perivascular histiocytic infiltrates, are rare in conjunction with segmental necrotizing vasculitis. When *Salmonella* Choleraesuis is present, morbidity varies and mortality is significant (Soliani et al., 2023).

While fecal shedding can occur often or intermittently, even for prolonged periods, without any sign of clinical illness, pigs infected with uncontrolled *Salmonella* frequently show no symptoms. After infection with S. Typhimurium, similar clinical symptoms can be seen in sick pigs. These signs include fever, decreased feed intake, dehydration, inanition, as well as yellow diarrhea, which seldom contains blood (Hoelzer et al., 2011). Debilitating conditions include inadequate hygiene and viral infections that impair immunity, like pig reproductive and respiratory virus (PRRSV) as well as porcine circovirus 2 (PCV2), which might trigger onset of diseases (Watanabe et al., 2011; Soliani et al., 2023). Pigs often have a low mortality rate and can function as carriers along intermittent shedders for at least 5 months following full clinical recovery (Luppi et al., 2023). The organism is especially persistent in the tonsils, large intestine, and submandibular and ileocolic lymph nodes. In addition, stressful situations for the animals, such as handling, transportation, changing their diet, and lairage, can cause an increase in shedding. According to Massacci et al. (2020), some pigs may exhibit constipation and noticeable abdominal distension, while others may continue to be chronically wasted. According to a number of studies, *Salmonella* Typhimurium and its monophasic form, *Salmonella enterica* subsp. *enterica* serovar 1,4,[5],12:i:-, are more frequently implicated in human foodborne outbreaks than serotype S. Choleraesuis. This may be due to either host-adapted nature of S. Choleraesuis (Napoleoni et al., 2023).

Zoonotic Potential

Human salmonellosis is an emerging foodborne zoonosis. The burden of foodborne illnesses is enormous; it is believed that 550 million people, especially 220 million children under five (1 in 10) of the population, get sick each year as a result of eating tainted food (WHO, 2015). Most foodborne diseases cause self-limiting diarrhea in adults. However, they can cause serious systemic infection in young children, aged people, and immunocompromised individuals. Diarrheal infections are the most frequent ailment caused by consumption of improper food. A prominent foodborne pathogen is *Salmonella*. As to Wang et al. (2024), the Chinese CDC reports that *Salmonella* is responsible for 70–80% of bacterial foodborne infections. *Salmonella* lives in the intestinal tracts of many species, including cold-blooded animals, and serves as a reservoir for the pathogen without causing any symptoms. Although it can be transmitted from animals to people, direct or indirect contact between humans can also result in transmission. Figure 2 shows how *Salmonella* can spread from sick pigs to humans. The primary cause of human infection is believed to be ingesting food tainted with *Salmonella*, especially from animal sources. Eating food tainted with *Salmonella* is thought to cause about 80.3 million person cases of salmonellosis per year (Soliani et al., 2023). As pork consumption is highest compared to meat of other animals, swine acts as a potential reservoir of Salmonella to cause foodborne disease in humans. In recent decades, there have been numerous reports

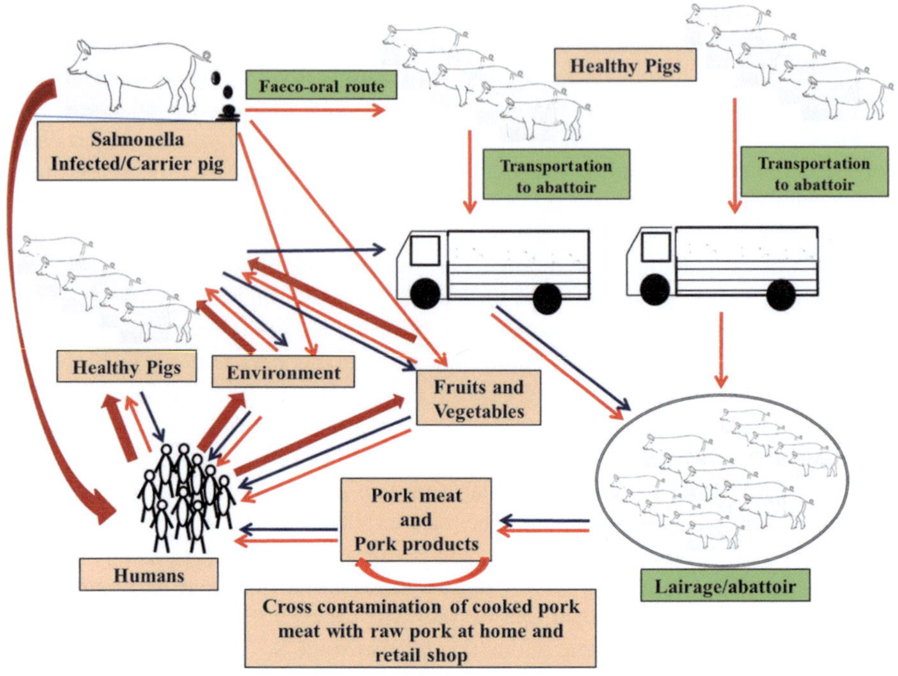

Fig. 2 Transmission of *Salmonella* from infected pigs to humans

of foodborne human salmonellosis outbreaks brought on by eating pig flesh tainted with *Salmonella*. During manufacturing and slaughter, fecal contact is typically the source of hog contamination. Pigs housed in abattoirs have been found to have a higher rate of *Salmonella* infection than pigs raised on farms. The reason may be the development of infection in carrier pigs and shedding of *Salmonella* in the feces, triggered by several stressful factors faced by carrier pigs during transportation and holding pens at abattoir. Additionally, these stressors make non-carrier pigs more vulnerable to emerging diseases (Martelli et al., 2021). Moreover, *Salmonella* infected workers can contaminate the pork during production and slaughtering (Bonardi, 2017). It is established that pork cooked at 165 °F or higher for at least 45 min is considered safer for consumption. However, cross-contamination by using the same knife and utensil to handle raw and cooked pork and improper storage may increase the number of *Salmonella* in cooked pork and pork meat products that may lead to human salmonellosis (Dang-Xuan et al., 2018).

CDC estimates that each year in the United States, salmonella infections result in 1.35 million illnesses, 26,500 hospitalizations, along 420 deaths. The main source of illnesses is contaminated food (Punchihewage-Don et al., 2022). In 2015, there were 902 foodborne disease cases reported in the United States, *Salmonella* is the second most common cause of foodborne illness, accounting for 34% of outbreaks alongside 39% of all infections. One of the top 3 main food categories in consideration had been found to be pork products (Dewey-Mattia, 2018). Serotypes

S. 1,4,[5],12:i:-, S. Derby as well as S. Typhimurium were responsible for 26.6%, 21.3%, as well as 14% *Salmonella* isolates from pig meat in European Union in 2019. Records from laboratory-based Enteric Disease Surveillance system show that since 2011, the incidence rate of S. 1,4,[5],12:i:-human infections has elevated by 580% in the United States (Roasto et al., 2023). S. Typhimurium (9.8%) along with S. 1,4,[5],12:i:- (4.7%) were two of the five most isolated serovars among 46,623 human salmonellosis cases that have been documented in the United States in 2016 (CDC, 2024). Additionally, foodborne salmonellosis is thought to cost the US $2.7 billion annually, with pig producers suffering losses of about $100 million. Human cases of salmonellosis and outbreaks associated with pork consumption in the United States as well as Europe are primarily caused by S. Typhimurium along with its monophasic variation *Salmonella enterica* subsp. *enterica* 1,4,[5],12:i:-, although S. Derby is also known to have a lower prevalence. In 2018, S. Typhimurium (9%), followed by S. 1,4,[5],12:i:- (1.6%), was the second most common serovar implicated in human outbreaks in Europe. Pork products accounted for the majority of human salmonellosis outbreaks in the European Union in 2020, followed by eggs and egg-derived products. The EU reports around 91,000 human cases of salmonellosis annually, with associated expenditures of up to €3 billion (EFSA, 2023), 10–20% of which are linked to pig intake (Soumet et al., 2022).

Clinical Manifestations and Treatment of Human Salmonellosis

Salmonella causes self-limiting gastroenteritis in the majority of cases. However, *Salmonella* enters the bloodstream in some situations and causes significant systemic infection (enteric fever). The result of human salmonellosis, whether self-limiting gastroenteritis or a major systemic infection, is usually determined by the competency of the host immune system and determinants of virulence factors present in *Salmonella* isolates (Worley, 2023).

The incubation duration for food poisoning caused by *Salmonella* depends on the bacterial dosage. Frequent symptoms include vomiting, nausea, diarrhea, as well as abdominal discomfort, and often appear 6–48 h after contaminated food or drink is consumed. Headache, abdominal cramping, and myalgia are common symptoms; nonetheless, diarrhea is the primary symptom. In addition, chills along with fever (38–39 °C) are typical. Fever, as well as diarrhea, can last anywhere from 2 to 7 days, though this is not always the case (CDC, 2024).

Serious systemic salmonellosis cases are known as enteric fevers. The symptoms appear after a 10- to 14-days incubation period. Gastroenteritis is a common precursor to enteric fevers and typically goes away before systemic illness manifests. Enteric fevers cause nonspecific symptoms such as anorexia, fever, myalgias, headache, as well as constipation. Enteric fevers can be fatal if not treated promptly with antibiotics (Neupane et al., 2021).

Rehydration and electrolyte replacement therapy are used to treat serious infections of *Salmonella*. Electrolytes, including sodium, potassium, and chloride ions that are lost through vomiting and diarrhea, are replaced by electrolyte replacement treatment. Because of the possibility of Salmonella strains becoming resistant to antibiotics, consistent antibiotic therapy is not recommended for mild to moderate infections in healthy individuals. In critically sick patients, treating these resistant bacteria is extremely challenging. However, antibiotic treatment should be provided promptly in case of systemic infection and those who fall into high-risk groups such as infants, aged persons, and immunocompromised patients.

Prevention of Transmission of *Salmonella* from Swine to Humans

As mentioned above, *Salmonella* is widely distributed in the environment. Moreover, many animal species, including cold-blooded animals, have *Salmonella* in their intestine. And, under favorable conditions, *Salmonella* can survive for several years in the environment. Therefore, *Salmonella* is particularly hard to eradicate. Reducing the amount of *Salmonella* in food animals can aid in the decrease of human salmonellosis cases and outbreaks because cattle and poultry serve as significant reservoirs of the pathogen. Here, we will focus on controlling *Salmonella* in pigs to reduce human exposure (Fig. 3).

The first and foremost thing is to prevent the introduction of *Salmonella* in farms. This can be achieved by taking strict biosecurity measures such as pigs being purchased from reputed and *Salmonella*-free farms, quarantine facilities for newly introduced pigs/piglets, testing of newly introduced pigs/piglets to confirm the *Salmonella*-negative status, foot bath at the entrance of pig farm, disinfection of vehicle before they enter into pig farms, outsider shouldn't be permitted to enter into farm, farm personnel must be provided with separate cloths for working in farm, and there must be regular testing of workers to confirm their *Salmonella* negative status. It is essential to observe the new piglets periodically for any illness indications during quarantine. The farm should be constructed to be rodent, wild animal, and vermin-proof; the equipment shouldn't be shared with other farms. The feed should be acquired from feed mills or sources with an effective bacterial control system to guarantee the *Salmonella*-free feed status. It is imperative that animals, both domestic and wild, are prohibited from entering feed stores. Feed should be kept dry to prevent the multiplication of *Salmonella* in feed. The mash feed is beneficial over pelleted feed as the pellets facilitate *Salmonella* colonization by stimulating the secretion of mucins. Feed sanitization is a good practice to control *Salmonella* in farms. Safe drinking water is equally crucial as safe animal feed free of Salmonella. This can be done through disinfecting drinking water. Regular cleaning and disinfection of the tanks, pipelines, and drinkers is essential. The percentage of pigs who shed *Salmonella* and the amounts of *Salmonella* in their guts may be decreased by adding esterified formic acid to the drinking water 5 days before slaughter (Bernad-Roche et al., 2023).

Despite various preventive measures, if *Salmonella* cases appear on farms, in that case, focus should be given to the segregation of infected pigs, treatment of infected pigs, and limiting the further spread of infection to healthy pigs by

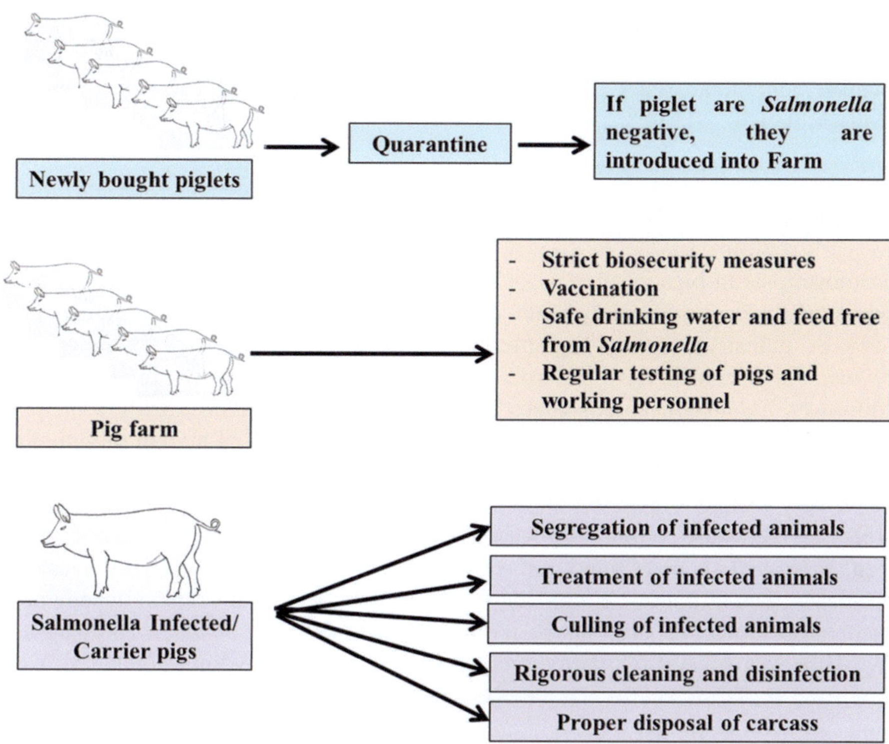

Fig. 3 Different ways to reduce the exposure of pigs to *Salmonella* to prevent the transmission of *Salmonella* to humans

slaughtering the infected pigs using the humane method of slaughter, and disposing of the carcass in a scientific manner. Everything that was in contact with infected pigs should be cleaned up and disinfected rigorously. The farm personnel and remaining healthy animals must be tested against *Salmonella* to confirm the *Salmonella*-negative status to limit infection within the farm. Vaccination is an effective method for reducing the prevalence of *Salmonella* in the pig population. A live attenuated S. Typhimurium strain vaccine is efficient in controlling S. Typhimurium infections in pig herds (Alborali et al., 2017). To prevent S. Choleraesuis infection, immunization with an attenuated S. Typhimurium strain followed by a booster vaccination with inactivated S. Choleraesuis outperformed inactivated S. Choleraesuis vaccine alone (Alborali et al., 2017). Treatment of salmonellosis in pigs using antibiotics is ineffective, as pigs recover from diseases after treatment with antibiotics, but they still shed *Salmonella* in their feces. Moreover, antibiotics used in human medicine are not recommended for use in food animals to prevent antibiotic resistance.

The stress factors that the pigs are subjected to during transportation and in the lairages alter the gut microbiome and the animal's immunity, possibly leading to Salmonella shedding in huge numbers. This makes it more likely that pigs from different farms may come into contact with one another in the lairages and during their transportation to the abattoir. As a result, thorough cleaning and proper hygiene management in abattoirs can help to prevent carcass and meat contamination (Massacci et al., 2020).

Conclusion

Salmonellosis in pigs is often associated with self-limiting gastroenteritis; it may occasionally lead to severe systemic infections. It has a serious economic impact on the pigs' industry due to its high morbidity rate, high mortality rate (in the case of *Salmonella* Choleraesuis), retarded growth, and treatment of infected pigs. Moreover, *Salmonella* is considered a major zoonotic foodborne pathogen. Pork and pork-derived items have been implicated in the majority of human salmonellosis infections and outbreaks. It is regarded as an emerging foodborne disease and has a very serious impact on human health. *S.* Typhimurium, *S.* 1,4,[5],12:i:-, as well as *S.* Derby are common serovars isolated from pork meat for human consumption. *Salmonella* is distributed in the environment and intestines of many livestock species as well as poultry. Moreover, it can survive for several years in the environment under ambient conditions. So, complete eradication of *Salmonella* is challenging. However, several mitigation techniques can be used to stop *Salmonella* from occurring on farms and in slaughterhouses, including farm biosecurity, the provision of uncontaminated feed, quarantine of recently introduced animals, lowering stress factors during transportation, vaccination, and cleaning and disinfection procedures. Besides, creating awareness can help prevent cross-contamination at retail shops and homes. Also, surveillance of *Salmonella* along the food chain allows us to link human cases to specific foodstuffs that enable us to identify the source of *Salmonella* and to adopt appropriate mitigation strategies. Human salmonellosis is an emerging foodborne zoonotic disease that can be effectively addressed by a coordinated effort among several stakeholders, including farmers, veterinarians involved in animal health, and food safety and regulatory organizations.

References

Alborali, G. L., Ruggeri, J., Pesciaroli, M., Martinelli, N., Chirullo, B., Ammendola, S., Battistoni, A., Ossiprandi, M. C., Corradi, A., & Pasquali, P. (2017). Prime-boost vaccination with attenuated salmonella Typhimurium ΔznuABC and inactivated salmonella Choleraesuis is protective against salmonella Choleraesuis challenge infection in piglets. *BMC Veterinary Research, 13*(1), 284.

Bernad-Roche, M., Marín-Alcalá, C. M., Vico, J. P., & Mainar-Jaime, R. C. (2023). Salmonella control in fattening pigs through the use of esterified formic acid in drinking water shortly before slaughter. *Animals, 13*(18), 2814.

Bonardi, S. (2017). Salmonella in the pork production chain and its impact on human health in the European Union. *Epidemiology & Infection, 145*(8), 1513–1526.

Centers for Disease Control and Prevention (CDC). (2024). National Salmonella Surveillance Annual Report, 2016. Atlanta, Georgia: US Department of Health and Human Services,

CDC. Available online: https://www.cdc.gov/nationalsurveillance/pdfs/2016-Salmonella-report-508.pdf. Accessed on 15 Mar 2024

Cheng, R. A., Eade, C. R., & Wiedmann, M. (2019). Embracing diversity: Differences in virulence mechanisms, disease severity, and host adaptations contribute to the success of nontyphoidal salmonella as a foodborne pathogen. *Frontiers in Microbiology, 10*, 439852.

Dang-Xuan, S., Nguyen-Viet, H., Pham-Duc, P., Grace, D., Unger, F., Nguyen-Hai, N., Nguyen-Tien, T., & Makita, K. (2018). Simulating cross-contamination of cooked pork with salmonella enterica from raw pork through home kitchen preparation in Vietnam. *International Journal of Environmental Research and Public Health, 15*(10), 2324.

De Jong, H. K., Parry, C. M., van der Poll, T., & Wiersinga, W. J. (2012). Host–pathogen interaction in invasive salmonellosis

Dewey-Mattia, D. (2018). Surveillance for foodborne disease outbreaks – United States, 2009–2015. *MMWR Surveillance Summaries, 67*, 1.

Diacovich, L., Lorenzi, L., Tomassetti, M., Méresse, S., & Gramajo, H. (2017). The infectious intracellular lifestyle of salmonella enterica relies on the adaptation to nutritional conditions within the salmonella-containing vacuole. *Virulence, 8*(6), 975–992.

EFSA (2023). "Salmonella." European Food Safety Authority. https://www.efsa.europa.eu/en/topics/topic/salmonella. Accessed 7 Aug 2023

Eng, S. K., Pusparajah, P., Ab Mutalib, N. S., Ser, H. L., Chan, K. G., & Lee, L. H. (2015). Salmonella: A review on pathogenesis, epidemiology and antibiotic resistance. *Frontiers in Life Science, 8*(3), 284–293.

Galán-Relaño, Á., Valero Díaz, A., Huerta Lorenzo, B., et al. (2023). Salmonella and salmonellosis: An update on public health implications and control strategies. *Animals, 13*(23), 3666.

Grantcharova, N., Peters, V., Monteiro, C., Zakikhany, K., & Römling, U. (2010). Bistable expression of CsgD in biofilm development of salmonella enterica serovar typhimurium. *Journal of Bacteriology, 192*(2), 456–466.

Harrell, J. E., Hahn, M. M., D'Souza, S. J., Vasicek, E. M., Sandala, J. L., Gunn, J. S., & McLachlan, J. B. (2021). Salmonella biofilm formation, chronic infection, and immunity within the intestine and hepatobiliary tract. *Frontiers in Cellular and Infection Microbiology, 10*, 624622.

Heredia, N., & García, S. (2018). Animals as sources of food-borne pathogens: A review. *Animal Nutrition, 4*(3), 250–255.

Hoelzer, K., Moreno Switt, A. I., & Wiedmann, M. (2011). Animal contact as a source of human non-typhoidal salmonellosis. *Veterinary Research, 42*, 1–28.

Hoffmann, S. A., Maculloch, B., & Batz, M. (2015). Economic burden of major foodborne illnesses acquired in the United States

Ibarra, J. A., & Steele-Mortimer, O. (2009). Salmonella–the ultimate insider. Salmonella virulence factors that modulate intracellular survival. *Cellular Microbiology, 11*(11), 1579–1586.

Kuria, J. K. (2023). Salmonellosis in food and companion animals and its public health importance. In *Salmonella-perspectives for low-cost prevention, control and treatment*. IntechOpen.

Lamichhane, B., Mawad, A. M., Saleh, M., Kelley, W. G., Harrington, P. J., Lovestad, C. W., Amezcua, J., Sarhan, M. M., El Zowalaty, M. E., Ramadan, H., & Morgan, M. (2024). Salmonellosis: An overview of epidemiology, pathogenesis, and innovative approaches to mitigate the antimicrobial resistant infections. *Antibiotics, 13*(1), 76.

Lou, L., Zhang, P., Piao, R., & Wang, Y. (2019). Salmonella pathogenicity Island 1 (SPI-1) and its complex regulatory network. *Frontiers in Cellular and Infection Microbiology, 9*, 270.

Luppi, A., D'Annunzio, G., Torreggiani, C., & Martelli, P. (2023). Diagnostic approach to enteric disorders in pigs. *Animals, 13*(3), 338.

Lyu, N., Feng, Y., Pan, Y., Huang, H., Liu, Y., Xue, C., Zhu, B., & Hu, Y. (2021). Genomic characterization of salmonella enterica isolates from retail meat in Beijing, China. *Frontiers in Microbiology, 12*, 636332.

Martelli, F., Oastler, C., Barker, A., Jackson, G., Smith, R. P., & Davies, R. (2021). Abattoir-based study of salmonella prevalence in pigs at slaughter in Great Britain. *Epidemiology & Infection, 149*, e218.

Massacci, F. R., Morelli, A., Cucco, L., Castinel, A., Ortenzi, R., Tofani, S., Pezzotti, G., Estellé, J., Paniccià, M., & Magistrali, C. F. (2020). Transport to the slaughterhouse affects the salmonella shedding and modifies the fecal microbiota of finishing pigs. *Animals, 10*(4), 676.

Napoleoni, M., Villa, L., Barco, L., Lucarelli, C., Tiengo, A., Baggio, G., Dionisi, A. M., Angellotti, A., Ferretti, E., Ruggeri, S., & Staffolani, M. (2023). Monophasic variant of salmonella Typhimurium 4,[5], 12: I:-(ACSSuGmTmpSxt type) outbreak in Central Italy linked to the consumption of a roasted pork product (Porchetta). *Microorganisms, 11*(10), 2567.

Neupane, D. P., Dulal, H. P., & Song, J. (2021). Enteric fever diagnosis: Current challenges and future directions. *Pathogens, 10*(4), 410.

Pradhan, D., & Negi, V. D. (2019). Stress-induced adaptations in salmonella: A ground for shaping its pathogenesis. *Microbiological Research, 229*, 126311.

Punchihewage-Don, A. J., Hawkins, J., Adnan, A. M., Hashem, F., & Parveen, S. (2022). The outbreaks and prevalence of antimicrobial resistant salmonella in poultry in the United States: An overview. *Heliyon, 8*(11), e11571.

Roasto, M., Bonardi, S., Mäesaar, M., Alban, L., Gomes-Neves, E., Vieira-Pinto, M., Vågsholm, I., Elias, T., Lindegaard, L. L., & Blagojevic, B. (2023). Salmonella enterica prevalence, serotype diversity, antimicrobial resistance and control in the European pork production chain. *Trends in Food Science & Technology, 131*, 210–219.

Ruby, T., McLaughlin, L., Gopinath, S., & Monack, D. (2012). Salmonella's long-term relationship with its host. *FEMS Microbiology Reviews, 36*(3), 600–615.

Shikov, A. E., Belousova, M. E., Belousov, M. V., Nizhnikov, A. A., & Antonets, K. S. (2022). Salmonella-based biorodenticides: Past applications and current contradictions. *International Journal of Molecular Sciences, 23*(23), 14595.

Singh, V. (2015). Host factors and compartments accessed by Salmonella Typhimurium for intracellular growth and survival

Sokaribo, A. S., Hansen, E. G., McCarthy, M., Desin, T. S., Waldner, L. L., MacKenzie, K. D., Mutwiri, G., Jr., Herman, N. J., Herman, D. J., Wang, Y., & White, A. P. (2020). Metabolic activation of CsgD in the regulation of salmonella biofilms. *Microorganisms, 8*(7), 964.

Soliani, L., Rugna, G., Prosperi, A., Chiapponi, C., & Luppi, A. (2023). Salmonella infection in pigs: Disease, prevalence, and a link between swine and human health. *Pathogens, 12*(10), 1267.

Soumet, C., Kerouanton, A., Bridier, A., Rose, N., Denis, M., Attig, I., Haddache, N., & Fablet, C. (2022). Report, Salmonella excretion level in pig farms and impact of quaternary ammonium compounds based disinfectants on Escherichia coli antibiotic resistance

Wang, M., Qazi, I. H., Wang, L., Zhou, G., & Han, H. (2020). Salmonella virulence and immune escape. *Microorganisms, 8*(3), 407.

Wang, Z., Huang, C., Liu, Y., Chen, J., Yin, R., Jia, C., Kang, X., Zhou, X., Liao, S., Jin, X., & Feng, M. (2024). Salmonellosis outbreak archive in China: Data collection and assembly. *Scientific Data, 11*(1), 244.

Watanabe, T. T. N., Zlotowski, P., Oliveira, L. G. S. D., Rolim, V. M., Gomes, M. J. P., Snel, G., & Driemeier, D. (2011). Rectal stenosis in pigs associated with salmonella Typhimurium and porcine circovirus type 2 (PCV2) infection. *Pesquisa Veterinária Brasileira, 31*, 511–515.

WHO. (2015). WHO's first ever global estimates of foodborne diseases find children under 5 account for almost one third of deaths. Retrieved from https://www.who.int/news/item/03-12-2015-who-s-first-ever-global-estimates-of-foodborne-diseases-find-children-under-5-account-for-almost-one-third-of-deaths

Worley, M. J. (2023). *Salmonella* bloodstream infections. *Infectious Diseases and Tropical Medicine, 8*(11), 487.

Hepatitis E Virus (HEV) Unveiled: A Comprehensive Examination from Genotypes, Epidemiology and Zoonotic Challenges to Public Health Strategies

Indu Reddy Bode, Abhilash Surakaram, and M. Gowtham

Abstract

Hepatitis E virus (HEV) is one of the significant global health problems, causing acute hepatitis with the potential for severe outcomes such as fulminant liver failure, particularly in pregnant women and individuals with underlying liver diseases. HEV exhibits genetic diversity, comprising four main genotypes with varying host ranges and transmission dynamics. Genotypes 1a and 2a are primarily human-restricted, while genotypes 3a and 4a circulate among animals like pigs, leading to zoonotic infections in humans. The epidemiology of HEV is complex, with waterborne transmission being a major route in developing regions and zoonotic transmission playing a significant role in developed nations. Recent evidence suggests a broader host range for HEV, including wildlife such as deer, bears, and camels, raising concerns about inter-species transmission and food safety. Transmission of HEV through blood transfusions and food products, especially undercooked or raw meat from infected animals, underscores the importance of robust surveillance and preventive measures. Control strategies focus on thorough cooking of meat, improved screening of blood donors, and enhancing food safety practices. Understanding the virology, genotypic variations, epidemiological patterns, zoonotic potentials, and transmission dynamics of HEV is crucial for developing targeted interventions and control strategies to reduce the burden of HEV-related diseases globally.

I. R. Bode
JRF, DBT-One Health Project, ICAR-National Meat Research Institute, Hyderabad, Telangana, India

A. Surakaram · M. Gowtham (✉)
Division of Veterinary Microbiology, ICAR-IVRI, Bareilly, Uttar Pradesh, India

R. Deb et al. (eds.), *Emerging Zoonotic Threats from Swine*,
https://doi.org/10.1007/978-981-96-7407-7_10

Keywords

Hepatitis E virus (HEV) · Epidemiology · Genotypes · Zoonoses

Introduction

Hepatitis E virus (HEV) is a significant cause of acute hepatitis globally, characterized by liver inflammation resulting from HEV infection. This hepatotropic virus is responsible for both epidemic outbreaks and sporadic cases, transmitted primarily through the enteric route. HEV exhibits genetic diversity, comprising at least eight distinct genotypes. Genotypes 1a and 2a are restricted to human hosts, while genotypes 3a and 4a circulate among various animals such as pigs, wild boars, and deer, occasionally infecting humans without causing clinical disease (Smith et al., 2020).

Globally, HEV is associated with approximately 20.0 million infections annually, leading to 3.3 million symptomatic cases and 57,000 deaths (WHO, 2024). The clinical spectrum of HEV infection can vary from mild to severe, potentially culminating in fulminant liver failure and mortality if left untreated. While initially considered an acute infection, chronic HEV cases have been identified in individuals with chronic liver disease (CLD) and recipients of kidney or liver transplants (Nan et al. 2017).

Despite advancements in awareness, the origins of HEV and its pathogenesis remain complex and not fully elucidated. HEV was first discovered in 1983 by a Russian virologist, who conducted electron microscopy examinations on a fecal extract from previously infected soldiers. Transmission of HEV primarily occurs via the gastrointestinal route, with infected individuals shedding the virus in their stools. Contaminated drinking water is a common mode of transmission (Turlewicz-Podbielska et al., 2023).

HEV infections typically resolve within 2–6 weeks, but in rare cases, they can progress to fulminant hepatitis or acute liver failure, which can be fatal (Azman et al., 2019). The prevalence of HEV has evolved, with once uncommon occurrences in developed nations now considered endemic, particularly due to zoonotic transmissions from genotypes 3 and 4. In developing nations, waterborne transmission of HEV-induced acute hepatitis is prevalent in areas with poor sanitation (Ferri & Vergara, 2021).

The single-stranded RNA structure of HEV contributes to its high mutation rate, exceeding 1.5 base substitutions per site per year, comparable to the hepatitis C virus (HCV). This rapid mutation rate leads to the diversification of HEV variants identified in various animal reservoirs, complicating disease management and control efforts (Nicot et al., 2018).

This comprehensive exploration will delve into the intricate virology, diverse genotypes, epidemiological patterns, zoonotic transmissions, diagnostic modalities, clinical manifestations, complications, and therapeutic interventions associated with HEV infection, drawing insights from current available scientific data and research.

Discovery of HEV

The discovery of hepatitis E gained prominence during the investigation of the 1978 Kashmir epidemic of hepatitis (Nicot et al., 2018). This region faced severe weather conditions, lacked basic healthcare infrastructure, and had limited advanced investigative facilities. The journey leading to this discovery unfolds a compelling narrative of human endeavour, encompassing complexities, challenges, successes, and setbacks (Khuroo et al., 2016).

Dr. Mohammad S. Khuroo began investigating a jaundice outbreak in a town 50 km from Srinagar, Kashmir, India, in November 1978. About 600,000 people lived in 200 villages that were impacted by the pandemic, which led to about 52,000 instances of icteric illness and 1700 deaths. Pregnant women were especially at risk, and numerous deaths were reported. An enterically transmitted Non-A, Non-B Hepatitis (NANBH) was discovered after a rigorous 14-year house-to-house research of this epidemic and subsequent isolated cases, which led to multiple outbreaks in Kashmir. The disease primarily afflicted young adults between the ages of 15 and 45. The link between this illness and pregnancy was an interesting discovery made during this study (Khuroo et al., 2016). There was a high rate of foetal and perinatal mortality due to the agent's vertical transmission (Wang & Meng, 2021). It is noteworthy that the illness was self-limiting and did not lead to cirrhosis, chronic hepatitis, or chronic viremia (Doceul et al., 2016). Furthermore, throughout the course of the 14 years, a sizable section of the population lost their IgG antibodies. An unnamed human hepatitis virus was thought to be the source of the illness. At the same time, it was discovered that a sporadic disease that contributed to almost half of the population's acute hepatitis cases had the same epidemiological and clinical characteristics as the epidemic disease (Khuroo et al., 2016).

According to Wang and Meng (2021), Russian military soldiers stationed in Afghanistan had a comparable outbreak of NANBH. The epidemiological features of this outbreak were similar to those of the Kashmir pandemic in 1978. In a self-experiment, Dr. Mikhail S. Balayan consumed a combination of stool extracts from nine individuals who were afflicted (Nan et al., 2017). He experienced jaundice, increased liver function tests, and severe acute hepatitis 36 days after consumption. Immunoelectron microscopy revealed the presence of virus-like particles (VLP) in stool samples taken on the 28th, 43rd, and 45th days. The suspected agent was then used to experimentally infect a number of monkeys, and the physicochemical characteristics of the virus were examined (Khuroo et al., 2016).

However, because of the poor yield of VLP in the infectious material, cloning the virus originally proved difficult. The discovery that significant quantities of VLPs could be extracted from bile extracted from infected primates helped to overcome this challenge. After Reyes et al. (1990) succeeded in partially cloning the virus, Tam et al. (1991) sequenced the 7.2 kb full-length HEV genome and developed an enzyme immunoassay-based diagnostic test.

Taxonomic Categorization of Varied HEV Strains

Hepatitis E virus (HEV) virions have a 7.2 kb poly-adenylated, capped mRNA-like genome. There are three main open reading frames (ORFs) in the HEV genome that are shared by all genotypes, and an extra ORF4 has only been found in genotype 1a HEV so far. HEV-ORF1 encodes non-structural proteins, primarily a replicase that is essential for replication, and is translated straight from its genome. Conversely, ORF2 and ORF3, which are translated from subgenomic RNA, partially overlap with one another (or, in certain Hepeviridae species, entirely overlap). While ORF3 encodes a multifunctional protein that is presumably a class I viroporin and necessary for virion release, ORF2 encodes the capsid protein, a key component of virion (Mori & Matsuura, 2011).

In the recent studies, it was discovered that genotype 1a HEV is the only one that synthesizes a novel ORF4 driven by a putative internal ribosome entry site (IRES)-like sequence (Nair et al., 2016). Additionally, two cis-reactive elements (CRE) that are essential for replication may be present in the HEV genome, according to sequence analysis (Cao et al., 2010; Parvez, 2015). The second CRE may act as a promoter for subgenomic RNA synthesis since it generates a stem-loop structure in the intergenic region between ORF1 and ORF2 (Cao et al., 2010).

The prototype strain SAR-55 from Pakistan was used as a primary sequence for comparison with other isolates, such as the Burmese strain from India and several Chinese isolates, after the hepatitis E virus (HEV) was confirmed to be the causative agent for hepatitis E (Aye et al., 1992; Tsarev et al., 1992; Bi et al., 1993). Referring to Fig. 1, these previous HEV isolates were categorized as genotype 1 HEV (now known as human HEV1a of Paslahepevirus balayani virus) because they shared more than 90% of their identities. The Asian HEV isolate was classified as "Old World" HEV, while the Mexican strain was initially regarded as the "New World" strain since it originated in Central America (Reyes et al., 1991). For ORF1, ORF2, and ORF3, the Mexican strain and the SAR-55 strain had 84%, 93%, and 87% amino acid similarity, respectively, when "Old World" and "New World" HEV sequences were analysed without nucleotide sequences within the ORF1 hypervariable region (Huang et al., 1992). Because they were more comparable to the Mexican strain, later investigation of more recent HEV isolates from Africa revealed that they were genotype 2 HEV, or HEV2a of the Paslahepevirus virus (Chatterjee et al., 1997). However, according to Kaiser et al. (2017), there are now just two full sequences of genotype 2 HEV accessible.

Identification of swine HEV linked to human hepatitis E was a major finding in 1997 (Meng et al., 1997). Phylogenetic investigations revealed a close yet unique relationship between swine HEV and earlier human HEV strains. The 1997 US swine HEV isolate, which represented another HEV genotype (genotype 3 HEV, now known as swine HEV3a of Paslahepevirus virus), shared close amino acid identity with novel HEV isolates (strains US-1 and US-2) recovered from acute hepatitis E patients in the United States (Kwo et al., 1997; Schlauder et al., 1998).

A heterogeneous genotype 4 HEV group was established in 1999 after fresh HEV isolates from Chinese patients were discovered to be a fourth HEV genotype

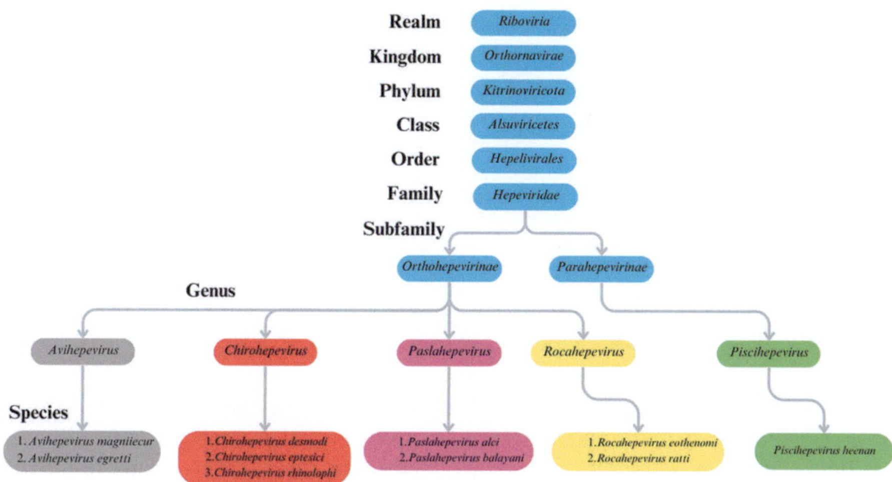

Fig. 1 ICTV classification of family *Hepeviridae*

based on phylogenetic analysis. At the same time, identical HEV isolates linked to Chinese genotype 4 were reported in Japan. The need for additional clarification in genotype descriptions is highlighted by the close sequence identity between swine HEV isolates and genotype 4 HEV, which has been demonstrated to be zoonotic (Takahashi et al., 2003, 2012; Nishizawa et al., 2003).

A new HEV classification system was proposed in 2020 under the Hepeviridae family to offer a single classification for a variety of HEV isolates (Smith et al., 2020).

The species Paslahepevirus was used to reclassify all four of the primary HEV genotypes (1–4) that infect people (Smith et al., 2020). Previously known as genotype 5 and genotype 6 HEVs, two new genotypes (5 and 6) were also discovered in Japanese wild boar. It's crucial to remember that not all HEV isolates from wild boar fall into genotypes 5 and 6; the majority are categorized as zoonotic potential HEVs with genotypes 3 and 4 (Sato et al., 2011). Moreover, genotype 7 of Paslahepevirus was assigned to HEV strains obtained from camels in the Middle East that showed notable nucleotide variations from the other genotypes (Smith et al., 2020; Woo et al., 2014). A Middle Eastern liver transplant recipient who contracted camel HEV showed signs of zoonotic transmission (Lee et al., 2016). Furthermore, because of their genetic differences from genotype 7 camel HEV, recently identified HEV isolates from Chinese bactrian camels were provisionally assigned to a new genotype 8 (Woo et al., 2016; Sridhar et al., 2017).

In addition to the HEV genotypes that infect mammals, two HEV-like virus isolates from chicken and cutthroat trout are currently classified under the genera Avihepevirus and Piscihepevirus and the species Avihepevirus magniiecurv and Piscihepevirus heenan (Huang et al., 2002; Batts et al., 2011; Smith et al., 2016, 2020). Less than 50% of the nucleotides of known human HEVs are shared by avian HEV-like viruses, or avian HEV. However, in contrast to mammalian HEVs, their viral capsid proteins have both common and unique antigenic epitopes, which can cause a variety of pathogenesis in chickens or hens, such as subclinical infection, reduced egg production, and hepatitis-splenomegaly syndrome (Haqshenas et al., 2001; Zhao et al., 2017; Gerber et al., 2015). Cutthroat trout virus (CTV) is another distant relative of HEV that belongs to the distinct genus Piscihepevirus and shows less sequence similarity to mammalian HEV than avian HEV (Batts et al., 2011; Smith et al., 2016). Even though there is no proof that avian HEV or CTV can infect people or animals, more investigation is required to fully comprehend the mechanics of their possible transmission.

Epidemiology of HEV

Globally, the HEV is a potential cause of hepatitis, responsible for over 50% of acute hepatitis cases in the endemic regions. Transmission primarily occurs via contaminated water in unsanitary conditions, facilitating the fecal-oral route transmission of both HEV1 and HEV2 resulting in large-scale outbreaks of HEV infection. While HEV infections are typically self-limiting, severe outcomes can occur, especially in pregnant individuals. Screening strategies for HEV infection have undergone significant advancements, leading to improved detection and surveillance. Zoonotic transmission of HEV3 and HEV4 through animal reservoirs has been identified as a source of periodic cases, further complicating the epidemiological landscape of HEV infection (Lozano et al., 2012).

The HEV is a common cause of acute liver infections. HEV exhibits characteristics with hepatitis A in its watery transmission mechanism and was originally classified as non-A non-B hepatitis. Epidemics are primarily associated with genotypes 1 and 2 in underdeveloped countries (Donnelly et al., 2017). However, HEV has now become a leading cause of acute liver failure and icteric hepatitis in underdeveloped regions globally. Its estimated annual occurrence of HEV infections is around 20 million, leading to 56,600 deaths approximately. In Western countries, locally acquired HEV infections have been associated with genotypes 3, 4, and 5 over the past decade (Lozano et al., 2012).

In developed countries, HEV is gaining recognition as an important pathogen, with increasing reports of confirmed cases. This underscores the necessity of considering HEV in the differential diagnosis of liver diseases, as diagnostic capabilities and surveillance efforts continue to improve.

Zoonotic Transmission of HEV

Initially, the understanding was that HEV infection was exclusive to humans, with average range of 0.5–3.0% mortality rates, but rising to approximately 30% among pregnant women. While initially hepatitis E is predominantly prevalent in developing nations (Khuroo et al., 2016), subsequent evidence of sporadic hepatitis E infections in developed countries challenged this notion, indicating a wider global distribution and host range (Anheyer-Behmenburg et al., 2017).

HEV-induced hepatitis E has become a prominent and powerful zoonotic viral illness. Cross-species transmission from animals is the main way that HEV is spread to humans in many areas. Sporadic occurrences of hepatitis E in affluent countries can be caused by contact with people who have travelled from endemic areas or by transmission from those regions, rather than the traditional feco-oral route. Additionally, compared to registered blood donors in Spain and Germany, those working with pigs, such as veterinary officers, pig labourers, and abattoir workers, had greater prevalences of serum antibodies reactive to HEV (Galiana et al., 2008; Krumbholz et al., 2012). This implies that people who have direct or indirect contact with pigs are more likely to be exposed to and infected with HEV.

HEV sequences from hepatitis E patients are very similar to those from swine HEV isolates (Widen et al., 2011). Eating pork products, especially those that contain pig liver, is linked to the high incidence of HEV infections, which are known to occur in pig farms. Hunting and consuming game meat are associated with exposure to HEVs, and wild boars are also known to contain HEV. Contact exposure with infected animals is another possible mode of transmission, since specialized occupations with animal reservoirs, such as hunters, forestry workers, veterinarians, and pig farmers, have a higher seroprevalence than the equivalent general population. The maintenance and spread of HEV in both reservoirs may be influenced by interactions between domestic and wild suids (Pavio et al., 2017). This raises the possibility of a connection between swine and human HEV infections, emphasizes the role of zoonotic transmission in the disease's progression, and clarifies the causes of autochthonous HEV infection, which is depicted in Fig. 2.

Animal Reservoirs

The first experimental proof of HEV-3 infections in domestic pigs was shown using a human HEV-3 strain in a seminal work by Baleyan and his coworkers in 1990. HEV-3 was later discovered in farmed pigs in the United States in 1997. A wide variety of mammalian species may serve as zoonotic reservoirs for HEV-3 and HEV-4, despite pigs being recognized as the main reservoirs for these viruses. Evidence of HEV infection has also been observed in a variety of domestic and wild animals (Arnaboldi et al., 2021). However, the entire range of species acting as HEV reservoirs is still not entirely known. Goats, sheep, and cattle have all been found to carry HEV-3 and HEV-4. Furthermore, HEV-3 and HEV-4 tests in rabbits have been positive. Although there have been signs of seroprevalence among zoo and captive pet animals, HEV RNA has not been found in these species, making it more difficult to identify their genotype with certainty (Li et al., 2022; Caballero-Gomez et al., 2022).

Additionally, HEV has been detected in a number of species of the Bovidae family, including yak and bison, as well as the Cervidae family, including moose and Sika deer. HEV detection in cetaceans has also been reported. Interestingly, more and more reports are being made about novel animal species that test positive for HEV RNA and have the ability to spread the virus zoonotically. For example, a

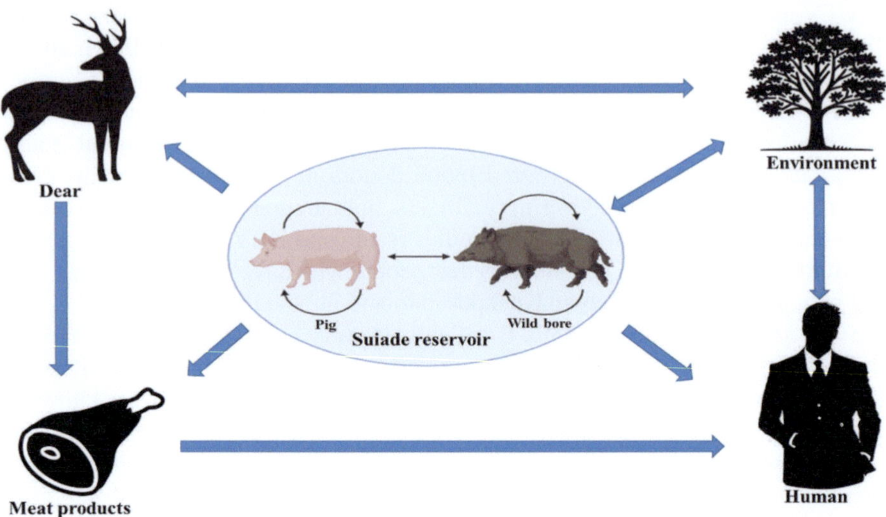

Fig. 2 Routes of zoonotic HEV transmission and exposure to humans by pigs

number of HEV strains have been found in lynxes, leopards, and bears in China and Europe (Spahr et al., 2017).

Transmission Pathways of Zoonotic HEV

Since swine HEV was discovered, there have been worries about possible zoonotic HEV transmission and its effects on public health. Additionally, three more case reports that showed how HEV is spread by consuming contaminated food sources provide more concrete proof that the virus is a zoonosis (Hofmeister et al., 2019). Figure 3 shows a schematic illustration of the zoonotic transmission paths of HEV.

Multiple reports have linked the consumption of raw or inadequately cooked swine or wild boar products, such as meat, liver, or liver-based stuffing, to sporadic cases or outbreaks of hepatitis E in Japan, France, Spain, and Australia. Nevertheless, there isn't any concrete proof that these foods are the actual causes of infection. Numerous studies have reported the detection of HEV-3 and HEV-4 RNA at different stages of the hog food chain globally. In the UK and Spain, HEV RNA has been found in a variety of pork products, including sausages (Nan et al. 2017).

A number of investigations have shown that commercially available hog livers and pork-derived products, particularly those that contain raw liver, can harbour infectious viruses and could be a source of foodborne HEV. For example, HEV was contracted by pigs that received intravenous injections of homogenates from tainted pig livers that were bought from supermarkets in the United States. Additionally, human cell lines exposed to extracts from raw pig liver purchased from Japanese grocery stores or Locatelli sausages made in France were able to successfully cultivate HEV (Ricci et al., 2017).

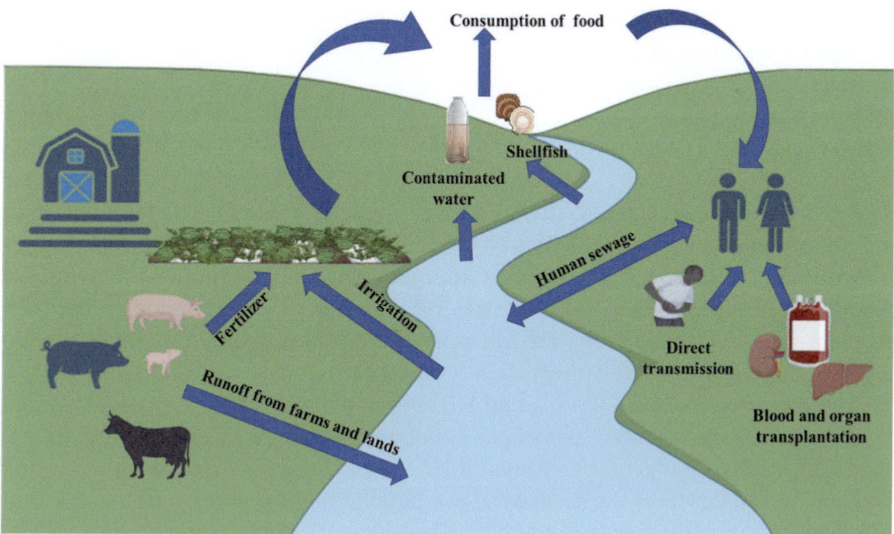

Fig. 3 Schematic representation of zoonotic transmission pathways in HEV

Oysters from Korea's coastal regions have been shown to have HEV-3 or HEV-4 RNA, suggesting that non-animal-based items may also be tainted with HEV and could be a source of foodborne illness. The contamination of surface and irrigation water by animal faeces is most likely the cause of the occurrence of HEV in fruits, vegetables, and seafood. As previously stated, HEV RNA has been found in a wide range of foods, including fruits, vegetables, meat, and seafood. It is yet unknown, though, if these objects could contain contagious living viruses. It is imperative that a reliable cell culture technology be developed quickly in order to alleviate this uncertainty. A model like this would be helpful in clarifying whether infectious viruses can exist in liverless swine products like cured gammon (Turlewicz-Podbielska et al., 2023).

The use of items containing raw hog liver is not the only factor contributing to the considerable prevalence of HEV seropositivity seen in some regions. Standardized techniques for quality control of products considered at risk must also be established. Many novel HEV strains have appeared in different animal species in recent decades, suggesting that there may be more HEV variants out there. Pork-derived meat and products have been the main focus of screening efforts for HEV in food, despite the fact that pigs have been thoroughly investigated as the main HEV reservoir since its discovery in the late 1990s. Other animal reservoirs, however, might exist and present serious hazards for the zoonotic spread of HEV (Hofmeister et al., 2019). In order to check for the presence of HEV RNA in a larger range of food products made from various animal species, such as camels, rabbits, and others, more research is necessary. To successfully prevent and control the disease in the future, a thorough grasp of the variety of animal reservoirs and possible routes of transmission that provide hazards for zoonotic hepatitis E infection is essential (Turlewicz-Podbielska et al., 2023).

Inter-Species Transmission of HEV

As was previously mentioned, studies on HEV natural reservoirs and research using animal models have provided important new information about the interspecies transmission of various HEV species and genotypes. According to the compiled results of multiple studies, HEV-1a and HEV-2a are primarily found in humans, whereas HEV-3a and HEV-4a are naturally present in a variety of animal species and are capable of surviving transplants across species boundaries (Nan et al., 2017).

The zoonotic event of HEV-3a and HEV-4a transfer from swine, wild boar, and deer to humans through the ingestion of contaminated meat has also been verified. Phylogenetic and molecular analyses of HEV-3a and HEV-4a sequences from pig and human sources have shown that the two populations are very similar, suggesting that there is no clear species grouping. This suggests that adaptation may not be necessary for swine HEV-3a and HEV-4a to promote interspecies transmission (Hofmeister et al., 2019).

Assessing the risk of zoonotic transmission from other strains, such as wild boar HEV-5a and HEV-6a, will require more research. Possible zoonotic transmission from camels to people is implied by the advent of HEV-7a, which has been linked to a human case connected to camel transmission. It is necessary to clarify the precise role that HEV-7a plays in zoonotic hepatitis E, nevertheless (Ricci et al., 2017).

Experimentally determining whether HEV-7a may infect other species is important because zoonotic genotypes such as HEV-3a and HEV-4a can infect different animal species. This will help determine whether there are secondary reservoirs of this possible zoonotic genotype or if they could form as a result of human meddling or direct camel transmission.

Zoonotic Transmission by Farm Animals and Meat

It is generally acknowledged that eating pork is frequently linked to acute hepatitis E infections that arise from local sources of infection; this trend is particularly evident in Japan (Miyashita et al., 2012). Cases of HEV infection by eating raw or undercooked pork have also been reported in a number of other nations. As a result, in affluent countries, pigs are acknowledged as the main risk factor for HEV gearbox.

Furthermore, eating wild boar meat and pork liver sausage is known to increase the risk of contracting HEV infection in European nations (La Rosa et al., 2011). The possible health concerns connected with consuming hog liver sausages are further highlighted by the worry that HEV infection spread through these products may cause hepatocarcinoma in humans (Berto et al., 2013).

According to Reuter et al. (2009), there is evidence that HEV-3a strains have been found in animals other than pigs, such as deer, wild boars, and other species in Hungary. Interestingly, roe deer and humans have been found to have very identical HEV infection sequences (Takahashi et al., 2004). These results suggest the possibility of HEV transmission between species, with wild animals like deer and boars contributing to the spread of HEV to people.

It was initially believed that the fecal-oral pathway was the main way that HEV was spread between humans and animals. Consuming shellfish is another important cause of HEV infections in people, as evidenced by several HEV infection cases in developed countries (La Rosa et al., 2011). These and other findings indicate that eating animal meat, meat products, and seafood, especially in developed nations, may be responsible for a significant percentage of human HEV infections.

Transmission of HEV Through Blood Donors

It has been suggested that in regions where HEV is endemic, blood transfusions play a role in the transmission of the infection (Arankalle & Chobe, 2000). This is evidenced by the presence of HEV-specific antibodies and elevated levels of alanine aminotransferase (ALT) in individuals who were previously HEV-negative after receiving blood transfusions. This phenomenon was also demonstrated in a study involving rhesus monkeys, where acute hepatitis developed in monkeys following blood transfusion from donors with hepatitis E viremia.

While HEV infections are typically more prevalent in individuals aged 15–45 years in areas with high HEV prevalence, studies suggest that children can also acquire HEV through blood transfusion (Colson et al., 2010). Therefore, blood transfusion is now recognized as a novel risk factor for HEV transmission.

Importance of HEV in Food Safety

HEV's substantial role in foodborne transmission globally has raised concerns about its effects on agro-food safety. According to Ricci et al. (2017), HEV has been linked to a significant number of clinical cases in EU member states, most of which are caused by locally acquired infections and result in death. A common cause of hepatitis E infections worldwide is the consumption of raw or undercooked organs and tissues from infected pigs, underscoring the need of food safety precautions in halting the spread of HEV (Pallerla et al., 2021; Salines et al., 2019). Even though there is little chance of HEV transmission in Canada from contact with pigs or pork, ongoing monitoring and precautionary steps are crucial to reducing the risk of contracting a zoonotic HEV infection.

HEV has been found to inhabit the internal tissues of food items, including muscles and liver (Bouwknegt et al., 2009). Nevertheless, limited data are available regarding HEV persistence within food matrices, particularly in products like ready-to-eat and raw meat, which may contain swine meat or liver. Additionally, there is a need for additional research to elucidate the survival mechanisms of HEV and assess the effects of industrial processing methods on the virus.

Measures to Prevent HEV Transmission

A number of tactics have been put out to reduce the spread of HEV in the food supply chain, with careful cooking being the main focus (Cook & Van Der Poel, 2015). Properly boiling meat before eating is essential for ensuring food safety because commercial meat and game meat products, including HEV, may be contaminated. To lower the danger of contracting foodborne illnesses from eating raw or undercooked meat, several nations have set cooking standards. The U.S. Department of Agriculture (2017) and Canada.ca's Safe Cooking Temperatures recommend that pork be cooked to an internal temperature of 71 °C (160 °F) and then rested for 3 min before consuming.

However, considering the multifaceted nature of transmission mitigation, further exploration is warranted. While HEV detection and elimination in meat production chains have been extensively studied, there is potential for similar investigations in other food matrices, such as milk and molluscs (Ferri & Vergara, 2021). Consequently, generating detailed data on HEV survival and inactivation across various strain-matrix combinations is imperative to comprehend the heat stability of HEV in diverse food environments.

Conclusion

Hepatitis E virus (HEV) remains a significant global health concern due to its widespread prevalence, diverse genotypes, and complex transmission pathways. The discovery of HEV and its taxonomic categorization have paved the way for understanding its molecular structure and evolutionary dynamics. The epidemiology of HEV reflects a dual burden, with endemicity in developing regions and emerging cases in developed countries, highlighting the need for comprehensive surveillance and control measures. Zoonotic transmission plays a crucial role in HEV's epidemiology, with various animal reservoirs contributing to human infections through the consumption of contaminated food sources. The inter-species transmission of HEV underscores the dynamic nature of viral evolution and the potential for new variants to emerge. Blood transfusion has also been identified as a route of HEV transmission, necessitating stringent screening protocols for blood donors. In terms of food safety, proper cooking practices and quality control measures are essential to reduce the risk of HEV transmission through food products. Continued research efforts are needed to understand HEV persistence in different food matrices and develop effective prevention strategies.

Overall, a multidisciplinary approach encompassing virology, epidemiology, food safety, and public health interventions is crucial for mitigating the impact of HEV on human health and preventing future outbreaks.

References

Anheyer-Behmenburg, H. E., Szabo, K., Schotte, U., Binder, A., Klein, G., & Johne, R. (2017). Hepatitis E virus in wild boars and spillover infection in red and roe deer, Germany, 2013–2015. *Emerging Infectious Diseases, 23*(1), 130.

Arankalle, V. A., & Chobe, L. P. (2000). Retrospective analysis of blood transfusion recipients: Evidence for posttransfusion hepatitis E. *Vox Sanguinis, 79*, 72–74.

Arnaboldi, S., Righi, F., Carta, V., Bonardi, S., Pavoni, E., Bianchi, A., Losio, M. N., & Filipello, V. (2021). Hepatitis E virus (HEV) spread and genetic diversity in game animals in northern Italy. *Food and Environmental Virology, 13*(2), 146–153. https://doi.org/10.1007/s12560-021-09467-z

Aye, T. T., Uchida, T., Ma, X. Z., Iida, F., Shikata, T., Zhuang, H., & Win, K. M. (1992). Complete nucleotide sequence of a hepatitis E virus isolated from the Xinjiang epidemic (1986–1988) of China. *Nucleic Acids Research, 20*(13), 3512.

Azman, A. S., Ciglenecki, I., Wamala, J. F., Lynch, J., Aggarwal, R., Rahman, M., Wong, S., Serafini, M., Moussa, A. M., Dalton, H. R., & Shrestha, A. (2019). Hepatitis E should be considered a neglected tropical disease. *PLoS Neglected Tropical Diseases, 13*(7), e0007453.

Batts, W., Yun, S., Hedrick, R., & Winton, J. (2011). A novel member of the family Hepeviridae from cutthroat trout (Oncorhynchus clarkii). *Virus Research, 158*(1–2), 116–123.

Berto, A., et al. (2013). Hepatitis E virus in pork liver sausage, France. *Emerging Infectious Diseases, 19*, 264–266.

Bi, S. L., Purdy, M. A., McCaustland, K. A., Margolis, H. S., & Bradley, D. W. (1993). The sequence of hepatitis E virus isolated directly from a single source during an outbreak in China. *Virus Research, 28*(3), 233–247.

Bouwknegt, M., Rutjes, S. A., Reusken, C. B., Stockhofe-Zurwieden, N., Frankena, K., de Jong, M. C., de Roda Husman, A. M., & van der Poel, W. H. (2009). The course of hepatitis E virus infection in pigs after contact-infection and intravenous inoculation. *BMC Veterinary Research, 5*, 1–12.

Caballero-Gomez, J., et al. (2022). Hepatitis E virus in the endangered Iberian lynx (Lynx pardinus). *Transboundary and Emerging Diseases, 69*(5), e2745–e2756.

Cao, D., Huang, Y. W., & Meng, X. J. (2010). The nucleotides on the stem-loop RNA structure in the junction region of the hepatitis E virus genome are critical for virus replication. *Journal of Virology, 84*(24), 13040–13044.

Chatterjee, R., Tsarev, S., Pillot, J., Coursaget, P., Emerson, S. U., & Purcell, R. H. (1997). African strains of hepatitis E virus that are distinct from Asian strains. *Journal of Medical Virology, 53*(2), 139–144.

Colson, P., et al. (2010). Pig liver sausage as a source of hepatitis E virus transmission to humans. *Journal of Infectious Diseases, 202*, 825–834.

Cook, N., & Van Der Poel, W. H. M. (2015). Survival and elimination of hepatitis E virus: A review. *Food and Environmental Virology, 7*(3), 189–194. https://doi.org/10.1007/s12560-015-9196-2

Doceul, V., Bagdassarian, E., Demange, A., & Pavio, N. (2016). Zoonotic hepatitis E virus: Classification, animal reservoirs and transmission routes. *Viruses, 8*(10), 270.

Donnelly, M. C., et al. (2017). Hepatitis E – A concise review of virology, epidemiology, clinical presentation and therapy. *Aliment Pharmacology Therapeutics, 46*, 126–141.

Ferri, G., & Vergara, A. (2021). Hepatitis E virus in the food of animal origin: A review. *Foodborne Pathogens and Disease, 18*(6), 368–377.

Galiana, C., et al. (2008). Occupational exposure to hepatitis E virus (HEV) in swine workers. *American Journal of Tropical Medicine and Hygiene, 78*, 1012–1015.

Gerber, P. F., Trampel, D. W., Willinghan, E. M., Billam, P., Meng, X. J., & Opriessnig, T. (2015). Subclinical avian hepatitis E virus infection in layer flocks in the United States. *The Veterinary Journal, 206*(3), 304–311.

Haqshenas, G. S. H. L., Shivaprasad, H. L., Woolcock, P. R., Read, D. H., & Meng, X. J. (2001). Genetic identification and characterization of a novel virus related to human hepatitis E virus from chickens with hepatitis–splenomegaly syndrome in the United States. *Journal of General Virology, 82*(10), 2449–2462.

Hofmeister, M. G., Foster, M. A., & Teshale, E. H. (2019). Epidemiology and transmission of hepatitis A virus and hepatitis E virus infections in the United States. *Cold Spring Harbor Perspectives in Medicine, 9*(4), a033431.

Huang, R. T., Li, D. R., Wei, J., Huang, X. R., Yuan, X. T., & Tian, X. (1992). Isolation and identification of hepatitis E virus in Xinjiang, China. *Journal of General Virology, 73*(5), 1143–1148.

Huang, F. F., Haqshenas, G., Shivaprasad, H. L., Guenette, D. K., Woolcock, P. R., Larsen, C. T., Pierson, F. W., Elvinger, F., Toth, T. E., & Meng, X. J. (2002). Heterogeneity and seroprevalence of a newly identified avian hepatitis E virus from chickens in the United States. *Journal of Clinical Microbiology, 40*(11), 4197–4202.

Kaiser, M., Kamili, S., Hayden, T., Blümel, J., & Baylis, S. A. (2017). Genome sequence of a genotype 2 hepatitis E virus World Health Organization reference strain. *Genome Announcements, 5*(7), 10–1128.

Khuroo, M. S., Khuroo, M. S., & Khuroo, N. S. (2016). Hepatitis E: Discovery, global impact, control and cure. *World Journal of Gastroenterology, 22*(31), 7030.

Krumbholz, A., Mohn, U., Lange, J., Motz, M., Wenzel, J. J., Jilg, W., Walther, M., Straube, E., Wutzler, P., & Zell, R. (2012). Prevalence of hepatitis E virus-specific antibodies in humans with occupational exposure to pigs. *Medical Microbiology and Immunology, 201*, 239–244.

Kwo, P. Y., Schlauder, G. G., Carpenter, H. A., Murphy, P. J., Rosenblatt, J. E., Dawson, G. J., Mast, E. E., Krawczynski, K., & Balan, V. (1997). Acute hepatitis E by a new isolate acquired in the United States. *Mayo Clinic Proceedings, 72*(12), 1133–1136.

La Rosa, G., et al. (2011). Hepatitis E virus in Italy: Molecular analysis of travel-related and autochthonous cases. *Journal of General Virology, 92*, 1617–1626.

Lee, G.-H., Tan, B.-H., Teo, E. C.-Y., Lim, S.-G., Dan, Y.-Y., Wee, A., Aw, P. P. K., Zhu, Y., Hibberd, M. L., Tan, C.-K., et al. (2016). Chronic infection with camelid hepatitis E virus in a liver transplant recipient who regularly consumes camel meat and milk. *Gastroenterology, 150*, 355–357.

Li, P., Ji, Y., Li, Y., Ma, Z., & Pan, Q. (2022). Estimating the global prevalence of hepatitis E virus in swine and pork products. *One Health, 14*, 100362.

Lozano, R., et al. (2012). Global and regional mortality from 235 causes of death for 20 age groups. *The Lancet, 380*, 2095–2128.

Meng, X. J., Purcell, R. H., Halbur, P. G., Lehman, J. R., Webb, D. M., Tsareva, T. S., Haynes, J. S., Thacker, B. J., & Emerson, S. U. (1997). A novel virus in swine is closely related to the human hepatitis E virus. *Proceedings of the National Academy of Sciences, 94*(18), 9860–9865.

Miyashita, K., et al. (2012). Three cases of acute or fulminant hepatitis E caused by ingestion of pork meat and entrails in Hokkaido, Japan: Zoonotic food-borne transmission of hepatitis E virus and public health concerns. *Hepatology Research, 42*, 870–878.

Mori, Y., & Matsuura, Y. (2011). Structure of hepatitis E viral particle. *Virus Research, 161*(1), 59–64.

Nair, V. P., Anang, S., Subramani, C., Madhvi, A., Bakshi, K., Srivastava, A., Shalimar, N., & B., CT, R.K. and Surjit, M. (2016). Endoplasmic reticulum stress induced synthesis of a novel viral factor mediates efficient replication of genotype-1 hepatitis E virus. *PLoS Pathogens, 12*(4), e1005521.

Nan, Y., Wu, C., Zhao, Q., & Zhou, E. M. (2017). Zoonotic hepatitis E virus: An ignored risk for public health. *Frontiers in Microbiology, 8*, 322012.

Nicot, F., Jeanne, N., Roulet, A., Lefebvre, C., Carcenac, R., Manno, M., Dubois, M., Kamar, N., Lhomme, S., Abravanel, F., & Izopet, J. (2018). Diversity of hepatitis E virus genotype 3. *Reviews in Medical Virology, 28*(5), e1987.

Nishizawa, T., Takahashi, M., Mizuo, H., Miyajima, H., Gotanda, Y., & Okamoto, H. (2003). Characterization of Japanese swine and human hepatitis E virus isolates of genotype IV with 99% identity over the entire genome. *Journal of General Virology, 84*(5), 1245–1251.

Pallerla, S. R., Schembecker, S., Meyer, C. G., Linh, L. T. K., Johne, R., Wedemeyer, H., Bock, C. T., Kremsner, P. G., & Velavan, T. P. (2021). Hepatitis E virus genome detection in commercial pork livers and pork meat products in Germany. *Journal of Viral Hepatitis, 28*(1), 196–204.

Parvez, M. K. (2015). The hepatitis E virus ORF1 'X-domain' residues form a putative macrodomain protein/Appr-1″-pase catalytic-site, critical for viral RNA replication. *Gene, 566*(1), 47–53.

Pavio, N., Doceul, V., Bagdassarian, E., & Johne, R. (2017). Recent knowledge on hepatitis E virus in Suidae reservoirs and transmission routes to human. *Veterinary Research, 48*, 1–14.

Reuter, G., et al. (2009). Characterization and zoonotic potential of endemic hepatitis E virus (HEV) strains in humans and animals in Hungary. *Journal of Clinical Virology, 44*, 277–281.

Reyes, G. R., Purdy, M. A., Kim, J., Luk, K. C., Young, L. M., Fry, K. E., & Bradley, D. W. (1990). Isolation of a cDNA from the virus responsible for enterically transmitted non-a, non-B hepatitis. *Science, 247*(4948), 1335–1339.

Reyes, G. R., Yarbough, P. O., Tam, A. W., Purdy, M. A., Huang, C. C., Kim, J. S. P., Bradley, D. W., & Fry, K. E. (1991). Hepatitis E virus (HEV): The novel agent responsible for enterically transmitted non-A, non-B hepatitis. *Gastroenterologia Japonica, 26*(Suppl 3), 142–147.

Ricci, A., Allende, A., Bolton, D., Chemaly, M., Davies, R., Fernandez Escamez, P. S., Herman, L., Koutsoumanis, K., Lindqvist, R., Nørrung, B., Robertson, L., Ru, G., Sanaa, M., Simmons, M., Skandamis, P., Snary, E., Speybroeck, N., Ter Kuile, B., Threlfall, J., & Girones, R. (2017). Public health risks associated with hepatitis E virus(HEV) as a food-borne pathogen. *EFSA Journal, 15*(7).

Salines, M., Dumarest, M., Andraud, M., Mahé, S., Barnaud, E., Cineux, M., Eveno, E., Eono, F., Dorenlor, V., Grasland, B., & Bourry, O. (2019). Natural viral co-infections in pig herds affect hepatitis E virus (HEV) infection dynamics and increase the risk of contaminated livers at slaughter. *Transboundary and Emerging Diseases, 66*(5), 1930–1945.

Sato, Y., Sato, H., Naka, K., Furuya, S., Tsukiji, H., Kitagawa, K., Sonoda, Y., Usui, T., Sakamoto, H., Yoshino, S., & Shimizu, Y. (2011). A nationwide survey of hepatitis E virus (HEV) infection in wild boars in Japan: Identification of boar HEV strains of genotypes 3 and 4 and unrecognized genotypes. *Archives of Virology, 156*, 1345–1358.

Schlauder, G. G., Dawson, G. J., Erker, J. C., Kwo, P. Y., Knigge, M. F., Smalley, D. L., Rosenblatt, J. E., Desai, S. M., & Mushahwar, I. K. (1998). The sequence and phylogenetic analysis of a novel hepatitis E virus isolated from a patient with acute hepatitis reported in the United States. *Journal of General Virology, 79*(3), 447–456.

Smith, D. B., Simmonds, P., Izopet, J., Oliveira-Filho, E. F., Ulrich, R. G., Johne, R., Koenig, M., Jameel, S., Harrison, T. J., Meng, X. J., & Okamoto, H. (2016). Proposed reference sequences for hepatitis E virus subtypes. *Journal of General Virology, 97*(3), 537–542.

Smith, D. A., Wang, T., Freeman, O., Crichton, C., Salih, H., Matthews, P. C., Davies, J., et al. (2020a). National Institute for Health Research health informatics collaborative: Development of a pipeline to collate electronic clinical data for viral hepatitis research. *BMJ Health & Care Informatics, 27*(3), e100145.

Smith, D. B., Izopet, J., Nicot, F., Simmonds, P., Jameel, S., Meng, X. J., Norder, H., Okamoto, H., van Der Poel, W. H., Reuter, G., & Purdy, M. A. (2020b). Update: Proposed reference sequences for subtypes of hepatitis E virus (species Orthohepevirus A). *Journal of General Virology, 101*(7), 692–698.

Spahr, C., Ryll, R., Knauf-Witzens, T., Vahlenkamp, T. W., Ulrich, R. G., & Johne, R. (2017). Serological evidence of hepatitis E virus infection in zoo animals and identification of a rodent-borne strain in a Syrian brown bear. *Veterinary Microbiology, 212*, 87–92.

Sridhar, S., Teng, J. L., Chiu, T. H., Lau, S. K., & Woo, P. C. (2017). Hepatitis E virus genotypes and evolution: Emergence of camel hepatitis E variants. *International Journal of Molecular Sciences, 18*(4), 869.

Takahashi, M., Nishizawa, T., Miyajima, H., Gotanda, Y., Iita, T., Tsuda, F., & Okamoto, H. (2003). Swine hepatitis E virus strains in Japan form four phylogenetic clusters comparable with those of Japanese isolates of human hepatitis E virus. *Journal of General Virology, 84*(4), 851–862.

Takahashi, K., Kitajima, N., Abe, N., & Mishiro, S. (2004). Complete or near-complete nucleotide sequences of hepatitis E virus genome recovered from a wild boar, a deer, and four patients who ate the deer. *Virology, 330*(2), 501–505.

Takahashi, H., Tanaka, T., Jirintai, S., Nagashima, S., Takahashi, M., Nishizawa, T., Mizuo, H., Yazaki, Y., & Okamoto, H. (2012). A549 and PLC/PRF/5 cells can support the efficient propagation of swine and wild boar hepatitis E virus (HEV) strains: Demonstration of HEV infectivity of porcine liver sold as food. *Archives of Virology, 157*, 235–246.

Tam, A. W., Smith, M. M., Guerra, M. E., Huang, C. C., Bradley, D. W., Fry, K. E., & Reyes, G. R. (1991). Hepatitis E virus (HEV): Molecular cloning and sequencing of the full-length viral genome. *Virology, 185*(1), 120–131.

Tsarev, S. A., Emerson, S. U., Reyes, G. R., Tsareva, T. S., Legters, L. J., Malik, I. A., Iqbal, M., & Purcell, R. H. (1992). Characterization of a prototype strain of hepatitis E virus. *Proceedings of the National Academy of Sciences, 89*(2), 559–563.

Turlewicz-Podbielska, H., Augustyniak, A., Wojciechowski, J., & Pomorska-Mól, M. (2023). Hepatitis E virus in livestock – Update on its epidemiology and risk of infection to humans. *Animals, 13*(20), 3239.

U.S Department of Agriculture. (2017). Export requirements for Japan. https://www.fsis. usda.gov/inspection/import-export/import-export-library/japan

Wang, B., & Meng, X. J. (2021). Hepatitis E virus: Host tropism and zoonotic infection. *Current Opinion in Microbiology, 59*, 8–15.

Widén, F., Sundqvist, L., Matyi-Toth, A., Metreveli, G., Belák, S., Hallgren, G., & Norder, H. (2011). Molecular epidemiology of hepatitis E virus in humans, pigs and wild boars in Sweden. *Epidemiology & Infection, 139*(3), 361–371.

Woo, P. C., Lau, S. K., Teng, J. L., Tsang, A. K., Joseph, M., Wong, E. Y., Tang, Y., Sivakumar, S., Xie, J., Bai, R., & Wernery, R. (2014). New hepatitis E virus genotype in camels, the Middle East. *Emerging Infectious Diseases, 20*(6), 1044.

Woo, P. C., Lau, S. K., Teng, J. L., Cao, K. Y., Wernery, U., Schountz, T., Chiu, T. H., Tsang, A. K., Wong, P. C., Wong, E. Y., & Yuen, K. Y. (2016). New hepatitis E virus genotype in Bactrian camels, Xinjiang, China, 2013. *Emerging Infectious Diseases, 22*(12), 2219.

World Health Organization. (2024). Available online: https://www.who.int/news-room/fact-sheets/detail/hepatitis-e. Accessed on 2 Jan 2024

Zhou, X., Huang, F., Xu, L., Lin, Z., de Vrij, F. M., Ayo-Martin, A. C., van Der Kroeg, M., Zhao, M., Yin, Y., Wang, W., & Cao, W. (2017). Hepatitis E virus infects neurons and brains. *The Journal of Infectious Diseases, 215*(8), 1197–1206.

Swine-Associated Parasites and Their Impact on Human Health

Prabodh Kumar Hembram and Gatchanda Shravan Kumar

Abstract

Pigs are vital to worldwide farming efforts and are not only valuable food sources but also reservoirs for a range of parasites such as protozoa, nematodes, cestodes, and trematodes, which can infect humans through the consumption of contaminated pork or direct contact with infected environments. This chapter explores the significant health implications of swine-associated parasitic infections on humans, focusing on the transmission, epidemiology, and management of diseases such as trichinellosis, cysticercosis, toxoplasmosis, Sarcocystosis and other parasitic zoonoses. The goal is to mitigate the risks associated with these zoonotic infections, thereby improving public health outcomes and ensuring food safety in swine-consuming communities worldwide.

Keywords

Pork · Trichinellosis · Cysticercosis · Toxoplasmosis · Sarcocystosis · Zoonotic infections

P. K. Hembram
Animal Resources Development Department, Government of West Bengal, Kolkata, West Bengal, India

G. S. Kumar (✉)
Department of Veterinary Parasitology, Shourabh College of Veterinary Science, Hindaun, Rajasthan, India

R. Deb et al. (eds.), *Emerging Zoonotic Threats from Swine*,
https://doi.org/10.1007/978-981-96-7407-7_11

Introduction

Domestic pigs, or swine, are central to global agriculture and food production, providing a significant source of protein, essential nutrients, and livelihood for millions globally. The role of pork in cultural traditions underscores its socioeconomic and nutritional importance (Zhang et al., 2023). However, the close contact between humans and swine, especially in intensive farming environments, introduces challenges, particularly with zoonotic diseases—those transmissible from animals to humans (Godwin et al., 2022). Swine are key carriers of various pathogens, including viruses, bacteria, and parasites, which can lead to serious health problems in humans ranging from mild gastrointestinal issues to life-threatening conditions (Thapaliya et al., 2023). Among these, infections caused by parasites such as protozoa, nematodes (roundworms), cestodes (tapeworms), and trematodes (flukes) are particularly concerning. These parasites naturally infect swine and can be transmitted to humans mainly through the ingestion of contaminated pork or via direct contact with infected animals or their environments. Major pig parasites having zoonotic importance and their transmission routes are listed in Table 1. Research into swine-associated parasites is crucial for public health due to its implications for understanding parasite life cycles and transmission routes, which are essential for devising effective prevention and control strategies (Mathew, 2018). This is especially vital in areas with prevalent pork consumption and certain farming practices that may elevate zoonotic transmission risks. Moreover, the global health burden from these parasites calls for sustained research and public health initiatives to lessen their impact. The socio-economic effects are significant, influencing the productivity of individuals and exerting pressure on healthcare systems, particularly in under-resourced areas. Thus, studying swine-associated parasites is not just a health issue

Table 1 Major pig parasites with zoonotic potential: transmission routes from pigs to humans

Parasite	Pork borne infection	Feco-oral infection (waterborne, contaminated food, etc.)	References
Toxoplasma gondii	+	–	Solaymani-Mohammadi and Petri (2006)
Sarcocystis suihominis	+	–	Solaymani-Mohammadi and Petri (2006)
Balantidium coli	–	+	Solaymani-Mohammadi and Petri (2006)
Taenia solium	+	–	Olson and Guselle (2000)
Taenia asiatica	+	–	Conlan et al. (2011)
Ascaris suum	–	+	Roepstorff et al. (2011)
Trichinella spiralis	+	–	Olson and Guselle (2000)
Fasciolopsis buski	–	+	Mas-Coma et al. (2005)
Gastrodiscoides hominis	–	+	Kumar (1999)

but also a matter of food security, economic resilience and addressing global health inequalities.

This chapter delves into the intricate relationships between swine-associated parasites and human health. It begins by exploring the biology and life cycles of key parasitic species such as *Taenia solium, Trichinella spiralis, Sarcocystis suihominis, Toxoplasma gondii, Fasciolopsis buski, Gastrodiscoides hominis, Balantidium coli,* and *Ascaris suum*. The discussion extends to the epidemiological pathways through which these parasites are transmitted from swine to humans, highlighting the roles of agricultural practices, food consumption habits and environmental factors.

Taenia Solium

The parasite *Taenia solium* ranks at the forefront of the global multicriteria-based evaluation of foodborne parasites, as outlined by the FAO/WHO (Torgerson et al., 2015), and is the primary cause behind cysticercosis in both humans and pigs, creating significant health and economic impacts (Dixon et al., 2020). In the United States, the Centers for Disease Control and Prevention (CDC) has identified cysticercosis as one of five parasitic diseases to focus on for public health initiatives as part of its effort to address neglected parasitic infections. Remarkably, neurocysticercosis caused by *T. solium* stands as the leading preventable factor for acquired epilepsy, accounting for over 30% of epilepsy cases in endemic regions (Wagner & Newton, 2009) and is considered a major cause globally (Rajshekhar et al., 2006). In 2010, the Foodborne Disease Burden Epidemiology Reference Group (FERG) made an estimation indicating that epilepsy linked to neurocysticercosis (NCC) was responsible for roughly 2.8 million disability-adjusted life years (DALYs) on a global scale (Dixon et al., 2020).

Transmission and Hosts

The life cycle of *Taenia solium* involves two hosts, humans and pigs. "Humans serve as both definitive and intermediate hosts for *Taenia solium*, with pigs also acting as intermediate hosts." In humans, who are the definitive hosts, ingestion of undercooked pork containing cysticerci leads to taeniasis, with the tapeworm maturing in the intestine. The tapeworm releases eggs that are excreted in feces. Pigs, the intermediate hosts, ingest these eggs, which develop into cysticerci in their tissues (heart, tongue, masseter muscle, diaphragm, shoulder muscles, intercostal muscles, esophagus, whereas lymph nodes, liver, spleen, lungs, and the brain are rare localizations). Humans then consume these infected pork tissues, continuing the cycle. Additionally, humans can also become accidental intermediate hosts if they ingest *T. solium* eggs directly from contaminated hands, food, or water, leading to cysticercosis, including neurocysticercosis when cysticerci develop in the brain (Del Brutto et al., 2014).

Clinical Manifestation

Human taeniasis generally results in minimal clinical issues, typically causing slight inflammation where the parasite implants. Often, individuals show no symptoms, or they may experience mild, vague symptoms such as abdominal pain, bloating, nausea, and variations in bowel habits including diarrhea or constipation. Nevertheless, the real concern with taeniasis is the dispersal of parasitic eggs. When these eggs are consumed, they can develop into cysticercosis, a condition that is clinically significant and poses serious health risks. Neurocysticercosis stands as the foremost neurological parasitic ailment in regions endemic to *Taenia solium* (Maudlin et al., 2009). It commonly presents as epilepsy and increased intracranial pressure, yet it can manifest a range of neurological symptoms and is the primary cause of epilepsy starting in adulthood in these areas (Maudlin et al., 2009; Del Brutto & Sotelo, 1988). The development of intracranial hypertension and hydrocephalus can lead to significant mortality rates (Garcia & Del Brutto, 2003; Fleury et al., 2011). Additionally, *Taenia solium* ranks as the most frequent parasite found within the orbit, affecting 3–3.5% of those infected (Madigubba et al., 2007). Vision loss can result from complications such as damage to the retinal tissue, chronic uveitis, papilledema, or pressure on the optic chiasm from cerebral cysticercosis.

Prevalence and Economic Impact

The rate of infection is influenced by economic development levels and sanitary practices (Morales et al., 2008). Regions where traditional pig farming is common, particularly in developing countries across South and Central America, sub-Saharan Africa, and the Asia-Pacific region excluding Islamic nations, often report human cysticercosis. The phenomenon of economic migration from endemic regions to developed countries, coupled with increased travel to developing nations, positions *T. solium* as a parasite with significant international health implications (Pawlowski et al., 2005).

Diagnosis and Challenges

For diagnosing taeniasis, analyzing stool samples for *Taenia solium* eggs represents a foundational approach; but for differential diagnosis within the Taenia species, coproantigen detection by ELISA or PCR is required (Mahanty et al., 2010). Identifying *Taenia solium* infection in pigs often involves methods such as tongue palpation and serological testing. However, these approaches may lack sensitivity, particularly in endemic regions where pigs typically harbor only mild infections (da Silva et al., 2012). Routine meat/carcass inspection is of low sensitivity too, as only 11–18% of cysticerci were located in organs indicated for routine meat inspection (heart, tongue, and masseter muscle) (da Silva et al., 2012; Boa et al., 2002). In the case of cysticercosis, diagnostic imaging is pivotal for accurately assessing the quantity, location, and developmental stage of lesions. Serological tests are the most common diagnostic method, but it must be noted that they may be positive in patients who have been exposed to the adult parasite without developing cysticercosis (Garcia et al., 2005), whereas even highly sensitive variants including enzyme-linked immunoelectrotransfer with highly purified cysticercus antigens may give false-negative results in up to 50% of patients with a single cerebral cyst or in those with calcifications alone (Singh et al., 2010).

Treatment Strategies

Treatment for taeniasis involves a one-time administration of niclosamide, with praziquantel or albendazole serving as alternative options. For cysticercosis, however, a single therapeutic approach is not useful and management includes antiparasitic drugs (albendazole, praziquantel), symptomatic therapy (analgesics, antiepileptics, anticonvulsant drugs), anti-inflammatory drugs (corticosteroids), and surgery (Nash et al., 2006).

Prevention and Vaccination

Proper cooking of pork, improved sanitation to prevent fecal-oral transmission, and health education on the risks of consuming undercooked pork. Recent advancements have been made in creating vaccines aimed at pigs, the intermediary hosts for *Taenia solium*, to curb the parasite's spread to humans. The TSOL18 vaccine, in particular, has demonstrated success in lowering the occurrence of cysticercosis in pigs, which in turn helps protect humans by minimizing the chances of transmission via the consumption of inadequately cooked or raw pork.

Trichinellosis

Trichinellosis, formerly known as trichinosis, is a zoonotic disease transmitted to humans through the consumption of meat or meat products contaminated with the larvae of Trichinella nematodes. This condition can be particularly severe in older adults, potentially leading to fatal outcomes due to complications such as myocarditis (heart inflammation) or encephalitis (brain inflammation).

Epidemiology and Transmission

Since the nineteenth century, *Trichinella* spp. have been documented worldwide, except in Antarctica. In the last 20 years, infections have been reported in 95 countries, encompassing wild, domestic, and human cases (Borhani et al., 2023). The majority of trichinellosis outbreaks are linked to consuming undercooked pork infected with *Tr. spiralis* larvae, although meats from wild animals and horsemeat have also been implicated. Other species, including *Tr. britovi*, *Tr. nativa*, *Tr. pseudospiralis*, *Trichinella zimbabwensis* and *Tr. papuae*, have been identified as causes of the disease in various regions and hosts. Estimates suggest that the yearly incidence rate of trichinellosis ranges from 469.2 to 985.3 cases per billion people, with a worldwide mortality rate falling between 0.3 and 0.8 deaths per billion individuals annually. In 2010, the global burden of this disease, measured in disability-adjusted life years (DALYs), was calculated at 523 (Devleesschauwer et al., 2015). While the majority of *Trichinella* sp. infections are found in wildlife, the transmission of these parasites from wild to domestic animals poses a significant obstacle for managing the disease in regions where it is endemic.

Life Cycle

The life cycle of the parasite includes two main phases: the enteral (intestinal) phase and the parenteral (muscular) phase. Contamination results from ingesting raw or undercooked meat infested with tiny, 0.5 mm coiled larvae. The life cycle of the parasite encompasses two distinct stages: an initial intestinal (or enteral) phase followed by a muscular (parenteral or systemic) phase, both of which may overlap, extending from several days to a few weeks in duration. When infected meat is digested in the stomach, the larvae emerge, burrow through the small intestine's mucosa, and grow into adult worms within 5 days post-infection. This invasion of the intestinal wall leads to changes in the epithelial cells, particularly affecting the brush border of villi, the lamina propria, and the smooth muscles of the jejunum. Following reproduction in the intestines, adult female worms release newborn larvae (NBL), measuring about 100 micrometer in length, into the bloodstream and lymphatic system. These larvae then circulate, eventually settling in skeletal muscle fibers, their ultimate habitat. During their journey, the larvae cause parasitic vasculitis in the host. Once inside the muscle fiber, the larvae manipulate the host cell, prompting the formation of a collagen capsule for most Trichinella species, encapsulating the larva. Within 2 weeks, the NBL grows 600 times in size, becoming capable of causing infection. Encased within what is now termed a "nurse cell," the larvae can survive for months or even years. Adult females continue to release NBL for 3–4 weeks, after which they either die or are eliminated through an immune response-triggered increase in smooth muscle contractions (Djurkovic-Djakovic et al., 2013).

Clinical Manifestations

In swine, *Trichinella* infections are typically asymptomatic, showing no noticeable clinical signs. In contrast, humans may experience an initial intestinal phase of 3–7 days, marked by abdominal discomfort and diarrhea, followed by the more severe invasive phase. This phase, starting roughly a week post-infection, is characterized by symptoms such as significant fever, swelling of the face, and muscle soreness as larvae move from the intestines to muscle and other tissues. The symptoms can escalate to include muscle aches and debility, elevated body temperature, swelling, skin rash, eye inflammation, headaches, feeling cold, and respiratory issues, alongside an increase in eosinophils, a type of white blood cell. In its more extreme form, trichinellosis can progress to life-threatening conditions, including inflammation of the heart (myocarditis), brain (encephalitis), lungs (pneumonia), and brain and its membranes (meningoencephalitis) (Dupouy-Camet & Murrell, 2007).

Diagnosis

In pigs, diagnosing involves identifying larvae through chlorhydropeptic digestion of a significant quantity of meat. The method of trichinoscopy, which can detect approximately one larva per gram, is generally not advised. Serological methods are available to identify infections, but they may yield false-positive results. Regulatory standards differ by country, and comprehensive details are provided in the guidelines developed through a collaboration between the Food and Agriculture Organization, the World Organization for Animal Health, and the WHO, all of which are accessible online (Dupouy-Camet & Murrell, 2007).

In humans, diagnosis may be suspected when there are clustered cases of individuals exhibiting fever, facial swelling, and muscle pain. If cases are isolated or the symptoms do not follow typical patterns, suspecting an infection becomes more challenging. When an infection is suspected, it is crucial to gather details about the consumption of raw or undercooked meat, including where and when the meat was purchased and consumed, as noted in source (Dupouy-Camet & Murrell, 2007). Elevated eosinophil counts along with high levels of muscular enzymes such as creatine phosphokinase and aldolase strongly suggest this diagnosis. Initially, antibody tests like ELISA and indirect fluorescence may return negative results and should therefore be repeated after a few days. Western blot analysis can identify specific antibodies sooner. Antibodies remain detectable in the serum for months or even years following the acute phase of the disease. During the acute stage, muscular biopsy is not effective because the larvae are not yet encapsulated and are difficult to detect. However, changes in muscle fibers, such as the disappearance of myofibrils and enlarged nuclei with prominent nucleoli, may indicate the disease. One month post-onset, larvae become visible in muscle tissue and can be precisely identified to determine the parasite's genotype. Although PCR testing of parasitic DNA in blood is effective in experimental settings, its sensitivity and specificity in human infections remain unverified (Dupouy-Camet & Murrell, 2007).

Treatment

Treatment involves antiparasitic medications like albendazole or mebendazole, and symptomatic care for pain and inflammation. Early treatment initiation is crucial to minimize cardiovascular and neurological complications. The regimen usually consists of administering albendazole (preferably) or mebendazole at a dosage of 15 mg twice daily with a fat-rich meal for a duration of 10–15 days. To mitigate symptoms and avert further complications, a course of prednisolone at a dose of 1 mg/kg once daily is recommended for a few days (Dupouy-Camet & Murrell, 2007).

Sarcocystosis

In pigs, three distinct types of Sarcocystis are identified: *S. miescheriana*, *S. porcifelis*, and *S. suihominis*. Of these, only *S. suihominis* has the potential to infect human intestines if raw pork containing the parasite is consumed.

Life Cycle

The life cycle of *Sarcocystis suihominis* involves two hosts: the definitive host and the intermediate host. *Sarcocystis suihominis* is a protozoan parasite that can affect humans and pigs, with pigs serving as the intermediate host and humans (or potentially other primates) as the definitive host. Here's a detailed look at its life cycle: The life cycle begins when the definitive host, a human, ingests undercooked or raw pork containing Sarcocystis cysts, also known as sarcocysts, within the muscle tissue. Once ingested, the sarcocysts release bradyzoites in the small intestine of the human host. These bradyzoites invade the intestinal epithelium and develop into sexual stages of the parasite, producing oocysts. Within these oocysts, sporogony occurs, leading to the formation of sporocysts containing sporozoites. The oocysts are eventually shed in the feces of the definitive host. This shedding into the environment is crucial for the transmission to the intermediate host. Pigs become infected by ingesting food or water contaminated with these oocysts. Once ingested, the sporocysts release sporozoites, which invade the pig's intestinal wall and eventually the bloodstream, disseminating throughout the body. The sporozoites undergo asexual replication (schizogony) and eventually develop into sarcocysts within the pig's muscle tissues. These sarcocysts mature over time and become infective to the definitive host when ingested. The cycle is completed when humans consume infected pork containing these mature sarcocysts, starting the process anew (Fayer, 2004).

Clinical Manifestation

Infection may present with or without symptoms. Individuals who consumed pork infected with *S. suihominis* experienced severe symptoms ranging from bloat and nausea to vomiting, diarrhea, stomach pain, respiratory difficulties, and accelerated heart rate within 6–48 h. Conversely, a researcher who self-administered the parasite started to pass sporocysts after 12 days, continuing for more than 120 days, yet exhibited no symptoms during this period, according to source (Li & Lian, 1986).

Diagnosis

For Definitive Hosts (Humans with Intestinal Sarcocystosis)

Microscopic Examination of Feces: This involves the detection of oocysts or sporocysts in fecal samples. However, because Sarcocystis oocysts can be difficult to differentiate from those of other coccidian parasites, this method may not always provide a definitive diagnosis.

Molecular Methods: PCR (Polymerase Chain Reaction) and other molecular techniques can be used to detect Sarcocystis DNA in fecal samples. These methods offer higher specificity and sensitivity than microscopic examination and can differentiate *Sarcocystis* species.

Serological Tests: Serological methods like ELISA (Enzyme-Linked Immunosorbent Assay) can detect antibodies against *Sarcocystis* in blood samples. However, serology can indicate exposure rather than an active infection and may cross-react with other parasites.

For Intermediate Hosts (Pigs with Muscular Sarcocystosis)

Histological Examination: Muscle tissues, often from the esophagus, diaphragm, or other striated muscles, are examined under a microscope for the presence of *sarcocysts*. This method can directly show the parasitic cysts within the muscle fibers.

Molecular Diagnosis: As with humans, PCR and other molecular techniques can identify Sarcocystis DNA in tissue samples. These methods can confirm the presence of the parasite and specify the species.

Immunohistochemistry (IHC): IHC can be used on muscle tissue samples to detect Sarcocystis antigens with specific antibodies, providing both localization and identification of the parasite.

Serological Tests for Animals: These tests can detect antibodies against Sarcocystis in the blood of infected animals, indicating exposure to the parasite. However, like in humans, they cannot confirm active muscular sarcocystosis without additional evidence.Sarcocystosis is a self-limiting infection, and prophylaxis and treatment are not known.

Toxoplasmosis

Toxoplasmosis, recognized as a prevalent zoonotic disease, impacts roughly one-third of the global population, positioning *Toxoplasma gondii* as the most significant protozoan transmitted through food, especially meat.

Life Cycle

The life cycle of *Toxoplasma gondii*, a protozoan parasite, involves two main stages: the sexual phase (occurring only in the definitive hosts, which are members of the Felidae family, such as domestic cats and other wild cats) and the asexual phase (occurring in a wide range of intermediate hosts, including humans and other mammals).

Sexual Phase in Definitive Hosts (Cats)

T. gondii enters its sexual phase in the intestines of cats, the definitive hosts. Here, the parasites undergo sexual reproduction, producing oocysts that are shed in the cat's feces.

These oocysts are highly resilient and can survive in the environment for months. Asexual Phase in Intermediate Hosts (Including Humans):

Intermediate hosts, such as humans, pigs, rodents, and birds, can become infected by ingesting soil, water, or food contaminated with these oocysts. Once ingested, the oocysts release sporozoites that invade the host's cells, converting into tachyzoites. Tachyzoites are the rapidly multiplying form of the parasite, spreading throughout the body and causing acute infection. As the host's immune system responds, tachyzoites convert into bradyzoites, forming tissue cysts primarily in the brain, muscles, and other tissues. These cysts can remain in the host for life, potentially reactivating if the immune system is compromised.

Transmission to Humans

Humans can become infected through several routes: by ingesting undercooked meat containing tissue cysts, consuming food or water contaminated with oocysts shed by cats, via congenital transmission from an infected mother to her fetus, or through organ transplantation or blood transfusion from an infected donor. This cycle allows *T. gondii* to spread and maintain itself within populations of both its definitive and intermediate hosts, making it one of the most successful parasitic organisms worldwide.

Globally, infection rates of *T. gondii* vary significantly, spanning from 8% to 92% (Alvarado-Esquivel et al., 2006; Figueiro-Filho et al., 2005). The prevalence is typically greater in regions that are warmer and more humid but also varies based on the dietary practices of different populations, leading to differences even within nearby locations (Bobic et al., 2011). Pork is typically regarded as the meat with the highest risk due to its global seroprevalence rate in pigs and its dominance as the most consumed meat worldwide. The likelihood of infection in pigs escalates with their age due to ongoing exposure to infection, which in turn raises the risk associated with consuming pork products, particularly those made from older animals (Dubey et al., 1991, 1995; Damriyasa et al., 2004; Klun et al., 2006, 2011).

Clinical Signs in Humans

In humans, the clinical signs of *T. gondii* infection (toxoplasmosis) can vary widely, from asymptomatic to severe, depending on the individual's immune status and the timing of the infection:

Asymptomatic: The majority of infected individuals are asymptomatic, with the immune system usually keeping the parasite under control.

Acute Toxoplasmosis: In some cases, especially in individuals with weakened immune systems, acute infection can cause flu-like symptoms such as body aches, fever, fatigue, and sometimes sore throat or swollen lymph nodes.

Congenital Toxoplasmosis: If a woman gets infected for the first time during pregnancy, the parasite can be transmitted to the fetus, potentially causing miscarriage, stillbirth, or congenital defects such as chorioretinitis (inflammation of the retina and choroid of the eye), intracranial calcifications, and hydrocephalus.

Ocular Toxoplasmosis: In both congenital and acquired cases, *T. gondii* can affect the eyes, leading to reduced vision, eye pain, redness, and blurred vision due to retinitis.

Severe Toxoplasmosis: In immunocompromised patients (such as those with HIV/AIDS, organ transplant recipients, or individuals undergoing chemotherapy), the infection can cause more severe complications, including encephalitis (brain inflammation), myocarditis (heart muscle inflammation), pneumonitis (lung inflammation), and potentially death.

Clinical Signs in Pigs

In pigs, *Toxoplasma gondii* infection is often subclinical, meaning that infected pigs rarely show noticeable symptoms. However, the presence of the parasite in pigs is primarily a concern due to the risk of transmission to humans through consumption of undercooked or raw pork. Clinical signs, when present, might be non-specific and could include:

Poor Growth: Infected pigs may exhibit reduced growth rates or poor feed efficiency.

Reproductive Issues: In some cases, *T. gondii* infection can lead to reproductive problems, such as abortions or mummified fetuses, although these are more commonly observed in sheep.

Neurological Signs: Rarely, severe infections might cause neurological signs, but this is not commonly reported.

Diagnosis

For both humans and pigs, the diagnosis of toxoplasmosis relies on a combination of clinical signs, serological tests (detecting antibodies against *T. gondii*), and molecular techniques (such as PCR for detecting the parasite's DNA). In humans, particularly pregnant women and immunocompromised patients, early diagnosis and treatment are crucial to prevent severe disease and complications.

Treatment

Currently, there is no vaccine available for humans (with a localized exception for sheep), and existing treatments cannot remove the parasite's cysts from an infected individual. Thus, treatment is restricted to managing acute and reactivated infections, marked by the parasite's proliferative stage, utilizing traditional medications such as pyrimethamine and sulfa drugs, along with newer options like clindamycin, azithromycin, and atovaquone. Although atovaquone has been noted to have efficacy against cysts, prevention remains the most effective strategy against toxoplasmosis.

Fasciolopsiasis

Etiology

Fasciolopsis buski, the largest fluke that impacts humans, is responsible for the occurrence of the disease.

Epidemiology

The parasite is widespread across several South and East Asian countries, such as Thailand, China, Taiwan, Vietnam, Bangladesh, and India (Mas-Coma et al., 2005; Lo & Lee, 1996; Wiwanitkit et al., 2002; Gilman et al., 1982; Le et al., 2004).

Reservoir

Pigs act as important reservoirs of infection.

Transmission

People contract the infection by consuming metacercariae, either through drinking water that has been contaminated or by eating infected plants. The occurrence of fasciolopsiasis is commonly associated with areas close to freshwater environments, especially those with stagnant or gently flowing water (Mas-Coma et al., 2005). The growth of freshwater vegetation along with contamination from both human and animal waste, particularly from pigs, plays a crucial role in the spread of this disease (Mas-Coma et al., 2005).

Life Cycle

In both humans and pigs, the adult form of the parasite resides in the intestine, specifically within the duodenum and jejunum, though it can also spread to other sections of the intestinal tract during severe infections. According to Weng et al. (1989), the eggs that are expelled in the feces take 3–7 weeks to develop in water. Subsequently, the emerging miracidia infect certain snail species, including those from the *Segmentina*, *Hippeutis*, and *Gyraulus* genera. These snails then release cercariae within 4–6 weeks (Graczyk et al., 2000). These cercariae form cysts on the surfaces of freshwater plants, and the cycle of infection to humans and pigs continues with the consumption of these metacercariae.

Disease in Man

High morbidity occurs due to fasciolopsiasis in endemic areas and the disease may become fatal in heavy infections (Graczyk et al., 2001; Weng et al., 1989). Mild infections may present symptoms such as anemia, headaches, dizziness, stomach pains, gastric discomfort, and diarrhea (Gilman et al., 1982). More severe cases can lead to intense epigastric and abdominal pain, diarrhea or intestinal blockage, nausea, acute ileus, widespread swelling (anasarca), and significant increases in eosinophils and white blood cells (Gilman et al., 1982). Additionally, malnutrition has been identified as a critical factor linked to the severity of infections (Graczyk et al., 2001; Weng et al., 1989).

Diagnosis

Diagnosis of the disease can be achieved through the analysis of stool samples for the detection of eggs and adult parasites (Mas-Coma et al., 2005). Additionally, there is potential for the application of molecular methods in future diagnostics.

Control

Effective control measures include accurate diagnosis, treating both humans and livestock, preventing future infections, adopting contemporary practices in pig farming, and refraining from eating freshwater plants (Mas-Coma et al., 2005).

Gastrodiscoidosis

Etiology

Gastrodiscoides hominis is known to infect humans. This parasite is characterized by having a pharynx, lobed testes arranged in tandem, an ovary located behind the testes, an ascending uterus, and a genital pore on the ventral side (Kumar, 1999).

Epidemiology

Primarily documented in India, instances of the parasite have also been recorded in Bangladesh and various East Asian countries (Acha & Szyfres, 2006).

Transmission

Disease transmission takes place through the consumption of raw or insufficiently cooked plants, crustaceans, mollusks, or amphibians that are contaminated with encysted metacercariae.

Clinical Signs in Man and Animals

Pigs are considered the natural definitive hosts for this parasite. The condition caused by *G. hominis* is known as gastrodisciasis. Following ingestion, the flukes emerge from the metacercariae in the digestive tract and move to the cecum and colon, where they develop into mature adults (Kumar, 1999). The parasite affects both humans and swine, including cases reported in African and Indian swine (Goldsmid, 1975; Hira, 1983; Murty & Reddy, 1980). While the disease often presents without symptoms, it can lead to mucoid diarrhea (Strickland, 1991).

Diagnosis

Identifying the trematode fluke's morphology and finding parasite eggs in stool samples are key methods for diagnosing the disease.

Balantidiosis

Etiology

Balantidium coli, the largest ciliate protozoan, causes the disease and can infect a variety of hosts including swine, primates, humans, and, less commonly, rats, guinea pigs, and dogs.

Epidemiology

This disease is endemic and widespread globally, with higher prevalence in temperate and tropical regions (Arean & Koppisch, 1956).

Transmission

Pigs and rats are significant sources of infection for humans (Esteban et al., 1998). Water or food contaminated with cysts is a crucial source of infection for humans.

Life Cycle

Cysts expelled in the feces of infected hosts transmit infection to susceptible hosts via the fecal-oral route, following the ingestion of water or food contaminated with these cysts.

Clinical Signs in Man

Sometimes, balantidiosis can mimic intestinal amoebiasis. The acute version is marked by a sudden onset of diarrhea or dysentery (Castro et al., 1983) along with symptoms such as abdominal pain, nausea, and vomiting. The chronic version features periods of intermittent diarrhea that alternate with normal bowel movements or constipation. Additional symptoms may include headache, loss of appetite, weight reduction, or muscle weakness.

Clinical Signs in Animals

Typically, the parasite is either non-pathogenic or results in asymptomatic conditions in swine and primates.

Diagnosis

The disease can be identified by directly observing the parasite, including trophozoites and cysts, in feces or intestinal scrapings, particularly in wet mounts of fresh feces. Typically, trophozoites are found in diarrheal stools, while cysts appear in solid stools.

Control

Managing the disease involves preventing the contamination of food and water with infected feces and treating cases that are infected.

Ascaris Suum

Epidemiology

A. suum, a parasite found worldwide, commonly infects pigs at high rates (Roepstorff et al., 1998; Nansen & Roepstorff, 1999). Cases of zoonotic ascariasis linked to *A. suum* have been reported in North America, Denmark (Anderson, 1995; Nejsum et al., 2005), and the UK (Nejsum et al., 2010). Additionally, molecular analysis has revealed infections of *A. suum* in chimpanzees at the Copenhagen Zoo, originating from pigs (Nejsum et al., 2005).

Transmission

Humans can become infected by accidentally consuming Ascaris eggs present in contaminated food, water, or soil.

Life Cycle

The disease spreads through the fecal-oral route. Upon ingestion, the infective eggs release L3 larvae in the intestine. These larvae then travel from the small intestine to the large intestine, penetrating the mucosa. Subsequently, the larvae enter the bloodstream, travel to the liver where they shed the L2 cuticle, and then migrate to the lungs. In the lungs, the larvae break through into the alveolar spaces, ascend to the pharynx, and are swallowed. Returning to the small intestine, the larvae grow to full maturity and reach reproductive age. Eggs are then excreted in the feces and develop into infective larvae under suitable environmental conditions.

Clinical Signs in Man and Animals

Clinical manifestations can vary from no symptoms to severe coughing and wheezing, with younger age groups typically being more susceptible. Ascaris pneumonia can occur due to lung damage inflicted by the larvae. In children, a heavy burden of worms may cause intestinal blockage and obstruction. Additional complications might include intussusception, perforation, and bowel gangrene. In regions where the disease is common, complications related to biliary and pancreatic involvement may include biliary colic, acute cholecystitis, acute cholangitis, acute pancreatitis, and hepatic abscess.

Diagnosis

The disease is diagnosable through the identification of parasitic eggs in the intestinal stage. Symptoms like labored breathing and stunted growth can also assist in diagnosing the condition. During the larvae's migratory phase, serological and molecular methods can be useful in detection (Zhu et al., 1999).

Control

Measures to prevent and control the disease encompass enhancing personal hygiene, providing health education, upgrading sanitation, and administering chemotherapy (Hotez et al., 2006).

Conclusion

Swine-associated parasitic infections represent a complex and significant global health issue, intertwined with economic, social, and cultural factors. The role of domestic pigs as reservoirs for zoonotic parasites exposes human populations to a variety of health risks, manifesting from mild to severe and sometimes life-threatening conditions. The transmission of these parasites from swine to humans, primarily through the consumption of contaminated pork or direct contact with infected animals, underscores the critical need for stringent food safety and animal husbandry practices.

Effective management and mitigation of these parasitic infections require a multifaceted approach, including enhanced surveillance, improved diagnostic techniques, and widespread public health education to promote safe cooking practices and hygiene. Furthermore, intersectoral collaboration between veterinary and public health sectors is essential to develop and implement strategies that control the spread of these parasites across the borders of farms and into the human population.

Addressing swine-associated parasitic infections not only aims to reduce the direct health burdens but also seeks to alleviate the broader socio-economic impacts.

This involves safeguarding the livelihoods of those dependent on swine agriculture, maintaining the stability of pork markets, and ensuring the nutritional security provided by pork products. Ultimately, the challenge of swine-associated parasitic worms is a reminder of our interconnectedness with animal health and the environment, urging ongoing research, policy-making, and community engagement to create resilient public health systems capable of confronting these zoonotic threats effectively.

References

Acha, P. N., & Szyfres, B. (2006). *Zoonoses and communicable diseases common to man and animals* (Vol. III). (Parasitosis), Pan American Health Organisation.

Alvarado-Esquivel, C., Sifuentes-Álvarez, A., Narro-Duarte, S. G., Estrada-Martínez, S., Díaz-García, J. H., Liesenfeld, O., et al. (2006). Seroepidemiology of *toxoplasma gondii* infection in pregnant women in a public hospital in northern Mexico. *BMC Infectious Diseases, 6*, 1–7.

Anderson, T. J. C. (1995). Ascaris infections in humans from North America: Molecular evidence for cross-infection. *Parasitology, 110*, 215–219.

Arean, V. M., & Koppisch, E. (1956). Balantidiasis: A review and report of cases. *The American Journal of Pathology, 32*, 1089–1115.

Boa, M. E., Kassuku, A. A., Willingham Iii, A. L., Keyyu, J. D., Phiri, I. K., & Nansen, P. (2002). Distribution and density of cysticerci of Taenia solium by muscle groups and organs in naturally infected local finished pigs in Tanzania. *Veterinary Parasitology, 106*(2), 155–164.

Bobic, B., Nikolić, A., Klun, I., & Djurkovic-Djakovic, O. (2011). Kinetics of toxoplasma infection in the Balkans. *Wiener Klinische Wochenschrift, 123*, 2–6.

Borhani, M., Fathi, S., Harandi, M. F., Simsek, S., Ahmed, H., Wu, X., & Liu, M. (2023). *Trichinella* infections in animals and humans of Iran and Turkey. *Frontiers in Medicine, 10*, 1088507.

Castro, J., Vazquez-Iglesias, J. L., & Arnal-Monreal, F. (1983). Dysentery caused by *Balantidium coli* – Report of two cases. *Endoscopy, 15*, 272–274.

Conlan, J. V., Sripa, B., Attwood, S., & Newton, P. N. (2011). A review of parasitic zoonoses in a changing Southeast Asia. *Veterinary Parasitology, 182*(1), 22–40.

da Silva, M. R., Uyhara, C. N., Silva, F. H., Espindola, N. M., Poleti, M. D., Vaz, A. J., et al. (2012). Cysticercosis in experimentally and naturally infected pigs: Parasitological and immunological diagnosis. *Pesquisa Veterinária Brasileira, 32*, 297–302.

Damriyasa, I. M., Bauer, C., Edelhofer, R., Failing, K., Lind, P., Petersen, E., et al. (2004). Cross-sectional survey in pig breeding farms in Hesse, Germany: Seroprevalence and risk factors of infections with toxoplasma gondii, Sarcocystis spp. and Neospora caninum in sows. *Veterinary Parasitology, 126*(3), 271–286.

Del Brutto, O. H., & Sotelo, J. (1988). Neurocysticercosis: An update. *Clinical Infectious Diseases, 10*(6), 1075–1087.

Del Brutto, O. H., García, H. H., Del Brutto, O. H., & García, H. H. (2014). *Taenia solium*: Biological characteristics and life cycle. In *Cysticercosis of the human nervous system* (pp. 11–21).

Devleesschauwer, B., Praet, N., Speybroeck, N., Torgerson, P. R., Haagsma, J. A., De Smet, K., et al. (2015). The low global burden of trichinellosis: Evidence and implications. *International Journal for Parasitology, 45*(2–3), 95–99.

Dixon, M. A., Winskill, P., Harrison, W. E., Whittaker, C., Schmidt, V., Sarti, E., et al. (2020). Force-of-infection of *Taenia solium* porcine cysticercosis: A modelling analysis to assess global incidence and prevalence trends. *Scientific Reports, 10*(1), 17637.

Djurkovic-Djakovic, O., Bobić, B., Nikolić, A., Klun, I., & Dupouy-Camet, J. (2013). Pork as a source of human parasitic infection. *Clinical Microbiology and Infection, 19*(7), 586–594.

Dubey, J. P., Leighty, J. C., Beal, V. C., Anderson, W. R., Andrews, C. D., & Thulliez, P. (1991). National seroprevalence of *Toxoplasma gondii* in pigs. *The Journal of Parasitology, 77*, 517–521.

Dubey, J. P., Weigel, R. M., Siegel, A. M., Thulliez, P., Kitron, U. D., Mitchell, M. A., et al. (1995). Sources and reservoirs of *Toxoplasma gondii* infection on 47 swine farms in Illinois. *The Journal of Parasitology, 81*, 723–729.

Dupouy-Camet, J., & Murrell, K. D. (2007). FAO/WHO/OIE Guidelines for the surveillance, management, prevention and control of trichinellosis, pp. 1–108. Available at: http://www.oie.int/doc/ged/D11303.PDF. Accessed 3 Dec 2012

Esteban, J. G., Aguirre, C., Angles, R., Ash, L. R., & Mas-Coma, S. (1998). Balantidiasis in Aymara children from the northern Bolivian Altiplano. *The American Journal of Tropical Medicine and Hygiene, 59*, 922–927.

Fayer, R. (2004). Sarcocystis spp. in human infections. *Clinical Microbiology Reviews, 17*(4), 894–902.

Figueiro-Filho, E. A., Lopes, A. H. A., Senefonte, F. R. D. A., Souza Júnior, V. G. D., Botelho, C. A., Figueiredo, M. S., & Duarte, G. (2005). Toxoplasmose aguda: estudo da freqüência, taxa de transmissão vertical e relação entre os testes diagnósticos materno- fetais em gestantes em estado da Região Centro-Oeste do Brasil. *Revista Brasileira de Ginecologia e Obstetrícia, 27*, 442–449.

Fleury, A., Carrillo-Mezo, R., Flisser, A., Sciutto, E., & Corona, T. (2011). Subarachnoid basal neurocysticercosis: A focus on the most severe form of the disease. *Expert Review of Anti-Infective Therapy, 9*(1), 123–133.

Garcia, H. H., & Del Brutto, O. H. (2003). Imaging findings in neurocysticercosis. *Acta Tropica, 87*(1), 71–78.

Garcia, H. H., Del Brutto, O. H., Nash, T. E., White, A. C., Tsang, V. C., & Gilman, R. H. (2005). New concepts in the diagnosis and management of neurocysticercosis (Taenia solium). *The American Journal of Tropical Medicine and Hygiene, 72*(1), 3–9.

Gilman, R. H., Mondal, G., Maksud, M., Alam, K., Rutherford, E., & Gilman, J. B. (1982). Endemic focus of *Fasciolopsis buski* infection in Bangladesh. *The American Journal of Tropical Medicine and Hygiene, 31*, 796–802.

Godwin, E. J. O., Chandrasekaran, V., Smah, A. C., & Faith, E. O. (2022). Emerging infectious food system related zoonotic foodborne disease–a threat to global food safety and nutrition security. In *Foodborne pathogens-recent advances in control and detection*. IntechOpen.

Goldsmid, J. M. (1975). Ecological and cultural aspects of human trematodiasis excluding schistosomiasis in Africa. *The Central African Journal of Medicine, 21*, 49–53.

Graczyk, T. K., Alam, K., Gilman, R. H., Mondal, G., & Ali, S. (2000). Development of Fasciolopsis buski (Trematoda; Fasciolidae) in Hippeutis umbilicalis and Segmentina trochoideus (Gastropoda: Pulmonata). *Parasitology Research, 86*, 324–326.

Graczyk, T. K., Gilman, R. H., & Fried, B. (2001). Fasciolopsiasis: Is it a controllable food borne disease? *Parasitology Research, 87*, 80–83.

Hira, P. R. (1983). Further spurious parasitic infestations of man in Zambia. *The Central African Journal of Medicine, 29*, 33–40.

Hotez, P. J., Bundy, D. A. P., Beegle, K., Brooker, S., Drake, L., de Silva, N. R., Montresor, A., Engels, D., & Jukes, M. (2006). Helminth infections: Soil-transmitted helminth infection and schistosomiasis. In D. T. Jamison, J. G. Breman, A. R. Measham, G. Alleyne, M. Claeson, D. B. Evans, P. Jha, A. Mills, & P. Musgrove (Eds.), *Disease control priorities in developing countries* (pp. 467–478). World Bank Group.

Klun, I., Djurković-Djaković, O., Katić-Radivojević, S., & Nikolić, A. (2006). Cross-sectional survey on *Toxoplasma gondii* infection in cattle, sheep and pigs in Serbia: Seroprevalence and risk factors. *Veterinary Parasitology, 135*(2), 121–131.

Klun, I., Vujanić, M., Yera, H., Nikolić, A., Ivović, V., Bobić, B., et al. (2011). *Toxoplasma gondii* infection in slaughter pigs in Serbia: Seroprevalence and demonstration of parasites in blood. *Veterinary Research, 42*, 1–6.

Kumar, V. (1999). *Trematode infections and diseases of man and animals*. Kluwer.

Le, T. H., Nguyen, V. D., Phan, B. U., Blair, D., & McManus, D. P. (2004). Case report: Unusual presentation of *Fasciolopsis buski* in a Vietnamese child. *Transactions of the Royal Society of Tropical Medicine and Hygiene, 98*, 193–194.

Li, Y. M., & Lian, Z. Q. (1986). Studies on man-pig cyclic infection of Sarcocystis suihominis found in Yunnan Province, China.

Lo, C. T., & Lee, K. M. (1996). Intestinal parasites among the southeast Asian laborers in Taiwan during 1993–1994. *Zhonghua Yi Xue Za Zhi (Taipei), 57*, 401–404.

Madigubba, S., Vishwanath, K., Reddy, G. B. K. G., & Vemuganti, G. K. (2007). Changing trends in ocular cysticercosis over two decades: An analysis of 118 surgically excised cysts. *Indian Journal of Medical Microbiology, 25*(3), 214–219.

Mahanty, S., Garcia, H. H., et al. (2010). Cysticercosis and neurocysticercosis as pathogens affecting the nervous system. *Progress in Neurobiology, 91*(2), 172–184.

Mas-Coma, S., Bargues, M. D., & Valero, M. A. (2005). Fascioliasis and other plant-borne trematode zoonoses. *International Journal for Parasitology, 35*, 1255–1278.

Mathew, A. (2018). Zoonoses associated with pigs Peter R. Davies, University of Minnesota, USA. In *Achieving sustainable production of pig meat* (Vol. 1, pp. 19–54). Burleigh Dodds Science Publishing.

Maudlin, I., Eisler, M. C., & Welburn, S. C. (2009). Neglected and endemic zoonoses. *Philosophical Transactions of the Royal Society B: Biological Sciences, 364*(1530), 2777–2787.

Morales, J., Martinez, J. J., Rosetti, M., Fleury, A., Maza, V., Hernandez, M., et al. (2008). Spatial distribution of Taenia solium porcine cysticercosis within a rural area of Mexico. *PLoS Neglected Tropical Diseases, 2*(9), e284.

Murty, C. V., & Reddy, C. R. (1980). A case report of Gastrodiscoides hominis infestation. *Indian Journal of Pathology & Microbiology, 23*, 303–304.

Nansen, P., & Roepstorff, A. (1999). Parasitic helminths of the pig: Factors influencing transmission and infection levels. *International Journal for Parasitology, 29*, 877–891.

Nash, T. E., Singh, G., White, A. C., Rajshekhar, V., Loeb, J. A., Proano, J. V., et al. (2006). Treatment of neurocysticercosis: Current status and future research needs. *Neurology, 67*(7), 1120–1127.

Nejsum, P., Bertelsen, M. F., Betson, M., Stothard, J. R., & Murrell, K. D. (2010). Molecular evidence for sustained transmission of zoonotic Ascaris suum among zoo chimpanzees (pan troglodytes). *Veterinary Parasitology, 171*, 273–276.

Nejsum, P., Parker, E. D., Frydenberg, J., Roepstorff, A., Boes, J., Haque, R., Astrup, I., Prag, J., & Sensen, U. B. S. (2005). Ascariasis is a zoonosis in Denmark. *Journal of Clinical Microbiology, 43*, 1142–1148.

Olson, M. E., & Guselle, N. (2000). Are pig parasites a human health risk. *Advances in Pork Production, 11*, 153–162.

Pawlowski, Z., Allan, J., & Sarti, E. (2005). Control of Taenia solium taeniasis/cysticercosis: From research towards implementation. *International Journal for Parasitology, 35*(11–12), 1221–1232.

Rajshekhar, V., Raghava, M. V., Prabhakaran, V., Oommen, A., & Muliyil, J. (2006). Active epilepsy as an index of burden of neurocysticercosis in Vellore district, India. *Neurology, 67*(12), 2135–2139.

Roepstorff, A., Nilsson, O., Oksanen, A., Gjerde, B., Richter, S. H., Örtenberg, E., Christensson, D., Martinsson, K. B., Bartlett, P. C., & Nansen, P. (1998). Intestinal parasites in swine in the Nordic countries: Prevalence and geographical distribution. *Veterinary Parasitology, 76*, 305–319.

Roepstorff, A., Mejer, H., Nejsum, P., & Thamsborg, S. M. (2011). Helminth parasites in pigs: New challenges in pig production and current research highlights. *Veterinary Parasitology, 180*(1–2), 72–81.

Singh, G., Rajshekhar, V., Murthy, J. M. K., Prabhakar, S., Modi, M., Khandelwal, N., & Garcia, H. H. (2010). A diagnostic and therapeutic scheme for a solitary cysticercus granuloma. *Neurology, 75*(24), 2236–2245.

Solaymani-Mohammadi, S., & Petri, W. A., Jr. (2006). Zoonotic implications of the swine- transmitted protozoal infections. *Veterinary Parasitology, 140*(3–4), 189–203.

Strickland, G. T. (1991). *Hunter's tropical medicine* (7th ed.). Saunders.

Thapaliya, D., Hanson, B. M., Kates, A., Klostermann, C. A., Nair, R., Wardyn, S. E., & Smith, T. C. (2023). Zoonotic diseases of swine: Food-borne and occupational aspects of infection. In *Zoonoses: Infections affecting humans and animals* (pp. 113–162). Springer International Publishing.

Torgerson, P. R., Devleesschauwer, B., Praet, N., Speybroeck, N., Willingham, A. L., Kasuga, F., et al. (2015). World Health Organization estimates of the global and regional disease burden of 11 foodborne parasitic diseases, 2010: A data synthesis. *PLoS Medicine, 12*(12), e1001920.

Wagner, R. G., & Newton, C. R. (2009). Do helminths cause epilepsy? *Parasite Immunology, 31*(11), 697–705.

Weng, Y. L., Zhuang, Z. L., Jiang, H. P., Lin, G. R., & Lin, J. J. (1989). Studies on ecology of Fasciolopsis buski and control strategy of fasciolopsiasis. *Chinese Journal of Parasitology and Parasitic Diseases, 7*, 108–111.

Wiwanitkit, V., Suwansaksri, J., & Chaiyakhun, Y. (2002). High prevalence of *Fasciolopsis buski* in an endemic area of liver fluke infection in Thailand. *Medgenmed: Medscape General Medicine, 4*, 6.

Zhang, H., Shi, Z., Zhou, H., & Hu, X. (2023). Pork Consumption Patterns among Rural Residents in China: A Regional and Cultural Perspective (2000–2020). *Agriculture, 13*(10), 1888.

Zhu, X., Chilton, N. B., Jacobs, D. E., Boes, J., & Gasser, R. B. (1999). Characterisation of Ascaris from human and pig hosts by nuclear ribosomal DNA sequences. *International Journal for Parasitology, 29*, 469–478.

Toxoplasmosis: Understanding the Swine and Human Transmission Cycle

Irtiqa Manzoor, D. Mohan Krishna, J. L. Singh, and Abhishek Pathak

Introduction

Toxoplasmosis is an infectious zoonotic parasitic disease caused by a protozoan parasite *Toxoplasma gondii*, infecting a wide range of mammals, birds, and humans (Scofano et al., 2023). It is considered as one of the major health concerns and ranks third worldwide for zoonosis (Hotea & Darabus, 2023). An estimated one-third of the global population has encountered this parasite (Rouba et al., 2019). Among foodborne illnesses in the USA, it is the second leading cause of death (Gao et al., 2016). Within the European Union, *T. gondii* stands as one of the most prevalent zoonotic agents in humans, with estimates suggesting it surpasses other parasitic infections such as salmonellosis and campylobacteriosis (Djurkovic-Djakovic et al., 2019). Traditionally, Toxoplasmosis has been attributed to cats, the only definitive host of the parasite have ability to release oocysts; however, 50% of cases in humans are foodborne (Herrero et al., 2016). Humans acquire infections mostly via ingestion of contaminated food and water containing sporulated oocysts, consuming raw or improperly cooked meat from infected or wild pigs with tissue cysts or by congenital route (Almeria & Dubey, 2021). Toxoplasmosis is more frequently reported among pigs and small ruminants within the livestock community, often manifesting as subclinical infections in pigs. This prevalence is notably observed in various settings, including free-ranging farms, outdoor or backyard small pig farms, as well as

I. Manzoor · J. L. Singh
Department of Veterinary Medicine, College of Veterinary & Animal Sciences, G.B. Pant University of Agriculture and Technology, Pantnagar, Uttarakhand, India

D. M. Krishna
Division of Animal Biotechnology, ICAR-NDRI, Karnal, Haryana, India

A. Pathak (✉)
Department of Veterinary Pharmacology & Toxicology, MJF College of Veterinary & Animal Sciences, Jaipur, Rajasthan, India

R. Deb et al. (eds.), *Emerging Zoonotic Threats from Swine*,
https://doi.org/10.1007/978-981-96-7407-7_12

among farmed or hunted wild boars. Globally, the average seroprevalence of *T. gondii* in pigs stands at 13% in Europe, 21% in Africa, 25% in North America, 21% in Asia, and 23% in South America. Serological surveys have revealed that *T. gondii* exposure rates among domestic pigs globally can reach up to 30% (Foroutan et al., 2019), with viable *T. gondii* isolated from pork tissues obtained during slaughter (Dubey, 2010). In humans, the diagnosis is performed using various methods like tissue culture isolation, molecular methods (PCR), serology, and histopathology. Traditionally, the gold standard for diagnosing Toxoplasma infection in food animals involved bioassays in mice or cats. However, epidemiological surveys commonly rely on serological methods including the modified agglutination test (MAT), enzyme-linked immunosorbent assay, indirect fluorescent assay (IFA), Latex agglutination tests (LAT), Sabin-Feldman dye test (SFDT), or a combination of methods (Elsalem, 2024). This chapter provides an overview of toxoplasmosis focusing mainly on etiology, transmission route, life cycle, potential risk factors supporting the *T. gondii* infections in human and animals and their prevention and control strategies. The chapter will also highlight the significance of one health approach in integrated swine and health perspectives.

Etiology

The disease is caused by *Toxoplasma gondii*, an obligate intracellular protozoan parasite, a member of the phylum Apicomplexa (Fig. 1).

T. gondii was thought to be the sole recognized species in the Toxoplasma genus for over past 30 years; however, recent research has revealed that only one clone line is virulent for mice among the two recognized clone lines of *T. gondii*. Type I, Type II, and Type III are the three prominent genotypes of *T. gondii* strains; however, no such correlates are found in higher animals (Dubey, 2010). Rodents (mice) primarily become infected with type I while as they are less susceptible for Type II and III. Type II has been identified as the infectious agent in small ruminants, however, infectious potential of Type III remains unconfirmed. Type IV, a lately identified genotype, is predominant in wildlife (Ahmad & Tasawar, 2015). The parasite exhibits significant diversity in pathogenicity and drug susceptibility across different genotypes throughout the world. In the USA and Europe, genotype II is found to be prevailing in cases of congenital toxoplasmosis (Hosseini et al., 2018). The parasite exists in three developmental stages: tachyzoite, bradyzoite, and sporozoite. Human infection is caused by all three kinds.

(a) *Tachyzoites*: A highly proliferative, and invasive form, predominantly found in intermediate hosts as pseudocysts during acute toxoplasmosis or early infection. It measures approximately 7 × 3 μm and is crescent-shaped.
(b) *Bradyzoites*: A form of slow multiplication, characteristic of chronic or late-stage infection in intermediate hosts remain as tissue cysts for extended periods of time. The terminal stage of life cycle in the intermediate stage is represented by tissue cysts. Depending on the number of organisms proliferated inside

Fig. 1 Taxonomy of T. gondii

Toxoplasma cyst, the size varies. A cyst of >100 μm dia. Can accommodate approximately 50–3000 organisms.

(c) *Sporozoites*: This form is produced during sexual reproduction in definitive host and is released in oocysts via cat feces only. The sporozoites are produced inside oocysts during the enteroepithelial phase of life cycle in the intestines. The diameter of each sporozoite ranges from 10 to 12 μm.

Epidemiology

The worldwide distribution of toxoplasmosis is disproportionate owing to different cultures, environmental conditions, and fauna structure. The hot and humid climate usually favors the increased incidence of toxoplasmosis than the dry and cold climate. The prevalence of disease for herbivores, and pigs is more during spring, and autumn and winter season, respectively. It is estimated that approximately one-third of human population are exposed to toxoplasmosis; however, the prevalence is quite varying in humans belonging to same or different countries, different areas of the same country. Generally speaking, in humans *T. gondii* infection is quite prevailing; however, the disease is clinically relevant only in immunocompromised individual's viz., AIDS, cancer, and organ transplant patients. The epidemiological investigation of clinical toxoplasmosis outbreaks in humans carried out for five decades by Dubey (2021) is presented in Table 1.

Transmission of *Toxoplasma gondii*

A wide range of hosts including terrestrial and aquatic mammals, and birds act as intermediate hosts harboring only the asexual stages of *T. gondii*, while the sexual stages are seen in domestic cats which act as a prime source of infection to humans. Humans get infected by ingesting food and water contaminated with *T. gondii* oocysts excreted by cats or handling infected cats or via accidental ingestion of oocysts from environment. The most important source of infection to humans in the USA include undercooked pork and consumption of hunted feral pigs for food as tissue cysts may remain viable in animals for more than 865 days (Kim & Weiss, 2004). As per Elsalem (2024), the various pathways by which intermediate hosts become infected include

(i) Ingestion of raw or undercooked contaminated meat (pork, mutton, or venison) containing tissue cysts or pseudocysts with bradyzoites or tachyzoites, respectively (Dubey & Jones, 2008).
(ii) Ingestion of raw fruits and vegetables contaminated with cat feces containing sporulated viable oocysts.
(iii) Accidental ingestion of oocysts from environment or via handling infected cats.
(iv) Accidental ingestion of tissue cysts during hand-to-mouth contact while handling undercooked contaminated meat or shellfish and not thoroughly washing hands.
(v) Congenital transmission (Mother-to-child transmission)—Transplacental transmission of tachyzoites (Pardini et al., 2018).
(vi) Consuming unpasteurized milk.
(vii) Tissue or organ transplants from a Toxoplasma-positive donor rarely transmit *T. gondii* (Robert-Gangneux & Darde, 2012).
(viii) Blood Transfusion, Bone marrow transplantation, ogeneic stem cell transplantation, sputum, and breast-feeding milk.
(ix) It can also be transmitted by knives, containers, utensils, cutting boards, or other preparation surfaces contaminated with raw meat or shellfish.

Life Cycle of *T. gondii*

According to Dubey (2009), the biological cycle of *T. gondii* is intricate and heterogenous, with an incredibly wide host range, including humans, livestock, birds, companion animals, and wildlife. The definitive hosts of *T. gondii* are domestic felines, which harbor both sexual (sporogony) and asexual (schizogony) cycles of *T. gondii*. Within this cycle, cats from the Felidae family play a crucial role by excreting resilient oocysts into the environment. Intermediate hosts, which support the parasite's asexual reproduction, include a wide array of warm-blooded animals, with over 30 bird species and 300 mammal species among them. Sheep are particularly susceptible to *T. gondii* infection.

Table 1 Worldwide scenario of clinical toxoplasmosis outbreaks in humans

Country	Outbreak	Year	Source of Infection	References
Brazil	Sao Paulo	1966	Ingestion of food/water contaminated with oocysts	
USA	New York City	1968	Ingestion of undercooked beef (hamburgers)	
USA	Pennsylvania	1974	Ingestion of undercooked beef (Kibbeh nayeh-Syrian dish)	
UK	London	NR	Lamb	
USA	New York City	1975	Ingestion of lamb	
USA	Alabama	1976	Ingestion of dirt contaminated with oocysts from cat feces	
USA	Georgia	1977	Ingestion of food or water contaminated with oocysts	
USA	Panama	1979	Ingestion of food or water contaminated with oocysts (drinking water from a contaminated stream)	
USA	South Carolina	1979	Ingestion of venison	
Brazil	Parana	1993	Lamb	
Australia	Brisbane	1994	Kangaroo meat	
South Korea	Kyongsang Buk-do	1995	Raw pork	
Canada	Greater Victoria	1995	Contamination of an open reservoir (municipal water supply) by feral cats.	
Brazil	Parana	2001	Ingestion of food or water contaminated with oocysts	
Turkey	Izmir	2002	No common source	
India	Coimbatore	2004	Contaminated water	
Brazil	Rio Grande do sul	2005	Processed pork	
Brazil	Sao Paulo	2006	Raw ground beef	
Brazil	Sao, Paulo	2009	Ingestion of food/water contaminated with oocysts	
France	Aveyron	2010	Lamb roast	
Brazil	Goias	2015	Ingestion of food/water contaminated with oocysts	

(continued)

Table 1 (continued)

Country	Outbreak	Year	Source of Infection	References
Brazil	Parana	2015, 2016	Ingestion of food/water contaminated with oocysts	
Brazil	French, Guiana	2017	Ingestion of food/water contaminated with oocysts	
USA	Tennessee	2017	Venison	
USA	Wisconsin	2017	Ingestion of undercooked venison	
USA	Illinois	2018	Venison	

Source: Author's compilation based on data from Dubey (2021), used with permission
NR not recorded

Life Cycle in Definitive Host

The cats of Felidae family only harbor the sexual cycle of *T. gondii*. A cat becomes infected primarily through consuming prey that contains tissue cysts or oocysts containing sporozoites excreted by another cat. After consumption, the low pH of stomach and proteolytic enzyme activity cause the cyst walls to rupture, releasing bradyzoites, or sporozoites. The first cells to invade in either scenario are the intestinal epithelial cells, which develop into schizonts, a stage of schizogony distinguished by the presence of many nuclei. The individualization of every cell in asexual reproduction occurs before a series of nuclear divisions. The inner membrane complex forms following successive rounds of nuclear division allowing each merozoite to form. The enterocytes rupture releasing numerous merozoites, which have the capacity to infect naive enterocytes and divide via schizogony, hence exponentially increasing the parasitic population. The schizonts and merozoites are primarily located in the ileum, and some of them differentiate into gametes, 10–15 days post-primary feline infection. Macrogametes are formed from a single merozoite and have an oval shape (8 μm long and 6 μm wide), while a schizogonic division produces elongated microgametes, measuring 6 μm in length and 2 μm in width. Following the union of microgamete with a macrogamete in the intestinal lumen of cat, the immature oocyst is released. The cats liberate resilient oocysts with the feces and maturation occurs in exposure to the aerated environment. The sporulation splits the oocyst into two sporocysts and upon subsequent maturation of oocyst, each sporocyst contains four sporozoites. The sporulated oocysts are highly resilient and remain viable both in dry and wet conditions.

Life Cycle in Intermediate Host

There are multiple ways for intermediate hosts to become infected. Digestive enzymes dissolve the walls of tissue cysts and oocysts, releasing bradyzoites or sporozoites, respectively, which glide through a special mechanism into their new host. The internalization of *T. gondii* is processed by interaction of protozoa with nucleated cells, especially epithelial cells, macrophages, muscle cells, and neurons.

The transport of Tachyzoites is mostly mediated by an effective Trojan horse (Macrophages). The tachyzoites initiates endodyogeny cycle in which daughter cells get attached to the residual body, creating rosettes (cluster of tachzoites). Tachzoites detach from residual body, rupture the host cells membrane, and release fresh tachyzoites that have potential to infect new host cells in the extracellular environment. Tachyzoites become localized in a Parasitophorus vacoule within a few days post infection, progressively slow down the rate of division by altering their metabolism and converting into bradyzoites dwelling in tissue cyst. The tissue cysts are usually found in central nervous system, muscles, and in the retina.

Role of Swine in Human Toxoplasmosis

Swine is considered as the significant meat source of *T. gondii* for humans in the USA (Dubey, 2009). The seropositive pigs can pose a zoonotic danger to humans consuming raw or undercooked pork and its products as tissue cysts remain viable in their flesh (Scofano et al., 2023) and DNA being detected in processed pork and uncured pig products over the last 10 years (Papatsiros et al., 2021; Dubey et al., 2020). An epidemiological study revealed that swine usually become infected by the ingestion of contaminated food containing oocysts, and close proximity of wild and domestic animals to barns. In developed nations, approximately 50% of infections are believed to originate from meat (Scallan et al., 2011), with pork implicated in 41% of food-borne toxoplasmosis cases in the USA. The transmission of *T. gondii* is epidemiologically valid for the increased seroprevalence in sows as compared to market age pigs. The risk of infection in processed pork products (salami and sausages) obtained from breeding sows is diminished compared to fresh unprocessed pork obtained from market age pigs due to measures that reduce or inactivate *T. gondii* tissue cysts. This distinction may serve as the risk of human toxoplasmosis related to the consumption of pork products (Papatsiros et al., 2021). The most important risk factors responsible for *T. gondii* prevalence in swine include origin, age, and stock density on farm, management system, water source and sanitary facilities, farm altitude, presence of rodents, and other favorable conditions for sporulation of oocysts (Scofano et al., 2023; Oliveria et al., 2018). The prevalence was lower on farms with <50 stocking density and located at higher altitudes of more than 200 meters. The intensive management system in the USA and other European countries has drastically reduced the seroprevalence of toxoplasmosis in pigs depicting the importance of rearing pigs indoors. As per, the exposure of Toxoplasma parasitism was higher in pigs reared in poorly managed non-confinement systems. Experimental studies have proved that pigs can become infected by ingesting oocysts or tissue cysts and by intravenous tachyzoites inoculation. In swine, *T. gondii* abortion is rarely seen, however, it is fatal for neonates. The modified agglutination test based on antibodies from fetal fluids can be used to diagnose abortion in sows. The use of intensive farm management combined with appropriate measures of confinement and hygiene, keeping meat-producing animals indoors and feeding them sterilized food, and keeping the sheds free of rodents, cats, and birds has significantly decreased the risk of Toxoplasma infection in livestock. As a result, the seroprevalence of *T. gondii* in pork has significantly decreased. In the USA, an investigation of *T. gondii* in meat purchased from retail outlets has shown a seroprevalence of around 0.57% as per a 2005 nationwide survey. Every industrialized nation has observed a decline of *T. gondii* seroprevalence in pigs, but the use of "organic" or "animal-friendly" outdoor production systems has been on the rise recently. The *T. gondii* seroprevalence in swine (Hotea and Darabus, 2023) is enlisted in Table 2.

Risk Factors of Toxoplasmosis

The potential risk variables detected in some of the studies conducted by Elsalem, 2024; Thebault et al., 2021 (Table 3) point towards the significant role of oocysts associated with toxoplasma transmission to humans.

Table 2 Seroprevalence of toxoplasmosis in swine from different countries (2000–2024)

Location	Species	Positive samples	References
Haryana, India	Pigs	24.7% (*n* = 106)	
Brazil	Commercial pigs	15.4% (*n* = 416)	Scofano et al. (2023)
Argentina	Domestic pigs	53.3% (*n* = 240)	
Cuba	Pigs	13.3% (*n* = 420)	
Myanmar	Backyard pigs	18.4% (*n* = 256)	
China	Pigs	13.8% (*n* = 1158)	
India/Chandigarh	Abattoir pigs	48.3% (*n* = 151)	
Chian/Jiangsu	Pigs	46.81% (*n* = 141)	
Indonesia/ Sulawesi	Farm pigs	2.3% (*n* = 310)	
Spain/Aragon	Fattening pigs	24.5% (*n* = 1200)	Herrero et al. (2016)
Finland/ nationwide	Abattoir pigs	3.2% (*n* = 1353)	
Japan/Gifu	Abattoir pigs	5.2% (*n* = 155)	
Nepal/Kathmandu	Abattoir pigs	11.7% (*n* = 742)	
Chile/Southern	Abattoir pigs	8.8% (*n* = 340)	
Romania/Arad	Outdoor pigs	16.28% (*n* = 700)	
China/Fujian	Sows	14.38% (*n* = 605)	
China/Yunnan	Pigs	16.97% (*n* = 831)	
Thailand	Farm pigs	7% (*n* = 322)	
Brazil/Parana	Pigs	8.54% (*n* = 117)	
USA	Pigs	56.52% (*n* = 69)	

Source: Author's compilation based on data from Hotea and Darabus (2023), used with permission

Table 3 Risk factors associated with toxoplasmosis in humans

S. no.	Risk variables	
1.	Geographical location	Humid climate and abundant rainfall
2.	Contact with animals	Exposure to domestic cats
		Direct contact with farm animals/or their products
		Environmental contamination (soil on fur)
		Contact with dogs, rodents, and flies
3.	Environmental factors	Contact with wastewater (lack of sanitation)
		Farm management
		Contact with contaminated soil
		Unfiltered water source/consuming inadequately treated water
4.	Food consumption	Undercooked meat (pork, mutton, beef), offal's or minced meat products
		Raw milk (goat/cow milk)
		Unwashed vegetables and fruits
		Shell fish (oysters, mussels, etc.)
5.	Lack of hygiene	Improper hand washing
6.	Blood transfusion	

Prevention and Control Strategies

Toxoplasmosis can pose severe risks, especially to immune-compromised individuals and pregnant women, leading to congenital infections. Prevention and control strategies play a crucial role in mitigating the burden of this disease on public health.

Prevention Strategies

1. *Public Awareness and Education*: Although there are doubts about its effectiveness, public education is a vital aspect. The need for practical, informative, and detailed communication skills to facilitate clear communication between medical professionals and patients, as well as measures and habits to reduce exposure to *T. gondii* oocysts and cysts, is especially important for pregnant women and immunc-compromised individuals. Freely accessible accurate and practical information about toxoplasmosis is advantageous for both medical professionals and the public (Smith et al., 2021).
2. *Food Safety and Hygiene Practices*: The consumption of food contaminated with *T. gondii* oocysts from cat feces, along with raw or undercooked meat and unpasteurized milk, is also associated with health risks. Some of the treatment options for *T. gondii* in foodstuffs intended for public consumption include thermal, non-thermal, and chemical methods that can be used to inactivate, infest, or kill the

bacteria (Shapiro et al., 2019). Pigs raised conventionally indoors are typically free from Toxoplasma infection, but there is a risk of reemergence in animal-friendly production systems. It is important to monitor pigs from these systems and implement prevention strategies to ensure the safety of meat products for consumers. The major prevention strategies of *T. gondii* are enlisted in Table 4.

Control Strategies

Controlling the population of intermediate hosts such as rodents and birds can help reduce the transmission and limit the spread of the parasite to humans and other animals. Including routine screening and treatment of domestic animals for toxoplasmosis implementing measures to reduce environmental contamination with Toxoplasma oocysts, such as covering sandboxes, maintaining clean water sources, and proper disposal can minimize the risk of human exposure to the parasite. Some other approaches are enlisted in Table 5 and Fig. 2.

Toxoplasmosis remains a significant public health concern worldwide, but with effective prevention and control strategies, its burden can be substantially reduced. By promoting awareness, improving food safety, implementing vector control measures, and targeting high-risk populations, concerted efforts can be made to prevent transmission and mitigate the impact of toxoplasmosis on human and animal health.

Table 4 Major prevention strategies for *T. gondii* infection

S. no.	Strategy/approach		References
1.	Public awareness and education	Reinforcement of health professionals, Completeness and accuracy of advice, Effectiveness of education efforts, integration of education, Regular screening, Timely treatment options, Special focus on pregnant women & immune-compromised people.	
2.	Food safety and hygiene practices	Ensure minimal contamination of land or fodder, Boil meat at 60 °C for 15 min or keep it at −20 °C for 2 days, Avoid contact with disease individuals, Wash hands thoroughly after contact with soil or sand, food preparation or contact with uncooked food, contact with pets or pet feces, and reinforce with children the importance of hand washing, Avoid drinking untreated water.	Shapiro et al. (2019), Smith et al. (2021)

Table 5 Control strategies of T. gondii infection

S. no	Methodology	Advantages	Disadvantages	References
1.	Pre-harvesting	Minimal contamination in farm or fodder, remove or inactivate oocysts, restrict intermediate hosts, controlling husbandry conditions.	Reduce the population of host, extremely difficult to remove oocysts, costly to initiate	
2.	Post-harvesting	Meat/food inactivated the tissue cysts by freezing, boiling, irradiation, high pressure	Reduce meat tenderness, texture, quality would be varying.	
3.	Chemical	Using anti-toxoplasma drugs, sulfadiazine, pyrimethamine derivatives, safe during pregnancy, actively target tachyzoites, bradyzoites.	Adverse side effects, fewer, bone marrow suppression, hepatic complications, toxicity for host system.	
4.	Immunological	Less prone to evergence of resistance, conceivably treatment for immune-suppressed people, target different antigens like tachyzoites, bradyzoites, cyst walls	Cost-effective while production (mAbs), modulate immune response of host, fewer side effects	
5.	Vaccines	Ideal, protect against both acute, chronic phages of infection, prevent primary infection pregnant women, latent parasite in immunosuppressed individual	Weak immune response (enzyme degradation), safety and regulatory issue with reversion of fully virulent parasite, immunogenicity issue like DNA vaccines.	
6.	Nanoparticle delivery	Improve diagnosis assays, especially immune-compromised conditions (weak serological PCR tests) best way to target chemotherapy and vaccine formulations	Toxicity due to metal nanoparticles, accumulation in organs, non-biodegradable nature	

One Health Interventions for Toxoplasmosis

The complexity of toxoplasmosis requires the development of a control panel of measures that are a combination of animal and human health and ecological factors, that is, an easy set of direction for quick reference to identify prevention and management. Using core elements like transdisciplinarity, integrative research, and capacity building are establishing One Health interventions that address toxoplasmosis (Aguirre et al., 2019). The effective control requires integrated efforts of multiple systems (Fig. 3). Some of them are listed below.

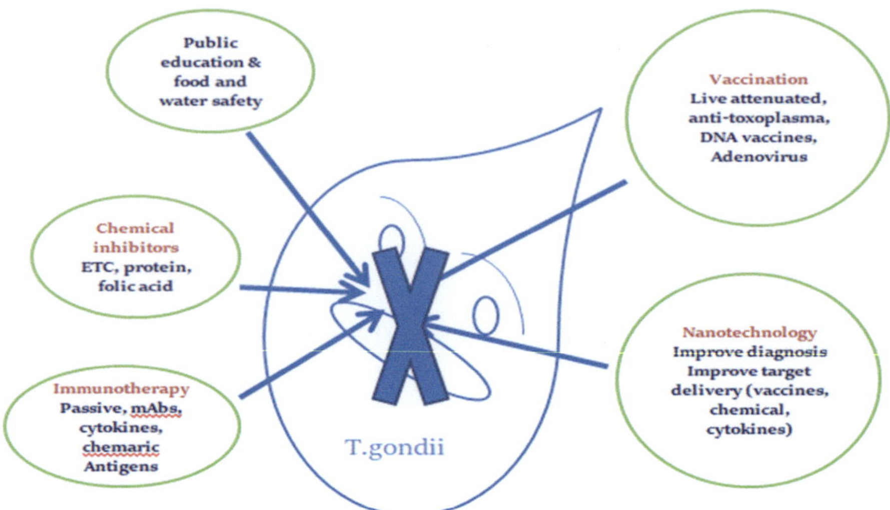

Fig. 2 Control approaches for Toxoplasmosis in humans and livestock

1. **Monitoring Systems**:

For early detection and intervention by sharing the data, information, educational approaches between veterinary and environment health sectors, its an easy way to identify and respond for the outbreak.

2. **Public Education and Awareness**:

Engage with communities to implement public health campaigns, surveys and raise awareness about toxoplasmosis, its transmission routes, and preventive measures. Instead of targeting all focus on high-risk groups such as pregnant women, weak immune, and those handling animals or soil environment.

3. **Animal Health Management**:

By implementing regular veterinary care, controlling intermediate host populations, improving the biosecurity in livestock farms including securing feed and water supplies, and keeping cats/transmission hosts away from farm animals.

4. **Food Management**:

Safety handling practices will help us to educate the importance of cooking meat, regular washing, and avoiding untreated products to reduce the foodborne

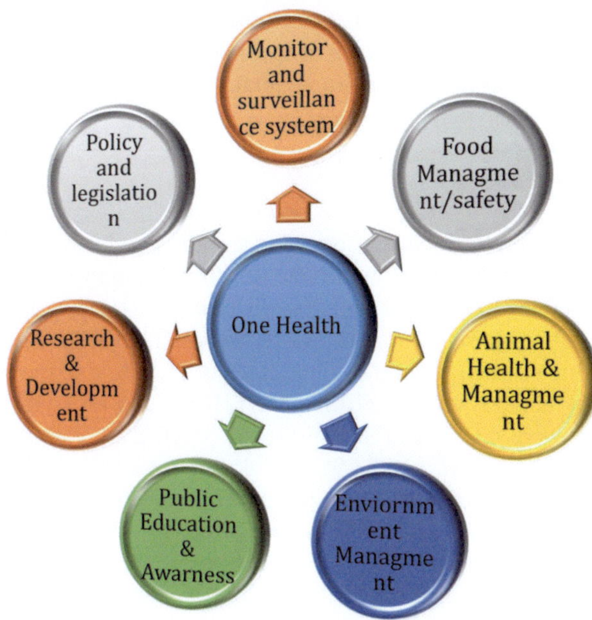

Fig. 3 The multidisciplinary One Health approach to Toxoplasmosis

transmission. In addition, regular inspections ensure safety standards in meat or food industries to reduce contamination.

5. **Environmental Management**:

In environment there is a high chance of *T. gondii* transmission among humans as well as animals, therefore by maintaining proper handling of soil, sand, and raw meat. Proper disposal of cat feces, treating drinking water, and managing stormwater runoff effectively can reduce environmental contamination.

6. **Research and Development**:

T. gondii has a complex life cycle and most of the signs are asymptomatic. However support research into developing better diagnosis, treatment, as well as vaccines for the animals to reduce the prevalence of *T. gondii.* In addition, conduct studies to understand *T. gondii* in different environments and how it spreads between hosts and the environment.

7. **Policy and Legislation**:

Finally develop the policies that support a one health approach with collaboration of interdisciplinaries such as health, agriculture, and environmental sectors. Implement regulations that require farms and food production.

By addressing the disease from these multiple angles, the One Health approach aims to reduce the burden of toxoplasmosis on human health while also considering animal welfare and environmental protection.

Conclusions

The overall global seroprevalence of *T. gondii* infection in pigs was almost 19%, slightly lower than wild boar (23%). Although seroprevalence rates for pigs and wild boar were 13% and 26% in Europe, 21% and 13% in Asia, 25% and 32% in North America, and 23% and 5% in South America, respectively, whereas pigs from China and Brazil show higher rates of *T. gondii* seroprevalence. The main serological methods such as ELISA, MAT, IFAT, and IHA yielded, sensitivity and specificity were 82.9% and 90.2% for the MAT, 29.4% and 98.3% for IHAT, 45.9% and 96.9% for LAT, and 72.9% and 85.9% for ELISA. It's known that the survival rate of Toxoplasma oocysts is higher in areas with moderate temperatures (15–30 °C) and damp soil and lower in case of colder climates. There is uncertainty regarding many aspects, such as assessment of risk factors while pig farming, e.g., about the role of general data, facilities, conversation while maintenance of farms, feeding conditions as well as intermediate host agents. In pigs, it seems clear that outdoor access is an important risk factor for *T. gondii* infection. The routes of infection in herbivores appear to be well understood, with oocysts presumed to be the primary source. However, the extent to which oocyst contamination or the presence and uptake of infected intermediate hosts contribute to infection remains unclear. Overall, globally, approximately one-fifth of domestic pigs are infected with *T. gondii* infection. Instead, it was shown that geographical and climate factors have a significant effect on the prevalence rate of infection in pigs. Since pork and pork products are one of the main human food sources, and the presence of infective *T. gondii* in pork meat. In addition, pigs sold for fresh pork consumption (feeder pigs, market pigs) are mostly raised indoors in well-managed facilities to prevent access to rodents and cats. In these well-managed facilities, the prevalence of *T. gondii* has declined drastically in the last decade but it's not enough to overcome *T. gondii* spreading, for this more prospective studies including the assessment of interventions are needed to confirm previous findings and to determine the feasibility and the efficiency of control measures. Furthermore, the economic impact of toxoplasmosis in livestock, e.g., in small ruminants, has never been assessed in most of the regions worldwide.

Future Directions

Future directions mainly focus on the advanced aspects, like research needs required for the development of standard diagnosis for the clearance of human and animal hosts, in addition to approaching modern farming techniques. Further, it is important to enhance the improved education of health professional and general people in monitoring programs to screen animal's food chain. By developing vaccines, detective protocols for *T. gondii* tissue cysts in meat, surrounding environment, soil, water, and food need to be thoroughly investigated with low cost and more effectiveness. In order to avoid exposure, more attention needs to be paid towards the disinfection of vegetables, quality of water, further genome level studies as well as epidemiologically relevant routes of *T. gondii* infection in livestock.

Acknowledgements The authors would like to thank Jitender P. Dubey, Ionela Hotea, and Gheorghe Darabus for their permission to access data and figures.

References

Aguirre, A. A., Longcore, T., Barbieri, M., Dabritz, H., Hill, D., Klein, P. N., et al. (2019). The one health approach to toxoplasmosis: Epidemiology, control, and prevention strategies. *EcoHealth, 16*(2), 378–390.

Ahmad, S., & Tasawar, Z. (2015). Seroprevalence of toxoplasma gondii in four ovine breeds of Cholistan desert of Pakistan. *Pakistan Journal of Life and Social Sciences, 13*(2), 91–96.

Almeria, S., & Dubey, J. P. (2021). Foodborne transmission of toxoplasma gondii infection in the last decade: An overview. *Research in Veterinary Science, 135*, 371–385.

Djurković-Djaković, O., Dupouy-Camet, J., Van der Giessen, J., & Dubey, J. P. (2019). Toxoplasmosis: Overview from a one health perspective. *Food and Waterborne Parasitology, 15*, e00054. https://doi.org/10.1016/j.fawpar.2019.e00054

Dubey, J. P. (2009). History of the discovery of the life cycle of toxoplasma gondii. *International Journal of Parasitology, 39*, 877–882.

Dubey, J. P. (2010). *Toxoplasmosis of animals and humans* (2nd ed., p. 133). CRC Press.

Dubey, J. P. (2021). Outbreaks of clinical toxoplasmosis in humans: Five decades of personal experience, perspectives and lessons learned. *Parasites & Vectors, 14*(1), 263. https://doi.org/10.1186/s13071-021-04769-4

Dubey, J. P., & Jones, J. L. (2008). Toxoplasma gondii infection in humans and animals in the United States. *International Journal for Parasitology, 38*, 1257–1278.

Dubey, J. P., Cerqueira-Cézar, C. K., Murata, F. H. A., Kwok, O. C. H., Hill, D., Yang, Y., & Su, C. (2020). All about toxoplasma gondii infections in pigs: 2009–2020. *Veterinary Parasitology, 288*, 109185.

Elsalem, R. (2024). A review of toxoplasmosis in humans and animals in Libya. *Journal of Pure & Applied Sciences, 23*(1), 64–71. https://doi.org/10.51984/jopas.v23i1.2447

Foroutan, M., Fakhri, Y., Riahi, S. M., Ebrahimpour, S., Namroodi, S., Taghipour, A., Spotin, A. H., Gamble, R., & Rostami, A. (2019). The global seroprevalence of toxoplasma gondii in pigs: A systematic review and meta-analysis. *Veterinary Parasitology, 269*, 42–52.

Gao, X., Wang, H., Wang, H., Qin, H., & Xiao, J. (2016). Land use and soil contamination with toxoplasma gondii oocysts in urban areas. *Science of the Total Environment, 568*, 1086–1091.

Herrero, L., Gracia, M. J., Pérez-Arquillué, C., Lázaro, R., Herrera, M., Herrera, A., & Bayarri, S. (2016). Toxoplasma gondii: Pig seroprevalence, associated risk factors and viability in fresh pork meat. *Veterinary Parasitology, 224*, 52–59.

Hosseini, S. A., Amouei, A., Sharif, M., Sarvi, S., Galal, L., Javidnia, J., Pagheh, A. S., Gholami, S., Mizani, A., & Daryani, A. (2018). Human toxoplasmosis: A systematic review for genetic diversity of toxoplasma gondii in clinical samples. *Epidemiology and Infection, 147*(36), 1–9.

Hotea, I., & Dărăbuş, G. (2023). *Toxoplasmosis: Epidemiology, prevention and control*. MDPI. https://doi.org/10.3390/books978-3-0365-2698-0

Kim, K., & Weiss, L. M. (2004). Toxoplasma gondii: The model apicomplexan. *International Journal for Parasitology, 34*, 423.

Oliveira, J. P., Casseb, A. R., Ramos, A. S., Rolim, S. T., et al. (2018). Risk factors associated with the epidemiology of toxoplasma gondii in cattle and buffaloes in the state of Pará, Brazil. *Semina: Ciênc Agrár, 39*(5), 2029–2038. https://doi.org/10.5433/1679-0359.2018v39n5p2029

Papatsiros, V. G., Athanasiou, L. V., Kostoulas, P., Giannakopoulos, A., Tzika, E., & Billinis, C. (2021). Toxoplasma gondii infection in swine: Implications for public health. *Foodborne Pathogens and Disease, 18*(12), 823–840.

Pardini, L., Bernstein, M., Carral, L. A., Kaufer, F. J., Dellarupe, A., Gos, M. L., Campero, L. M., Moré, G., Messina, M. T., Schneider, M. V., Freuler, C. B., Durlach, R. A., Unzaga, J. M., & Venturini, M. C. (2018). Congenital human toxoplasmosis caused by non-clonal toxoplasma gondii genotypes in Argentina. *Parasitology International, 68*, 48–52.

Robert-Gangneux, F., & Dardé, M. L. (2012). Epidemiology of and diagnostic strategies for toxoplasmosis. *Clinical Microbiology Reviews, 25*, 264–296.

Rouatbi, M., Amairia, S., Amdouni, Y., Boussaadoun, M. A., Ayadi, Q., Al-Hosary, A. A. T., Rekik, M., Abdallah, R. B., Aoun, K., Mohamed Aziz Darghouth, M. A., Salem, R. S., Mohamed, A. A., & Randa, M. E. (2019). Seroprevalence of Toxoplasma gondii among pregnant women in Misurata, Libya. In *Second symposium on theories and applications of basic and biosciences*.

Scallan, E., Hoekstra, R. M., Angulo, F. J., Tauxe, R. V., Widdowson, M. A., Roy, S. L., Jones, J. L., & Griffin, P. M. (2011). Foodborne illness acquired in the United States–major pathogens. *Emerging Infectious Diseases, 17*, 7–15.

Scofano, A. S., Arruda, I. F., Teixeira, J. N., Cunha, N. C., Nascimento, E. R., Amendoeira, M. R. R., et al. (2023). Toxoplasma gondii infection in pig intended for human consumption: Seroprevalence, risk factors and influence of biosecurity measures. *Brazilian Journal of Veterinary Parasitology, 32*(4), e008523.

Shapiro, K., Bahia-Oliveira, L., Dixon, B., Dumètre, A., de Wit, L. A., VanWormer, E., & Villena, I. (2019). Environmental transmission of toxoplasma gondii: Oocysts in water, soil and food. *Food and Waterborne Parasitology, 15*, e00049.

Smith, N. C., Goulart, C., Hayward, J. A., Kupz, A., Miller, C. M., & van Dooren, G. G. (2021). Control of human toxoplasmosis. *International Journal for Parasitology, 51*(2–3), 95–121. https://doi.org/10.1016/j.ijpara.2020.11.001

Thebault, A., Kooh, P., Cadavez, V., Gonzales-Barron, U., & Villena, I. (2021). Risk factors for sporadic toxoplasmosis: A systematic review and meta-analysis. *Microbial Risk Analysis, 17*, 100133.

Emerging Coronaviruses in Swine and Their Potential to Affect Humans

Tapan R. Kumbhani and Sejalben P. Antiya

Abstract

Coronaviruses, a significant group of RNA viruses, pose notable risks to both animal and human health. Swine coronaviruses, encompassing Alphacoronaviruses, Betacoronaviruses, and Deltacoronaviruses, notably impact pig populations globally. Key members like Transmissible Gastroenteritis Virus (TGEV), Porcine Epidemic Diarrhea Virus (PEDV), and Porcine Delta Coronavirus (PDCoV) have led to substantial economic losses in the swine industry due to high piglet mortality and reduced productivity. These viruses primarily cause gastrointestinal and respiratory illnesses in pigs, with some variants such as Porcine Hemagglutinating Encephalomyelitis Virus (PHEV) affecting the nervous system. Furthermore, the zoonotic potential of these coronaviruses underscores their relevance to human health. Genetic recombination and mutations increase the likelihood of interspecies transmission, potentially enabling novel strains with heightened virulence. Effective surveillance, biosecurity, and vaccination strategies are critical for managing outbreaks. This chapter emphasizes the importance of a One Health approach to understand the epidemiology, genetic diversity, and control measures for porcine coronaviruses. Enhanced collaborative efforts between veterinary and public health sectors are vital for mitigating risks associated with these emerging pathogens, safeguarding both agricultural livelihoods and global health security.

T. R. Kumbhani
Department of Veterinary Pathology, College of Veterinary Science and Animal Husbandry at Kamdhenu University (KU), Anand, Gujarat, India

S. P. Antiya (✉)
Department of Veterinary Microbiology, College of Veterinary Science and Animal Husbandry at Kamdhenu University (KU), Anand, Gujarat, India

R. Deb et al. (eds.), *Emerging Zoonotic Threats from Swine*,
https://doi.org/10.1007/978-981-96-7407-7_13

Keywords

Swine coronaviruses · Zoonosis · Transmissible Gastroenteritis Virus (TGEV) · Porcine Epidemic Diarrhea Virus (PEDV) · Porcine Delta Coronavirus (PDCoV) · One Health · Genetic recombination · Biosecurity · Veterinary epidemiology · Zoonotic diseases

Introduction

Recently, COVID-19 caused a huge socioeconomic loss in the world which shows that coronaviruses pose a great threat to human and animal health, as they can infect mammals and birds (Liu et al., 2020). Coronaviruses are a large family of viruses that can cause illness in both animals and humans. These viruses get their name from the spike-like glycoproteins known as spike (S) proteins that are found on their surfaces and resemble crowns.

Coronaviruses are widespread in animals and can cause a range of diseases, including gastrointestinal and respiratory infections. For instance, the bovine coronavirus (BCoV) and porcine epidemic diarrhea virus (PEDV) respectively infect cattle and pigs, resulting in significant economic losses for the livestock sector as a result of reduced production and mortality.

Numerous human outbreaks of severe respiratory illnesses have been linked to coronaviruses. Numerous outbreaks over the years, such as the Middle East respiratory disease (MERS) outbreak in 2012, the severe acute respiratory syndrome (SARS) outbreak in 2002–2003, and the COVID-19 pandemic brought on by the novel coronavirus SARS-CoV-2 have highlighted the importance of coronaviruses in human health (Dhama et al., 2020; Shaw et al., 2020). Hundreds of thousands of people have died and millions of illnesses have been caused by SARS-CoV-2 infection worldwide. The virus has produced extensive social and psychological effects, disrupted economies, and overwhelmed healthcare systems.

The aforementioned outbreaks underscore the persistent risk that coronaviruses offer to the health of pigs and the significance of proactive surveillance, biosecurity protocols, and research endeavors aimed at improving comprehension and management of these viruses. Furthermore, the resemblances between human and swine coronaviruses emphasize the critical importance of a One Health strategy to tackle emerging infectious diseases at the interface of humans, animals, and the environment. It is crucial to understand the biology and epidemiology of swine coronaviruses (CoVs) for the swine enterprise, veterinary medicine, and public health. These viruses can have a negative economic impact because of their influence on food production and trade, in addition to posing a serious threat to the health of pigs.

The likelihood of coronaviruses undergoing genetic recombination or mutation, which might result in the development of novel strains with higher virulence or the ability to infect new hosts, is one of the primary concerns regarding animal health (Wells et al., 2023). This could render it more difficult to prevent and control disease in both human and animal populations. Since coronaviruses can cause severe respiratory illnesses ranging from mild flu-like symptoms to severe pneumonia and acute respiratory distress syndrome (ARDS), they are important to human health. Some populations are more vulnerable to serious COVID-19 problems, including the elderly, immunocompromised individuals, and those with existing medical disorders.

The main reason swine coronaviruses have an influence on public health is due to the fact viruses can lead to outbreaks in swine populations, which can have significant financial effects on the swine business. Global food production depends heavily on the swine sector, and swine coronavirus epidemics may decrease swine productivity and raise piglet mortality rates, which in turn can impact the supply and price of pork. Furthermore, swine coronaviruses have the potential to infect humans, which is known as a zoonotic risk. Concerns are raised over the swine coronaviruses' potential to spread to humans through zoonotic transmission. Additionally, the possibility of new strains arising with the ability to infect humans more effectively is facilitated by the genetic diversity and inclination of coronaviruses to undergo genetic recombination (Wells et al., 2023). To mitigate the potential for future pandemics of swine coronaviruses, comprehensive surveillance programs are essential for the early detection of emerging strains in swine populations. Additionally, research efforts focused on understanding the genetic diversity, transmission dynamics, and pathogenesis of swine coronaviruses are crucial for developing effective control strategies and vaccines.

Structure and Classification of Porcine Coronaviruses

Coronaviruses are a family of viruses that infect a wide range of animals, including humans, birds, and various mammalian species such as swine. Coronaviruses belong to the family *Coronaviridae* and the order *Nidovirales* (Su et al., 2016). The viruses of the *coronaviridae* family have a positive-sense single-stranded RNA genome and are enveloped viruses. The genome of coronaviruses is the largest among all RNA viruses, ranging from about 26 to 32 kilobases in length (Alluwaimi et al., 2020; Chen et al., 2020). This large genome size allows for high mutation rates, which contribute to the ability of coronaviruses to adapt to new hosts and environments.

Coronaviruses are further classified into four genera: Alphacoronavirus, Betacoronavirus, Gammacoronavirus, and Deltacoronavirus. Alphacoronaviruses and Betacoronaviruses primarily infect mammals, including humans, while Gammacoronaviruses and Deltacoronaviruses typically infect birds and certain mammals (Chen et al., 2020).

Six members of the *Coronaviridae* family have been reported to affect the pigs (Decaro et al., 2020). There are four viruses under 3 subgenuses of alpha coronavirus that affect the pigs, i.e., Transmissible gastroenteritis virus (TGEV) (subgenus Tegacovirus), Porcine respiratory coronavirus (PRCV) (subgenus Tegacovirus), Porcine epidemic diarrhea virus (PEDV) (subgenus Pedacovirus), and Swine acute diarrhea syndrome coronavirus (SADSCoV) (subgenus Rhinacovirus). The beta coronavirus that affects the pigs is Porcine hemagglutinating encephalomyelitis virus (PHEV) (subgenus Embecovirus). Porcine delta coronavirus (PDCoV) (subgenus Buldecovirus) belongs to delta coronavirus that affect pigs (Thakor et al., 2022) (Table 1).

Four structural proteins are identified in porcine coronaviruses, i.e., spike protein (S), Integral membrane glycoprotein (M), envelope small membrane protein (E), and a nucleocapsid protein (N) (Song et al., 2019). The S protein is required for virus cellular entry (Wang et al., 2020a, b). M protein is essential to preserve the core structure of the virus (Kuo et al., 2016). The 'E' protein is needed for virus assembly. N protein forms a helical structure of capsid by the formation of a complex with the genome RNA (Asrani et al., 2020). Porcine coronaviruses genome schematic representation is summarized in Fig. 1.

Table 1 Porcine coronaviruses and diseases caused by coronaviruses in swine

Genus	Subgenus	Virus	Disease
Alpha	Tegacovirus	Transmissible Gastroenteritis Virus (TGEV)	Gastroenteritis
		Porcine Respiratory Coronavirus (PRCV)	Bronchointerstitial pneumonia
	Pedacovirus	Porcine Epidemic Diarrhea Virus (PEDV)	Gastroenteritis
	Rhinacovirus	Swine Acute Diarrhea Syndrome Coronavirus (SADS-CoV)	Gastroenteritis
Beta	Embecovirus	Porcine Hemagglutinating Encephalomyelitis Virus (PHEV)	Vomiting and Wasting Disease (VWD) and encephalomyelitis
Delta	Buldecovirus	Porcine Delta Coronavirus (PDCoV)	Gastroenteritis

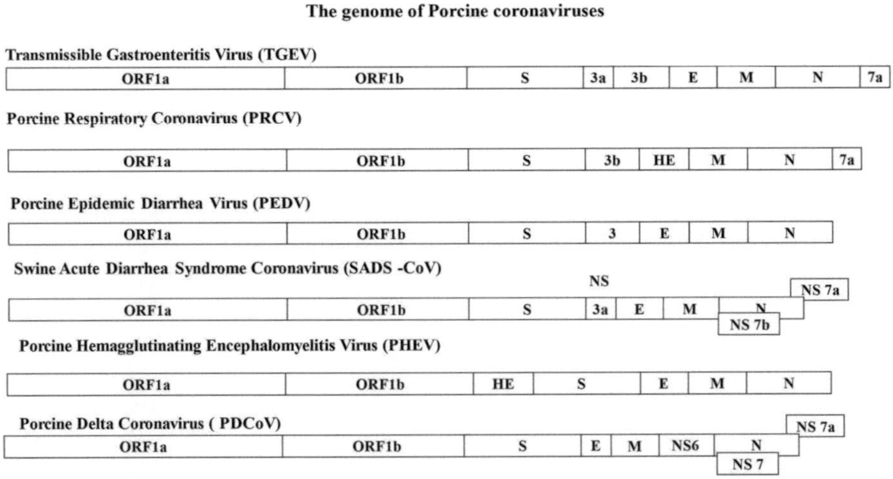

The genome of Porcine coronaviruses
Transmissible Gastroenteritis Virus (TGEV)
ORF1a ORF1b S 3a 3b E M N 7a
Porcine Respiratory Coronavirus (PRCV)
ORF1a ORF1b S 3b HE M N 7a
Porcine Epidemic Diarrhea Virus (PEDV)
ORF1a ORF1b S 3 E M N
Swine Acute Diarrhea Syndrome Coronavirus (SADS -CoV)
NS
NS 7a
ORF1a ORF1b S 3a E M N
NS 7b
Porcine Hemagglutinating Encephalomyelitis Virus (PHEV)
ORF1a ORF1b HE S E M N
Porcine Delta Coronavirus (PDCoV)
NS 7a
ORF1a ORF1b S E M NS6 N
NS 7

Fig. 1 Schematic representation of genome structure of different porcine coronaviruses. (S—Spike S structural gene, E—envelope, M—membrane, N—nucleoprotein, HE—hemagglutinin-esterase, Ns3a, Ns6, Ns7, Ns7a, Ns7b—accessory genes)

Transmissible Gastroenteritis Virus (TGEV)

TGEV is one of the earliest identified coronaviruses in pigs, first recognized in the 1940s. The virus is a member of the Alpha Coronavirus genus, specifically the Tegacovirus subgenus. It primarily infects the epithelial cells of the small intestine of young piglets, causing severe diarrhea, dehydration, and high mortality rates, particularly in piglets less than 2 weeks old (Garwes, 1988). TGEV has a significant economic impact on the swine industry due to mortality and reduced growth rates in surviving piglets.

Porcine Epidemic Diarrhea Virus (PEDV)

PEDV emerged in the 1970s but gained global attention during large-scale outbreaks in Asia in the 2010s and North America in 2013. The virus belongs to the subgenus Pedacovirus of the Alpha Coronavirus genus. Similar to TGEV, PEDV also targets the epithelial cells in the small intestine, resulting in symptoms including severe diarrhea and dehydration that can be fatal (Li et al., 2018). It poses a significant threat to pig populations, particularly neonatal piglets. Its introduction to naïve swine populations can lead to rapid spread and significant economic losses within the industry. Vaccines and improved biosecurity protocols have been developed to mitigate PEDV outbreaks.

Porcine Delta Coronavirus (PDCoV)

PDCoV was first identified in Hong Kong in 2012 and later detected in the United States in 2014. The virus belongs to the subgenus Buldacovirus of the Delta Coronavirus genus. Like PEDV, PDCoV primarily affects the digestive tract, resulting in vomiting, diarrhea, and dehydration in pigs (Song et al., 2015). It poses a challenge for swine producers due to its similarity in clinical signs and transmission routes to PEDV, complicating diagnosis and control efforts. However, clinical signs produced by PDCoV are less severe than those of PEDV. Control measures include strict biosecurity practices, vaccination, and enhanced surveillance.

Swine Acute Diarrhea Syndrome Coronavirus (SADS-CoV)

SADS-CoV was first reported in China in 2017, causing severe diarrhea and high mortality rates in pigs, particularly in neonatal piglets (Pan et al., 2017). The virus belongs to the subgenus Rhinacovirus of the Alpha Coronavirus genus. Although there have been no reports of human infections, SADS-CoV has caused significant financial losses and has generated concerns in the swine industry due to its potential for zoonotic diseases. It is believed that SADS-CoV can infect intestinal cells, fibroblasts, human nasal epithelial cells, and the primary human airway (Goldstein et al., 2021).

Porcine Respiratory Coronavirus (PRCV)

PRCV is an attenuated strain of TGEV that mainly infects the respiratory tract of pigs (Saif & Jung, 2020). Pigs typically experience mild respiratory symptoms like coughing and nasal discharge as a result of PRCV infection. The primary site of infection with PRCV is the lung, which typically manifests as bronchointerstitial pneumonia (Cui et al., 2020).

Porcine Hemagglutinating Encephalomyelitis Virus (PHEV)

PHEV belongs to the subgenus Embecovirus of the Beta Coronavirus genus. The virus primarily affects the central nervous system of pigs, causing symptoms like encephalomyelitis, vomiting, and ataxia. The virus causes vomiting and wasting disease (VWD) in pigs. It is relatively rare but can lead to significant neurological damage in affected animals. Cachexia, abdominal distension, and stomach dilatation are commonly seen as gross lesions in pigs with natural infections (Mora-Díaz et al., 2020).

The ability of coronaviruses to spread from animals to humans is referred to as zoonotic transmission. The enteric coronaviruses, which include TGEV, PEDV, PDCoV, and SADSCoV—also referred to as swine enteric alphacoronavirus (SeACoV) and pig enteric alphacoronavirus (PEAV)—are among the six members and have significance for public health due to their potential for cross-species transmission. These viruses can potentially mutate and adapt to infect humans, leading to outbreaks or even pandemics if they acquire efficient human-to-human transmission capabilities.

Transmission of Porcine Coronavirus of Porcine Coronaviruses

- *Direct Contact*: One common route that swine coronaviruses spread is through direct contact between susceptible and infected pigs. This can happen by aerosol transmission of respiratory secretions, oral-fecal contact, or nose-to-nose contact. Closely confined pigs, like those kept in the same barn or enclosure, are more vulnerable to direct infection (Niederwerder & Hesse, 2018). Infected pigs shed the virus in feces, saliva, and respiratory secretions, which can readily infect susceptible pigs upon contact.
- *Fomites*: Additionally, via means of fomites—inanimate items or materials that have the potential to contain and transfer infectious agents—porcine coronaviruses can also spread indirectly. Equipment that has been contaminated, such as waterers, feeders, clothes, boots, and cars, can act as channels for the spread of viruses among pigs and between places (Niederwerder & Hesse, 2018). This mode of transmission is particularly relevant in settings where biosecurity measures are inadequate or not rigorously enforced.
- *Contaminated Feed and Water*: Porcine coronavirus can spread through contaminated feed and water, especially when feeding ingredients or water supplies have

been contaminated with feces from pigs that are affected (Bowman et al., 2015). This mode of transmission highlights the importance of maintaining strict hygiene practices in feed manufacturing and delivery systems.
- *Airborne Transmission*: Porcine coronaviruses can also spread through the air by aerosols or respiratory droplets over short distances. This mechanism of transmission is especially important for viruses like PDCoV that cause respiratory illnesses in pigs (Niederwerder & Hesse, 2018). Factors such as ventilation systems, pig density, and environmental conditions can influence the extent of airborne transmission within swine populations.
- *Vertical Transmission*: It is possible for some porcine coronaviruses to spread vertically from sow to piglet. The virus can be transmitted by infected sows in their milk, feces, or respiratory secretions, which can infect young piglets during delivery or while nursing (Yuan et al., 2022). Vertical transmission can perpetuate the virus within a herd and contribute to its persistence over time.
- *Vectors*: This is a less common route for the coronavirus to spread. Some vectors, such as rodents or flies, might be involved in the spread of swine coronaviruses. These vectors can mechanically spread the virus among pigs or throughout premises, especially in less regulated or outdoor production systems where pigs are exposed to more environmental influences. The main transmission of porcine coronaviruses is summarized in Fig. 2.

Factors Affecting Coronavirus Spread

- *Biosecurity Measures*: The efficiency of biosecurity measures is one of the main variables determining the transmission of coronaviruses across swine herds. Strict biosecurity precautions are essential for preventing the entry and spread of coronaviruses (Albert et al., 2021). These measures include limiting access to

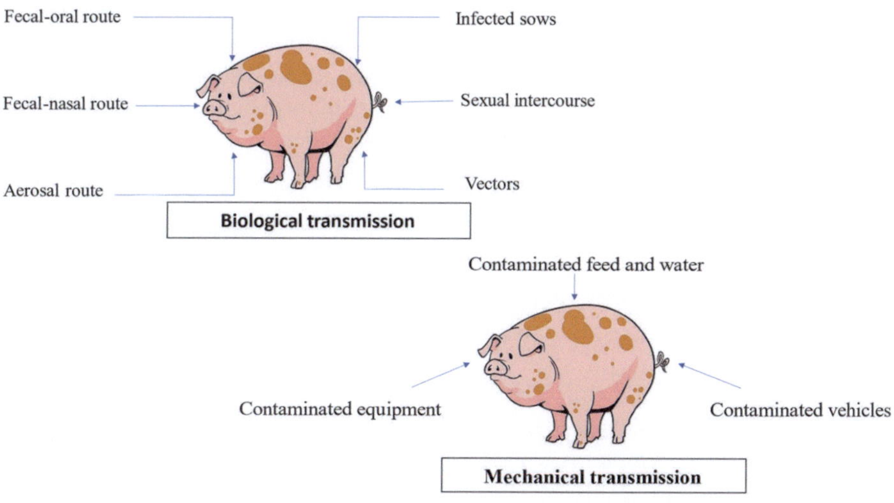

Fig. 2 Schematic representation of transmission route of porcine coronaviruses

farms, following proper cleaning and disinfection methods, and establishing quarantine procedures for incoming animals.

- *Herd Size and Density*: The size and density of swine herds can impact the spread of coronaviruses. Larger herds with higher animal densities may experience more rapid transmission due to increased opportunities for contact and exposure among animals.
- *Animal Movements*: Animal movement within and between swine herds can aid in the coronavirus's dissemination (Albert et al., 2021). Outbreaks can occur when the virus is introduced into susceptible populations through the introduction of contaminated equipment or infected animals from neighboring farms.
- *Environmental Factors*: Environmental conditions, such as ventilation, temperature, and humidity, can influence the transmission of coronaviruses within swine facilities (Weaver et al., 2022).
- *Presence of Carriers*: Within swine herds, asymptomatic coronavirus carriers can act as reservoirs of infection and aid in the virus's dissemination. Controlling outbreaks requires identifying and eliminating carriers from the herd, which can be difficult sometimes.
- *Stress Factors*: Swine's immune systems can be weakened by stress factors such as overcrowding, transportation, and changes to management methods, which make them more vulnerable to coronaviruses. Animals under stress may release more virus, which would boost the infection's spread across the herd.
- *Vaccination Status*: Vaccination can be quite effective in preventing coronaviruses from spreading throughout swine herds. Effective vaccinations may decrease viral shedding and reduce the severity of clinical illness, which helps stop the spread of the infection among animals.
- *Hygiene Practices*: Minimizing the spread of coronaviruses within swine herds requires good hygiene procedures, such as routine facility cleaning and disinfection, appropriate waste management, and maintenance of clean water and feed supplies.
- *Surveillance and Monitoring*: To detect outbreaks early and establish control measures in place as soon as possible, swine herds must be regularly inspected and monitored for the presence of coronaviruses. Identification and containment of the virus can be achieved through monitoring clinical signs, performing diagnostic testing, and keeping track of epidemiological data.

Clinical Manifestations of Porcine Coronavirus Infection

Clinical signs of coronavirus infections in swine can vary depending on the specific strain involved, the age and immune status of the animals, and environmental factors. Common clinical manifestations are as under.

Coronavirus-infected swine, particularly those with PRCV infection, may display respiratory signs such as sneezing, coughing, nasal discharge, and dyspnea. In young piglets, these symptoms tend to be more prominent and can lead to respiratory distress (Cui et al., 2020). Some coronaviruses, such as PEDV, PDCoV, TGEV, and SADS-CoV, primarily affect the gastrointestinal tract, leading to symptoms like reduced feed intake, diarrhea, vomiting, and dehydration (Yang et al., 2020). These symptoms can result in significant economic losses due to reduced growth rates and increased mortality in piglets. In severe cases, systemic signs such as fever, lethargy, and weight loss may be observed. These signs indicate a more widespread infection and can contribute to overall disease severity. Rarely, some coronaviruses, such as PHEV, can infect pigs and cause neurological symptoms such as ataxia, tremors, and paralysis (Mora-Díaz et al., 2019). These manifestations typically indicate a more severe and potentially fatal form of the disease.

Factors Affecting Disease Severity

The severity of coronavirus infections in swine can vary widely and depends on the following factors:

- Virulence: Certain coronavirus strains exhibit greater virulence than others, which can cause more severe clinical illness. The pathogenicity of the virus can be attributed to several factors, including its capacity for effective replication within host cells and immune response evasion.
- Age of the Animals: Young piglets are susceptible to severe coronavirus infections due to their less developed immune systems and lack of maternal antibodies. In outbreaks of diseases like PEDV, mortality rates can be highest in neonatal piglets, leading to significant losses in affected herds.
- Immune Status: The swine population's immune status is an important variable in determining the severity of the disease. The incidence and severity of coronavirus infections in swine herds can be reduced by herd immunity, which is obtained by vaccination or previous exposure.
- Environmental Factors: Swine coronavirus infections can vary in severity depending on several factors, including co-infections with other viruses, stress, and housing circumstances. Poor hygiene and overcrowding can accelerate the virus's spread among a herd and raise the risk of serious health consequences (Weaver et al., 2022).

Impact of Porcine Coronaviruses on Pig and Human Health

In addition to posing hazards to humans, swine coronaviruses have significant effects on the swine industry and agricultural economy. Pig farmers and other sectors may suffer significant financial losses as a result of diseases like PEDV and PDCoV, which can cause serious illness and high mortality rates in pig populations. Understanding the possibility of these viruses spreading to human populations can help develop preventive measures against infections in humans and animals, protecting public health and the agricultural economy.

Employees in the swine sector, such as farmers, veterinarians, and butchers, may come into proximity to swine coronaviruses. Occupational exposure to diseased animals or their bodily fluids can transmit zoonotic illnesses, which can make humans sick. Appropriate preventative measures can be undertaken to safeguard the health and safety of those employed in the swine industry by being aware of the potential for swine coronaviruses to impact human health.

The necessity of strong monitoring systems and quick reaction times to recognize and prevent the spread of emerging infectious diseases has been highlighted by the COVID-19 pandemic. Through the study of swine coronaviruses and their capacity to infect humans, scientists can recognize high-risk viral strains, evaluate their potential for pandemics, and create early warning systems to prevent the introduction of new viruses. This proactive strategy improves our ability to successfully respond to new health threats and improves global readiness for pandemics in the future.

Zoonotic Potential of Porcine Coronavirus

Porcine coronaviruses (CoVs) are a diverse group of viruses that primarily infect pigs but also have the potential to infect humans (Li et al., 2023). These viruses belong to the Coronaviridae family, which includes several well-known human pathogens such as SARS-CoV, MERS-CoV, and more recently, SARS-CoV-2. Understanding the zoonotic potential of porcine coronaviruses is crucial for assessing the risk of transmission from pigs to humans and for developing strategies to prevent and control outbreaks. Several mechanisms facilitate the cross-species transmission of these viruses:

- *Genetic Similarity*: Numerous studies have revealed that there are genetic similarities between some swine coronavirus strains and human coronavirus strains. For example, SADS-CoV and the bat coronavirus HKU2 of bats are closely related (Gong et al., 2017). This genetic resemblance raises concerns about the potential for cross-species transmission.
- *Genetic Diversity*: Numerous strains of porcine coronaviruses are circulating across pig populations globally, demonstrating the significant genetic diversity of these viruses (Mandary et al., 2019). This genetic variability increases the likelihood of viral adaptation to new hosts, including humans.
- *Receptor Binding Specificity*: The ability of a virus to infect a host cell depends on the interaction between viral surface proteins and specific cellular receptors. Porcine coronaviruses primarily use the angiotensin-converting enzyme 2 (ACE2) receptor for entry into host cells (Tiwari et al., 2020). While ACE2 is abundantly expressed in the respiratory tract of pigs, it also exists in humans, making them susceptible to infection by porcine coronaviruses.
- *Receptor Binding Domain (RBD) Mutations*: Mutations in the viral spike protein's receptor-binding domain (RBD) can increase the virus's affinity for the human ACE2 receptor, which makes cross-species transmission easier (Wang

et al., 2020a, b). These mutations may arise through natural selection or genetic recombination events between different strains of coronaviruses (Yan et al., 2020).
- *Host Range Expansion*: Porcine coronaviruses have shown evidence of a broad host range by their capacity to infect a variety of hosts, including humans. The risk of zoonotic transmission can be increased by things like eating contaminated pork products and having close contact with infected animals.
- *Viral Shedding and Environmental Persistence*: Porcine coronaviruses are excreted from infected pigs through their feces, respiratory secretions, and other body fluids that might contaminate the surrounding environment. Interspecies transmission is made possible by the environmental stability of these viruses as well as human activities including farming, transportation, and pig slaughter.

Potential Risk Factors of Porcine Coronaviruses to Human Health

- *Zoonotic Potential*: Coronaviruses are known to have zoonotic potential (Li et al., 2023). Although there isn't any evidence at this time that pig coronaviruses can infect people directly, cross-species transmission can be possible because of the genetic diversity and adaptability of coronaviruses (Guo et al., 2023).
- *Genetic Reassortment and Recombination*: Since coronaviruses can undergo genetic reassortment and recombination processes and have a high mutation rate, new strains with altered virulence, transmissibility, and host range may emerge (Yan et al., 2020). Pigs that are co-infected with various coronaviruses, such as porcine coronaviruses and other respiratory viruses, have the potential to exchange genetic material and generate hybrid viruses with undetermined characteristics (Wells et al., 2023). Genetic analysis of porcine coronaviruses has revealed similarities with human coronaviruses, raising concerns about the potential for genetic exchange and the emergence of novel zoonotic strains (Gong et al., 2017).
- *Occupational Exposure*: Direct contact with infected animals or their respiratory secretions, feces, or other body fluids may increase the risk of exposure to swine coronaviruses for those who deal directly with pigs, such as farmers, veterinarians, and slaughterhouse workers. Performing necropsies, handling sick animals, cleaning contaminated surfaces, and other normal animal husbandry procedures can expose workers to swine coronaviruses.
- *Transmission Pathways*: Although it is rare for swine coronaviruses to spread directly from pigs to human beings, it is possible for the viruses to do so indirectly through contaminated food items, air, or surfaces. Pigs that are infected can release porcine coronaviruses into their feces or respiratory secretions, which can contaminate agricultural land and possibly spread to individuals by ingestion or inhalation.
- *Potential for Viral Adaptation*: Porcine coronaviruses have the potential to evolve and adapt over time in pig populations, which may enhance their ability to replicate and infect human cells. Genetic changes that increase the affinity of porcine

coronaviruses for human cell receptors or facilitate efficient human-to-human transmission could increase the risk of zoonotic transmission and spark outbreaks in human populations.

Prevention and Control Strategies

- *Biosecurity Measures*: Strict biosecurity protocols are essential to prevent the introduction of the virus onto swine farms. This includes controlling access to farms, implementing disinfection procedures for vehicles, equipment, and personnel, and establishing a clear separation between different production areas (Vlasova et al., 2020). Quarantine protocols for incoming animals should be enforced to ensure they are free from infection before introduction to the herd.
- *Risk Assessment and Mitigation*: Conducting risk assessments to determine the factors that lead to the development and spread of porcine coronaviruses. This entails evaluating factors including agricultural practices, interactions with wildlife, human behavior, and environmental changes. Implementing targeted treatments to reduce hazards that have been identified, such as enhanced farm biosecurity protocols, swine vaccination campaigns, and methods to minimize human-wildlife conflict (Leopardi et al., 2020).
- *Surveillance and Monitoring*: Early identification of swine coronavirus infections depends on routinely testing and observing pig herds for symptoms of disease. Testing of nasal swabs, fecal samples, or serum samples may be used in surveillance programs to identify infected animals. Monitoring asymptomatic infections as well as clinical cases in swine herds should be part of this surveillance. Early warning indicators of viral circulation in swine herds can also be obtained by environmental surveillance techniques like testing wastewater for viral RNA. Preventing and managing the spread of disease requires the establishment of strong monitoring systems and early warning systems for identifying and handling swine CoV outbreaks. To enable quick response to outbreaks, research should focus on creating syndromic monitoring technologies, improving networks for data sharing and communication, and combining genetic and epidemiological data.
- *Vaccination*: Vaccination can be an effective tool for preventing swine coronavirus infections. However, the development of effective vaccines specific to swine coronaviruses is challenging due to the genetic diversity of these viruses.
- *Herd Management Practices*: Implementing good management practices can help to reduce stress on pigs, which can decrease the susceptibility of animals to infections. Good management practices include ensuring proper nutrition, maintaining optimal environmental conditions, and minimizing overcrowding (Tråvén et al., 1999). Segregating sick animals from healthy ones helps in preventing the spread of the virus within the herd.
- *Sanitation and Hygiene*: Proper sanitation and hygiene protocols are essential for controlling the spread of swine coronaviruses within and between farms. Regular

cleaning and disinfection of equipment, and water sources can help reduce the risk of transmission.

- *Education and Training*: Effective outbreak prevention and management depend on educating farm employees on biosecurity precautions, appropriate sanitation practices, and symptoms associated with swine coronavirus infection. Farm workers can be better prepared to prevent diseases by participating in training programs that provide them with the necessary knowledge and skills.
- *Collaboration and Communication*: Government organizations, veterinary professionals, researchers, and industry stakeholders can collaborate to effectively address the threat of emerging coronaviruses in swine, reduce the risk of zoonotic transmission, and safeguard public health and agricultural livelihoods by integrating the perspectives of human, animal, and environmental health. Open channels of communication make it easier to share information, resources, and best practices to successfully combat the problems caused by swine coronaviruses. Public health messaging should emphasize the importance of early detection, rapid response, and collaboration across sectors to prevent the spread of emerging coronaviruses.
- *Research and Development*: Continued investment in research is needed to improve our understanding of the epidemiology, genetics, and pathogenesis of emerging coronaviruses in swine for the development of more effective control strategies, including vaccines and diagnostic tools. Studies should be carried out to identify potential reservoir hosts, characterize viral evolution and transmission dynamics, and develop novel diagnostic tools and therapeutics. Innovation in vaccine development is critical for controlling emerging coronaviruses in swine and reducing the risk of spillover events. Research efforts should also focus on understanding the role of environmental factors, host immunity, and viral evolution in the transmission and persistence of swine coronaviruses.

One Health Approach

The concept of One Health emphasizes the significance of interdisciplinary collaboration in addressing health hazards at the human-animal-environment interface, acknowledging the interdependence of human, animal, and environmental health (Leroy et al., 2020). A comprehensive understanding of the factors affecting the emergence, transmission, and potential effects on human health is made possible by studying swine coronaviruses within the framework of One Health. To fully understand a variety of factors affecting virus development, transmission, and distribution, virologists, epidemiologists, veterinarians, ecologists, and other pertinent stakeholders must collaborate transdisciplinary. This method makes it easier to create surveillance, control, and preventative strategies that effectively lessen the hazards brought on by zoonotic coronaviruses (Cipolla et al., 2015). It is critical to understand how swine coronaviruses can influence human health in order to safeguard agricultural economies, prevent the spread of zoonotic diseases, and protect public health. We can more accurately predict and respond to new infectious diseases by implementing a One Health strategy and giving multidisciplinary research, surveillance, and preparedness initiatives a top priority. This would lessen the impact of future pandemics on both human and animal populations.

References

Albert, C., Baez, A., & Rutland, J. (2021). Human security as biosecurity. *Politics and the Life Sciences, 40*(1), 83–105. https://doi.org/10.1017/pls.2021.1

Alluwaimi, A. M., Alshubaith, I. H., Al-Ali, A. M., & Abohelaika, S. (2020). The coronaviruses of animals and birds: Their zoonosis, vaccines, and models for SARS-CoV and SARS-CoV2. *Frontiers in Veterinary Science, 7*, 582287. https://doi.org/10.3389/fvets.2020.582287

Asrani, P., Hasan, G. M., Sohal, S. S., & Hassan, M. I. (2020). Molecular basis of pathogenesis of coronaviruses: A comparative genomics approach to planetary health to prevent zoonotic outbreaks in the 21st century. *OMICS: A Journal of Integrative Biology, 24*(11), 634–644. https://doi.org/10.1089/omi.2020.0131

Bowman, A. S., Krogwold, R. A., Price, T., Davis, M., & Moeller, S. J. (2015). Investigating the introduction of porcine epidemic diarrhea virus into an Ohio swine operation. *BMC Veterinary Research, 11*(1), 38. https://doi.org/10.1186/s12917-015-0348-2

Chen, Y., Liu, Q., & Guo, D. (2020). Emerging coronaviruses: Genome structure, replication, and pathogenesis. *Journal of Medical Virology, 92*(4), 418–423. https://doi.org/10.1002/jmv.25681

Cipolla, M., Bonizzi, L., & Zecconi, A. (2015). From "one health" to "one communication": The contribution of communication in veterinary medicine to public health. *Veterinary Sciences, 2*(3), 135–149. https://doi.org/10.3390/vetsci2030135

Cui, T., Theuns, S., Xie, J., Broeck, W., & Nauwynck, H. (2020). Role of porcine aminopeptidase N and sialic acids in porcine coronavirus infections in primary porcine enterocytes. *Viruses, 12*(4), 402. https://doi.org/10.3390/v12040402

Decaro, N., Martella, V., Saif, L. J., & Buonavoglia, C. (2020). COVID-19 from veterinary medicine and one health perspectives: What animal coronaviruses have taught us. *Research in Veterinary Science, 131*, 21–23. https://doi.org/10.1016/j.rvsc.2020.04.009

Dhama, K., Khan, S., Tiwari, R., Sircar, S., Bhat, S., Malik, Y. S., Singh, K. P., Chaicumpa, W., Bonilla-Aldana, D. K., & Rodriguez-Morales, A. J. (2020). Coronavirus disease 2019–COVID-19. *Clinical Microbiology Reviews, 33*(4), e00028–e00020. https://doi.org/10.1128/CMR.00028-20

Garwes, D. (1988). Transmissible gastroenteritis. *Veterinary Record, 122*(19), 462–463. https://doi.org/10.1136/vr.122.19.462

Goldstein, S. A., Brown, J., Pedersen, B. S., Quinlan, A. R., & Elde, N. C. (2021). Extensive recombination-driven coronavirus diversification expands the pool of potential pandemic pathogens. *BioRxiv: The Preprint Server for Biology*. https://doi.org/10.1101/2021.02.03.429646

Gong, L., Li, J., Zhou, Q., Xu, Z., Chen, L., Zhang, Y., Xue, C., Wen, Z., & Cao, Y. (2017). A new bat-HKU2–like coronavirus in swine, China, 2017. *Emerging Infectious Diseases, 23*(9), 1607–1609. https://doi.org/10.3201/eid2309.170915

Guo, Z., Jin, Q., Li, P., Xing, G., Lu, Q., & Zhang, G. (2023). Potential cross-species transmission risks of emerging swine enteric coronavirus to human beings. *Journal of Medical Virology, 95*(7), e28919. https://doi.org/10.1002/jmv.28919

Kuo, L., Hurst-Hess, K. R., Koetzner, C. A., & Masters, P. S. (2016). Analyses of coronavirus assembly interactions with interspecies membrane and Nucleocapsid protein chimeras. *Journal of Virology, 90*(9), 4357–4368. https://doi.org/10.1128/JVI.03212-15

Leopardi, S., Priori, P., Zecchin, B., Zamperin, G., Milani, A., Tonon, F., Giorgiutti, M., Beato, M. S., & De Benedictis, P. (2020). Interface between bats and pigs in heavy pig production. *Viruses, 13*(1), 4. https://doi.org/10.3390/v13010004

Leroy, E. M., Ar Gouilh, M., & Brugère-Picoux, J. (2020). The risk of SARS-CoV-2 transmission to pets and other wild and domestic animals strongly mandates a one-health strategy to control the COVID-19 pandemic. *One Health, 10*, 100133. https://doi.org/10.1016/j.onehlt.2020.100133

Li, Y., Wu, Q., Huang, L., Yuan, C., Wang, J., & Yang, Q. (2018). An alternative pathway of enteric PEDV dissemination from nasal cavity to intestinal mucosa in swine. *Nature Communications, 9*(1), 3811. https://doi.org/10.1038/s41467-018-06056-w

Li, Q., Shah, T., Wang, B., Qu, L., Wang, R., Hou, Y., Baloch, Z., & Xia, X. (2023). Cross-species transmission, evolution and zoonotic potential of coronaviruses. *Frontiers in Cellular and Infection Microbiology, 12*, 1081370. https://doi.org/10.3389/fcimb.2022.1081370

Liu, Q., Xu, K., Wang, X., & Wang, W. (2020). From SARS to COVID-19: What lessons have we learned? *Journal of Infection and Public Health, 13*(11), 1611–1618. https://doi.org/10.1016/j.jiph.2020.08.001

Mandary, M. B., Masomian, M., & Poh, C. L. (2019). Impact of RNA virus evolution on Quasispecies formation and virulence. *International Journal of Molecular Sciences, 20*(18), 4657. https://doi.org/10.3390/ijms20184657

Mora-Díaz, J. C., Piñeyro, P. E., Houston, E., Zimmerman, J., & Giménez-Lirola, L. G. (2019). Porcine Hemagglutinating encephalomyelitis virus: A review. *Frontiers in Veterinary Science, 6*, 53. https://doi.org/10.3389/fvets.2019.00053

Mora-Díaz, J. C., Magtoto, R., Houston, E., Baum, D., Carrillo-Ávila, J. A., Temeeyasen, G., Zimmerman, J., Piñeyro, P., & Giménez-Lirola, L. (2020). Detecting and monitoring porcine Hemagglutinating encephalomyelitis virus, an Underresearched Betacoronavirus. *MSphere, 5*(3), e00199–e00120. https://doi.org/10.1128/mSphere.00199-20

Niederwerder, M. C., & Hesse, R. A. (2018). Swine enteric coronavirus disease: A review of 4 years with porcine epidemic diarrhoea virus and porcine deltacoronavirus in the United States and Canada. *Transboundary and Emerging Diseases, 65*(3), 660–675. https://doi.org/10.1111/tbed.12823

Pan, Y., Tian, X., Qin, P., Wang, B., Zhao, P., Yang, Y.-L., Wang, L., Wang, D., Song, Y., Zhang, X., & Huang, Y.-W. (2017). Discovery of a novel swine enteric alphacoronavirus (SeACoV) in southern China. *Veterinary Microbiology, 211*, 15–21. https://doi.org/10.1016/j.vetmic.2017.09.020

Saif, L. J., & Jung, K. (2020). Comparative pathogenesis of bovine and porcine respiratory coronaviruses in the animal host species and SARS-CoV-2 in humans. *Journal of Clinical Microbiology, 58*(8), e01355–e01320. https://doi.org/10.1128/JCM.01355-20

Shaw, P. D., Patel, N., Patil, S., Samuel, R., Khanna, P., Prajapati, B., Sharun, K., Tiwari, R., Dhama, K., & Natesan, S. (2020). Comparative evaluation of the origin, evolution, transmission, diagnosis, and vaccine development of three highly pathogenic human coronaviruses (SARS-CoV, MERS-CoV and SARS-CoV-2). *Journal of Experimental Biology and Agricultural Sciences, 8*(Spl-1-SARS-CoV-2), S103–S113. https://doi.org/10.18006/2020.8(Spl-1-SARS-CoV-2).S103.S113

Song, D., Zhou, X., Peng, Q., Chen, Y., Zhang, F., Huang, T., Zhang, T., Li, A., Huang, D., Wu, Q., He, H., & Tang, Y. (2015). Newly emerged porcine Deltacoronavirus associated with Diarrhoea in swine in China: Identification, prevalence and full-length genome sequence analysis. *Transboundary and Emerging Diseases, 62*(6), 575–580. https://doi.org/10.1111/tbed.12399

Song, Z., Xu, Y., Bao, L., Zhang, L., Yu, P., Qu, Y., Zhu, H., Zhao, W., Han, Y., & Qin, C. (2019). From SARS to MERS, thrusting coronaviruses into the spotlight. *Viruses, 11*(1), 59. https://doi.org/10.3390/v11010059

Su, S., Wong, G., Shi, W., Liu, J., Lai, A. C. K., Zhou, J., Liu, W., Bi, Y., & Gao, G. F. (2016). Epidemiology, genetic recombination, and pathogenesis of coronaviruses. *Trends in Microbiology, 24*(6), 490–502. https://doi.org/10.1016/j.tim.2016.03.003

Thakor, J. C., Dinesh, M., Manikandan, R., Bindu, S., Sahoo, M., Sahoo, D., Dhawan, M., Pandey, M. K., Tiwari, R., Emran, T. B., Dhama, K., & Chaicumpa, W. (2022). Swine coronaviruses (SCoVs) and their emerging threats to swine population, inter-species transmission, exploring the susceptibility of pigs for SARS-CoV-2 and zoonotic concerns. *Veterinary Quarterly, 42*(1), 125–147. https://doi.org/10.1080/01652176.2022.2079756

Tiwari, R., Dhama, K., Sharun, K., Iqbal Yatoo, M., Malik, Y. S., Singh, R., Michalak, I., Sah, R., Bonilla-Aldana, D. K., & Rodriguez-Morales, A. J. (2020). COVID-19: Animals, veterinary and zoonotic links. *Veterinary Quarterly, 40*(1), 169–182. https://doi.org/10.1080/01652176.2020.1766725

Tråvén, M., Carlsson, U., Lundén, A., & Larsson, B. (1999). Serum antibodies to bovine coronavirus in Swedish sheep. *Acta Veterinaria Scandinavica, 40*(1), 69–74. https://doi.org/10.1186/BF03547042

Vlasova, A. N., Wang, Q., Jung, K., Langel, S. N., Malik, Y. S., & Saif, L. J. (2020). Porcine Coronaviruses. *Emerging and Transboundary Animal Viruses, 2020*, 79–110. https://doi.org/10.1007/978-981-15-0402-0_4

Wang, J., Li, Y., Wang, S., & Liu, F. (2020a). Dynamics of transmissible gastroenteritis virus internalization unraveled by single-virus tracking in live cells. *The FASEB Journal, 34*(3), 4653–4669. https://doi.org/10.1096/fj.201902455R

Wang, Y., Liu, M., & Gao, J. (2020b). Enhanced receptor binding of SARS-CoV-2 through networks of hydrogen-bonding and hydrophobic interactions. *Proceedings of the National Academy of Sciences, 117*(25), 13967–13974. https://doi.org/10.1073/pnas.2008209117

Weaver, A. K., Head, J. R., Gould, C. F., Carlton, E. J., & Remais, J. V. (2022). Environmental factors influencing COVID-19 incidence and severity. *Annual Review of Public Health, 43*(1), 271–291. https://doi.org/10.1146/annurev-publhealth-052120-101420

Wells, H. L., Bonavita, C. M., Navarrete-Macias, I., Vilchez, B., Rasmussen, A. L., & Anthony, S. J. (2023). The coronavirus recombination pathway. *Cell Host & Microbe, 31*(6), 874–889. https://doi.org/10.1016/j.chom.2023.05.003

Yan, R., Zhang, Y., Li, Y., Xia, L., Guo, Y., & Zhou, Q. (2020). Structural basis for the recognition of SARS-CoV-2 by full-length human ACE2. *Science, 367*(6485), 1444–1448. https://doi.org/10.1126/science.abb2762

Yang, Y.-L., Yu, J.-Q., & Huang, Y.-W. (2020). Swine enteric alphacoronavirus (swine acute diarrhea syndrome coronavirus): An update three years after its discovery. *Virus Research, 285*, 198024. https://doi.org/10.1016/j.virusres.2020.198024

Yuan, C., Zhang, P., Liu, P., Li, Y., Li, J., Zhang, E., Jin, Y., & Yang, Q. (2022). A novel pathway for porcine epidemic diarrhea virus transmission from sows to neonatal piglets mediated by colostrum. *Journal of Virology, 96*(14), e0047722. https://doi.org/10.1128/jvi.00477-22

Japanese Encephalitis: An Arbovirus with Swine Reservoir

N. Ratnamrutha, M. S. Chandana, Annepu Revathi, and Abhishek Pathak

Abstract

Japanese encephalitis (JE) is caused by the Japanese encephalitis virus (JEV), transmitted through mosquito bites, and is the leading type of epidemic encephalitis in Asia. It is prevalent in much of South and Southeast Asia, with case numbers varying significantly across different regions. Although many JEV infections are asymptomatic, those that manifest symptoms can be severe and life-threatening. The natural reservoirs for JEV are ardeid wading birds, while pigs serve as crucial amplifying hosts during human outbreaks. Although safe and effective vaccines for JE exist, their usage remains limited in many endemic areas where they are needed most. Enhanced surveillance and diagnosis of JE are essential, especially as climate change and social disruption are likely to expand the geographical range of Culex mosquitoes and increase JE risk areas.

Introduction

JEV is a major contributor to viral encephalitis in humans in Asia (Campbell et al., 2011). As a zoonotic and vector-borne virus, it is predominantly transmitted by mosquitoes (Culex). Pigs are the major amplifying or maintenance hosts for JEV,

N. Ratnamrutha · M. S. Chandana
Division of Biological Standardization, ICAR- Indian Veterinary Research Institute, Bareilly, Uttar Pradesh, India

A. Revathi
Division of Biological Products, ICAR- Indian Veterinary Research Institute, Bareilly, Uttar Pradesh, India

A. Pathak (✉)
Department of Veterinary Pharmacology and Toxicology, MJF College of Veterinary and Animal Sciences, Jaipur, Rajasthan, India

R. Deb et al. (eds.), *Emerging Zoonotic Threats from Swine*,
https://doi.org/10.1007/978-981-96-7407-7_14

while a variety of avian species act as its natural reservoir. Human infection with JEV typically causes a mild febrile illness, though around 1% of cases progress to JE, which has a fatality rate nearing 30%. Additionally, among survivors, 25–30% experience long-term neurological issues or cognitive impairments (Solomon et al., 2000). The WHO estimates there are roughly 68,000 cases of JE globally each year (World Health Organization, 2021). This figure is thought to be understated, though, as the true illness burden is probably closer to 175,000 cases per year (Tarantola et al., 2014; Quan et al., 2020).

Humans are considered a dead-end host for Japanese encephalitis virus (JEV) because their viremia levels are too low to infect mosquitoes (Lord et al., 2015). The virus naturally cycles among various species, including wild wading birds, Culex mosquitoes, and pigs. While birds serve as the natural reservoir, pigs are significant hosts that amplify the JEV and are frequently linked to human outbreaks (Mulvey et al., 2021). However, outbreaks can also occur without pigs, indicating that avian or other species may sometimes act as amplifier hosts (Yap et al., 2019). Vaccination and eradication programs for JEV have been highly effective in virtually eliminating human cases in economically developed Asian nations such as Japan, Korea, and Taiwan (Yang et al., 2006). Despite vaccination campaigns in some countries, the geographical range of JEV has been expanding in Southeast Asian nations. This expansion is driven by the spread of mosquito vectors and a lack of comprehensive surveillance, which hampers understanding of JEV transmission (Hanna et al., 1999). Climate change further exacerbates the situation by potentially increasing mosquito habitats, allowing JEV to spread to previously unaffected areas.

Background and History

Japanese encephalitis virus (JEV) was initially identified and recognized as the public health problem in Japan. However, molecular research indicates that the ancestral JEV likely originated in the Indonesia/Malaysia region before spreading northward (Solomon et al., 2003). Currently, JEV is classified into 5 distinct genotypes: Genotype I (clades GI-a and GI-b), Genotype II, III, IV, and V (Schuh et al., 2013) (Fig. 1). These genotypes are differentiated by the sequence of nucleotides in the gene coding for E-protein, although all strains of JEV are members of the same serotype due to cross-reactive neutralizing antibodies (International Committee on Taxonomy of Viruses (ICTV), 2021). Up until the 1990s, genotype GIII was the most frequently isolated genotype in Asia and was the main cause of several Japanese encephalitis epidemics (Han et al., 2014; Gao et al., 2015). After being first isolated in 1967 in Cambodia, GI started to supplant GIII in the early to mid-1990s and has since taken over as the main source of outbreaks in the area (Schuh et al., 2013). Recent outbreaks have seen GI strains in Korea, Japan, India, China, Vietnam, Taiwan, Malaysia, Thailand, and Cambodia (Mulvey et al., 2021). In the Australian region, a GII strain was responsible for the first outbreak in 1995. However, from 2000 onwards, only GI viruses have been observed (Pyke et al., 2001). According to phylogeographic and phylodynamic studies, the GI-a strain

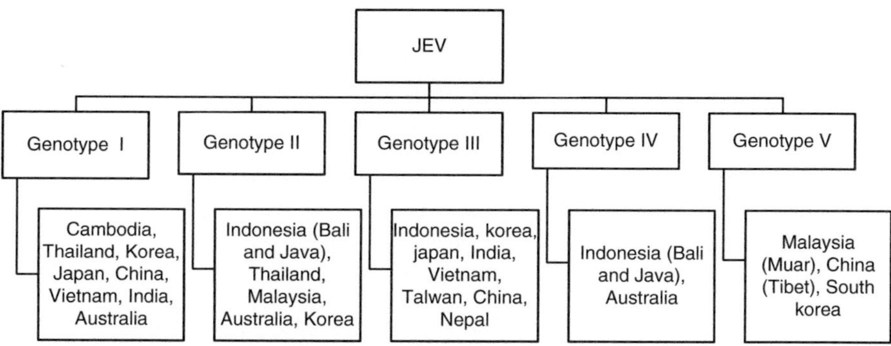

Fig. 1 Genotypes of JEV. A broad illustration of the countries and regions where JEV genotypes are most prevalent or have the biggest effects, as well as their place of origin. (The information shown was adapted from Srivastava et al. 2023)

emerged in Thailand during the 1940s, while the GI-b strain originated in Vietnam during the 1950s. By 1983, GI-b was spread widely across temperate Asian nations and exhibited increased genetic diversity, eventually becoming the most dominant genotype in both endemic and newly impacted regions of Asia by the 2000s.

Virology of JE

The JEV is an enclosed virus with a single-stranded positive-sense, RNA genome, approximately having a diameter of 40–50 nm, and exhibits symmetry of spheroid cubical (Fig. 2). Three structural proteins (capsid, precursor membrane, envelope) and seven non-structural proteins such as NS1, 2A, 2B, 3, 4A, 4B, and 5 are encoded by its about 11 kb RNA genome. The RNA does not have a poly-A tail at the 3′ end, but it does have a 5′ methylated cap. A single open reading frame in the genomic RNA forms the lengthy chain of 3432 amino acids that makes up all 10 proteins (Srivastava et al., 2023).

The capsid protein (C) of JEV forms dimers in a head-to-tail, anti-parallel manner, with multiple dimers assembling into spherical nucleocapsid that encloses the viral genome. Recent studies have unveiled crystal structure of this protein, revealing that it comprises four α-helices (α1–α4), which are similar to those found in the capsid proteins of WNV, DENV, and ZIKV (Poonsiri et al., 2019). Specifically, each capsid protein monomer includes 4 helices: α1 (29–38 amino acids), α2 (44–57aa), α3 (63–70aa), and the longest α4 (74–96aa), which are linked by short loops. The N-terminal of α-helix 1 can adopt both open and closed conformations, making it a promising target for antiviral drugs. Conversely, the C-terminal pairing of the α4 helices forms a coiled coil like, potentially aiding in binding of nucleic acids.

The virol precursor membrane protein (prM) is produced from the nascent polyprotein through cotranslational cleavage from signal peptide. It begins assembling around the viral RNA within vesicles of endoplasmic reticulum (ER). Once assembled, these vesicles bud from ER and travel to Golgi apparatus, where the prM

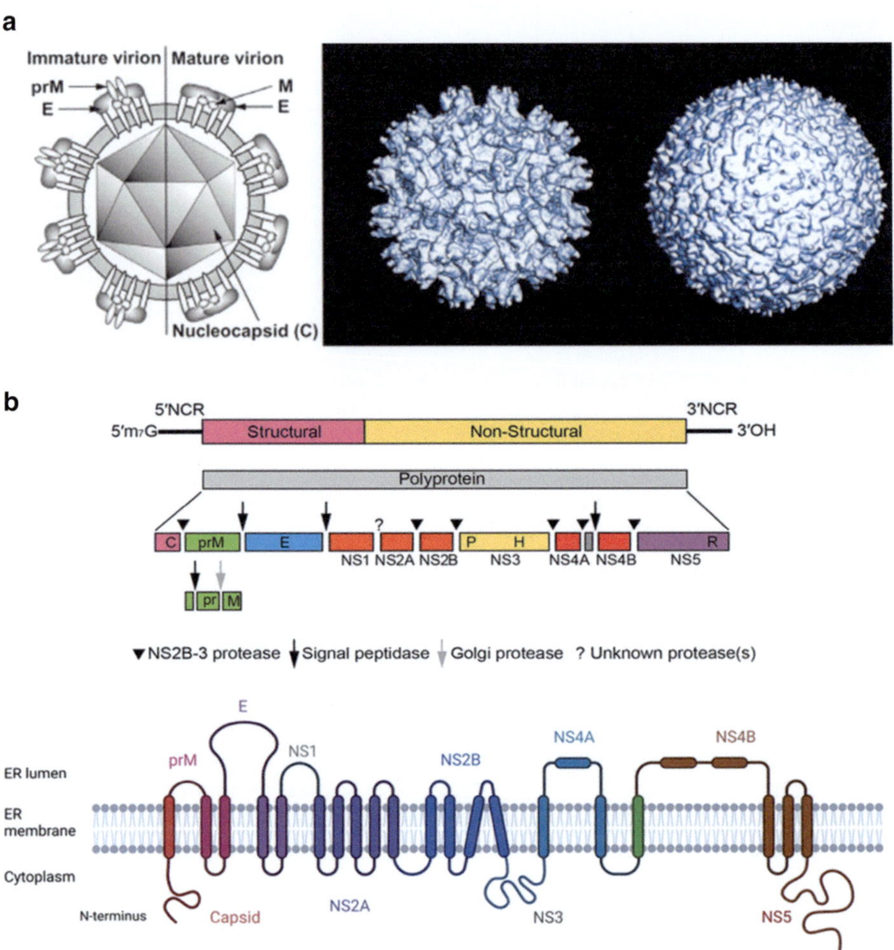

Fig. 2 Genus Flavivirus, family Flaviviridae. (**a**) (Left) Diagram depicting the virion's immature and mature stages. (Right and center) cryo-electron microscopic reconstructions of adult and immature particles in three dimensions. E stands for main spike protein, M for transmembrane protein, C for nucleocapsid protein, and prM for precursor glycoprotein. (**b**) Flavivirus genome arrangement and polyprotein processing. The 5′ and 3′ noncoding regions (NCR) and structural and nonstructural protein coding regions are found in the viral genomes. Viral proteins produced by the proteolytic processing cascade are indicated by boxes beneath the genomes. Protease cleavage sites are shown by arrows, arrowheads, and "?" in between the viral protein boxes. The location of the NS3 RNA helicase, NS3 protease, and NS5 RNA-dependent RNA polymerase is shown by the P, H, and R symbols, respectively. (Adapted from Fenner's Veterinary Virology Fenner et al., 2014)

undergoes cleavage by the enzyme furin, resulting in the formation of the M protein and the virus maturation before release from host cell. Although the precise role of prM/M is not fully understood, but in related viruses such as DENV and YFV, prM plays a role in the maturation of viral particles and ensures the correct folding of E protein. Additionally, the membrane protein is crucial for binding the E protein to the host receptor during infection. After the virus enters the cell, membrane protein aids in the fusion of the vesicles of virus with the endosome.

One essential element that envelops the virion, aids in attaching to host cell receptors, and helps in fusing with the plasma membrane of host is the envelope protein (E) of JEV. It is also the primary target for virus-neutralizing antibodies. The E protein consists of 3 domains: envelope domain I (EDI), EDII, and EDIII. The E protein's crystal structure demonstrates that, like other flaviviruses, it dimerizes in an antiparallel, head-to-tail arrangement, albeit with a smaller interface (Luca et al., 2012). The nine-stranded β-barrel that makes up EDI, the core domain, is situated between the globular EDIII and the expanded EDII. Two long loops that extend from EDI are held in place by three disulfide bonds, and have a conserved fusion peptide at the top are characteristics of EDII. The EDIII has an immunoglobulin-like structure at the c-terminus of ectodomain, which facilitates binding to host receptors during the internalization of virion. The features of EDIII domain make it an attractive target in developing antiviral drugs to combat JEV infections.

The JEV has 7 non-structural (NS) proteins that are translated from a single polyprotein and subsequently cleaved. These proteins aid in the formation of new virus particles and are principally engaged in viral replication. Among these, NS1 has received relatively little research, and its precise role is yet unknown. According to several studies, NS1 aids in the transcription of double-stranded intermediate RNA by being a component in the replication complex (Muller & Young, 2013). Furthermore, research has demonstrated that JEV replication can be inhibited in vitro by siRNA targeting NS1 (Liu et al., 2006). However, none of these siRNAs have advanced to clinical development. According to Yen et al., NS1 can function as heterologous epitope, triggering an immune response that is cross-reactive to different infections (Yen et al., 2016).

The production and assembly of the viral RNA genome are directly aided by NS2A, whereas NS2B combines with NS3 to support its protease activity. As a helicase, NS3 is essential to the replication of the genome. NS3 is also believed to be the reservoir for viral proteins during virus assembly and to originate from the transGolgi network or the endoplasmic reticulum. Highly hydrophobic NS4 proteins, such as NS4A and NS4B, are thought to aid in the formation of membrane constituents. This characteristic suggests they may be crucial for the virus's adaptability to various environments, although their exact roles remain unclear (Srivastava et al., 2023).

The multipurpose protein NS5 is necessary for the replication complex of viral RNA. NS5 has an RNA-dependent RNA polymerase (RdRp) domain at the C-terminus and a methyltransferase domain at the N-terminus, similar to NS and cellular proteins found in other flaviviruses (Lu & Gong, 2013). While the RdRp domain directly participates in the replication of RNA, methyltransferase domain mostly controls the formation of 5′ cap of genomic viral RNA (Vannice et al., 2021).

Epidemiology

The annual incidence of disease varies significantly within and across endemic regions, rates can range from fewer than 1 to more than 10 cases per 100,000 people, and potentially higher during outbreaks. Globally, it is estimated to cause between 13,600 and 20,400 deaths each year, with an estimated 68,000 clinical cases occurring each year (World Health Organisation, n.d.). Due to widespread pesticide use and the advent of JEV vaccinations in wealthier countries, the JEV burden in Asia decreased in the late 1960s (Yang et al., 2006). However, in recent decades, factors such as growth in population, enhanced pork production, and the expansion of irrigated paddy agriculture throughout Southeast Asia have contributed to the additional spread of JEV and a subsequent rise in the burden of Japanese Encephalitis (Poonsiri et al., 2019).

A latest study (Moore, 2021), conducted prior to the Australian epidemics, assessed the current burden and the effects of vaccination against Japanese encephalitis (JE) in Asia using the force of infection estimations and spatial analysis. Significant underreporting was brought to light in this study, along with the possibility that raising vaccination rates could reduce the burden of disease. There are about 1.54 billion individuals living in regions where JEV transmission is possible. Important elements that support virus transmission were found by the spatial analysis, including rice production, closeness to wetlands, and the existence of particular mosquitoes as vectors. Significant differences in the intensity of transmission among nations were shown by the force of infection analysis.

With the Western Pacific islands at the east to the India-Pakistan border at the west, and the China-Russia border at the north to Australia at the south, JE is thought to be the most common cause of viral encephalitis among Asian nations. In certain nations, the prevalence of JE has dramatically declined during the last few decades, whereas in others, it has increased. In Asia, there are two different epidemiological models for JE: in temperate parts, there are significant outbreaks during summer, while in tropics, cases are more sporadic, with peaks being observed during the rainy season (Erlanger et al., 2009).

JEV first appeared in Torres Strait islands during the late 1990s, and it later moved to northern Australia's Cape York Peninsula, where it posed a major risk to public health and sparked worries about future spread. These concerns proved valid as the virus later spread to continental Australia and 25 other countries in the Western Pacific and Asia (Duong et al., 2017). In 2022, Australia experienced an unprecedented outbreak of JEV following extensive rainfall. The resulting flooding created conditions conducive to mosquito proliferation, providing suitable habitats for water birds—the main virus carriers. This outbreak sparked worries about the possible effects of climate change and brought to light the intricate interactions between illness, wildlife, and weather.

Transmission

An enzootic cycle involving mosquitoes and vertebrates as hosts, especially birds and pigs, is how the JEV, an arbovirus (arthropod-borne virus), is spread (Fig. 3). When a human is bitten by a mosquito carrying the virus, they contract it. Dead-end hosts for JEV include a variety of domestic animals, including dogs, chickens, cows, goats, and horses, along with wildlife, including frogs, flying foxes, ducks, and snakes. This is because they produce low levels of viremia, insufficient to infect mosquitoes (Mansfield et al., 2017). Domestic pigs are a major source of JEV transmission to humans, despite the fact that the virus can infect a wide variety of vertebrates. This is due to the fact that pigs frequently reside on farms near human habitations, which contributes to the development of high viral titers and extended viremia following a natural infection. Since they don't create enough viremia to infect new mosquitoes, horses, humans, and other non-avian vertebrates are inadvertent dead-end hosts (Auerswald et al., 2021). Besides horizontal transmission via mosquito bites, there is also possibility for vertical transmission of JEV from female-infected mosquitoes to their youngs via their eggs. Attempts to manage and eradicate the disease are made more difficult by this vertical transmission, which aids the virus's persistence and maintenance within mosquito populations.

The cell tropism for JEV is likely influenced by the virus's ability to attach and enter host cells. The initial interaction involves virion attaching non-specifically to host cell, followed by binding of the envelope (E) protein to an unidentified receptor specifically (Yun & Lee, 2014). While the viral mechanisms of attachment and entry are relatively well understood, the cellular components of this process remain largely unknown. Mammals, avians, and insects are among the animal species in

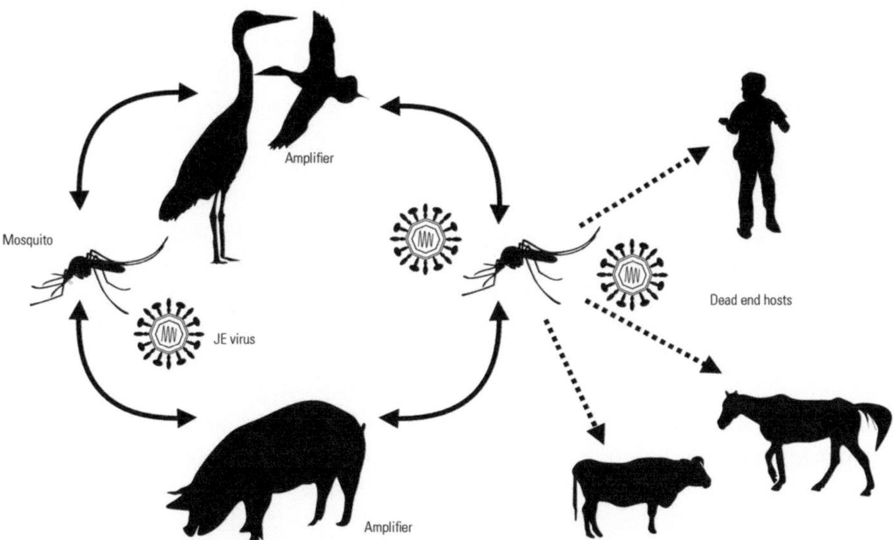

Fig. 3 JEV transmission cycle

which JEV can infect and multiply in a variety of cell types. This suggests that multiple cellular factors are likely involved in virus attachment to cell and entry. Understanding these virus-host interactions is essential for developing possible therapeutics for JEV infection.

JEV in Mosquitoes

At least 14 species of mosquitoes have been identified as JEV vectors, and 11 more species have demonstrated experimental vector competence (Auerswald et al., 2021). In particular, Cx. Tritaeniorhynchus (Simpson et al., 1970) is a member of the Culex vishnui subgroup, which includes the major vectors. In some regions, other Culex species, including Culex fuscocephala, Culex bitaeniorhynchus, Culex gelidus, Culex quinquefasciatus, and Culex annulirostris, may function as primary vectors and are important secondary vectors. These species have all adapted to different types of groundwater habitats, including semi-permanent, permanent, and transitory ones. Puddles, ponds, little streams, rice fields and man-made water containers are examples of these habitats. The transmission cycle is supported by migratory wading avians and Culex mosquitoes, which nest in irrigated areas (Yang et al., 2006). Additionally, Cx. tritaeniorhynchus larvae have been found in urban storage containers, ponds, wells, and ditches. The possibility of JEV transmission is increased by the availability of human blood meals in metropolitan settings.

JEV in Birds

The main wildlife reservoirs of JEV and important hosts in its transmission have been found to be wild ardeid aquatic birds, including herons and egrets. While various other bird species can be infected with JEV, they are considered less significant as virus reservoirs compared to pigs, egrets, and herons. In ardeid birds, JEV infection is asymptomatic but leading to seroconversion (Boyle et al., 1983). Experimental infections have demonstrated that herons and egrets with high levels of viremia can transmit JEV to mosquitoes. The importance of ardeid birds in JEV transmission is supported by surveillance studies conducted in villages close to rice fields, both without and with herons. In villages without herons, seroconversion rates of JEV neutralizing antibody were 0–13% and 5–12%, in children of age 0–5 years and 6–15 years respectively, compared to 50% and 56% in villages with herons present (Mani et al., 1991). With the exception of Antarctica, ardeid birds migrate seasonally across all continents. They are particularly active in southern, eastern, central, and northern Asia, which may increase the range of JEV and aid in its spread. Due to their low viremia levels, which are insufficient for transferring to feeding mosquito, domestic birds, such as adult ducks and chickens, are thought to have a very minimal role in the ecology of JEV.

Swine as Reservoir Host

In epidemic regions, pigs act as primary amplifier hosts for Japanese encephalitis virus, while in endemic regions, they act as the maintenance hosts. The concentration of pig farming in parts of Eastern and Southeastern Asia has made pigs the central element of the domestic transmission cycle of JEV (Ladreyt et al., 2019; Ren et al., 2017). In Southeastern Asia, particularly in Myanmar, Thailand, and Vietnam, pig farming has industrialized leading to intensified JEV amplification in dense pig herds, thereby elevating the risk levels of JEV transmission (Le Flohic et al., 2013). Consequently, being close to pig populations increases the danger of transmission of JEV to people. Swine epidemics are difficult to identify because JEV infection in pigs typically causes asymptomatic or moderate illness (Ricklin et al., 2016a).

Immunologically naïve sows may experience increased rates of abortion and stillbirth (Takashima et al., 1988), while sows exposed to viruses prior to pregnancy often had fewer pregnancy-related problems (Lindahl et al., 2012). Boars infected with JEV can also suffer from infertility (Ogasa et al., 1977), and encephalitis has been observed in experimentally infected piglets (Williams et al., 2019; Yamada et al., 2004). Pigs in endemic areas usually have a very high seroprevalence of JEV (98–100%), and usually they have high level of viremia for 3–5 days after infection, that is sufficient to infect Culex mosquitoes that bite (Hurlbut & Thomas, 1950). The transmission cycle can then be continued by these infected mosquitoes spreading JEV to further immunocompromised pigs.

According to preliminary data, there are two cycles of virus amplification in pigs: the first cycle starts when mosquito bite pigs and infect them at a rate of about 20%, and the second cycle occurs when mosquitoes feed on pigs having viremia and subsequently spread JEV to other naive pigs, resulting in almost complete seroconversion among the pig's population (Van den Hurk et al., 2009a). It was recently discovered that direct contact between pigs through the oronasal route can result in vector-less JEV transmission. Pig tonsils were found to contain JEV RNA and live virus for 6 weeks, indicating that this is the main location for JEV replication and transmission (Ricklin et al., 2016b). The high sero-conversion rates of neonatal pigs to JEV may be explained by this vector-less transmission (Ogasa et al., 1977). According to a study conducted in Cambodia, piglets began to seroconvert within a month of weaning, with 28 out of 29 piglets (96.6%) seroconverting before 6 months of age, indicating intense virus transmission. In the same investigation, only a pool of Culex tritaeniorhynchus mosquitoes tested positive for JEV, despite this high degree of circulation (Di Francesco et al., 2018). This and previous studies' low prevalence rates of mosquitoes positive for JEV (Diallo et al., 2018), however, raise the possibility that transmission without vector among pigs represents a substantial but little-known component of JEV epidemiology.

Vaccination of pig populations can mitigate the risk of JEV outbreaks in humans. Pigs are shielded against injected JEV challenges and other feeding mosquitoes by the quick systemic IgM and IgG responses that are often elicited by JEV vaccination (Sasaki et al., 1982). However, there are challenges to widespread swine vaccination. Vaccination is costly and impractical since commercial farms have large turnover rates and the majority of pigs are killed between the ages of 6 and 8 months. Furthermore, the duration of effective immunity in production pigs is limited by maternal antibodies, which lessen the efficiency of the live-attenuated vaccination in pigs under 3 months of age. However, vaccination may assist lower human risk for JE and decrease losses in sow reproductivity in JEV endemic regions and pigs live for long duration (Khan et al., 2014). Due to the limited adverse effects of JEV infection in pigs, economically disadvantaged farmers have little incentives for vaccination of swine, leading to low vaccine uptake in developing countries endemic to JE.

Removing pigs from densely populated areas in JEV-endemic regions had proven effective in decreasing JE incidence. For instance, during a JV outbreak in Malaysia from 1998–1999, culling approximately 50% of swine halted further clinical infections of JEV (Wong et al., 2008). The decrease in JE cases in Taiwan, Korea, and Japan may also partly result from relocating piggeries away from populated areas (Solomon et al., 2000). Following a JEV epidemic in 1995, pigs were relocated 2.5 km from the settlement on Badu Island in Australia's Torres Strait. Even at that time, JEV was still found later in community, presumably due to the piggery being inside the vectors' flight path and the possibility of infection by nearby viremic waterbirds (Wang et al., 2017). Between 1991 and 2000, JEV decreased from 14 cases per year to three imported cases as a result of Singapore's 1992 ban on pig farms (Yap et al., 2019). However, recent findings have demonstrated that a variety of domestic and migratory birds, including eagles, redshanks, plovers, and egrets, as well as wild boars, can transmit zoonotic JEV (Ting et al., 2004). Therefore, in situations where domestic swine populations are small or nonexistent, JEV amplification in ardeid birds (such as egrets and herons) may be extremely important.

JEV in Other Hosts

Other domestic animals like cattle, horses, buffalo, and goats, as well as wild animals such as marsupials, are classified as dead-ends for JEV transmission. Although they can contract the virus, these animals have low viremia levels, which prevents them from transmitting virus to mosquitoes (Shimizu et al., 1951; Ilkal et al., 1988; Gulati et al., 2011; Ellis et al., 2000; Carey et al., 1969). When hosts which act as dead-ends are prevalent and vectors prefer them for blood, this may help to reduce the activity of JEV by diverting vectors far from amplifier hosts. A study conducted recently in Cambodia found evidence that this virus circulates among multiple hosts, like dogs, chickens, and ducks, with neutralizing antibodies found in a variety of animals (Ladreyt et al., 2020; Auerswald et al., 2020).

In horses and cattle, the majority of JEV infections are asymptomatic. Although JE is uncommon in cattle, it is widely known in horses, and epidemics in horses sometimes resemble human outbreaks (Ellis et al., 2000). Places like Hong Kong (China), Malaysia, Japan, and Singapore require horses to be vaccinated against JEV, which lowers the prevalence of JEV infection there (Lam et al., 2005). Very little is known regarding JEV viremia in newly born calves or foals, or whether these animals may develop greater levels of viremia. Maternal antibodies, on the other hand, may shield calves and foals from JEV till they are weaned. Cattle and goats are regarded as suitable animals for surveillance because of their high seropositivity. Because the vector prefers to feed on goats and cattle rather than pigs, seroprevalence in these animals has been determined to be a better indicator of human risk of JE infection in Sri Lanka than swine seroprevalence (Peiris et al., 1993).

Antibodies for JEV have also been detected in a wide variety of bat species in Eastern Asia (Cui et al., 2008; Wang et al., 2009). Virus transmission by transplacental route has also been demonstrated experimentally, suggesting a potential mechanism for JEV maintenance in nature. In infections done experimentally to megabat species (*Pteropus alecto*), animals infected either by inoculation or by infected mosquitoes developed viremia which are capable to infect recipient mosquitoes (van den Hurk et al., 2009b). Bats are also thought to play an important role in overwintering of JEV in its north range, with reactivation of viremia in infected bats next to hibernation. Further research is needed to fully understand the role of bats in natural cycle of JEV transmission.

In Eastern Asia, JEV antibodies also have been found in a large number of bat species (Cui et al., 2008; Wang et al., 2009). In China, Japan, and Taiwan, the virus had been isolated from bats (Sulkin et al., 1970; Cross, 1971; Liu et al., 2013). Experiment studies have focused mainly on microbats, where viremia has been observed to last up to 25–30 days at levels higher enough to infect mosquitoes. Experimental evidence of transmission of virus via the transplacental channel also points to a possible mechanism for JEV maintenance in the natural world. Animals infected by inoculation or infected mosquitoes acquired viremia that might infect recipient mosquitoes in experimental infections to megabat species (*Pteropus alecto*) (van den Hurk et al., 2009b). With viremia-infected bats reactivating after hibernation, bats are also believed to be crucial to JEV's overwintering in its northern distribution. To completely comprehend bats' participation in the natural transmission cycle, more research is required.

Clinical Picture

Generally, most Japanese encephalitis (JE) infections are mild, often presenting as subclinical febrile illness with flu-like symptoms lasting 5–15 days, or with no apparent symptoms. JE mainly affects children under 14 years old in endemic areas, though in epidemic areas, adults are being at risk. However, some patients experience encephalitis-related clinical disease, which can be deadly in up to 30% of cases. The severity and clinical results of this neurotropic viral infection are greatly influenced by the virus's capacity to pass the blood-brain barrier (Ghosh & Basu, 2009). Approximately 30–50% of individuals who survived the severe JE infection suffer from neurological or behavioral sequelae, such as frequent seizures, paralysis, or speech impairments (Tiwari et al., 2012; World Health Organisation, n.d.).

Table 1 Clinical phases of JE

Transmission stage	Prodromal stage	Acute stage	Late stage	Sequelae stage
Incubation time: 5–15 days Majority of human infections are asymptomatic	Fever Headache Exhaustion Nausea Chills Vomiting	Acute encephalopathy Mental status changes Mild disorientation that progresses to agitation or coma Parkinsonian syndrome Lower and upper paralysis Seizures	Gradual recovery Possible persistence of some CNS signs and symptoms	Cognitive and memory impairments Neuromuscular dysfunction Psychiatric and behavioral disturbances Seizures Impairment of daily activities

Adapted from Lopalco and Biasio (2024)

The disease progression in patients who develop neurological disease can be characterized into 3 stages (Table 1). Symptoms of the first stage, referred to as the prodromal stage, include chills, a low-grade fever, muscle aches, diarrhea, vomiting, and meningitis Reduced consciousness, seizures, and Parkinsonian syndrome are among the symptoms of the second phase, often known as the acute phase, which can progress to encephalitis. Cogwheel stiffness, widespread hypertonia, tremors, and other abnormalities that could result in coma are possible symptoms of this stage. In certain cases, the illness progresses quickly and can be lethal. Either recovery or protracted neurological sequelae are the outcomes of the last stage, or the late stage (Unni et al., 2011). Severe JE affects the thalamus, hippocampus, basal ganglia, parenchyma, temporal lobes, cerebral cortex, midbrain, substantia nigra, brain stem, and anterior horn cells of the spinal cord, with the hippocampus suffering the most damage. Perivascular cuffing, gliomesenchymal nodules, vascular leakage, microglial nodule development, necrolytic lesions, cerebral edema, scarred ramified foci, and congested leptomeninges are among the histopathological alterations (Unni et al., 2011).

Prevention and Control

Japanese encephalitis (JE) has no known treatment, hence the only long-term, effective control method is immunization. For populations that are at risk, the WHO advises vaccination. Numerous nations in the Western Pacific and Asia have immunization programs in place (Vannice et al., 2021). Non-immune travelers and expatriates are nevertheless susceptible to infection because the virus is maintained by an enzootic cycle that involves mosquitoes and various host animals (Hills et al., 2014; Lopalco & Biasio, 2024). Protection from mosquito bites can be achieved through the use of skin repellents, wearing proper clothing, staying indoors during peak mosquito activity hours, and employing other personal protective measures.

While these methods are important and help prevent various mosquito-borne diseases, they aren't completely successful. The most effective form of prevention is still vaccination (Rogers et al., 2016).

Numerous JE vaccines, such as live attenuated vaccines, live recombinant (chimeric) vaccines, inactivated mouse brain-derived vaccines, and inactivated Vero cell-derived vaccines, have been developed as a result of research into JEV, a significant emerging and reemerging pathogen (Ginsburg et al., 2017). Despite being used extensively for active vaccination for decades, the inactivated mouse brain-derived vaccine has lately been phased out of manufacture in favor of new cell culture-derived vaccines that are now accessible worldwide. Adults and children as young as 2 months old are advised to receive the authorized inactivated Vero cell-derived vaccination (strain SA14–14-2) in Europe. Significant protection against the main JEV genotypes present in endemic areas is offered by this vaccination (Erra et al., 2013).

Two doses spaced 4 weeks apart make up the standard vaccination schedule; people ages 18–65 can opt for an expedited schedule with a one-week gap. Other travel vaccinations, such as those for rabies and hepatitis A, can be given alongside the vaccine. The Summary of Product Characteristics states that seroconversion rates after the first vaccination cycle are 97.3% in individuals aged 18–76 on day 35 (using the conventional schedule with the second dose on day 28), 99% in individuals aged 18–65 on day 14 (using the rapid schedule with the second dose on day 7 and co-administration with rabies vaccine), and ≥99% in child and adolescents. If possible re-exposure to JEV is expected, a third dose is advised 12–24 months following the initial immunization. After immunization, the majority of side effects are minor and go away in a few days. Seroconversion rates ranged from 93% to 100%, according to a 2020 systematic review (Kling et al., 2020) that comprised roughly 32 research from 16 nations on the immunogenicity and safety of this vaccination in adults. Less than 5% of people of all ages experienced serious side effects, the majority of which were not directly linked to the vaccine (Table 2).

Although vaccination campaigns have made a substantial contribution to the reduction of JEV, improved surveillance is required to improve the estimates of the burden of JE. Understanding the local and global effects of JE and identifying at-risk locations are still significantly hampered by underreporting. To address this issue, WHO surveillance guidelines are published (World Health Organization (WHO), 2018). However, the majority of JE-endemic nations have weak JEV diagnostic capability.

The WHO has created a JEV laboratory network to address this, based on the measles and polio laboratory networks (World Health Organization (WHO), 2018; Centers for Disease Control and Prevention (CDC), 2012). Through a variety of trainings and development initiatives, this network seeks to increase its capability for surveillance and diagnosis. The network has already increased monitoring in the Asian region, with 92% of endemic nations currently doing JE surveillance, up from 75%. While some of these monitoring programs are subnational or sentinel, over half of them are national in scope (Heffelfinger, 2017). Despite a 60% overall reduction in JE cases from 2011 to 2015, Vietnam and Nepal reported a two-fold and

Table 2 JEV vaccines licenced so far

Licensed Vaccines (types)	Viral strain used	Trade name	Licensing year	Required doses	Age at vaccination	Administration route
JE-MB (inactivated mouse brain-derived JE vaccine)	Nakayama-NH Beijing-1	JE-VAX	1954 1993	3	≥12 months	S/C
JE-VC (inactivated Vero cell culture-derived JE vaccine)	SA14–14-2 (with adjuvant)	IXIARO®/JESPECT®/ JEEV®	2009 2013	2	≥17 year ≥2 months	I/M
	Bejing-I (without Adjuvant)	JEBIK-V ENCEVAC TC-JEV	2009 2011 2013	3	≥36 months	S/C
IMOJEV (recombinant chimeric virus vaccine	SA14–14-2	IMOJEV	2010	1	≥1 year	S/C
JE-LV (live attenuated Japanese encephalitis vaccine)	SA14–14-2	CD.JEVAX	1988	1	≥8 months	S/C
JENVAC	821564XY (Indian Kolar strain)	JENVAC	2013	2	≥6 months	I/M

Adapted from Srivastava et al. (2023)

11-fold increase in cases, respectively. These increases are likely due to improved surveillance practices and previously inconsistent reporting (Heffelfinger, 2017).

Conclusion

Japanese encephalitis (JE) is a dangerous illness spread by mosquitoes that frequently goes unnoticed. The risk of JE is rising and spreading to new areas due to climate change and intensive pig farming. Prevention is possible through proper counseling and enhanced vaccination access. In addition to raising awareness in non-endemic nations and, when required, recommending immunization, it is imperative to strengthen disease surveillance and control in areas where JE is prevalent.

References

Auerswald, H., Ruget, A. S., Ladreyt, H., et al. (2020). Serological evidence for Japanese encephalitis and West Nile virus infections in domestic birds in Cambodia. *Frontiers in Veterinary Science, 7*, 15.

Auerswald, H., Maquart, P. O., Chevalier, V., & Boyer, S. (2021). Mosquito vector competence for Japanese encephalitis virus. *Viruses, 13*(6), 1154.

Boyle, D. B., Dickerman, R. W., & Marshall, I. D. (1983). Primary viraemia responses of herons to experimental infection with Murray Valley encephalitis, Kunjin and Japanese encephalitis viruses. *Australian Journal of Experimental Biology and Medical Science, 61*(6), 655–664.

Campbell, G. L., Hills, S. L., Fischer, M., Jacobson, J. A., Hoke, C. H., Hombach, J. M., et al. (2011). Estimated global incidence of Japanese encephalitis: A systematic review. *Bulletin of the World Health Organization, 89*(10), 766–774.

Carey, D. E., Reuben, R., & Myers, R. M. (1969). Japanese encephalitis studies in Vellore, South India. Pt. V. Experimental infection and transmission. *Indian Journal of Medical Research, 57*(2), 282–289.

Centers for Disease Control and Prevention (CDC). (2012). Expanding poliomyelitis and measles surveillance networks to establish surveillance for acute meningitis and encephalitis syndromes-Bangladesh, China, and India, 2006-2008. *MMWR: Morbidity & Mortality Weekly Report, 61*(49).

Cross, J. H. (1971). Japanese encephalitis virus surveillance in Taiwan. II. Isolations from mosquitoes and bats in Taipei area 1969-1970. *Journal of the Formosan Medical Association, 70*(12), 681–686.

Cui, J., Counor, D., Shen, D., Sun, G., He, H., Deubel, V., & Zhang, S. (2008). Detection of Japanese encephalitis virus antibodies in bats in southern China. *American Journal of Tropical Medicine and Hygiene, 78*(6), 1007–1011.

Di Francesco, J., Choeung, R., Peng, B., Pring, L., Pang, S., Duboz, R., et al. (2018). Comparison of the dynamics of Japanese encephalitis virus circulation in sentinel pigs between a rural and a peri-urban setting in Cambodia. *PLoS Neglected Tropical Diseases, 12*(8), e0006644.

Diallo, A. O. I., Chevalier, V., Cappelle, J., Duong, V., Fontenille, D., & Duboz, R. (2018). How much does direct transmission between pigs contribute to Japanese encephalitis virus circulation? A modelling approach in Cambodia. *PLoS One, 13*(8), e0201209.

Duong, V., Choeung, R., Gorman, C., Laurent, D., Crabol, Y., Mey, C., et al. (2017). Isolation and full-genome sequences of Japanese encephalitis virus genotype I strains from Cambodian human patients, mosquitoes and pigs. *Journal of General Virology, 98*(9), 2287–2296.

Ellis, P. M., Daniels, P. W., & Banks, D. J. (2000). Japanese encephalitis. *Veterinary Clinics of North America: Equine Practice, 16*(3), 565–578.

Erlanger, T. E., Weiss, S., Keiser, J., Utzinger, J., & Wiedenmayer, K. (2009). Past, present, and future of Japanese encephalitis. *Emerging Infectious Diseases, 15*(1), 1.

Erra, E. O., Askling, H. H., Yoksan, S., Rombo, L., Riutta, J., Vene, S., et al. (2013). Cross-protective capacity of Japanese encephalitis (JE) vaccines against circulating heterologous JE virus genotypes. *Clinical Infectious Diseases, 56*(2), 267–270.

Fenner, F. J., Bachmann, P. A., & Gibbs, E. P. J. (2014). *Veterinary virology*. Academic Press.

Gao, X., Liu, H., Li, M., Fu, S., & Liang, G. (2015). Insights into the evolutionary history of Japanese encephalitis virus (JEV) based on whole-genome sequences comprising the five genotypes. *Virology Journal, 12*, 1–7.

Ghosh, D., & Basu, A. (2009). Japanese encephalitis – A pathological and clinical perspective. *PLoS Neglected Tropical Diseases, 3*(9), e437.

Ginsburg, A. S., Meghani, A., Halstead, S. B., & Yaich, M. (2017). Use of the live attenuated Japanese encephalitis vaccine SA 14–14–2 in children: A review of safety and tolerability studies. *Human Vaccines & Immunotherapeutics, 13*(10), 2222–2231.

Gulati, B. R., Singha, H., Singh, B. K., Virmani, N., Khurana, S. K., & Singh, R. K. (2011). Serosurveillance for Japanese encephalitis virus infection among equines in India. *Journal of Veterinary Science, 12*(4), 341.

Han, N., Adams, J., Chen, P., Guo, Z. Y., Zhong, X. F., Fang, W., et al. (2014). Comparison of genotypes I and III in Japanese encephalitis virus reveals distinct differences in their genetic and host diversity. *Journal of Virology, 88*(19), 11469–11479.

Hanna, J. N., Ritchie, S. A., Hills, S. L., van den Hurk, A. F., Phillips, D. A., Pyke, A. T., et al. (1999). Japanese encephalitis in North Queensland, Australia, 1998. *Medical Journal of Australia, 170*(11), 533–536.

Heffelfinger, J. D. (2017). Japanese encephalitis surveillance and immunization – Asia and Western Pacific regions, 2016. *MMWR. Morbidity and Mortality Weekly Report, 66*.

Hills, S. L., Stoltey, J., Martínez, D., Kim, P. Y., Sheriff, H., Zangeneh, A., et al. (2014). A case series of three US adults with Japanese encephalitis, 2010–2012. *Journal of Travel Medicine, 21*(5), 310–313.

Hurlbut, H. S., & Thomas, J. I. (1950). Observations on the experimental transmission of Japanese encephalitis by mosquitoes. *American Journal of Tropical Medicine, 30*(5), 683.

Ilkal, M. A., Dhanda, V., Rao, B. U., George, S., Mishra, A. C., Prasanna, Y., et al. (1988). Absence of viraemia in cattle after experimental infection with Japanese encephalitis virus. *Transactions of the Royal Society of Tropical Medicine and Hygiene, 82*(4), 628–631.

International Committee on Taxonomy of Viruses (ICTV). (2021). Genus: Flavivirus. Available online: https://talk.ictvonline.org/ictv-reports/ictv_online_report/positive-sense-rna-viruses/w/flaviviridae/360/genus-flavivirus

Khan, S. U., Salje, H., Hannan, A., Islam, M. A., Bhuyan, A. M., Islam, M. A., et al. (2014). Dynamics of Japanese encephalitis virus transmission among pigs in Northwest Bangladesh and the potential impact of pig vaccination. *PLoS Neglected Tropical Diseases, 8*(9), e3166.

Kling, K., Harder, T., Younger, Z., Burchard, G., Schmidt-Chanasit, J., & Wichmann, O. (2020). Vaccination against Japanese encephalitis with IC51: Systematic review on immunogenicity, duration of protection and safety. *Journal of Travel Medicine, 27*(2), taaa016.

Ladreyt, H., Durand, B., Dussart, P., & Chevalier, V. (2019). How central is the domestic pig in the epidemiological cycle of Japanese encephalitis virus? A review of scientific evidence and implications for disease control. *Viruses, 11*(10), 949.

Ladreyt, H., Auerswald, H., Tum, S., Ken, S., Heng, L., et al. (2020). Comparison of Japanese encephalitis force of infection in pigs, poultry and dogs in cambodian villages. *Pathogens, 9*(9), 719.

Lam, K. H. K., Ellis, T. M., Williams, D. T., Lunt, R. A., Daniels, P. W., Watkins, K. L., & Riggs, C. M. (2005). Japanese encephalitis in a racing thoroughbred gelding in Hong Kong. *Veterinary Record, 157*(6), 168–173.

Le Flohic, G., Porphyre, V., Barbazan, P., & Gonzalez, J. P. (2013). Review of climate, landscape, and viral genetics as drivers of the Japanese encephalitis virus ecology. *PLoS Neglected Tropical Diseases, 7*(9), e2208.

Lindahl, J., Boqvist, S., Ståhl, K., Thu, H. T. V., & Magnusson, U. (2012). Reproductive performance in sows in relation to Japanese encephalitis virus seropositivity in an endemic area. *Tropical Animal Health and Production, 44*, 239–245.

Liu, X., Cao, S., Zhou, R., Xu, G., Xiao, S., Yang, Y., et al. (2006). Inhibition of Japanese encephalitis virus NS1 protein expression in cell by small interfering RNAs. *Virus Genes, 33*, 69–75.

Liu, S., Li, X., Chen, Z., Chen, Y., Zhang, Q., Liao, Y., et al. (2013). Comparison of genomic and amino acid sequences of eight Japanese encephalitis virus isolates from bats. *Archives of Virology, 158*, 2543–2552.

Lopalco, P. L., & Biasio, L. R. (2024). Japanese encephalitis can be devastating. *Annali di Igiene, Medicina Preventiva e di Comunità, 36*(3).

Lord, J. S., Gurley, E. S., & Pulliam, J. R. (2015). Rethinking Japanese encephalitis virus transmission: A framework for implicating host and vector species. *PLoS Neglected Tropical Diseases, 9*(12), e0004074.

Lu, G., & Gong, P. (2013). Crystal structure of the full-length Japanese encephalitis virus NS5 reveals a conserved methyltransferase-polymerase interface. *PLoS Pathogens, 9*(8), e1003549.

Luca, V. C., AbiMansour, J., Nelson, C. A., & Fremont, D. H. (2012). Crystal structure of the Japanese encephalitis virus envelope protein. *Journal of Virology, 86*(4), 2337–2346.

Mani, T. R., Rao, C. M., Rajendran, R., Devaputra, M., Prasanna, Y., et al. (1991). Surveillance for Japanese encephalitis in villages near Madurai, Tamil Nadu, India. *Transactions of the Royal Society of Tropical Medicine and Hygiene, 85*(2), 287–291.

Mansfield, K. L., Hernández-Triana, L. M., Banyard, A. C., Fooks, A. R., & Johnson, N. (2017). Japanese encephalitis virus infection, diagnosis and control in domestic animals. *Veterinary Microbiology, 201*, 85–92.

Moore, S. M. (2021). The current burden of Japanese encephalitis and the estimated impacts of vaccination: Combining estimates of the spatial distribution and transmission intensity of a zoonotic pathogen. *PLoS Neglected Tropical Diseases, 15*(10), e0009385.

Muller, D. A., & Young, P. R. (2013). The flavivirus NS1 protein: Molecular and structural biology, immunology, role in pathogenesis and application as a diagnostic biomarker. *Antiviral Research, 98*(2), 192–208.

Mulvey, P., Duong, V., Boyer, S., Burgess, G., Williams, D. T., Dussart, P., & Horwood, P. F. (2021). The ecology and evolution of Japanese encephalitis virus. *Pathogens, 10*(12), 1534.

Ogasa, A., Yokoki, Y., Fujisaki, Y., & Habu, A. (1977). Reproductive disorders in boars infected experimentally with Japanese encephalitis virus.

Peiris, J. S. M., Amerasinghe, F. P., Arunagiri, C. K., Perera, L. P., Karunaratne, S. H. P. P., Ratnayake, C. B., et al. (1993). Japanese encephalitis in Sri Lanka: Comparison of vector and virus ecology in different agro-climatic areas. *Transactions of the Royal Society of Tropical Medicine and Hygiene, 87*(5), 541–548.

Poonsiri, T., Wright, G. S., Solomon, T., & Antonyuk, S. V. (2019). Crystal structure of the Japanese encephalitis virus capsid protein. *Viruses, 11*(7), 623.

Pyke, A. T., Williams, D. T., Nisbet, D. J., Van den Hurk, A. F., Taylor, C. T., Johansen, C. A., et al. (2001). The appearance of a second genotype of Japanese encephalitis virus in the Australasian region. *American Journal of Tropical Medicine and Hygiene, 65*(6), 747–753.

Quan, T. M., Thao, T. T. N., Duy, N. M., Nhat, T. M., & Clapham, H. (2020). Estimates of the global burden of Japanese encephalitis and the impact of vaccination from 2000-2015. *eLife, 9*, e51027.

Ren, X., Fu, S., Dai, P., Wang, H., Li, Y., Li, X., et al. (2017). Pigsties near dwellings as a potential risk factor for the prevalence of Japanese encephalitis virus in adult in Shanxi, China. *Infectious Diseases of Poverty, 6*, 1–11.

Ricklin, M. E., Garcìa-Nicolàs, O., Brechbühl, D., Python, S., Zumkehr, B., Posthaus, H., et al. (2016a). Japanese encephalitis virus tropism in experimentally infected pigs. *Veterinary Research, 47*, 1–11.

Ricklin, M. E., García-Nicolás, O., Brechbühl, D., Python, S., Zumkehr, B., Nougairede, A., et al. (2016b). Vector-free transmission and persistence of Japanese encephalitis virus in pigs. *Nature Communications, 7*(1), 10832.

Rogers, B., Bunn, W. B., & Connor, B. A. (2016). An update on travel vaccines and issues in travel and international medicine. *Workplace Health & Safety, 64*(10), 462–468.

Sasaki, O., Karoji, Y., Kuroda, A., Karaki, T., Takenokuma, K., & Maeda, O. (1982). Protection of pigs against mosquito-borne Japanese encephalitis virus by immunization with a live attenuated vaccine. *Antiviral Research, 2*(6), 355–360.

Schuh, A. J., Guzman, H., Tesh, R. B., & Barrett, A. D. (2013). Genetic diversity of Japanese encephalitis virus isolates obtained from the Indonesian archipelago between 1974 and 1987. *Vector-Borne and Zoonotic Diseases, 13*(7), 479–488.

Shimizu, T., Mochizuki, H., Sugawa, Y., Okazaki, K., & Matumoto, M. (1951). Studies on Japanese encephalitis of cattle. I. Bovine encephalitis caused by natural infection with Japanese encephalitis virus.

Simpson, D. I. H., Smith, C. G., Bowen, E. T. W., Platt, G. S., Way, H., McMahon, D., et al. (1970). Arbovirus infections in Sarawak: Virus isolations from mosquitoes. *Annals of Tropical Medicine & Parasitology, 64*(2), 137–151.

Solomon, T., Dung, N. M., Kneen, R., Gainsborough, M., Vaughn, D. W., & Khanh, V. T. (2000). Japanese encephalitis. *Journal of Neurology, Neurosurgery & Psychiatry, 68*(4), 405–415.

Solomon, T., Ni, H., Beasley, D. W., Ekkelenkamp, M., Cardosa, M. J., & Barrett, A. D. (2003). Origin and evolution of Japanese encephalitis virus in Southeast Asia. *Journal of Virology, 77*(5), 3091–3098.

Srivastava, K. S., Jeswani, V., Pal, N., Bohra, B., Vishwakarma, V., Bapat, A. A., et al. (2023). Japanese encephalitis virus: An update on the potential antivirals and vaccines. *Vaccine, 11*(4), 742.

Sulkin, S. E., Allen, R., Miura, T., & Toyokawa, K. (1970). Studies of arthropod-borne virus infections in chiroptera. VI. Isolation of Japanese B encephalitis virus from naturally infected bats.

Takashima, I., Watanabe, T., Ouchi, N., & Hashimoto, N. (1988). Ecological studies of Japanese encephalitis virus in Hokkaido: Interepidemic outbreaks of swine abortion and evidence for the virus to overwinter locally. *The American Journal of Tropical Medicine and Hygiene, 38*(2), 420–427.

Tarantola, A., Goutard, F., Newton, P., De Lamballerie, X., Lortholary, O., Cappelle, J., & Buchy, P. (2014). Estimating the burden of Japanese encephalitis virus and other encephalitides in countries of the mekong region. *PLoS Neglected Tropical Diseases, 8*(1), e2533.

Ting, S. H. L., Tan, H. C., Wong, W. K., Ng, M. L., Chan, S. H., & Ooi, E. E. (2004). Seroepidemiology of neutralizing antibodies to Japanese encephalitis virus in Singapore: Continued transmission despite abolishment of pig farming? *Acta Tropica, 92*(3), 187–191.

Tiwari, S., Singh, R. K., Tiwari, R., & Dhole, T. N. (2012). Japanese encephalitis: A review of the Indian perspective. *The Brazilian Journal of Infectious Diseases, 16*(6), 564–573.

Unni, S. K., Růžek, D., Chhatbar, C., Mishra, R., Johri, M. K., & Singh, S. K. (2011). Japanese encephalitis virus: From genome to infectome. *Microbes and Infection, 13*(4), 312–321.

Van den Hurk, A. F., Ritchie, S. A., & Mackenzie, J. S. (2009a). Ecology and geographical expansion of Japanese encephalitis virus. *Annual Review of Entomology, 54*, 17–35.

van den Hurk, A. F., Smith, C. S., Field, H. E., Smith, I. L., Northill, J. A., Taylor, C. T., et al. (2009b). Transmission of Japanese encephalitis virus from the black flying fox, Pteropus alecto, to Culex annulirostris mosquitoes, despite the absence of detectable viremia. *The American Journal of Tropical Medicine and Hygiene, 81*(3), 457–462.

Vannice, K. S., Hills, S. L., Schwartz, L. M., Barrett, A. D., Heffelfinger, J., Hombach, J., et al. (2021). The future of Japanese encephalitis vaccination: Expert recommendations for achieving and maintaining optimal JE control. *NPJ Vaccines, 6*(1), 82.

Wang, J. L., Pan, X. L., Zhang, H. L., Fu, S. H., Wang, H. Y., Tang, Q., et al. (2009). Japanese encephalitis viruses from bats in Yunnan, China. *Emerging Infectious Diseases, 15*(6), 939.

Wang, S., Liu, Y., Guo, J., Wang, P., Zhang, L., Xiao, G., & Wang, W. (2017). Screening of FDA-approved drugs for inhibitors of Japanese encephalitis virus infection. *Journal of Virology, 91*(21), 10–1128.

Williams, D. T., Mackenzie, J. S., & Bingham, J. (2019). Flaviviruses. In *Diseases of swine* (pp. 530–543).

Wong, S. C., Ooi, M. H., Abdullah, A. R., Wong, S. Y., Krishnan, S., Tio, P. H., et al. (2008). A decade of Japanese encephalitis surveillance in Sarawak, Malaysia: 1997–2006. *Tropical Medicine & International Health, 13*(1), 52–55.

World Health Organisation. (n.d.). Available online: https://www.who.int/news-room/fact-sheets/detail/japanese-encephalitis

World Health Organization. (2018). Japanese encephalitis: Vaccine preventable diseases, surveillance standards.

World Health Organization. (2021). Available online: https://www.who.int/publications/i/item.WHO-2019-nCoV-therapeutics-2023.1. Accessed on 1 Feb 2023

Yamada, M., Nakamura, K., Yoshii, M., & Kaku, Y. (2004). Nonsuppurative encephalitis in piglets after experimental inoculation of Japanese encephalitis flavivirus isolated from pigs. *Veterinary Pathology, 41*(1), 62–67.

Yang, S. E., Pan, M. J., Tseng, H. F., & Liau, M. Y. (2006). The efficacy of mouse-brain inactivated Nakayama strain Japanese encephalitis vaccine – Results from 30 years experience in Taiwan. *Vaccine, 24*(14), 2669–2673.

Yap, G., Lim, X. F., Chan, S., How, C. B., Humaidi, M., Yeo, G., et al. (2019). Serological evidence of continued Japanese encephalitis virus transmission in Singapore nearly three decades after end of pig farming. *Parasites & Vectors, 12*, 1–7.

Yen, L. C., Liao, J. T., Lee, H. J., Chou, W. Y., Chen, C. W., Lin, Y. L., & Liao, C. L. (2016). The C terminus of the Core β-ladder domain in Japanese encephalitis virus nonstructural protein 1 is flexible for accommodation of heterologous epitope fusion. *Journal of Virology, 90*(3), 1178–1189.

Yun, S. I., & Lee, Y. M. (2014). Japanese encephalitis: The virus and vaccines. *Human Vaccines & Immunotherapeutics, 10*(2), 263–279.

Leptospirosis: Investigating Swine as a Reservoir for Human Infections

Priyanshi Yadav, Santanu Pal, P. Manoj Kumar Goud, Shivali Khandelwal, and Dumala Naveen

Abstract

Leptospirosis, a globally re-emerging zoonotic illness, presents significant challenges to public health, particularly in tropical and subtropical regions. Environmental and social factors contribute to its spread, with outbreaks frequently associated with flooding and natural disasters. The disease, caused by the pathogen *Leptospira*, is traditionally linked to various animal hosts and is now observed in both tropical and temperate climates. While leptospirosis is commonly underestimated and underreported, its impact on human and animal health is substantial. This chapter investigates the role of swine as potential reservoirs for human infections with leptospirosis. Swine, among various animal species, harbor *Leptospira* asymptomatically, shedding the bacteria into the environment. The intensification and expansion of swine farming contribute to disseminating *Leptospira* globally. Additionally, wild pig populations serve as reservoirs for various serovars, posing risks to human health through environmental contamination. Understanding the epidemiology, transmission dynamics, and pathogenesis of leptospirosis is crucial for effective prevention and control strategies. One Health approach, emphasizing the interconnectedness of human, animal, and environmental health, are essential for mitigating the spread of leptospirosis. Furthermore, social, and occupational factors, such as agricultural practices and inadequate sanitation, significantly influence the transmission of leptospires. This chapter explores the complex interplay between swine, humans, and the environment in transmitting leptospirosis, highlighting the importance of interdisciplinary collaboration and comprehensive surveillance efforts in addressing this global public health concern.

P. Yadav (✉) · S. Pal · P. M. K. Goud · S. Khandelwal · D. Naveen
ICAR-Indian Veterinary Research Institute (ICAR-IVRI), Izatnagar, Bareilly, India

R. Deb et al. (eds.), *Emerging Zoonotic Threats from Swine*,
https://doi.org/10.1007/978-981-96-7407-7_15

Keywords

Leptospirosis · Zoonotic disease · Swine reservoirs · Transmission dynamics · One Health approach

Introduction

Leptospirosis is a re-emerging illness found worldwide, particularly prevalent in tropical and subtropical nations where environmental and social factors facilitate its spread, resulting in morbidity of approximately 1.03 million individuals annually (Costa et al., 2015). Over the past few years, numerous outbreaks of leptospirosis have been documented in various locations, as leptospires are sustained in nature by a diverse array of animal hosts, encompassing both wild and domestic species (Vijayachari et al., 2008). Leptospirosis is primarily endemic in countries characterized by humid tropical or subtropical climates. While traditionally associated with tropical regions, leptospirosis is now being observed in temperate areas as well, attributed to factors like climate change and human migration coupled with inadequate sanitation and waste management practices. Transmission tends to be more favorable in tropical regions (Holla et al., 2018). Endemic leptospirosis is linked to several factors, including tropical climates, stagnant water, inadequate sanitation, occupational or recreational activities, and the proximity of potential mammalian reservoirs to human communities. Epidemics often coincide with flooding caused by heavy rainfall or natural calamities such as hurricanes, typhoons, or earthquakes (Guerra, 2013).

Leptospirosis is referred to by various names in different regions before its formal identification. For instance, the Chinese called it "rice field jaundice," while in Japan, it was known as "autumn fever" or "seven-day fever." Occupationally related syndromes such as "cane-cutter's disease," "swine-herd's disease," and "mud fever" were associated with specific professions. In general, leptospirosis is commonly recognized by names like Weil's disease, canicola fever, nanukayami fever, 7-day fever, harvest fever, field fever, cane-field fever, mild fever, and rat catcher's yellows, among others. The actual burden and prevalence of leptospirosis are often underestimated and underreported, leading to noticeable reemergence in various parts of the world. For instance, in South India, there has been a rise in *Leptospira* infections over the past two decades, particularly in regions like Kerala, Tamil Nadu, and the Andaman Islands (John, 1996).

Leptospira measures around 0.15 μm in diameter, with lengths varying between 6 and 20 μm. These organisms exhibit remarkable motility facilitated by its two periplasmic axial flagella present beneath the cell membrane and are characterized by their slender, spiral-shaped morphology, featuring elongated hair-like structures. These periplasmic endoflagellum not only enable their distinctive corkscrew movement but also play a role in their pathogenicity (Karpagam & Ganesh, 2020). Unique hooked ends of these flagella distinguish *Leptospira* from other spirochetes. *Leptospira* exhibits robust growth within a temperature range of 28 °C to 30 °C, although it can also survive at 37 °C. The optimal pH for its growth lies between 7.2 and 7.4. Despite being a microaerophile, it can thrive even in environments devoid of oxygen.

The traditional classification of the genus *Leptospira* categorized it into two species: *L. interrogans*, which comprises pathogenic strains, and *L. biflexa*, which includes saprophytic strains. Serovars within both species are further distinguished based on antigenic agglutination reactions and cross-absorption. *L. biflexa* encompasses over 60 serovars, whereas *L. interrogans* encompasses more than 200 serovars (Rathinam, 2002). Serovars are distinguished by the surface epitopes, expressed within the mosaic of lipopolysaccharide antigens (LPS) determined by the arrangement and composition of carbohydrates (Adler & de la Peña Moctezuma, 2010).

The *Leptospira* genus has recently been reclassified using genomic methods, leading to the discovery of 13 new species, bringing the total number of identified species to 64, beyond the previously known ones. Genomic analysis has revealed over 260 serovars, categorized as pathogenic, intermediate, and saprophytic. Pathogenic *Leptospira* causes moderate to severe disease, while intermediate strains lead to milder infections. Saprophytic serovars, found in the environment, are not pathogenic unless they undergo genetic recombination with pathogenic strains (Balamurugan et al., 2013; Cilia et al., 2021).

The existing evidence regarding the involvement of micronutrients in leptospirosis is limited and diverse. Laboratory investigations indicate a potential association between micronutrients like iron, calcium, and magnesium with leptospirosis. However, there is a scarcity of prospective studies and no randomized trials have been conducted thus far to ascertain the significance of micronutrients in *Leptospira* infection. Research in laboratory settings has revealed the necessity of iron for leptospires growth and survival, and both animal and human studies have suggested a link between leptospirosis and compromised host hematological status. Moreover, calcium appears to impact host macrophage apoptosis and binding to a key *Leptospira* lipoprotein, LipL32, indicating that increased calcium levels might signal disease progression in leptospirosis. However, there is relatively limited investigation into the role of other micronutrients in *Leptospira* infection and its pathogenesis (Herman et al., 2016). Hypomagnesemia has been linked to *Leptospira* infection and the severity of the disease in both laboratory studies and observational research involving humans. It frequently occurs in hospitalized individuals and has been recognized as a contributing factor to renal failure in cohort investigations among patients with leptospirosis (Khositseth et al., 2007).

Epidemiology and Transmission Dynamics

Occurrences of leptospirosis outbreaks in animals and humans are shaped by a combination of management methods, human actions, and notably, environmental conditions and weather events such as floods, which contribute to the prevalence of this zoonotic disease in tropical and subtropical regions.

Table 1 Leptospirosis outbreaks worldwide and in India

Year	Location	Probable cause	References
1996	Brazil	Heavy rainfall and flooding	Ko (1999)
2003	Jakarta, Indonesia	Flooding and contaminated water	Okatini et al. (2007)
2008	Sri Lanka	Environmental factors and occupational exposure	Agampodi et al. (2011)
2009	Philippines	Flooding and poor sanitation	Amilasan et al. (2012)
2010	Nicaragua	Contaminated water sources	Bacallao et al. (2014)
2017	Fiji	Widespread damage and contaminated water	Reid et al. (2017)
2022	Kerala, India	Monsoon-related flooding	Ifejube et al. (2023) and James et al. (2018)
2023	Andaman and Nicobar Islands, India	Environmental factors and occupational exposure	Fatema et al. (2023)

One Health is a holistic approach that underscores the interdependence of human, animal, and environmental health. It acknowledges the interconnectedness of humans, animals, and the environment, encompassing various living organisms like plants, to achieve comprehensive well-being. This approach advocates for collaborative efforts across different disciplines at local, national, and global levels to attain optimal health outcomes for humans, animals, and the environment (Roberts, 2019). The comprehensive "One Health" approach is essential for comprehending the interplay between *Leptospira* spp. infections in humans and animals, along with the environmental factors influencing its transmission. Due to increased interaction between humans and animals, along with human encroachment into natural habitats, leptospirosis is recognized as an emerging zoonotic disease of significant global public health concern. Zoonotic pathogens like *Leptospira* spp. are found in rural areas where community members may lack awareness of the associated risks and necessary preventive measures. Therefore, it is imperative to collect data on this pathogen's prevalence in both humans and animals, as well as its transmission through water. This approach relies on the collaboration between human, animal, and environmental health for the well-being of all individuals and ecosystems (Mazet et al., 2009; Allan et al., 2015) (Table 1).

Abiotic Factors Influencing the Transmission of *Leptospira*

Inadequate public hygiene contributes to the transmission of diseases, with approximately 1.9 million deaths globally and 4.2% of the total disease burden attributed to substandard sanitation. Leptospirosis is common in impoverished urban regions that suffer from inadequate sanitation. Urban poverty stems from disparities in wealth and development, resulting in economic inequalities even within areas. The challenges of managing sanitation are exacerbated by large population sizes, leading to inadequate waste management and heightened proliferation of leptospirosis vectors (Soo et al., 2020).

The global occurrence of leptospirosis varies widely due to specific climatic factors such as from 4 to 40 °C temperature, humidity exceeding 20%, and precipitation patterns unique to each geographic location. This disease is more prevalent in tropical and subtropical regions, where it is present year-round, whereas, in temperate zones, it tends to occur seasonally during periods of elevated temperatures and rainfall. *Leptospira* can endure in natural environments, surviving in soil and water with pH levels between 5.5 and 7.6, and even persisting in cattle urine for 6–18 h at a pH of 7–8 (Thiermann, 1982). Furthermore, certain serovars exhibit the ability to endure for as long as 344 days in water, retaining their virulence through the regulation of crucial genes that support survival even in harsh environmental conditions such as temperature and osmolarity extremes. This adaptation includes interactions with environmental bacteria and the formation of biofilms, enabling them to persist in urine and enhance their resistance against antibiotics (Bierque et al., 2020). Nevertheless, the comprehensive understanding of the external and internal factors enabling *Leptospira's* survival in the environment remains a subject of ongoing investigation.

Animals become infected with leptospirosis through contact with contaminated urine. During the acute phase of the disease, the bacteria are found in the bloodstream, urine, as well as various tissues and organs of the affected animal. In chronic cases, the organisms are primarily localized in the kidneys and are excreted in the urine. Chronic cases pose the greatest risk for spreading the disease as they often do not exhibit visible symptoms and are frequently overlooked. Nevertheless, they persist in excreting viable organisms for many days or months following "recovery". Another common route of transmission is inhaling infected urine droplets from the air, which occurs in situations where animals are closely confined and urinate on concrete floors. The primary modes of transmission involve direct contact with infected urine and indirect contact with urine-contaminated materials, including bedding, poorly drained pastures, or ponds. Additionally, inhaling urine tiny droplets from the surroundings, particularly in situations where animals are closely confined and urinate on concrete floors, represents another route of infection. It is believed that infection can be caused by a single leptospire.

Biotic Factors Influencing the Transmission of *Leptospira*

Animals susceptible to leptospirosis are categorized as natural or maintenance reservoirs and incidental hosts. In natural reservoirs, the infection is prevalent and often acquired early in life, typically through direct contact with infected animals. Incidental hosts contract the infection either directly from natural reservoirs or indirectly via contaminated water or soil. Certain species may act as natural hosts for specific serovars while serving as incidental reservoirs for others. Furthermore, the same species may function as a natural reservoir for distinct serovars across different geographic regions (Putz & Nally, 2020). Wild and synanthropic species serve as the primary natural reservoirs for pathogenic leptospires, with the bacteria residing in their kidneys. These animals typically do not exhibit clinical symptoms of the disease (Montalvo Corral, 2021). In incidental hosts, leptospirosis can lead to various acute clinical symptoms such as fever, respiratory issues, reproductive issues, decreased milk production, systemic failure, and kidney and liver insufficiency. Conversely, in reservoir hosts like swine, *Leptospira* may be present without significant adverse effects but can be shed through oral, renal, and reproductive routes. The risk of transmission from pigs to humans is further elevated due to the absence of noticeable clinical symptoms and specific indicators. Swine commonly harbor serovars such as Lora, Icterohaemorrhagiae, Pomona, and Tarassovi (Petrakovsky et al., 2014). Given their proximity to individuals involved in food production, livestock animals serve as a pivotal link in the interface between humans, animals, and the environment for *Leptospira* transmission, potentially serving as a source of natural or incidental infection to humans (Montalvo Corral, 2021).

Infection can occur due to direct or indirect contact with urine from reservoir host like swine infected with the pathogen, which is harbored in their renal tubules and excreted as pathogenic leptospires, contaminating soils, surface waters, streams, and rivers and through contact with mucous membranes, cuts, or abrasions in the skin. Prolonged exposure to, or ingestion of, contaminated water can also lead to infection (Pedersen et al., 2017). The release of leptospires in urine can occur intermittently or consistently, with bacterial concentrations in urine reaching levels as high as 10^8/mL. Leptospires exhibit reduced viability in acidic urine but can remain viable in alkaline urine. As a result, herbivores and animals with diets that lead to alkaline urine production are comparatively more significant as sources of shedding than those producing acidic urine (Adler & de la Peña Moctezuma, 2010).

Social and Occupational Factors Influencing the Transmission of *Leptospira*

Leptospirosis is classified as an occupational hazard for individuals engaged in agricultural, livestock, meat processing, abattoir, and rice cultivation activities, as well as for veterinarians, hunters, wildlife caretakers, and farmers. This is primarily because of their proximity to animals, which heightens the likelihood of exposure to potentially infected carcasses or live animals carrying *Leptospira* bacteria (Bengis et al., 2004). Epidemiological assessments suggest that around 30% of leptospirosis cases stem from occupational exposure (Richard & Oppliger, 2015). Furthermore, engaging in activities such as milk product formation and coming into contact with cattle drinking water sources may pose risks. Additionally, individuals involved in livestock handling and waste management, particularly without proper personal protection face an increased risk of infection. Individuals who own cattle or work with pigs or bovine tissues are also at heightened risk. In farms, typical activities include managing obstetrics in sows and performing necropsies after mortality occurrences. Because leptospirosis frequently shows no symptoms, workers are seriously in danger from these activities (Delbem et al., 2002) (Fig. 1).

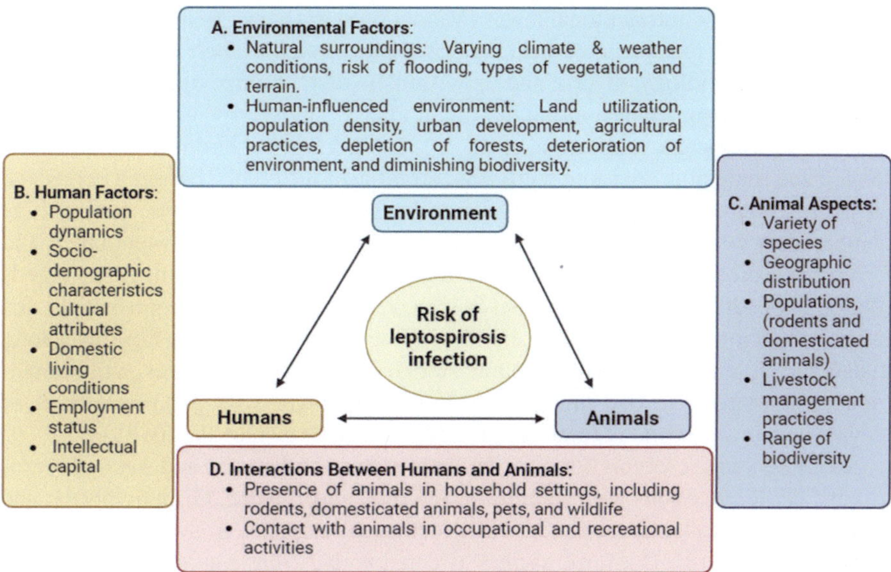

Fig. 1 Leptospirosis: key factors contributing to infection risk and transmission dynamics

Swine as Potential Reservoirs

Leptospires can infect various animal species such as cattle, dogs, horses, pigs, small ruminants, and wild animals. Many of these animals harbor the bacteria asymptomatically, with leptospires residing in the kidneys and being excreted into the environment. Given suitable environmental conditions, the bacteria can persist for extended periods, ranging from weeks to months. Animals are traditionally categorized as either maintenance hosts or susceptible hosts. Susceptible hosts typically develop varying degrees of illness after infection, which can sometimes be fatal. Populations of maintenance hosts serve as reservoirs for leptospirosis. However, while a particular animal population may act as a reservoir for a specific strain of *Leptospira*, individual animals within that population may still be susceptible to other strains of the bacterium.

Swine are an abundant invasive species and their existence poses substantial risks to native subpopulations, ecological environments, agricultural activities, and the transmission of zoonotic diseases. In pigs, the pathogen has been documented to induce fetal infections during the acute phase and genital lesions in the chronic phase of the disease (Fernandes et al., 2020). Pig farming plays a crucial role in ensuring global food security, supporting agricultural values, and facilitating local and international trade. However, infectious diseases pose a significant threat to pig health and can adversely affect the stability and productivity of the global swine industry. The intensification and expansion of the swine sector on a global scale have led to the emergence and dissemination of swine pathogens worldwide. This trend is fueled by the frequent transportation of pigs, feed, and pork commodities at local, national, and international levels (VanderWaal & Deen, 2018). Numerous factors contribute to the spread of wild pig populations, such as their fast reproductive pace, adaptable biology, diverse and opportunistic diet, absence of predators in certain regions, capability to flourish in human-altered landscapes, and human-driven activities at the local level (Baroch et al., 2015). Additionally, seropositivity between female and male pigs are same there is no significant difference between males and females. Mature pigs are found to be significantly more likely to be seropositive compared to young pigs. Additionally, no association is found between breed and *Leptospira* seropositivity in exotic/cross-breed pigs compared to indigenous breeds (Ngugi et al., 2019). It is thought that human actions significantly contribute to this range expansion, as evidenced by hunting activities prompting pigs to travel long distances, regional movement for game stocking/restocking purposes, and human-induced alterations to the environment that either favor wild pig populations or elevate densities beyond natural carrying capacities (Brown et al., 2018).

Swine serve as reservoir hosts for serovars within the *Pomona* and Australis serogroups, while infections with serogroups Icterohaemorrhagiae, Grippotyphosa, and Tarassovi are frequently observed as incidental occurrences in swine (Strutzberg-Minder et al., 2018). Domestic swines affected with *L. interrogans* are recognized to enter a “carrier state,” where they periodically release the bacterium after an outbreak. Carrier pigs can retain the leptospiral organism within the anterior convoluted tubules of their kidneys, even when antibodies are present in the blood (Meng et al., 2009). Seroprevalence of *Leptospira* infection varies widely among countries, with low rates (5–13%) observed in pigs in Trinidad (Suepaul et al., 2011), Thailand (Chadsuthi et al., 2017), and feral swine in the USA (Pedersen et al., 2015), intermediate rates (20.2–25%) in Portugal (Rocha, 1998), and high rates (55.9%) in Córdoba, Colombia (Calderón et al., 2014). Infection caused by serovar *Pomona* was linked to stillborn piglets and mummified fetuses, while Icterohaemorrhagiae infection was associated with stillborn piglets as well (Ramos et al., 2006). Serological evidence of positivity for various serovars was reported in different regions: Castellonis and Icterohaemorrhagiae in Argentina; Icterohaemorrhagiae, Australis, and Ballum in Trinidad; and Bratislava in Jamaica. Additionally, serological positivity for Bratislava, Castellonis, and Icterohaemorrhagiae was observed in both Mexico and Argentina (Petrakovsky et al., 2014).

Porcine leptospirosis is frequently reported in regions such as Southeast Asia and South America, primarily due to the favorable weather conditions that support the environmental survival and transmission of leptospires (Desvars et al., 2011). Pigs raised on farms alongside other livestock species showed a higher likelihood of being seropositive, indicating the potential for transmission between various animal species. The pathogens can penetrate the body through cuts in the skin, contact with mucous membranes or the eyes, inhalation of airborne particles, or ingestion of food or drinks contaminated with the bacteria (Musso & La Scola, 2013). Leptospirosis leads to reproductive issues in sows, including abortions, resorption, stillbirths, the delivery of underdeveloped piglets, as well as reduced litter size, weakness, muscle contraction, and rigidity. The disease documented in both domestic and wild pig populations across numerous countries (Niwetpathomwat et al., 2006). However, the disease's effects can extend to other stages as well, manifesting in symptoms like diarrhea, jaundice, and hemoglobinuria in nursing piglets, or subclinical infections in pigs during pre-fattening and fattening stages, resulting in the shedding of the microorganism into the environment (Ospina-Pinto & Hernández-Rodríguez, 2021).

Ellis identified domestic pigs as maintenance hosts for the a*ustralis* serogroup, while Jansen et al. categorized them as maintenance hosts for the Pomona serogroup. Conversely, wild boars were classified as accidental hosts for the Grippothyphosa serovar in Treml et al.'s study and for the Pomona and Bratislava serogroups in Jansen et al.'s research (Ellis, 2015; Jansen et al., 2007; Treml et al., 2003). In a study conducted by Slavica et al., wild boars in Croatia were subjected to serological analysis using the MAT technique. The study revealed that the most prevalent serovars were Australis (33.3%), Pomona (21.8%), and Tarassovi (14.3%) out of a total of 351 serum samples. The highest recorded titer was 1/3200 for the Pomona serovar. Similarly, a recent serological investigation of wild boars in Poland involved the analysis of 3621 blood samples for various *Leptospira* serovars/serogroups (Slavica et al., 2010; Żmudzki et al., 2015). This study found that serovars Pomona and Sejore, which are typically prevalent in domestic pigs in Poland, were less common in their study. Additionally, they highlighted the growing population of free-living wild boars in urban and suburban regions of Europe, posing a potential risk for the spread of pathogenic leptospiral strains. This increase in population also raises concerns about hunters being exposed to *Leptospira* spp., emphasizing the importance of population control measures (Jansen et al., 2006; Richard & Oppliger, 2015). The expanding human presence in non-urbanized regions has led to closer interaction between wildlife animals and inhabitants of these areas. For instance, in 2006, a case of leptospirosis in Berlin was associated with potential exposure to freshwater contaminated with wild boar urine. This highlights the role of wild boars as potential sources of infections in both humans and livestock (Jansen et al., 2006; Meng et al., 2009).

Pathogenesis and Clinical Manifestations

Leptospirosis was first documented two centuries ago, yet its pathogenesis and mechanisms remain poorly understood to this day. Recent research utilizing molecular techniques and bioinformatics has aimed to elucidate the function of various genes and their role in the pathogenicity and immunogenicity of the causative agent. Leptospiral virulence genes are distinct and do not share homology with genes found in other bacterial species, underscoring a unique virulence mechanism. Comparative genetic analysis between pathogenic and saprophytic *Leptospira* strains has identified approximately 900 genes exclusive to pathogenic strains. These genes encode proteins associated with virulence, including outer membrane proteins (OMP), lipopolysaccharides (LPS), flagellar components, motility-related proteins, chemotaxis factors, extracellular matrix-binding proteins like laminin, sphingomyelinase, hemolysins, and others (Picardeau et al., 2008; Adler et al., 2011).

The entry of *Leptospira* into the body can occur through skin lesions, even minor ones, mucous membranes such as the conjunctiva and oral mucosa, and by contact with moist skin or inhalation (Adler & de la Peña Moctezuma, 2010). After entering a new host, leptospires move through the peritubular capillaries or glomeruli to reach the kidneys through the bloodstream. Once within the renal tubular lumen, they infiltrate the brush border of the proximal tubule, which is the pathway for urine excretion (Haake & Levett, 2015). The chemoattractants for *Leptospira* bacteria bind to the extracellular matrix (ECM) and fibrinogen network, facilitating the invasion of the host's defense mechanisms. Many studies indicate that the pathogen generates certain toxic substances or proteins that disrupt vascular integrity by damaging the host cell membrane (Martinez-Lopez et al., 2010; Evangelista et al., 2014) (Fig. 2).

Once inside, infiltrated microorganisms enter the bloodstream, leading to bacteremia lasting approximately 5–7 days. The onset of initial symptoms coincides with the proliferation of bacteria in the blood and their migration across endothelial barriers. While the exact pathogenic mechanism of *Leptospira* remains incompletely understood, it is hypothesized that virulence factors such as toxins, adhesins, and other surface proteins play crucial roles (Levett & Haake, 2010).

Numerous leptospiral adhesins have demonstrated the capacity to bind to various host components and exhibit evasion tactics against the host immune response. For instance, leptospires can circumvent the complement system by incapacitating complement proteins and recruiting host complement regulators. This evasion

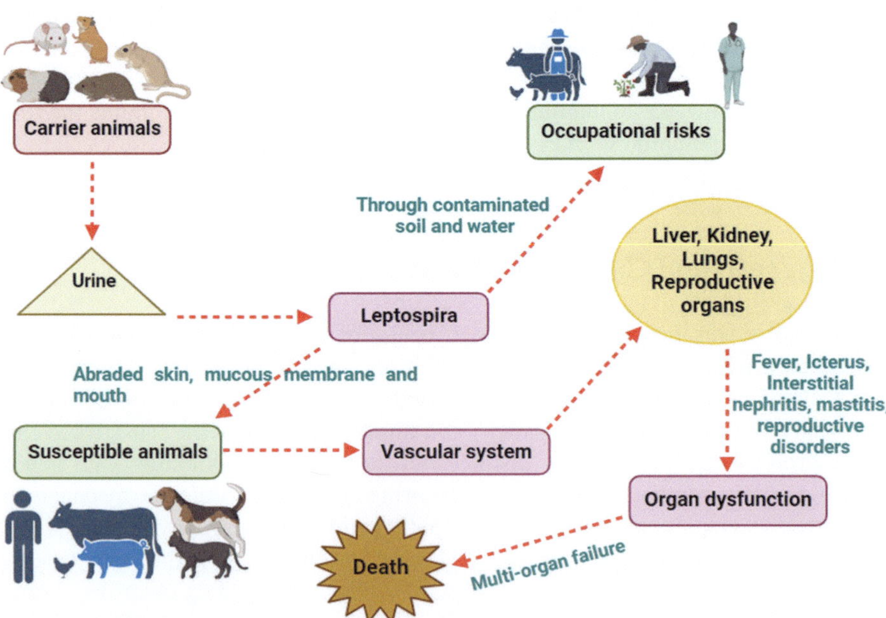

Fig. 2 An overview of the transmission pathways, disease development process, and the clinical symptoms observed in cases of leptospirosis

mechanism involves leptospires either deactivating the proteins through self-produced proteases or cleaving them with host proteases acquired by the bacteria (Fraga et al., 2016). Leptospires employ a strategy of binding to host complement regulators, responsible for regulating complement initiation, using surface proteins. This interaction enables leptospires to disrupt the host's complement system pathways (Fraga et al., 2016). Additionally, leptospires may evade macrophages and neutrophils until the production of anti-leptospiral antibodies. Research suggests that leptospires can conceal themselves within macrophages and subsequently exit through apoptosis (Fraga et al., 2016; Soo et al., 2020).

Leptospirosis manifests in two stages of infection: (i) a mild anicteric phase and (ii) a classical icteric phase. During the mild anicteric phase, the infection is typically mild and self-limiting, with some cases resolving without treatment. Approximately 80–90% of leptospirosis cases present with this mild phase without jaundice (Levett et al., 2001). The icteric phase is another typical presentation of severe form leptospirosis also known as Weil's disease, which affects approximately 5–10% of patients. During this phase, leptospires invade the liver, altering the activity of aminotransferases. Leukocytes and erythrocytes may be detected in the urine, leading to symptoms such as reduced urine output (oliguria) and the absence of urine (anuria) (Karpagam & Ganesh, 2020). Initial lesions impact the endothelium of small blood vessels, leading to ischemic injury in multiple systems such as the renal, hepatic, respiratory, brain, and muscles. Despite the severity of tissue damage, it can either fully heal or result in scar tissue formation, akin to the frequently observed "white spots" in pig kidneys (Cilia et al., 2021).

In humans, the typical initial clinical symptoms consist of a sudden onset fever, profound overall discomfort, muscle pain, and redness of the eyes. Conversely, jaundice and hemorrhage are clinical manifestations observed in individuals with severe leptospirosis. In animals, the initial stage of *Leptospira* infection often presents as subclinical, with few observable symptoms. However, chronic infections lead to reproductive losses and significant economic impacts (Ellis, 2015; Kobayashi, 2001).

Host Immune Response Against Leptospirosis

The primary defense against leptospirosis involves the humoral response, as documented by several studies. Antibodies generated during infection with species exhibit agglutinating properties, akin to those observed with other Gram-negative bacteria (Jost et al., 1986). The primary target of the antibodies is the leptospiral lipopolysaccharide (LPS). When guinea pigs were infected experimentally, monoclonal antibodies produced against leptospiral LPS in infected mice offered passive protection. However, immunity mediated by anti-LPS antibodies is restricted to serovars that match, unlike whole leptospiral protein preparations, which have shown protection against both matching and different serovars upon challenge (Palaniappan et al., 2007). Combining leptospiral outer membrane proteins (OMPs) such as OmpL1 and LipL41 has shown promising results as protective immunogens, indicating the potential for developing subunit vaccines with enhanced efficacy and reduced adverse effects. While some other surface-exposed proteins also demonstrate potential immunoprotective properties, their evaluation has been limited to a small number. For instance, immunization with both conserved and variable regions of LigB, followed by challenge with *Leptospira interrogans* serovar *Pomona*, induces protective responses in hamsters. Discovering additional protective antigens involved in leptospirosis immunity will not only aid in improving diagnostic methods but also enable early detection of *Leptospira* infections (Yan et al., 2009).

Effective innate immune defense against *Leptospira* requires the presence of both TLR2 and TLR4. Mice lacking both TLR2 and TLR4 are highly susceptible to leptospire infection compared to those lacking only one of these receptors. However, the absence of TLR4 results in severe leptospirosis characterized by clinical symptoms (Viriyakosol et al., 2006; Chassin et al., 2009). Leptospiral LPS, which typically triggers the TLR4 pathway in response to Gram-negative bacteria, was found to activate the TLR2 pathway in human monocytic cell lines. Mice lacking TLR2 did not exhibit a response to intraperitoneal inoculation of leptospiral LPS, failing to produce TNF-α and IL-6. These findings suggest potential variations in the response to leptospires among different species. Additionally, human monocytic TLR4 did not show activation by LPS or heat-killed leptospires, providing further support for this notion.

Human infection typically originates from contact with urine from infected animals. As a result, the considered hazardous factors and activities revolve around exposure to animal reservoirs or contaminated environments. These activities include coming into contact with various animal species, handling animal tissues, being exposed to animal urine, navigating water bodies, and engaging in occupational or recreational activities that involve exposure to a contaminated wet environment (Vijayachari et al., 2008). Advanced illness can result in various systemic complications, including acute kidney or liver failure, as well as severe lung hemorrhage, which can be fatal (Levett et al., 2001). Chronic renal carriers in both domestic and wild animals harbor viable leptospires in their kidneys, which can be shed in urine, thereby serving as a potential source of infection for humans. Humans have the potential to contract any strain of *Leptospira* from any animal or environmental setting, primarily through exposure to fluids from infected animals (Guerra, 2013; Calderón et al., 2014). Susceptibility levels vary among domestic species, with each serovar typically being maintained within a specific animal species. Within the same geographical region, animals may acquire serovars maintained by either their species or other animal species (Ngugi et al., 2019). Leptospirosis is recognized as an occupational hazard, particularly impacting individuals involved in agriculture, fishing, veterinary medicine, and occupations in sewage and abattoirs. Another potential source of infection for humans is exposure during recreational water activities (Agampodi et al., 2014) (Table 2).

Table 2 Virulence factors of Leptospira organisms

Virulence factor	Function/role	References
Outer membrane proteins	Adhesion to host cells, evasion of host immune response	Picardeau (2017)
Lipopolysaccharides (LPS)	Structural component of outer membrane, antigenic variation	Eshghi et al. (2009).
Flagellar components	Facilitate motility	Lourdault et al. (2011)
Extracellular matrix-binding proteins	Bind to host components, facilitate invasion	Stevenson et al. (2007)
Toxins	Disrupt vascular integrity, damage host cell membranes	Matsunaga et al. (2007)
Hemolysins	Induce hemolysis	Matsunaga et al. (2003)
Sphingomyelinase	Promote tissue invasion, contribute to pathogenesis	Choy et al. (2007)
Complement evasion factors	Disable complement proteins, recruit host complement regulators	Fraga et al. (2016)
Macrophage evasion	Concealment within macrophages, exit through apoptosis	Hu et al. (2017)

Various Diagnostic Techniques

Diagnosing leptospiral infection can be challenging and complex as it requires specialized laboratory facilities and skilled personnel, which may not be available in all endemic regions. Additionally, the infection presents symptoms similar to those of other diseases such as hepatitis, dengue, and scrub typhus, further complicating the diagnostic process. Various specimens including blood, urine, cerebrospinal fluid (CSF), infected tissues, and body fluids can be utilized for diagnosis. A standardized testing method for detecting leptospiral infection at all stages is currently unavailable, which poses challenges in diagnosing the disease effectively. *Leptospira* can be detected in the blood during the starting stage of infection when early diagnosis is crucial for prompt treatment. Subsequently, they are found in the urine during later stages, often after antibiotic therapy has begun. Antibody tests conducted on blood samples can provide epidemiological insights, particularly in endemic areas.

Numerous diagnostic assays have been devised to accurately detect leptospirosis, categorized into those targeting the bacteria, their antigens, or genomic material, and those detecting antibodies to the infecting bacteria. However, interpreting results from natural infections can be challenging due to factors such as intermittent shedding and discrepancies between taxonomic and antigenic classifications of the infecting genus. Dark-field microscopy of blood and urine is a rapid method for detecting leptospires, especially in resource-limited settings. However, its sensitivity is limited, it demands skilled operators, and it does not offer insights into the specific serovar causing the infection (O'Keefe, 2002) (Fig. 3).

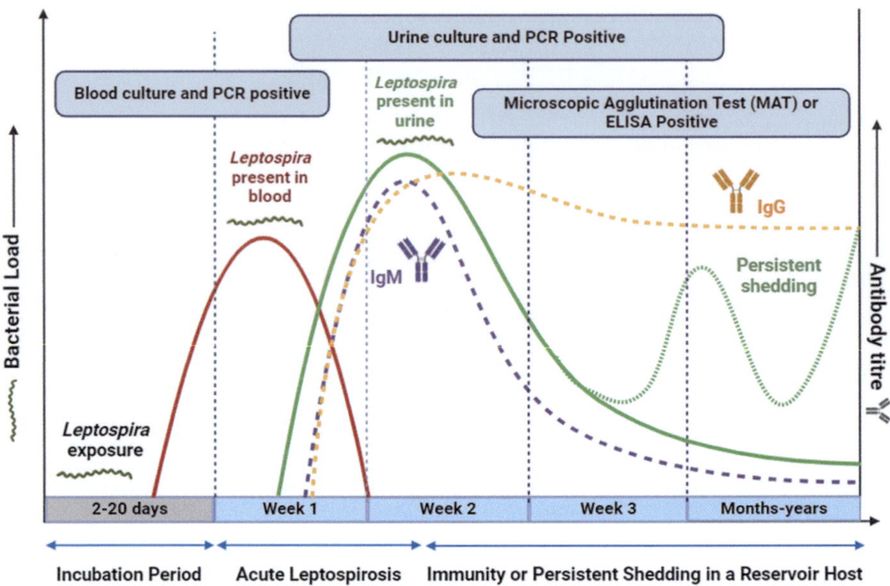

Fig. 3 The dynamics of leptospiral infection progression and associated diagnostic methodologies

Microscopic Agglutination Test

Isolation of the *Leptospira* is the most preferred method for the diagnosis of leptospirosis. While isolation is the most precise method for diagnosing *Leptospira* infections, its practicality is limited due to its complexity and time-consuming nature. Isolation typically involves the use of liquid mediums like Ellinghausen–McCullough–Johnson–Harris (EMJH) or Fletcher media, supplemented with albumin, serum, and Tween 80 or 40 to promote *Leptospira* growth (Kędzierska-Mieszkowska & Arent, 2020; Cilia et al., 2021).

The main diagnostic method and survey tool for *Leptospira* infections is the microscopic agglutination test (MAT). MAT involves using a panel of live antigens representing the predominant serogroups in the area of interest, mixed with serum at a starting dilution of 1:100 and further diluted as needed. The concentration of *Leptospira* should match that of the negative control, which is a culture diluted 1:2 with saline solution. The optimal cutoff value for MAT remains debatable as chronic and subclinical infections, particularly those caused by host-specific strains, might exhibit low titers, while acute illness typically presents with high titers (Pinto et al., 2017). Additionally, establishing the endemic status of a particular area may also influence the selection of an appropriate cutoff threshold, as proposed by Picardeau in 2013, indicating that cutoff values could differ depending on the species or regions under investigation (Picardeau, 2013; Pinto et al., 2017).

PCR-Based Diagnosis

Genomic techniques for detecting *Leptospira* include different conventional PCR, real-time PCR, and RT-PCR. These methods, known for their high sensitivity, rely on amplifying genes present in leptospires, such as the 16S ribosomal RNA gene, the B subunit of DNA gyrase and secY, as well as genes unique to pathogenic species like LipL32, lfb1, and ompL1. PCR is the recommended method for detecting and identifying nucleic acids of *Leptospira* serovars. PCR can be particularly valuable in cases where the host's immune response to the infecting serovar is weak, such as in cattle infected with serovar hardjo, or when sample quality compromises the viability of bacteria. However, PCR assays have limitations in identifying isolates as specific serovars, often categorizing them into genotypic groups rather than serovar-specific ones. Moreover, recent protocols may not be sensitive potent to find all serovars without generating false-positive results from unintended bacterial contaminants (O'Keefe, 2002).

Diagnosis by Other Molecular Methods

Various molecular techniques serve as supplementary typing systems in epidemiological research, enabling the differentiation of strains at a sub-specific level. These methods encompass restriction endonuclease analysis of chromosomal DNA using fixed-field electrophoresis or PFGE, RFLPs, and ribotyping. However, accurately identifying leptospires at the species level remains challenging, as DNA-DNA hybridization is not practical for routine identification. PCR-based approaches have been developed to address this limitation, allowing for the classification of new *Leptospira* species. Mapped restriction site polymorphisms (MRSPs) in PCR-amplified ribosomal genes effectively group reference strains based on their genetic relatedness. Arbitrarily primed PCR (AP-PCR) produces distinct genetic patterns useful for molecular epidemiology and rapid species-level strain identification (Perolat et al., 1998).

Implications for Public Health

The recognition of swine as potential reservoirs for human leptospirosis infections has significant implications for public health surveillance and control strategies. Integrated approaches that consider both animal and human health aspects are essential for effectively managing and preventing leptospirosis transmission at the human-animal interface. Brazil operates a National Program for Swine Health (Programa Nacional de Sanidade Suídea—PNSS), overseen by a public agency, but its adoption is not obligatory for all establishments (Bharti et al., 2003). It is recommended that farms that house healthy animals alongside sick ones modify their management practices to reduce the risk of infection, particularly those situated near flooded areas. Special emphasis should be placed on monitoring water sources, as stagnant water has been identified as a leptospirosis risk factor. Farmers with stagnant water sources are strongly encouraged to make necessary changes (dos Santos et al., 2019). The Council of State and Territorial Epidemiologists (CSTE) sanctioned the inclusion of leptospirosis as a Nationally Notifiable Condition in the United States in 2012. This decision to reinstate national surveillance aims to enable the evaluation of leptospirosis incidence, geographic spread, patterns over time, and the factors contributing to human cases. Additionally, it will aid in detecting outbreaks and identifying potential new animal hosts (Guerra, 2013).

Leptospirosis poses a threat to both swine producers and slaughterhouse employees but can be mitigated by practicing proper hygiene, maintaining sanitation standards, and implementing sound animal husbandry practices. Educating individuals handling animals or animal products is crucial for minimizing the risk of exposure to zoonotic pathogens (Campagnolo et al., 2000). However, there remains a deficiency in research assessing the true epidemiological landscape of the disease in domestic animals, particularly in tropical regions, which could hinder control efforts. Strategies for controlling leptospirosis primarily involve antibiotic treatment for carriers, environmental management practices, and predominantly, systematic immunization of vulnerable animals. However, antibiotic usage is restricted in numerous countries for combating swine leptospirosis (Verma et al., 2012).

Vaccination is a potential strategy to prevent leptospirosis in both humans and animals. However, there are challenges due to the diversity of leptospiral strains, which can limit the effectiveness of vaccines. Currently, only one nation in Latin America, Cuba routinely vaccinates humans against *Leptospira* (Pereira et al., 2017). Vaccines are rarely accessible, and their usage is often insufficient. Vaccines need to target the prevalent leptospiral serovars specific to the species or region, while environmental strategies may vary based on the infecting strain. Implementing effective management strategies is challenging and, in many instances, economically unfeasible. Therefore, comprehensive diagnosis is crucial for the effectiveness of control programs (Subharat et al., 2011). Vaccines are mainly bacterins made from whole dead cells, but they have limitations such as high production costs, short duration of immunity, and limited protection against specific serovars. Polyvalent vaccines are used in animals, providing immunity for up to 3 years (Koizumi & Watanabe, 2005). Recombinant DNA vaccines offer advantages like lower production costs and stability, with the potential to induce long-term immune responses against multiple serovars. Genes like LipL32, OmpL1, and LipL41 have been investigated for their vaccine potential in animal models (Montalvo Corral, 2021).

An additional option for preventing leptospirosis is chemoprevention prophylaxis, typically employed in situations of heightened infection risk and inevitable exposure. Weekly oral administration of 200 mg doxycycline has demonstrated efficacy in lowering the incidence of clinical infection, although it does not completely prevent infection. Nonetheless, it notably diminishes both morbidity and mortality associated with the disease (Sehgal et al., 2000). Managing leptospirosis presents challenges, particularly due to its variation across host species and infecting serogroups. Tailoring control measures to specific strains is essential, underscoring the importance of understanding prevalent serogroups in each host population. Reducing the risk of infection entails minimizing contact with carrier hosts or environments contaminated with the pathogen. Raising awareness among susceptible populations, particularly those at higher risk, regarding leptospirosis is crucial for facilitating early detection and appropriate treatment. This objective can be accomplished through educational initiatives or interventions aimed at fostering preventive health practices among vulnerable groups.

Conclusion

Leptospirosis is a zoonotic ailment with global significance, and witnessing a rise in both human and animal cases across various rural and urban locales. The intricate interplay of serovar distribution, host diversity, and socio-environmental factors shapes its ecology and epidemiology in this region. While systematic diagnosis of leptospirosis is not universally implemented, active surveillance utilizing appropriate diagnostic tools in humans and animals could prove pivotal in averting and managing leptospirosis outbreaks. Swine represents a potential reservoir for human leptospirosis infections, highlighting the importance of comprehensive surveillance and control measures at the human-animal interface. By elucidating the role of swine in the epidemiology of leptospirosis, this chapter contributes to our understanding of zoonotic disease transmission dynamics and informs strategies for mitigating the risk of human infection.

References

Adler, B., & de la Peña Moctezuma, A. (2010). Leptospira and leptospirosis. *Veterinary Microbiology, 140*(3–4), 287–296. https://doi.org/10.1016/j.vetmic.2009.03.012

Adler, B., Lo, M., Seemann, T., & Murray, G. L. (2011). Pathogenesis of leptospirosis: The influence of genomics. *Veterinary Microbiology, 153*(1–2), 73–81. https://doi.org/10.1016/j.vetmic.2011.02.055

Agampodi, S. B., Peacock, S. J., Thevanesam, V., Nugegoda, D. B., Smythe, L., Thaipadungpanit, J., Craig, S. B., Burns, M. A., Dohnt, M., Boonsilp, S., Senaratne, T., Kumara, A., Palihawadana, P., Perera, S., & Vinetz, J. M. (2011). Leptospirosis outbreak in Sri Lanka in 2008: Lessons for assessing the global burden of disease. *American Journal of Tropical Medicine and Hygiene, 85*(3), 471–478. https://doi.org/10.4269/ajtmh.2011.11-0276

Agampodi, S. B., Karunarathna, D., Jayathilala, N., Rathnayaka, H., Agampodi, T. C., & Karunanayaka, L. (2014). Outbreak of leptospirosis after white-water rafting: Sign of a shift from rural to recreational leptospirosis in Sri Lanka? *Epidemiology and Infection, 142*(4), 843–846. https://doi.org/10.1017/S0950268813001465

Allan, K. J., Biggs, H. M., Halliday, J. E. B., Kazwala, R. R., Maro, V. P., Cleaveland, S., & Crump, J. A. (2015). Epidemiology of leptospirosis in Africa: A systematic review of a neglected zoonosis and a paradigm for 'One Health' in Africa. *PLoS Neglected Tropical Diseases, 9*(9), e0003899. https://doi.org/10.1371/journal.pntd.0003899

Amilasan, A. S. T., Ujiie, M., Suzuki, M., Salva, E., Belo, M. C. P., Koizumi, N., Yoshimatsu, K., Schmidt, W. P., Marte, S., Dimaano, E. M., Villarama, J. B., & Ariyoshi, K. (2012). Outbreak of leptospirosis after flood, The Philippines, 2009. *Emerging Infectious Diseases, 18*(1), 91–94. https://doi.org/10.3201/eid1801.101892

Bacallao, J., Schneider, M. C., Najera, P., Aldighieri, S., Soto, A., Marquiño, W., Sáenz, C., Jiménez, E., Moreno, G., Chávez, O., Galan, D. I., & Espinal, M. A. (2014). Socioeconomic factors and vulnerability to outbreaks of leptospirosis in Nicaragua. *International Journal of Environmental Research and Public Health, 11*(8), 8301–8318. https://doi.org/10.3390/ijerph110808301

Balamurugan, V., Gangadhar, N. L., Mohandoss, N., Thirumalesh, S. R. A., Dhar, M., Shome, R., Krishnamoorthy, P., Prabhudas, K., & Rahman, H. (2013). Characterization of leptospira isolates from animals and humans: Phylogenetic analysis identifies the prevalence of intermediate species in India. *Springerplus, 2*(1), 362. https://doi.org/10.1186/2193-1801-2-362

Baroch, J. A., Gagnon, C. A., Lacouture, S., & Gottschalk, M. (2015). Exposure of feral swine (Sus scrofa) in the United States to selected pathogens. *Canadian Journal of Veterinary Research = Revue Canadienne de Recherche Veterinaire, 79*(1), 74–78.

Bengis, R. G., Leighton, F. A., Fischer, J. R., Artois, M., Mörner, T., & Tate, C. M. (2004). The role of wildlife in emerging and re-emerging zoonoses. *Revue Scientifique et Technique (International Office of Epizootics), 23*(2), 497–511.

Bharti, A. R., Nally, J. E., Ricaldi, J. N., Matthias, M. A., Diaz, M. M., Lovett, M. A., Levett, P. N., Gilman, R. H., Willig, M. R., Gotuzzo, E., & Vinetz, J. M. (2003). Leptospirosis: A zoonotic disease of global importance. *The Lancet Infectious Diseases, 3*(12), 757–771. https://doi.org/10.1016/S1473-3099(03)00830-2

Bierque, E., Thibeaux, R., Girault, D., Soupé-Gilbert, M.-E., & Goarant, C. (2020). A systematic review of Leptospira in water and soil environments. *PLoS One, 15*(1), e0227055. https://doi.org/10.1371/journal.pone.0227055

Brown, V. R., Bowen, R. A., & Bosco-Lauth, A. M. (2018). Zoonotic pathogens from feral swine that pose a significant threat to public health. *Transboundary and Emerging Diseases, 65*(3), 649–659. https://doi.org/10.1111/tbed.12820

Calderón, A., Rodríguez, V., Máttar, S., & Arrieta, G. (2014). Leptospirosis in pigs, dogs, rodents, humans, and water in an area of the Colombian tropics. *Tropical Animal Health and Production, 46*(2), 427–432. https://doi.org/10.1007/s11250-013-0508-y

Campagnolo, E. R., Warwick, M. C., Marx, H. L., Cowart, R. P., Donnell, H. D., Bajani, M. D., Bragg, S. L., Esteban, J. E., Alt, D. P., Tappero, J. W., Bolin, C. A., & Ashford, D. A. (2000). Analysis of the 1998 outbreak of leptospirosis in Missouri in humans exposed to infected swine. *Journal of the American Veterinary Medical Association, 216*(5), 676–682. https://doi.org/10.2460/javma.2000.216.676

Chadsuthi, S., Bicout, D. J., Wiratsudakul, A., Suwancharoen, D., Petkanchanapong, W., Modchang, C., Triampo, W., Ratanakorn, P., & Chalvet-Monfray, K. (2017). Investigation on predominant Leptospira serovars and its distribution in humans and livestock in Thailand, 2010-2015. *PLoS Neglected Tropical Diseases, 11*(2), e0005228. https://doi.org/10.1371/journal.pntd.0005228

Chassin, C., Picardeau, M., Goujon, J.-M., Bourhy, P., Quellard, N., Darche, S., Badell, E., d'Andon, M. F., Winter, N., Lacroix-Lamandé, S., Buzoni-Gatel, D., Vandewalle, A., & Werts, C. (2009). TLR4- and TLR2-mediated B cell responses control the clearance of the bacterial pathogen, Leptospira interrogans. *The Journal of Immunology, 183*(4), 2669–2677. https://doi.org/10.4049/jimmunol.0900506

Choy, H. A., Kelley, M. M., Chen, T. L., Møller, A. K., Matsunaga, J., & Haake, D. A. (2007). Physiological osmotic induction of Leptospira interrogans adhesion: LigA and LigB bind extracellular matrix proteins and fibrinogen. *Infection and Immunity, 75*(5), 2441–2450. https://doi.org/10.1128/IAI.01635-06

Cilia, G., Bertelloni, F., Albini, S., & Fratini, F. (2021). Insight into the epidemiology of leptospirosis: A review of Leptospira isolations from "unconventional" hosts. *Animals, 11*(1), 191. https://doi.org/10.3390/ani11010191

Costa, F., Hagan, J. E., Calcagno, J., Kane, M., Torgerson, P., Martinez-Silveira, M. S., Stein, C., Abela-Ridder, B., & Ko, A. I. (2015). Global morbidity and mortality of leptospirosis: A systematic review. *PLoS Neglected Tropical Diseases, 9*(9), e0003898. https://doi.org/10.1371/journal.pntd.0003898

Delbem, Á. C. B., de Freitas, J. C., Bracarense, A. P. F. R. L., Müller, E. E., & de Oliveira, R. C. (2002). Leptospirosis in slaughtered sows: Serological and histopathological investigation. *Brazilian Journal of Microbiology, 33*(2). https://doi.org/10.1590/S1517-83822002000200016

Desvars, A., Cardinale, E., & Michault, A. (2011). Animal leptospirosis in small tropical areas. *Epidemiology and Infection, 139*(2), 167–188. https://doi.org/10.1017/S0950268810002074

dos Santos, C. V. B., Mathias, L. A., da Silva Feitosa, P. J., Oliveira, J. M. B., Pinheiro Júnior, J. W., & Brandespim, D. F. (2019). Risk factors associated with leptospirosis in swine in state of Pernambuco, Brazil. *Arquivos do Instituto Biológico, 86*. https://doi.org/10.1590/1808-1657000632017

Ellis, W. A. (2015). *Animal leptospirosis* (pp. 99–137). https://doi.org/10.1007/978-3-662-45059-8_6

Eshghi, A., Cullen, P. A., Cowen, L., Zuerner, R. L., & Cameron, C. E. (2009). Global proteome analysis of Leptospira interrogans. *Journal of Proteome Research, 8*(10), 4564–4578. https://doi.org/10.1021/pr9004597

Evangelista, K., Franco, R., Schwab, A., & Coburn, J. (2014). Leptospira interrogans binds to Cadherins. *PLoS Neglected Tropical Diseases, 8*(1), e2672. https://doi.org/10.1371/journal.pntd.0002672

Fatema, A., Ramu, M., Thiruvengadam, K., Sunish, I. P., & Vijayachari, P. (2023). Knowledge, attitude, and preventive practices of leptospirosis affected populations in South Andaman, India: A cross-sectional study. *Journal of Health Sciences, 13*(2), 105–112. https://doi.org/10.17532/jhsci.2023.2145

Fernandes, J. J., Araújo Júnior, J. P., Malossi, C. D., Ullmann, L. S., da Costa, D. F., Silva, M. L. C. R., Alves, C. J., de Azevedo, S. S., & Dos Santos Higino, S. S. (2020). High frequency of seropositive and carriers of Leptospira spp. in pigs in the semiarid region of northeastern Brazil. *Tropical Animal Health and Production, 52*(4), 2055–2061. https://doi.org/10.1007/s11250-020-02203-y

Fraga, T. R., Isaac, L., & Barbosa, A. S. (2016). Complement evasion by pathogenic Leptospira. *Frontiers in Immunology, 7*. https://doi.org/10.3389/fimmu.2016.00623

Guerra, M. A. (2013). Leptospirosis: Public health perspectives. *Biologicals, 41*(5), 295–297. https://doi.org/10.1016/j.biologicals.2013.06.010

Haake, D. A., & Levett, P. N. (2015). Leptospirosis in humans (Vol. 387, pp. 65–97). https://doi.org/10.1007/978-3-662-45059-8_5

Herman, H. S., Mehta, S., Cárdenas, W. B., Stewart-Ibarra, A. M., & Finkelstein, J. L. (2016). Micronutrients and leptospirosis: A review of the current evidence. *PLoS Neglected Tropical Diseases, 10*(7), e0004652. https://doi.org/10.1371/journal.pntd.0004652

Holla, R., Darshan, B., Pandey, L., Unnikrishnan, B., Kumar, N., Thapar, R., Mithra, P., & Kulkarni, V. (2018). Leptospirosis in coastal South India: A facility based study. *BioMed Research International, 2018*, 1–5. https://doi.org/10.1155/2018/1759125

Hu, W. L., Dong, H. Y., Li, Y., Ojcius, D. M., Li, S. J., & Yan, J. (2017, November). Bid-induced release of AIF/EndoG from mitochondria causes apoptosis of macrophages during infection with Leptospira interrogans. *Frontiers in Cellular and Infection Microbiology, 7*. https://doi.org/10.3389/fcimb.2017.00471

Ifejube, O. J., Kuriakose, S. L., & Blanford, J. I. (2023). Analysing the outbreaks of leptospirosis after floods in Kerala, India. https://doi.org/10.21203/rs.3.rs-3673273/v1

James, S., Sathian, B., Van Teijlingen, E., & Asim, M. (2018). Outbreak of leptospirosis in Kerala. *Nepal Journal of Epidemiology, 8*(4), 745–747. https://doi.org/10.3126/nje.v8i4.23876

Jansen, A., Nöckler, K., Schönberg, A., Luge, E., Ehlert, D., & Schneider, T. (2006). Wild boars as possible source of hemorrhagic leptospirosis in Berlin, Germany. *European Journal of Clinical Microbiology & Infectious Diseases, 25*(8), 544–546. https://doi.org/10.1007/s10096-006-0174-3

Jansen, A., Luge, E., Guerra, B., Wittschen, P., Gruber, A. D., Loddenkemper, C., Schneider, T., Lierz, M., Ehlert, D., Appel, B., Stark, K., & Nöckler, K. (2007). Leptospirosis in urban wild boars, Berlin, Germany. *Emerging Infectious Diseases, 13*(5), 739–742. https://doi.org/10.3201/eid1305.061302

John, T. J. (1996). Emerging & re-emerging bacterial pathogens in India. *The Indian Journal of Medical Research, 103*, 4–18.

Jost, B. H., Adler, B., Vinh, T., & Faine, S. (1986). A monoclonal antibody reacting with a determinant on leptospiral lipopolysaccharide protects Guinea pigs against leptospirosis. *Journal of Medical Microbiology, 22*(3), 269–275. https://doi.org/10.1099/00222615-22-3-269

Karpagam, K. B., & Ganesh, B. (2020). Leptospirosis: A neglected tropical zoonotic infection of public health importance—An updated review. *European Journal of Clinical Microbiology & Infectious Diseases, 39*(5), 835–846. https://doi.org/10.1007/s10096-019-03797-4

Kędzierska-Mieszkowska, S., & Arent, Z. (2020). AAA+ molecular chaperone ClpB in Leptospira interrogans: Its role and significance in leptospiral virulence and pathogenesis of leptospirosis. *International Journal of Molecular Sciences, 21*(18), 6645. https://doi.org/10.3390/ijms21186645

Khositseth, S., Sudjaritjan, N., Tananchai, P., Ong-ajyuth, S., Sitprija, V., & Thongboonkerd, V. (2007). Renal magnesium wasting and tubular dysfunction in leptospirosis. *Nephrology Dialysis Transplantation, 23*(3), 952–958. https://doi.org/10.1093/ndt/gfm698

Ko, A. I., Reis, M. G., Ribeiro Dourado, C. M., Johnson, W. D., Jr., Riley, L. W., & Salvador Leptospirosis Study Group. (1999). Urban epidemic of severe leptospirosis in Brazil. *The Lancet, 354*(9181), 820–825.

Kobayashi, Y. (2001). Clinical observation and treatment of leptospirosis. *Journal of Infection and Chemotherapy, 7*(2), 59–68. https://doi.org/10.1007/s101560100011

Koizumi, N., & Watanabe, H. (2005). Leptospirosis vaccines: past, present, and future. *Journal of Postgraduate Medicine, 51*(3), 210–214.

Levett, P. N., & Haake, D. A. (2010). Leptospira species (leptospirosis). https://doi.org/10.1016/B978-0-443-06839-3.00240-X

Levett, P. N., Branch, S. L., Whittington, C. U., Edwards, C. N., & Paxton, H. (2001). Two methods for rapid serological diagnosis of acute leptospirosis. *Clinical Diagnostic Laboratory Immunology, 8*(2), 349–351. https://doi.org/10.1128/CDLI.8.2.349-351.2001

Lourdault, K., Cerqueira, G. M., Wunder, E. A., & Picardeau, M. (2011). Inactivation of clpB in the pathogen Leptospira interrogans reduces virulence and resistance to stress conditions. *Infection and Immunity, 79*(9), 3711–3717. https://doi.org/10.1128/IAI.05168-11

Martinez-Lopez, D. G., Fahey, M., & Coburn, J. (2010). Responses of human endothelial cells to pathogenic and non-pathogenic Leptospira species. *PLoS Neglected Tropical Diseases, 4*(12), e918. https://doi.org/10.1371/journal.pntd.0000918

Matsunaga, J., Barocchi, M. A., Croda, J., Young, T. A., Sanchez, Y., Siqueira, I., Bolin, C. A., Reis, M. G., Riley, L. W., Haake, D. A., & Ko, A. I. (2003). Pathogenic Leptospira species express surface-exposed proteins belonging to the bacterial immunoglobulin superfamily. *Molecular Microbiology, 49*(4), 929–946. https://doi.org/10.1046/j.1365-2958.2003.03619.x

Matsunaga, J., Medeiros, M. A., Sanchez, Y., Werneid, K. F., & Ko, A. I. (2007). Osmotic regulation of expression of two extracellular matrix-binding proteins and a haemolysin of Leptospira interrogans: Differential effects on LigA and Sph2 extracellular release. *Microbiology, 153*(10), 3390–3398. https://doi.org/10.1099/mic.0.2007/007948-0

Mazet, J. A. K., Clifford, D. L., Coppolillo, P. B., Deolalikar, A. B., Erickson, J. D., & Kazwala, R. R. (2009). A "One Health" approach to address emerging zoonoses: The HALI project in Tanzania. *PLoS Medicine, 6*(12), e1000190. https://doi.org/10.1371/journal.pmed.1000190

Meng, X. J., Lindsay, D. S., & Sriranganathan, N. (2009). Wild boars as sources for infectious diseases in livestock and humans. *Philosophical Transactions of the Royal Society B: Biological Sciences, 364*(1530), 2697–2707. https://doi.org/10.1098/rstb.2009.0086

Montalvo Corral, M. (2021). Leptospirosis at human-animal-environment interfaces in Latin-America: Drivers, prevention, and control measures. *Biotecnia, 23*(3). https://doi.org/10.18633/biotecnia.v23i3.1442

Musso, D., & La Scola, B. (2013). Laboratory diagnosis of leptospirosis: A challenge. *Journal of Microbiology, Immunology and Infection, 46*(4), 245–252. https://doi.org/10.1016/j.jmii.2013.03.001

Ngugi, J. N., Fèvre, E. M., Mgode, G. F., Obonyo, M., Mhamphi, G. G., Otieno, C. A., & Cook, E. A. J. (2019). Seroprevalence and associated risk factors of leptospirosis in slaughter pigs; a neglected public health risk, western Kenya. *BMC Veterinary Research, 15*(1), 403. https://doi.org/10.1186/s12917-019-2159-3

Niwetpathomwat, A., Luengyosluechakul, S., & Geawduanglek, S. (2006). A serological investigation of leptospirosis in sows from Central Thailand. *The Southeast Asian Journal of Tropical Medicine and Public Health, 37*(4), 716–719.

O'Keefe, J. (2002). A brief review on the laboratory diagnosis of leptospirosis. *New Zealand Veterinary Journal, 50*(1), 9–13. https://doi.org/10.1080/00480169.2002.36242

Okatini, M., Purwana, R., & Made Djaja, I. (2007). Hubungan faktor lingkungan dan karakteristik individu terhadap kejadian penyakit leptospirosis di Jakarta, 2003–2005. *Makara Journal of Health Research, 11*(1), 17–24.

Ospina-Pinto, M. C., & Hernández-Rodríguez, P. (2021). Identification of Leptospira spp. in the animal-environment interface (swine-water) in pig production cycle. *Tropical Animal Health and Production, 53*(1), 155. https://doi.org/10.1007/s11250-021-02567-9

Palaniappan, R. U., Ramanujam, S., & Chang, Y.-F. (2007). Leptospirosis: Pathogenesis, immunity, and diagnosis. *Current Opinion in Infectious Diseases, 20*(3), 284–292. https://doi.org/10.1097/QCO.0b013e32814a5729

Pedersen, K., Pabilonia, K. L., Anderson, T. D., Bevins, S. N., Hicks, C. R., Kloft, J. M., & Deliberto, T. J. (2015). Widespread detection of antibodies to *Leptospira* in feral swine in the United States. *Epidemiology and Infection, 143*(10), 2131–2136. https://doi.org/10.1017/S0950268814003148

Pedersen, K., Anderson, T. D., Bevins, S. N., Pabilonia, K. L., Whitley, P. N., Virchow, D. R., & Gidlewski, T. (2017). Evidence of leptospirosis in the kidneys and serum of feral swine (*Sus scrofa*) in the United States. *Epidemiology and Infection, 145*(1), 87–94. https://doi.org/10.1017/S0950268816002247

Pereira, M. M., Schneider, M. C., Munoz-Zanzi, C., Costa, F., Benschop, J., Hartskeerl, R., Julio Martinez, J., Jancloes, M., & Bertherat, E. (2017). A road map for leptospirosis research and health policies based on country needs in Latin America. *Revista Panamericana de Salud Pública, 41*, 1–9. https://doi.org/10.26633/RPSP.2017.131

Perolat, P., Chappel, R. J., Adler, B., Baranton, G., Bulach, D. M., Billinghurst, M. L., Letocart, M., Merien, F., & Serrano, M. S. (1998). Leptospira fainei sp. nov., isolated from pigs in Australia. *International Journal of Systematic Bacteriology, 48*(3), 851–858. https://doi.org/10.1099/00207713-48-3-851

Petrakovsky, J., Bianchi, A., Fisun, H., Nájera-Aguilar, P., & Pereira, M. (2014). Animal leptospirosis in Latin America and the Caribbean countries: Reported outbreaks and literature review (2002–2014). *International Journal of Environmental Research and Public Health, 11*(10), 10770–10789. https://doi.org/10.3390/ijerph111010770

Picardeau, M. (2013). Diagnosis and epidemiology of leptospirosis. *Médecine et Maladies Infectieuses, 43*(1), 1–9. https://doi.org/10.1016/j.medmal.2012.11.005

Picardeau, M. (2017). Virulence of the zoonotic agent of leptospirosis: Still terra incognita? *Nature Reviews Microbiology, 15*(5), 297–307. https://doi.org/10.1038/nrmicro.2017.5

Picardeau, M., Bulach, D. M., Bouchier, C., Zuerner, R. L., Zidane, N., Wilson, P. J., Creno, S., Kuczek, E. S., Bommezzadri, S., Davis, J. C., McGrath, A., Johnson, M. J., Boursaux-Eude, C., Seemann, T., Rouy, Z., Coppel, R. L., Rood, J. I., Lajus, A., Davies, J. K., et al. (2008). Genome sequence of the saprophyte Leptospira biflexa provides insights into the evolution of Leptospira and the pathogenesis of leptospirosis. *PLoS One, 3*(2), e1607. https://doi.org/10.1371/journal.pone.0001607

Pinto, P. S., Libonati, H., & Lilenbaum, W. (2017). A systematic review of leptospirosis on dogs, pigs, and horses in Latin America. *Tropical Animal Health and Production, 49*(2), 231–238. https://doi.org/10.1007/s11250-016-1201-8

Putz, E. J., & Nally, J. E. (2020). Investigating the immunological and biological equilibrium of reservoir hosts and pathogenic Leptospira: Balancing the solution to an acute problem? *Frontiers in Microbiology, 11*. https://doi.org/10.3389/fmicb.2020.02005

Ramos, A. C. F., Souza, G. N., & Lilenbaum, W. (2006). Influence of leptospirosis on reproductive performance of sows in Brazil. *Theriogenology, 66*(4), 1021–1025. https://doi.org/10.1016/j.theriogenology.2005.08.028

Rathinam, S. R. (2002). Ocular leptospirosis. *Current Opinion in Ophthalmology, 13*(6), 381–386. https://doi.org/10.1097/00055735-200212000-00007

Reid, S. A., Rodney, A., Kama, M., & Hill, P. S. (2017). A process for developing multisectoral strategies for zoonoses: The case of leptospirosis in Fiji. *BMC Public Health, 17*(1), 671. https://doi.org/10.1186/s12889-017-4673-1

Richard, S., & Oppliger, A. (2015). Zoonotic occupational diseases in forestry workers—Lyme borreliosis, tularemia and leptospirosis in Europe. *Annals of Agricultural and Environmental Medicine, 22*(1), 43–50. https://doi.org/10.5604/12321966.1141368

Roberts, M. C. (2019). One Health approach for identification of sources/reservoir of multidrug resistant bacteria in wild animals and their environment. *Journal of Integrated OMICS, 9*(2). https://doi.org/10.5584/jiomics.v9i2.297

Rocha, T. (1998). A review of leptospirosis in farm animals in Portugal. *Revue Scientifique et Technique de l'OIE, 17*(3), 699–712. https://doi.org/10.20506/rst.17.3.1128

Sehgal, S. C., Sugunan, A. P., Murhekar, M. V., Sharma, S., & Vijayachari, P. (2000). Randomized controlled trial of doxycycline prophylaxis against leptospirosis in an endemic area. *International Journal of Antimicrobial Agents, 13*(4), 249–255. https://doi.org/10.1016/S0924-8579(99)00134-X

Slavica, A., Cvetnić, Ž., Konjević, D., Janicki, Z., Severin, K., Dežđek, D., Starešina, V., Sindičić, M., Antić, J., & Alen Slavica, A. (2010). Detection of Leptospira spp. serovars in wild boars (Sus scrofa) from continental Croatia. *Veterinarski Arhiv, 80*(2), 247–257.

Soo, Z. M. P., Khan, N. A., & Siddiqui, R. (2020). Leptospirosis: Increasing importance in developing countries. *Acta Tropica, 201*, 105183. https://doi.org/10.1016/j.actatropica.2019.105183

Stevenson, B., Choy, H. A., Pinne, M., Rotondi, M. L., Miller, M. C., DeMoll, E., Kraiczy, P., Cooley, A. E., Creamer, T. P., Suchard, M. A., Brissette, C. A., Verma, A., & Haake, D. A. (2007). Leptospira interrogans endostatin-like outer membrane proteins bind host fibronectin, laminin and regulators of complement. *PLoS One, 2*(11), e1188. https://doi.org/10.1371/journal.pone.0001188

Strutzberg-Minder, K., Tschentscher, A., Beyerbach, M., Homuth, M., & Kreienbrock, L. (2018). Passive surveillance of Leptospira infection in swine in Germany. *Porcine Health Management, 4*(1), 10. https://doi.org/10.1186/s40813-018-0086-5

Subharat, S., Wilson, P., Heuer, C., & Collins-Emerson, J. (2011). Vaccination for leptospirosis improved the weaning percentage of 2-year-old farmed red deer hinds in New Zealand. *New Zealand Veterinary Journal, 59*(4), 191–196. https://doi.org/10.1080/00480169.2011.579554

Suepaul, S. M., Carrington, C. V., Campbell, M., Borde, G., & Adesiyun, A. A. (2011). Seroepidemiology of leptospirosis in livestock in Trinidad. *Tropical Animal Health and Production, 43*(2), 367–375. https://doi.org/10.1007/s11250-010-9698-8

Thiermann, A. B. (1982). Experimental leptospiral infections in pregnant cattle with organisms of the Hebdomadis serogroup. *American Journal of Veterinary Research, 43*(5), 780–784.

Treml, F., Pikula, J., & Holešovská, Z. (2003). Prevalence of antibodies against leptospires in the wild boar (Sus scrofa L., 1758). *Veterinární Medicína, 48*(3), 66–70. https://doi.org/10.17221/5751-VETMED

VanderWaal, K., & Deen, J. (2018). Global trends in infectious diseases of swine. *Proceedings of the National Academy of Sciences, 115*(45), 11495–11500. https://doi.org/10.1073/pnas.1806068115

Verma, A. K., Kumar, A., Dhama, K., Deb, R., Rahal, A. M., & Chakrabort, S. (2012). Leptospirosis-persistence of a dilemma: An overview with particular emphasis on trends and recent advances in vaccines and vaccination strategies. *Pakistan Journal of Biological Sciences, 15*(20), 954–963. https://doi.org/10.3923/pjbs.2012.954.963

Vijayachari, P., Sugunan, A. P., & Shriram, A. N. (2008). Leptospirosis: An emerging global public health problem. *Journal of Biosciences, 33*(4), 557–569. https://doi.org/10.1007/s12038-008-0074-z

Viriyakosol, S., Matthias, M. A., Swancutt, M. A., Kirkland, T. N., & Vinetz, J. M. (2006). Toll-like receptor 4 protects against lethal *Leptospira interrogans* Serovar Icterohaemorrhagiae infection and contributes to in vivo control of leptospiral burden. *Infection and Immunity, 74*(2), 887–895. https://doi.org/10.1128/IAI.74.2.887-895.2006

Yan, W., Faisal, S. M., McDonough, S. P., Divers, T. J., Barr, S. C., Chang, C.-F., Pan, M.-J., & Chang, Y.-F. (2009). Immunogenicity and protective efficacy of recombinant Leptospira immunoglobulin-like protein B (rLigB) in a hamster challenge model. *Microbes and Infection, 11*(2), 230–237. https://doi.org/10.1016/j.micinf.2008.11.008

Żmudzki, J., Jabłoński, A., Nowak, A., Zębek, S., Arent, Z., Bocian, Ł., & Pejsak, Z. (2015). First overall report of Leptospira infections in wild boars in Poland. *Acta Veterinaria Scandinavica, 58*(1), 3. https://doi.org/10.1186/s13028-016-0186-7

Swine Erysipelas: Unveiling the Risks and Strategies for Control

Pankaj Kumar, Mukul, Kritika Dhial, and Abhishek Pathak

Abstract

Clinical symptoms of the infectious disease erysipelas include fever, arthritis, skin lesions, and abrupt death. It primarily affects growing pigs. The disease could be subacute, acute, or chronic. A particular microorganism called *Erysipelothrix rhusiopathiae*, a zoonotic, prevalent, gram-positive bacterium is the cause of erysipelas in swine, birds, and mammals as well as Erysipeloid in humans. Those who come into contact with animals, animal byproducts, or animal waste are most vulnerable. Some pig infections, including African swine fever, that present with acute symptoms like abrupt mortality could have been mistaken for the acute form of swine erysipelas. Clinical indications, necropsy findings, antimicrobial response, bacteriology, and molecular and serological tests can all be used to diagnose it. It is advised to increase awareness of the disease among animal and human practitioners as treatment is easy and readily available and vaccination is possible. However, local lab workers, butchers, meat inspectors, clinical physicians, and veterinarians are still unaware of the disease. Promoting good cleanliness, routine pork inspections, and the use of protective

P. Kumar
Department of Veterinary Physiology, College of Veterinary and Animal Science, Bikaner, Rajasthan, India

Mukul
Department of Veterinary Public Health, Indian Veterinary Research Institute (IVRI), Izatnagar, Bareilly, Uttar Pradesh, India

K. Dhial
Department of Veterinary Microbiology, Apollo College of Veterinary Medicine, Jaipur, Rajasthan, India

A. Pathak (✉)
Department of Veterinary Pharmacology & Toxicology, Apollo College of Veterinary Medicine, Jaipur, Rajasthan, India

R. Deb et al. (eds.), *Emerging Zoonotic Threats from Swine*,
https://doi.org/10.1007/978-981-96-7407-7_16

gear by anyone who deals with or comes into touch with animals is important. Being a serious zoonotic disease, the disease has a negative impact on public health and generates significant economic losses in pig-producing areas. Therefore, the chapter aims to improve understanding of this disease to properly handle and prevent it from spreading.

Keywords

Zoonotic · Erysipelas · Erysipeloid · Zoonotic · Pig production · Diamond skin disease

Introduction

It is anticipated that population on the Earth will increase from 7.2 billion to 9.6 billion by the end of 2050 (United Nations, 2013). So, a 33% increase in population size will also witness around 70% increased demand for agricultural goods due to an increase in global living standards (Food and Agriculture Organization of the United Nations (FAO), 2009). Worldwide pig production has been improving in tandem with the number of pigs. Despite the high production, several challenges prevent the demand from being met, such as inadequate nutrition, poor health, and inadequate technical inputs in the pig production system. Both Erysipelas and African Swine Fever (ASF) are disease concerns that cause significant losses because of outbreaks that happen practically yearly in the majority of the world's countries (Habte et al., 2021). "Erysipelas" originates from the Latin words "Eruthros," which means "Red," and "Pella" which means "Skin" highlighting the characteristic red lesions that appear on the skin during the acute phase of the illness, termed "Diamond Skin Disease." Erysipelas is among the oldest known infectious diseases of swine discovered by Robert Koch in 1876 which is worldwide distributed and ubiquitous. There are eight species of erysipelas and primarily *Erysipelothrix rhusiopathiae* (*E. rhusiopathiae*) a gram-positive bacillary bacterium that causes disease in swine. Until now, 28 serotypes of *E. rhusiopathiae* have been identified; most of them belong to serotypes 1 and 2. The major clinical manifestations of erysipelas are fever, skin lesions, arthritis, and sudden mortality in growing piglets and adult swine. The major forms of the disease are classified as subacute, acute, or chronic. Primary reservoir of bacteria is swine and up to 30–50% healthy swine population are carriers of *E. rhusiopathiae.* The organism is located in the tonsillar tissue. These healthy carriers can excrete the organism in their oronasal secretion or faeces, so these act as a major source of infection for other pigs as well (To et al., 2012). The mode of transmission is intrauterine infection, natural infection via wounded skin, ingestion, biting flies, and contaminated soil-containing organisms and water contaminated with the organism (Vikaspedia Domains, n.d.). Both acute and chronic disease outbreaks as well as infections that don't show symptoms clinically can happen. Painful joints, sudden and unexpected deaths, skin lesions, and febrile episodes ranging widely from diamond skin (rhomboid urticaria) to generalised cyanosis are the hallmarks of acute outbreaks. Lameness and swollen joints are the hallmarks of chronic erysipelas, which usually follow acute outbreaks. Vegetative valvular endocarditis represents another variation of chronic erysipelas (Uddin Khan et al., 2013). Disease in swine rarely shows any clinical signs except for the acute stage of illness, therefore, the true burden of Erysipelas cannot be determined as it is underdiagnosed.

Swine erysipelas is a common and significant reason for carcass contamination as they can infect swine at any stage of life imposing a huge economic burden (Eriksson et al., 2014; Kwok et al., 2014). The disease can be effectively treated with penicillin and prevented by following vaccination schedules, good management practices, and cleanliness standards. However, the fact that the disease affects pigs of all ages on various farms and that carriers exist makes control challenging (Habte et al., 2021).

Aetiology

The bacillus bacteria *E. rhusiopathiae* is small gram-positive (0.2–0.4 × 0.8–2.5 μm), facultatively anaerobic, pleomorphic, nonmotile, non-acid fast, nonsporulated, filaments (rough form) or small rods (smooth form) and encapsulated. It is widely found in nature and can cause systemic infection or self-limited illnesses in a variety of animals, including humans. When bacteria are grown on non-enriched media, they can form small colonies with partial haemolysis after 48 h and pinpoint, non-haemolytic colonies after 24 h of incubation. Greyish translucent colonies are formed in agar media.

The ideal growth temperature is found between 30 °C and 37 °C, although the temperature range for growth is between 5 °C and 44 °C. The ideal pH range for growth is 7.6–7.2. In addition to causing erysipelas in pigs, it is also linked to a variety of diseases in sheep, chickens, birds, and wild animals. Humans are susceptible to bacterial infections as well. Erysipeloid, a localised skin lesion in humans caused primarily by *E. rhusiopathiae*, is an occupational disease that primarily affects those who handle and process meat (Bender et al., 2011; Wang et al., 2002).

E. tonsillarum and *E. rhusiopathiae* are the two main species that make up the genus *Erysipelothrix* (Table 1). At least 28 serotypes may be distinguished among the strains of *E.* spp. (2,3). The majority of field cases of erysipelas are caused by serotypes 1a, 1b, or 2 of *E. rhusiopathiae. E. tonsillarum* appeared to be avirulent for pigs at first. In a recent investigation, 3.4% of the carcass with typical swine erysipelas lesions, which tested negative for *E. rhusiopathiae*, had *E. tonsillarum* isolated from them. *E. tonsillarum* is a nonpathogenic form that is similar to *E. rhusiopathiae* in both morphology and biochemistry, but it has a significantly different genetic profile and is located in the tonsil.

Serotypes 1 and 2 of *E. rhusiopathiae* are frequently identified in clinically affected pigs, however, other serotypes have occasionally been connected to clinical disease. While no other species of *E.*, other than *E. rhusiopathiae*, has been shown to cause disease in pigs through experimentation, several strains of the species have

Table 1 Erysipelas species that are usually isolated from pigs (Opriessnig & Coutinho, 2019) with respective serotypes. *Erysipelothrix rhusiopathiae* species have maximum number of serotypes

Species	Serotype	Surface protective antigen
Erysipelothrix rhusiopathiae	1a, 1b, 2, 4, 5, 6, 8, 9, 11, 12, 15, 16, 17, 19, 21, N	A, B, C, or combinations
Erysipelothrix tonsillarum	3, 7, 10, 14, 20, 22, 23, 25, 26	None
Erysipelothrix sp. *strain 1*	13	None
Erysipelothrix sp. *strain 2*	9, 10, 18	C
Erysipelothrix sp. *strain 3*	7	None

been discovered from clinical cases and condemned carcasses at slaughterhouses (Harada et al., 2014).

Cell wall integrity can be lost by older colonies, giving the impression that they are gram-negative or gram-variable. The bacterium grows easily using conventional blood culture techniques and on a standard medium. On blood agar, colonies are observed to be both smooth and rough. Granular, non-branching filaments can be seen in smears from rough colonies. After 48 to 72 h, certain strains can induce α-haemolysis. So, we can easily identify *E. rhusiopathiae* from other gram-positive bacteria that have similar morphology, such as diphtheroid and *Listeria* species, by producing hydrogen sulphide (H_2S), having a negative catalase reaction, and lacking motility. *E. rhusiopathiae* is both oxidase-negative and urease-negative; it breaks down lactose and glucose into acid. A pipe cleaner or a test-tube brush shape is a peculiar growth pattern in gelatin stab cultures (Grainger et al., 2011).

In healthy pigs, the upper respiratory tract and digestive system are home to the commensal microbe *E. rhusiopathiae* found in swine flora. Long-term soil survival is a characteristic of *E. rhusiopathiae*, which can also be detected in fish, birds, sheep, and other mammalian species. It is considered that *E. rhusiopathiae* is a zoonotic agent (Dwight & Zee, 1999; Haesebrouck et al., 2004).

Epidemiology

Swine erysipelas is ubiquitous and its incidence level has been reached sufficient enough to cause serious economic losses due to mortality and devaluation of carcass because of arthritis in most of the countries. Despite it has been observed in a wide range of vertebrate and invertebrate species (wild mammals, different poultry species, fish, and shellfish, as well as domestic animals such as pigs, sheep, cattle, and horses) as a commensal as well as a pathogen, it is generally believed that domestic swine are the main reservoirs of *E. rhusiopathiae.* Healthy pigs' faeces have been found to include pathogenic strains of *E. rhusiopathiae*, which is frequently present in the tonsils and other lymphoid tissues of asymptomatic swine (Wood, 1974). Usually, diseases occur in unvaccinated swine from 3 months of age until adulthood.

Pigs older than 3 years or younger than 3 months are typically less susceptible to swine erysipelas. Age-related vulnerability may be explained as swine below the age of 8 weeks are usually protected because of maternal immunity through colostrum (Coutinho et al., 2011), i.e., passive immunity that young animals naturally acquire and active immunity that older animals gain after subclinical infection. After the birth, the immune sows' suckling pigs are protected from infection for a few weeks. The sow's immunological condition affects the extent and duration of passive immunity. It has been documented that parasitic infestations exacerbate clinical cases of swine erysipelas. Aflatoxin in the feed leads to subclinical toxicity which can increase swine's vulnerability to acute swine erysipelas. A combined effect of virulence due to causative organisms and susceptibility of animals can lead to sudden acute swine erysipelas epidemics (Zhu et al., 2018).

It has been observed that indoor confinement of swine has led to a decrease in the occurrence of the disease due to the decreased pig's contact with contaminated soil. This would not apply to outdoor units where vaccination is not performed. Contaminated soil is thought to be one of the sources. The infection has been confirmed with serotypes 1a or 2 present in wild boars, so these should be considered as a reservoir. Variations in the virulence of particular strains located in a particular area can lead to variations in economic losses and mortality from place to place. Morbidity and case fatality rates in pigs also vary from area to area. This is a result of virulence variation of the particular strain of the infectious organism. Infection is spread via carrier animals (Swine) urine, excreta-faeces, contaminated water and feed, body secretions-saliva, nasal, via skin abrasions most often in a sub-clinical manner and failures in external biosecurity (entry of animals such as birds, rodents, dogs, etc. carrying the organism).

Most likely, bacteria in contaminated soil lose their ability to spread the disease after 35 days. Surface water can carry resistant organisms to nearby localities. *E. rhusiopathiae* can occasionally be spread among swine by biting flies and ticks. Eradication of the disease is a challenging task due to the large number of carriers of *E. rhusiopathiae.*

Managemental conditions like nutrition, fatigue, ambient temperature, and surrounding environment conditions causing stress, and other factors like genetics, non-infectious diseases, age, infestation of worms, concurrent infection, and soil alkalinity are some of the disposing factors for disease occurrence. After ingestion, the organism may endure the hostile circumstances of the stomach and intestine and can even endure for several months in the faeces. Both chronically infected and recovered pigs have the potential to harbour *E. rhusiopathiae.* Asymptomatic carriers can also be healthy pigs.

In this scenario, it is essential to remember the zoonotic nature of the disease. Usually, a higher number of human cases are reported in the summer months. Higher occupational exposure has been seen in the case of men (4:1) (Duizer, 2015). Animal products that have been contaminated or occupational exposure to infectious animals can frequently result in human diseases. Slaughterhouse workers, veterinarians, poultry operations, butchers, fishermen, farmers, fish traders, and housewives are among those who are at risk (Forde et al., 2016). Therefore, control measures should not only be implemented for the productive animal but also to protect farmers and the general public health interest.

Human and animal infections have been reported from Africa, Australia, many American countries, China, Japan, and all over Europe. Animals or the environment can be the source of human diseases (Brooke & Riley, 1999). It's interesting to note that vegetative endocarditis outbreaks can happen even in the absence of other clinical symptoms. Numerous stressors, including heat, aflatoxin, and inadequate nutrition, have been suggested to be involved in triggering epidemics in older, more vulnerable pigs (Stokholm et al., 2010).

Modes of Transmission

The primary reservoir host and carrier of swine erysipelas is pigs. The organism in the tonsils and oropharynx is present in many healthy pigs. Indirect transmission of *E. rhusiopathiae* can happen when contaminated food or water is consumed, or it can happen directly when infected animals' faeces, urine, saliva, and nasal secretions are consumed. Other herd animals become sick when a pig is sub-clinically diseased or infected. Abrasions on the skin or mechanical vectors like insect bites can also result in infection.

Both chronically infected and recovered pigs may be lifelong carriers of the pathogen. Both ingesting and cutaneous abrasions are possible entrance points. After consumption, through the tonsils and lymphoid tissue of the gastrointestinal tract, the organism most preferably enters the body. Birds and rodents have easy access to small populations housed in backyards, orchards, or paddocks, and the organism's persistence in the soil encourages the spread of disease (Constable et al., 2016).

Erysipelas is prevalent in environments that permit or encourage: Exposure to solid waste, rodent contamination, and bird droppings. This means that, although the disease can occur at any time of the year, it is more prevalent in systems based on straw, particularly in open barns (i.e., systems thought to be welfare-friendly for raising pigs). It is most prevalent in the summer (Pomorska-Mól et al., 2012).

Pathogenicity

The ability of *E. rhusiopathiae* to persist in macrophages, an antiphagocytic capsule, a surface protein (Spa A), and the enzyme neuraminidase are some of the elements that are thought to contribute to virulence. However, the precise methods are still up for discussion.

When contaminated feed and water are consumed, *E. rhusiopathiae* generally enters the organism's body via tonsils present in the digestive tract or other lymphoid tissue. In rarer cases, infected cuts on the skin could provide access. In acute erysipelas, a bacteraemia causes organisms to spread throughout the body. There is speculation on the exact method by which *E. rhusiopathiae* produces disease. The organism secretes the enzyme neuraminidase, which cleaves cell wall mucopolysaccharides and may be responsible for the extensive vascular damage associated with swine erysipelas. Within 24 h of exposure, septicaemia sets in and causes the potentially lethal disseminated intravascular coagulation that is a hallmark of an acute disease. Animals who survive the acute phase are thereafter subjected to diseases such as endocarditis, polyarthritis, and cutaneous necrosis, which can vary from sub-acute to chronic infections. Pregnant sows may abort due to infection: bacteria from stillborn and aborted foetuses have been discovered.

Septicaemia, hyaline thrombi, and disseminated intravascular coagulation are all consequences of acute infection. After 4 days of infection, the bacterium has penetrated the endothelium, causing erythrocytic diapedesis. Usually, congestion and occasionally thrombosis of dermal vessels cause purple skin. One possible cause of fibrinoid necrosis in vessels is an Arthus-type hypersensitivity reaction. The "diamond skin" lesions are believed to be caused by arteriolar fibrinoid necrosis, which may not be evident in our piglets since the infection progressed quickly, possibly leaving little time for the development of full hypersensitivity vasculitis. One can use skin discolouration as a prognosticator. Pigs with lesions on their skin that are pink to red normally heal, but those with dark reddish-purple lesions usually pass away. The ears and limbs were the primary sites of dermal and hypodermal haemorrhage in piglets with acute erysipelas. Acute erysipelas can cause muscle degeneration, but locally a unique severe pattern of haemorrhagic infarction is experienced by pigs. Lesions less particular in nature, such as bacterial emboli or leukothrombi, can occur in any organ. Diseases that are acute or chronic may cause synovitis. Similar to the acute condition, but less severe, is the sub-acute type (Shankar et al., 2009).

In cases of chronic arthritis, vasculitis and fibrin exudate into perivascular tissues and joint(s) occurs. A notable proliferation of synovial membrane villi is also observed. More proliferative than exudative joint lesions are seen. Joint capsule thickening may occur as perivascular fibrin appears to induce the production of connective tissue surrounding joints. A small number of active bacteria in the joint or hypersensitivity to any leftover bacterial antigen could cause ongoing inflammation surrounding an affected joint (Shankar et al., 2009).

Another indication of chronic erysipelas is vegetative, valvular endocarditis, which occurs less frequently than joint involvement. It is believed that *E. rhusiopathiae* emboli trigger blood vessel inflammation in heart valves. The endocardium breaks down during the inflammatory process, forming bacterial colonies. There, fibrin is deposited and progressively arranges itself to create nodular vegetation. Emboli that emerge from plants can quickly result in death.

Clinical Signs

Hyperacute Form Usually seen in pigs getting close to market weight, but rare in sows. Sudden and unexpected deaths, lethargy, depression, and increased body temperature up to 42 °C (106–109 °F) are its distinctive features.

Acute Form After an incubation period of one to 7 days, this type is defined by a fast onset of a febrile phase with body temperatures reaching 42 °C (108 °F). Severe prostration, complete anorexia, thirst, and sporadic vomiting occurred. Swine that are affected may first exhibit high body temperatures, a strong appetite, and a high level of activity. Severely affected pigs exhibit ventral surface discoloration, whole-body cyanosis, or pronounced red to purple discoloration of the skin. Even while skin lesions are nearly usually indicative of this disease, this may not always be the case. These skin sores go away without causing any problems after roughly 10 days. In more severe situations, the plaques tend to expand and coalesce across the back, which results in the development of the chronic type. The skin lesions can appear as a more diffuse oedematous eruption or as red, diamond-shaped, urticarial plaques that are 2.5–5 cm^2. The lesions often emerge 24 h after the first symptoms of the disease and are most frequently found on the belly, inside the thighs, throat, neck, and ears. After 2–4 days, the pig either recovers or passes away, exhibiting final signs of dyspnoea, cyanosis, and diarrhoea. When an animal is pregnant and has a temperature and direct foetal action, abortion (Fig. 1) may occur.

Chronic Form Despite the possibility of typical joint lesions, this type of swine erysipelas is unusual. The elbow, hip, hock, stifle, and knee joints are more commonly impacted by these joint diseases, which cause lameness and stiffness in the affected joints. Usually hot and painful when they first appear, enlarged joints harden and lose their heat after 2–3 weeks. There may be a subclinical form of synovitis, which could impact feed intake and slow down growth. Growth retardation may be seen in conjunction with alopecia, sloughing of the tail and tips of the ears, and hyperkeratosis of the skin on the back, shoulders, and legs. In the chronic form of this erysipelas, vegetative endocarditis frequently develops. Following significant valve injury, there is a noticeable loud murmur on auscultation, a considerably elevated cardiac impulse, and quicker heart rates.

Risk Factors

As an opportunistic pathogen, *E. rhusiopathiae* enhances the likelihood that pasteurellosis may spread in favourable environmental conditions (Bender et al., 2011). High temperature can influence *E. rhusiopathiae* transmission through certain routes, with its optimal survival (Table 2) and reproduction occurring between 30 °C and 37 °C (Wang et al., 2010). Heavy rainfall is probably a significant factor

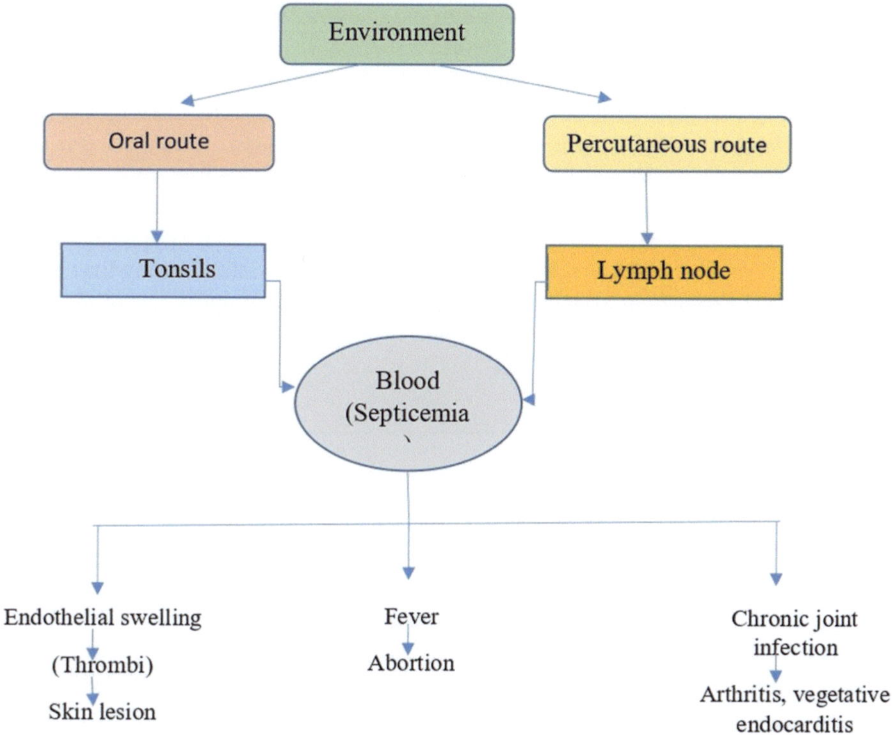

Fig. 1 Various routes of swine erysipelas and related clinical signs

Table 2 Number of days an Erysipelas species can survive on different inanimate objects at different temperatures

Temperature	Days of survival
3 °C	35
12 °C	18
20 °C	10
30 °C	2

Erysipelas (n.d.-b)

contributing to outbreaks, as monthly precipitation levels during these periods are substantially higher than historical averages (Risco et al., 2011). High wind speed and O_3 have shown a negative effect on the prevalence of swine erysipelas.

Economic Impact

Swine erysipelas is an economical important disease that might be re-emerging worldwide in the swine industry. The economic impact of the disease is not well understood since its clinical signs are not very peculiar except for acute illness (diamond skin lesion) and can be confused with other diseases or are often not even identified in sub-clinical, sub-acute, or chronic phases. Swine erysipelas cause significant economic losses throughout North America, Europe, Asia, and Australia. Increased morbidity and mortality, treatment and vaccination costs, the decline in the growth rate of pigs with clinical illness, and feed costs are some major factors associated with economic losses due to the disease (Wood, 1974). *E. rhusiopathiae*, together with parvovirus and leptospirosis, is one of the main infectious causes of reproductive loss in swine. An acute illness characterised by diamond skin lesions making it unfit for human consumption and total condemnation. Whereas several conditions classified as septicaemia or arthritis occur due to infections by Erysipelas in its chronic form, which certainly reinforces the economic importance of this bacterium. Bacterium accounted for more than 37% of causes of carcass condemnations during slaughter in Tuscany (Italy) (Guardone et al., 2020).

Zoonotic Potential

One of the leading causes of diseases and death is zoonotic diseases (Jaffry et al., 2009). The pathogenesis of a disease is set in motion by the transfer of infectious agents from animals to humans (Waltzek et al., 2012). Because erysipelas infections can spread from swine to humans, they pose a risk to public health. The primary risk groups for human infection with *E. rhusiopathiae* are veterinarians, domestic and farm-level piggery workers, and abattoir workers. Occupational exposure or professional related is one of the causes of *E. rhusiopathiae* infection in humans. These workers can become infected both directly and indirectly, especially during evisceration and carcass preparation without the use of appropriate protective devices. Worldwide, *E. rhusiopathiae* is enzootic and typically spreads to humans by direct contact, contaminated food and water, the faecal-oral pathway, and on rare occasions, vectors (Uddin Khan et al., 2013). Despite the organism's extensive presence in decomposing organic matter, contaminated soils, food scraps, and water are all important environmental sources of infection (Principe et al., 2016). As a result, human zoonotic *E. rhusiopathiae* infections are marked by severe systemic sickness, lymphadenopathy, redness, erythema, and localised pain. They can also be complicated with or without endocarditis. Since zoonotic erysipelas are becoming more common, it is crucial to diagnose and treat them because they present special challenges that call for the knowledge of physicians, veterinarians, and wildlife biologists (Waltzek et al., 2012).

Clinical Signs and Management in Humans

An erythematous, well-demarcated cutaneous lesion known as Erysipeloid is often present 10 days following inoculation. It is localised to the upper extremities, mainly the fingers, and is characterised by painful itching and burning. It is common to see lymphadenopathy (30%) and localised lymphangitis (30%), a skin and soft tissue disease that spreads from the original site of infection and is diffuse in nature, usually seen in people with systemic diseases who are immunocompromised.

A widespread illness that is typically endocarditis-complicated sepsis. About 40% of cases additionally have an Erysipeloid lesion. A persistent fever and many skin lesions on the trunk or extremities are common symptoms of the disease. Traditional underlying factors include corticosteroid use or chemotherapy, chronic liver disease, or alcohol misuse. The death rate that is linked to this is quite significant (38%). Renal failure, septic arthritis, persistent meningitis, and pneumonia are among the other clinical symptoms that have been seen in people.

The management of simple Erysipeloid skin lesions (with another active medication, such as clindamycin, fluoroquinolones, or another ß-lactam) or oral penicillin (500 mg q6h) for a week. The recommended therapy for severe cutaneous disease or disseminated disease is intravenous ciprofloxacin (400 mg q12h), ceftriaxone (2 g q24h), or benzylpenicillin (2–4 million units q4h) for a duration of 2–4 weeks. Because there are currently no human vaccinations against the pathogen, workplace exposure to it should be avoided.

Diagnosis of Disease

There have been various advancements in the diagnosis of swine erysipelas in the past few years. Clinical signs, gross lesions, necropsy findings, isolation of organisms, susceptibility to antibiotics, various molecular techniques, and serological methods can be applied for the diagnosis of erysipelas in swine.

It might be challenging to detect acute erysipelas in individual pigs exhibiting merely fever, low appetite, and listlessness. On the other hand, skin lesions and lameness are likely to be present in at least some cases in outbreaks involving multiple animals and would support a clinical diagnosis. When present, rhomboid urticaria or diamond skin lesions are nearly always indicative of swine fever virus infection; however, comparable lesions can also be observed in cases of classical infection. The clinical presentation and isolation of the organism which is simple to cultivate in a lab determine the diagnosis. It is thought to be pathognomonic when skin lesions shaped like diamonds appear (Wang et al., 2010).

For diagnosing localised Erysipeloid lesions, the best clinical specimens are deep tissue biopsies or liquid from vesicles. For systemic disease, blood cultures are used. Thin gram-positive bacilli may occasionally be visible under tissue biopsies' microscopy. After 2 days on blood agar, *E. rhusiopathiae* develops smooth or rough a-haemolytic colonies. At 33–37 °C, growth is accelerated in 5–10% CO_2. Initial identification is based on colony appearance and Gram stain. On either TSI or Kligler slant agar, *E. rhusiopathiae* exhibits H_2S positivity but is catalase-negative, nonmotile, and non-β-haemolytic.

Acute cases of *E. rhusiopathiae* can be diagnosed from the blood of affected swine, especially after enrichment or through animal inoculation (e.g., mouse inoculation). Molecular methods like PCR assays can detect *E. rhusiopathiae* DNA in tissues or blood. Immunohistochemical methods are useful for detecting the organism in formalin-fixed tissues, especially after antimicrobial treatment. As the organism is penicillin-sensitive, so acute erysipelas diagnosis can be performed via a rapid positive response to penicillin therapy (Kebede, 2005).

Chronic erysipelas diagnosis is challenging and often based on arthritis, lameness, and vegetative valvular endocarditis observed postmortem. Valvular vegetations positive culture or detection of *E. rhusiopathiae* DNA with the help of PCR confirms chronic erysipelas.

The organism grows easily from an array of body parts (heart, lungs, liver, spleen, kidneys, joints) following the necropsy of a pig that has died in the acute phase. However, after a few days, the organism is usually no longer viable to be grown from internal organs, while it can still be detected in the joints. Because the organisms may be sparse and localised, it is important to collect many samples of fluid and synovial tissue from as many synovial sacs of a joint as possible under such conditions. Chronic cases are more challenging to diagnose with precision. Attempts to culture several joints frequently fail. However, in erysipelas, the appearance of various cases of arthritis in growing pigs is more evident than of other diseases (Vandepitte, 2003).

There are a variety of serological tests applied to diagnose swine erysipelas including plate and tube agglutination, hemagglutination, hemagglutination inhibition, immunofluorescence, complement fixation test, and ELISA. Serologic tests can be used to verify vaccine success or prior exposure, but they are not a valid means of diagnosing erysipelas. Following vaccination, antibody titres usually rise; selected laboratories offer ELISAs and complement fixation assays for this purpose.

Following isolating *E. rhusiopathiae* from the acutely diseased animal, a definitive laboratory diagnosis of Swine Erysipelas is accomplished. Haemoculture is an effective diagnostic approach when applied to living animals; however, specimens should be taken from several diseased animals in the herd because the organism may not always be present in a single animal's blood. Whenever a pig dies in the acute phase, the organism can be easily grown from a variety of body components, including the heart, and lungs, liver, spleen, kidneys, and joints. Though the bacterium may still be present in the joints, it is usually no longer able to be cultivated from internal organs if the disease has lasted for several days. Because the organisms may be few and localised, it is crucial to collect numerous samples of synovial tissue from numerous synovial sacs of a joint and fluid that are accessible under such conditions (Riviere & Papich, 2013).

E. rhusiopathiae can be easily cultured from tissue specimens using only culture media, such as tryptose or meat infusion media and standard laboratory tools, that can be added with or without blood or serum. Because the bacterium is hazardous to humans, caution should be exercised to prevent unintentional skin infections. There are several places where selective culture techniques are explained for separating the organism from contaminated specimens.

Differential Diagnosis

There are various diseases and their causative organisms (Table 3) whose clinical signs, gross lesions, and necropsy findings are similar to those of swine erysipelas which are needed to be differentiated (Ogawa et al., 2017; Sawada & Takahashi, 1987).

Treatment, Control, and Prevention of Disease

It is best to promote vaccination against *E. rhusiopathiae* as it is highly successful in reducing disease outbreaks on swine farms (Table 4). However, it might not be as successful in avoiding chronic arthritis. On certain farms, the removal of vaccinations has been connected to outbreaks of disease. There are injectable bacterins and live, attenuated vaccinations that are administered through water that offer longer-lasting immunity. The best time to vaccinate could differ from farm to farm. In a production environment where *E. rhusiopathiae* is endemic, immunisation should

Table 3 Causative organism of diseases various diseases whose clinical signs, gross lesions, and necropsy findings are similar to those of swine erysipelas

Disease	Causative organism
Classical swine fever	Pestivirus infection
Septicaemic salmonellosis	*Salmonella choleraesuis*
Septicaemia and endocarditis	*Streptococcus suis*
Glasser's disease	*Haemophilus parasuis*
Mycoplasmal arthritis	*Mycoplasma hyosynoviae*

Table 4 Type of vaccine and its serovar used against swine Erysipelas

Vaccine	Serovar	Type	Availability
ERY VAC FD	1a	Attenuated	USA
ERY VAC 100	1a	Attenuated	USA
Ingelvac^{R}	1a	Attenuated	USA
Suvaxyn^{R} E-Oral	1a	Attenuated	USA, Canada
Swine erysipelas live	1a	Attenuated	Japan
Ruvax^{R}	2	Lysate bacterin	EU
Parvoruvax^{R}	2	Lysate bacterin	EU, Brazil, Mexico, Russia, Middle East
ERYGUARD^{R}	2	Bacterin	Australia
Suvaxyn^{R} Parvo/E	2	Bacterin	USA, Canada, EU
Swivac ERA	1a (SpaA)	Subunit	Japan
SUIMMUGEN^{R} Rart2/ER	2 (SpaA)	Subunit	Japan

Opriessnig et al. (2020)

occur before outbreaks are predicted. Pigs that are susceptible to vaccinations might receive them weeks before, during, or following their weaning. Three to five weeks after being chosen for the breeding herd, male and female pigs should receive a booster shot. Breeding stock should thereafter receive two annual vaccinations.

Antibiotic therapy animals shouldn't receive vaccinations since the antibiotics can affect the vaccine's future immunological response.

Some herds may experience vaccination failures as a result of management stressors that weaken vaccinated pigs' immune systems. Live vaccinations have the potential to cause clinical disease, especially chronic erysipelas. Though this is an uncommon occurrence, antigenic mismatches between the serotypes in vaccines and serotypes circulating on farms may also lead to partial immunity and disease outbreaks. This is because the main *E. rhusiopathiae* strains infecting pigs are believed to have high cross-protection.

Apart from immunisation, pig farms can also effectively control the disease by implementing measures such as maintaining cleanliness and hygiene, eliminating pigs exhibiting clinical signs of erysipelas infection, and other feasible approaches.

The conventional treatment consists of antimicrobial therapy with penicillin and anti-erysipelas serum. Penicillin is frequently administered in combination by dissolving it in the serum. Penicillin therapy is the recommended course of action for acute erysipelas. This antibiotic has a high sensitivity to *E. rhusiopathiae*, and when it is administered early in an acute epidemic, it typically produces a strong response in 24–36 hours. Penicillin can be given either alone or in combination with other antibiotics or antiserum (or often both) as part of specific treatment regimens to have a longer-acting effect (Eamens et al., 2006).

It is quite the usual procedure to treat suckling pigs with antiserum. When outbreaks arise, it is highly advised that vaccination programmes be started in herds that have never received vaccinations before. The serum needs to be administered early in the course of the disease for best results. For pigs under 50 pounds (23 kg), the advised therapeutic dose, administered S/C, ranges from 5 to 10 mL. For pigs over 100 pounds (45 kg), use 20–40 mL. When the strain exhibits only low virulence, penicillin alone is typically sufficient. A standard dosage of 50,000 IU/kg Body Weight (BW) of procaine penicillin I/M for 3 days is recommended.

Due to the organism's inaccessibility in endocardial lesions and the structural damage that occurs in joints, chronic cases do not respond well to treatment. Therefore, there is no workable cure for chronic Swine Erysipelas. Anti-inflammatory medications have been shown in experiments to partially mitigate the symptoms of chronic arthritis, and they may be utilised to treat particularly important individual animals (Jeon et al., 2018).

Aspirin can be dissolved in water or administered as NSAIDs (nonsteroidal anti-inflammatory drugs) such as flunixin meglumine, to treat fever related to acute illnesses. Although it is not widely accessible, erysipelas antiserum is said to be a useful addition to antibiotic therapy in the treatment of acute outbreaks. Chronic infection treatment is typically inefficient and expensive (Mekuriaw & Asmare, 2014).

General management techniques, excellent hygiene, biosecurity, stress reduction, an efficient 6-month vaccination policy—ideally two doses—for all animals—including boars older than 3 months—as well as prompt diagnosis, isolation, and treatment are all necessary for successful control. Usually, antimicrobials added to the drinking water and the administration of penicillin and/or Erysipelas antiserum to diseased pigs can control acute outbreaks of Swine Erysipelas until no sick pigs are seen for at least 3 days.

Conclusion and Key Points (Table 5)

Swine erysipelas is a prevalent infectious disease that can affect pigs of all ages. It can be particularly problematic in small populations where immunisations are not accessible. Although the acute form of the disease is potentially fatal, it is usually easily controlled with a normal vaccination schedule and responds well to appropriate antibiotic treatment. High death rates and significant financial losses are possible outcomes of the disease.

The high number of "carrier" species, such as birds and rodents, along with the large number of "carrier" pigs make it impractical to eradicate erysipelas on individual piggeries. Precautions regarding overall hygiene should be taken. Animals that are clinically affected should be put down right away, and every new animal should be quarantined and checked for endocarditis and arthritis. If an animal dies from a disease, it should be appropriately incinerated to prevent environmental pollution. A combination of routine vaccination, good hygiene, removing carriers with skin and joint lesions, and appropriate quarantine procedures for purchased animals may usually be used to control swine erysipelas (Straw et al., 2013; Birhan et al., 2015).

To effectively prevent disease outbreaks on swine farms, vaccination against *E. rhusiopathiae* should be promoted. Utilising low-virulence strains of bacteria or attenuated vaccines made by serial passage for pig vaccination. Growing pigs are often protected from the effect of acute disease until they reach market age by the immunity provided by the formalin-killed, aluminium hydroxide-adsorbed bacterin. Additionally, a low-virulence oral vaccination is utilised.

Before joining the breeding herd, all young boars and gilt should be twice vaccinated, scheduled between 2 and 4 weeks apart, as directed by the manufacturer to prevent swine erysipelas. 3–4 weeks before they give birth, sows should receive

Table 5 Important key points related to swine erysipelas

Key points	
Aetiological agent	*Erysipelothrix rhusiopathiae*
Clinical manifestations	Acute, subacute, and chronic
Clinical signs	Characteristic diamond-shaped skin lesions, diffuse erythema, septicaemia, and/or arthritis
Vaccination	Effective in preventing acute diseases, including abattoir condemnations and loss of animals

Note: Pigs are often healthy carriers of the bacterium

their vaccinations. Boars need to receive vaccinations every 6 months. Young stock can be vaccinated against high-risk diseases starting at 6 weeks of age, either with a single dose or, if required, a double-dose course.

Apart from immunisation, pig farms can also effectively control the disease by implementing measures such as maintaining cleanliness and hygiene, eliminating pigs exhibiting clinical signs of erysipelas infection, and other feasible approaches.

So overall following recommendations can be drawn:

To control the disease on swine farms, it is recommended that attention be focused on sanitation and hygiene, as well as eliminating pigs exhibiting clinical indications.

The best course of action would seem to be to educate and raise farmers' understanding of zoonosis's transmission, severity, control, measures for prevention, and early treatment.

To facilitate the development of an effective control strategy, a comprehensive study of seasonal variations and other risk variables should be conducted.

References

Bender, J. S., Irwin, C. K., Shen, H. G., Schwartz, K. J., & Opriessnig, T. (2011). Erysipelothrix spp. genotypes, serotypes, and surface protective antigen types associated with abattoir condemnations. *Journal of Veterinary Diagnostic Investigation, 23*(1), 139–142.

Birhan, M., Tamene, G., & Betelhem, G. (2015). Challenges and opportunities of pig farming and feeding strategy in Gondar town, Ethiopia. *Academic Journal of Nutrition, 4*(2), 84–89.

Brooke, C. J., & Riley, T. V. (1999). Erysipelothrix rhusiopathiae: Bacteriology, epidemiology and clinical manifestations of an occupational pathogen. *Journal of Medical Microbiology, 48*(9), 789–799.

Constable, P. D., Hinchcliff, K. W., Done, S. H., & Grünberg, W. (2016). *Veterinary medicine: A textbook of the diseases of cattle, horses, sheep, pigs and goats*. Elsevier Health Sciences.

Coutinho, T. A., Imada, Y., Barcellos, D. E., Oliveira, S. J., & Moreno, A. M. (2011). Phenotypic and molecular characterization of recent and archived Erysipelothrix spp. isolated from Brazilian swine. *Diagnostic Microbiology and Infectious Disease, 69*(2), 123–129.

Duizer, G. (2015). *Syndrome classification through a retrospective analysis of porcine submissions to a regional animal health laboratory*. University of Prince Edward Island.

Dwight, C. H., & Zee, Y. C. (1999). *Veterinary microbiology*. Blackwell Science.

Eamens, G. J., Chin, J. C., Turner, B., & Barchia, I. (2006). Evaluation of Erysipelothrix rhusiopathiae vaccines in pigs by intradermal challenge and immune responses. *Veterinary Microbiology, 116*(1–3), 138–148.

Eriksson, H., Bagge, E., Båverud, V., Fellström, C., & Jansson, D. S. (2014). Erysipelothrix rhusiopathiae contamination in the poultry house environment during erysipelas outbreaks in organic laying hen flocks. *Avian Pathology, 43*(3), 231–237.

Erysipelas | Iowa State University. (n.d.-b). https://vetmed.iastate.edu/vdpam/FSVD/swine/index-diseases/erysipelas

Food and Agriculture Organization of the United Nations (FAO). (2009). *Global agriculture towards 2050. High level expert forum issues paper*. FAO.

Forde, T. L., Orsel, K., Zadoks, R. N., Biek, R., Adams, L. G., Checkley, S. L., et al. (2016). Bacterial genomics reveal the complex epidemiology of an emerging pathogen in arctic and boreal ungulates. *Frontiers in Microbiology, 7*, 1759.

Grainger, J., Hurst, J., & Burdass, D. (2011). Basic Practical Microbiology. In *Microbiology*. Microbiology Society.

Guardone, L., Vitali, A., Fratini, F., Pardini, S., Cenci Goga, B. T., Nucera, D., & Armani, A. (2020). A retrospective study after 10 years (2010–2019) of meat inspection activity in a domestic swine abattoir in tuscany: The slaughterhouse as an epidemiological observatory. *Animals, 10*(10), 1907.

Habte, D., Tamir, D., & Tilahun, T. (2021). Swine erysipelas; it's epidemiology, diagnosis, treatment and control and preventive measures, comprehensive review. *Journal of Clinical Epidemiology & Toxicology, 2*(2), 1–7.

Haesebrouck, F., Pasmans, F., Chiers, K., Maes, D., Ducatelle, R., & Decostere, A. (2004). Efficacy of vaccines against bacterial diseases in swine: What can we expect. *Veterinary Microbiology, 100*(3–4), 255–268.

Harada, T., Ogawa, Y., Eguchi, M., Shi, F., Sato, M., Uchida, K., et al. (2014). Phosphorylcholine and SpaA, a choline-binding protein, are involved in the adherence of Erysipelothrix rhusiopathiae to porcine endothelial cells, but this adherence is not mediated by the PAF receptor. *Veterinary Microbiology, 172*(1–2), 216–222.

Jaffry, K. T., Ali, S., Rasool, A., Raza, A., & Gill, Z. J. (2009). Zoonoses. In *Encyclopedia of microbiology*. Elsevier.

Jeon, W., Kim, Y. C., Hong, M., Rejinold, S., Park, K., Yoon, I., et al. (2018). Microcrystalline cellulose for delivery of recombinant protein-based antigen against erysipelas in mice. *BioMed Research International, 2018*, 7670505.

Kebede, F. (2005). Standard veterinary laboratory diagnostic manual. *Bacteriology, Ministry of Agriculture and Rural Development Animal Health Department, Addis Ababa, Ethiopia, 2*, 1–175.

Kwok, A. H., Li, Y., Jiang, J., Jiang, P., & Leung, F. C. (2014). Complete genome assembly and characterization of an outbreak strain of the causative agent of swine erysipelas – Erysipelothrix rhusiopathiae SY1027. *BMC Microbiology, 14*, 1–12.

Mekuriaw, Y., & Asmare, B. (2014). Assessment of pig production and constraints in Mecha district, Amhara region, Northwestern Ethiopia. *Advances in Agriculture, 2014*, 1.

Ogawa, Y., Shiraiwa, K., Ogura, Y., Ooka, T., Nishikawa, S., Eguchi, M., et al. (2017). Clonal lineages of Erysipelothrix rhusiopathiae responsible for acute swine erysipelas in Japan identified by using genome-wide single-nucleotide polymorphism analysis. *Applied and Environmental Microbiology, 83*(11), e00130-17.

Opriessnig, T., & Coutinho, T. A. (2019). Erysipelas. In *Diseases of swine* (pp. 835–843). Wiley.

Opriessnig, T., Forde, T., & Shimoji, Y. (2020). Erysipelothrix spp.: Past, present, and future directions in vaccine research. Frontiers in veterinary. *Science, 7*. https://doi.org/10.3389/fvets.2020.00174

Pomorska-Mól, M., Markowska-Daniel, I., & Pejsak, Z. (2012). Effect of age and maternally-derived antibody status on humoral and cellular immune responses to vaccination of pigs against Erysipelothrix rhusiopathiae. *The Veterinary Journal, 194*(1), 128–130.

Principe, L., Bracco, S., Mauri, C., Tonolo, S., Pini, B., & Luzzaro, F. (2016). Erysipelothrix rhusiopathiae bacteremia without endocarditis: Rapid identification from positive blood culture by MALDI-TOF mass spectrometry. A case report and literature review. *Infectious Disease Reports, 8*(1), 6368.

Risco, D., Llario, P. F., Velarde, R., García, W. L., Benítez, J. M., García, A., et al. (2011). Outbreak of swine erysipelas in a semi-intensive wild boar farm in Spain. *Transboundary and Emerging Diseases, 58*(5), 445–450.

Riviere, J. E., & Papich, M. G. (Eds.). (2013). *Veterinary pharmacology and therapeutics*. Wiley.

Sawada, T., & Takahashi, T. (1987). Cross protection of mice and swine inoculated with culture filtrate of attenuated Erysipelothrix rhusiopathiae and challenge exposed to strains of various serovars. *American Journal of Veterinary Research, 48*(2), 239–242.

Shankar, B. P., Chauhan, S., Madhusudan, H. S., & Ranjith, D. (2009). Pathology of Erysipelas infection in piglets. *Veterinary World, 2*(6), 234.

Stokholm, N. M., Permin, A., Bisgaard, M., & Christensen, J. P. (2010). Causes of mortality in commercial organic layers in Denmark. *Avian Diseases, 54*(4), 1241–1250.
Straw, B. E., Zimmerman, J. J., D'Allaire, S., & Taylor, D. J. (Eds.). (2013). *Diseases of swine*. Wiley.
To, H., Sato, H., Tazumi, A., Tsutsumi, N., Nagai, S., Iwata, A., & Nagano, T. (2012). Characterization of Erysipelothrix rhusiopathiae strains isolated from recent swine erysipelas outbreaks in Japan. *Journal of Veterinary Medical Science, 74*(7), 949–953.
Uddin Khan, S., Atanasova, K. R., Krueger, W. S., Ramirez, A., & Gray, G. C. (2013). Epidemiology, geographical distribution, and economic consequences of swine zoonoses: A narrative review. *Emerging Microbes & Infections, 2*(1), 1–11.
United Nations. (2013). *World population projected to reach 9.6 billion by 2050*. United Nations (UN), Department of Economy and Social Affairs.
Vandepitte, J. (2003). *Basic laboratory procedures in clinical bacteriology*. World Health Organization.
Vikaspedia Domains. (n.d.). https://vikaspedia.in/agriculture/livestock/general-management-practices-of-livestock/common-animal-diseases-and-their-prevention-and-treatments
Waltzek, T. B., Cortés-Hinojosa, G., Wellehan, J. F., Jr., & Gray, G. C. (2012). Marine mammal zoonoses: A review of disease manifestations. *Zoonoses and Public Health, 59*(8), 521–535.
Wang, Q., Fidalgo, S., Chang, B. J., Mee, B. J., & Riley, T. V. (2002). The detection and recovery of Erysipelothrix spp. in meat and abattoir samples in Western Australia. *Journal of Applied Microbiology, 92*(5), 844–850.
Wang, Q., Chang, B. J., & Riley, T. V. (2010). Erysipelothrix rhusiopathiae. *Veterinary Microbiology, 140*(3–4), 405–417.
Wood, R. L. (1974). Isolation of pathogenic Erysipelothrix rhusiopathiae from feces of apparently healthy swine. *American Journal of Veterinary Research, 35*, 41–43.
Zhu, W., Wu, C., Kang, C., Cai, C., Wang, Y., Li, J., et al. (2018). Evaluation of the protective efficacy of four newly identified surface proteins of Erysipelothrix rhusiopathiae. *Vaccine, 36*(52), 8079–8083.

The Role of Vaccination in Controlling Swine Zoonosis

S. Arutkumaran, S. Shanmathi, and A. Hemavathi

Abstract

In today's scenario of climate change, pathogens that were previously less virulent have gained increased virulence through mutations. Additionally, pathogens that once infected only specific species and organ system have evolved to infect a number of species and other organ systems, potentially leading to epidemics or pandemics. Pigs, acting as maintenance or amplification hosts for various pathogens, and the widespread pork consumption, along with close human contact, facilitate the cross-species transmission of zoonotic diseases. Lessons from past outbreaks highlight the importance of vaccines for the control and prevention of diseases. So, accelerated development of vaccines, therapeutic antibodies, and antivirals or antibiotics are required to control and treat infections during outbreaks. Vaccinating pigs can stop the disease at the animal level, boosting productivity, increasing farmers' income, and protecting human health. Various vaccine approaches, including inactivated, live attenuated, subunit vaccines, recombinant and vectored vaccines, DNA and RNA vaccines, peptide-based vaccines, reverse genetics, and virus-like particles, have been used to prevent zoonotic transmission from pigs to humans. This review focuses on different vaccination strategies for countering various swine zoonotic diseases, including swine influenza, Nipah virus, Japanese encephalitis, swine coronavirus, brucellosis, salmonellosis, *E. coli*, leptospirosis, streptococcosis, erysipelas, taeniasis, trichinellosis, toxoplasmosis, and ascaris infection.

Keywords

Swine zoonosis · Emerging and re-emerging diseases · Multivalent vaccines · Reverse genetics

---

S. Arutkumaran (✉) · S. Shanmathi · A. Hemavathi
ICAR-Indian Veterinary Research Institute, Bareilly, Uttar Pradesh, India

R. Deb et al. (eds.), *Emerging Zoonotic Threats from Swine*,
https://doi.org/10.1007/978-981-96-7407-7_17

Viral Diseases

Influenza a Virus-Swine (IAV-S)

Influenza A virus is a single-stranded RNA with a negative sense genome belonging to Orthomyxoviridae family (Van Reeth & Vincent, 2019). They are more prone for mutations at their antigenic domains of surface proteins thereby resulting in antigenic drift or antigenic shift (Chen & Holmes, 2006; Taubenberger & Kash, 2010) and creating novel virus carrying a different hemagglutinin (HA) and/or neuraminidase (NA) protein. This poses unwavering threat to animal as well as human population and also in generation of commercially effective vaccines (Li & Chen, 2014). H1N1, H3N2, and H1N2 were the subtypes found in swine throughout the world but differing in their origin and antigenic characteristics (Lewis et al., 2016). Recent research underscores the importance of transmission from human to pig in understanding influenza diversity in pigs rather than pig-to-human transmission (Nelson & Vincent, 2015), emphasizing the need for a One Health approach in order to avoid unfairly blaming pigs as sources of human viruses. Vaccination tends to be a productive approach for controlling and preventing IAV-S (swine influenza A) infection. In the 1980s Europe introduced a bi-valent vaccine carrying H1avN1 and H3N2 subtypes, followed by a trivalent vaccine including H1huN2 in 2010, which remains the primary vaccine in most European countries. Another bi-valent vaccine from human-derived A/New Jersey/1976 (H1N1) and A/Port Chalmers/1973 (H3N2) strains showed protection against unrelated H1avN1 and recent H3N2 IAVS isolates (De Vleeschauwer et al., 2015). However, none of these vaccines were effective against H1N1pdm09. So, H1N1pdm09 vaccine (monovalent) was produced but could not provide complete protection against other viral strains (Everett et al., 2019). In North America, around 70% of pigs are vaccinated against IAV-S (Vincent et al., 2008), with the first vaccine targeting α-H1N1 virus. Subsequent vaccines, H3N2 (monovalent) and H1N1/H3N2 (bivalent) addressed the emergence of triple-reassortant H3N2 viruses. Additionally, a monovalent vaccine targeting H1N1pdm09 was approved in December 2009 (Sandbulte et al., 2015). In Latin America, primarily in Argentina and Brazil, IAV-S vaccines are utilized, with Flusure Pandemic being the only vaccine commercialized in Brazil. Cluster IV H3N2 strain vaccine provided better immunity than cluster I H3N2 strain vaccine against cluster IV H3N2 viruses (Kitikoon et al., 2013; Loving et al., 2013). Recombinant vaccine from HA of cluster IV H3N2 IAV-S and Venezulan-equine encephalitis virus showed reduced viral RNA and lung damage post-challenge. Vaccine expressing NP gene of cluster IV H3N2 showed reduced viral load and shedding in pigs upon challenge with H1N1pdm09. Pigs vaccinated with replication-defective human adenovirus serotype 5Ad5 possessing HA and NP genes of cluster I H3N2 were fully protected against heterologous challenge. Recombinant vaccine expressing IAV-S HA genes in the vectors of swinepox or equine herpes virus-1 protected the pigs against a homologous challenge (Said et al., 2013). European H1N1 NP gene expressed in classical swine fever or vesicular stomatitis virus elicited strong immune responses and was effective against homologous challenge (Ricklin et al., 2017). Live-attenuated influenza virus (LAIV) vaccines were created using reverse genetics to genetically modify the virus in order to reduce their replication and one such vaccine with truncated NS1 protein has been approved to use in pigs from day 1 of age (Solorzano et al., 2005). Altering IAV HA protein's cleavage site that is, it gets activated only by elastase and not by trypsin, has substantially reduced viral virulence due to the reduced availability of elastase in host tissues. Immense cell-mediated and mucosal immunity has been produced by elastase-dependent strains upon intratracheal or intranasal doses (Masic et al., 2009). A chimeric H1-H3 vaccine lacking functional neuraminidase induced antigen-specific cell-mediated and humoral immunity in the respiratory tract (Masic et al., 2013). Effective prevention and control of IAV-S benefits both swine and human health. LAIVs offer humoral immunity and are promising for IAV-S prevention. However, they can replicate and reassort with field strains.

Japanese Encephalitis

Japanese encephalitis (JE) was documented in Japan in 1871 and its prevalence was found across Asia, northern Australia, and western Pacific (Solomon, 2004). JEV belongs to the family Flaviviridae with five genotypes but one serotype and the virus is single-stranded RNA with a positive sense genome ranging between 40 and 50 nm in diameter. Primarily the transmission occurs through the bite of the infected mosquitoes to humans, specifically from infected Culex sp. (Solomon, 2004; Batchelor & Petersen, 2015). Ardeid wading birds, bats, domestic poultry, and possums are primary maintenance hosts, while pigs are principal amplifying hosts for JEV. Horses and humans are dead-end hosts, with no human-to-human transmission (Erlanger et al., 2009; Batchelor & Petersen, 2015; Hameed et al., 2021). Immunization stands out as the most efficacious preventive measure (Burchard et al., 2009). The initial vaccine was developed from mouse brain-derived formalin inactivated virus. Human vaccination with Nakayama-NIH strain commenced in 1954, later transitioning to the Beijing-1 strain in 1988 (Hegde & Gore, 2017). The effectiveness of early immunization varies between 91% and 97.5%. China developed an inactivated JEV vaccine derived from primary hamster kidney cells using Beijing-3 or P-3 strain (Yun et al., 2015; Hegde & Gore, 2017; Chanthavanich et al., 2018). Live attenuated vaccine named CD.JEVAX®, an attenuated SA 14-14-2 virus, produced an effectiveness rate of 94.5% at 6 months and 96.2% at 5 years (Tandan et al., 2007; Kumar et al., 2009). The other vaccine, IMOJEV®, a recombinant chimeric vaccine combining yellow fever vaccine 17D-204 (CV-JE) with the component of JE, introduced in 2012. 99% of vaccinated individuals exhibited neutralizing antibodies 28 days post-vaccination, with a seroprotection rate of 93%, enduring up to 5 years (Nasveld et al., 2010). An inactivated vaccine utilizing the attenuated SA-14-14-2 strain was marketed as IXIARO® in the USA, JEEV® in India, and JESPECT® in Australia and New Zealand (Li et al., 2014). Seroprotection rates ranged from 86% to 98% at various time intervals following the regimen (U.S. FDA, 2018; Schuller et al., 2008). Since 2014, India has produced its own inactivated JEV vaccine named JENVAC, manufactured from Vero cells and utilizing the Kolar-821564XY strain of JEV. Following a two-dose regimen with a 28-day interval provided a seroprotection rate of approximately 90% (Singh et al., 2015). Virus-like particles (VLPs) produced through *Pichia pastoris* expressing the envelope structural protein of JEV showcased a strong humoral and cellular immunity, in mouse and pig models. This vaccine completely protected the immunodeficient mice when challenged with a lethal strain of JEV (Yang et al., 2022). Following the incorporation of Japanese encephalitis (JE) vaccines into national immunization programs (NIP), reported cases of JEV infection have seen a remarkable decline. In India, vaccine coverage escalated from 9% in 2009 to 82% in 2021, while in Thailand, it rose from 87.4% in 2006 to 95.08% in 2019 (JE vaccine coverage, 2023). Continued research and coordinated efforts in mosquito control, antiviral drug development, and vaccine improvement are vital for managing and controlling JE, which remains a significant global public health issue.

Nipah Virus

Nipah virus (NiV) belongs to Paramyxoviridae family and the virus is single-stranded non-segmented RNA with negative sense genome with an envelope. In 1998, the first outbreak was reported in Kampung Sungai Nipah village, Malaysia where about 93% of infected cases had a history of contact with pigs, which showed the involvement of pig as intermediate and amplifying host (Parashar et al., 2000). Nipah viral disease gets transmitted via fruit bats of *Pteropus* spp. in various countries of South and Southeast Asia (Halpin et al., 2000; Daszak et al., 2013; Vandali & Biradar, 2018). Multiple vaccine candidates have been studied including live attenuated, viral vectors, subunit vaccines, peptide-based vaccines, virus-like particles, and DNA vaccines (Satterfield et al., 2016a). Different viral vectors have been used to develop vaccine for NiV like adeno-associated virus (AAV), Newcastle disease virus (NDV), Venezuelan equine encephalitis virus, measles virus, rhabdovirus, canary pox virus (ALVAC strain), and vesicular stomatitis virus glycoprotein (VSVΔG) (Weingartl et al., 2006; Chattopadhyay & Rose, 2011; Satterfield et al., 2016b). A subunit vaccine developed from Hendra virus (HeV) sG protein (Equivac® HeV, Zoetis) was approved to use in horses in Australia, but cannot able to protect pigs after challenge with NiV which might be because of decreased T cell responses (Pickering et al., 2016). In silico epitope prediction of G and F protein of NiV showed that either GPKVSLIDTSSTITI or EWISIVPNFILVRNT peptides could be used as an effective vaccine component which might provoke both cell-mediated and humoral-mediated immunity (Sakib et al., 2014). Further, VPATNSPEL, NPTAVPFTL, and LLFVFGPNL epitopes of NiV proteins N, V, and F respectively have been predicted to bind well with HLA-B7, HLA-B*2705, and HLA-A2 MHC class-I alleles, respectively inducing cell-mediated immunity (Kamthania & Sharma, 2015). M (GKLEFRRNNAIAFKG) and G (VDPLRVQWRNNSVIS) protein's epitope of HeV and NiV were predicted to develop epitope-based vaccines (Saha et al., 2017). Experimental studies with Nipah virus-like particles

(NiV-VLPs) possessing NiV proteins G, F, and M induced the antibody titer and also completely protected Golden Syrian hamsters upon viral challenge (Walpita et al., 2017). Phosphoprotein's "ELRSELIGY" and nucleocapsid protein's "YPLLWSFAM" epitopes of NiV RNA polymerase have been shown to be a promising candidate for T-cell epitopes, and phosphoprotein (positions 421–471), nucleocapsid protein (496-517), and polymerase enzyme gene (606–640) were predicted to be B-cell epitopes. These findings highlight potential vaccine targets for Nipah virus (Ravichandran et al., 2018). DNA-G (DNA vaccine) and AdC68-(recombinant chimpanzee adenovirus vaccine) provided in a heterologous regimen produced higher mucosal and T-cell responses than homologous AdC68-G immunization (Lu et al., 2023). ChAdOx1 NiV vaccines have protected hamster and African Green Monkey against lethal NiV disease by inducing high antibody titer (Lu et al., 2023). Despite the intensive research on NiV vaccine candidates, no vaccines were approved for use either in pigs or humans. Given the high risks posed by bat-borne viruses, a "One Health" approach is critical, requiring collaboration among medical doctors, veterinarians, public health officials, vector biologists, ecologists, and phylogeneticists to prevent major outbreaks (Zumla et al., 2016; Glennon et al., 2018).

Coronavirus

Coronaviruses (CoVs) are single-stranded RNA with positive sense genome and an enveloped virus belonging to the family Coronaviridae (Ma, 1993; Peiris et al., 2003). They are more prone for transmission across species because of genetic recombination and mutation leading to global pandemic condition (Alluwaimi et al., 2020; Edwards et al., 2020). Severe acute respiratory syndrome coronavirus 2 (SARS-CoV-2) (2019), Middle East respiratory syndrome coronavirus (MERS-CoV) (2012), and severe acute respiratory syndrome coronavirus (SARS-CoV) (2003) were the pandemic-causing coronaviruses transmitted to humans in the last two decades (Ksiazek et al., 2003; Berger et al., 2004; Dhama et al., 2020). Till date six swine coronaviruses have been reported. They are porcine respiratory coronavirus (PRCV), transmissible gastroenteritis virus (TGEV), porcine delta coronavirus (PDCoV), porcine hemagglutinating encephalomyelitis virus (PHEV), swine acute diarrhea syndrome coronavirus (SADS-CoV), and porcine epidemic diarrhea virus (PEDV). Human cases of porcine delta coronavirus have been discovered (Lednicky et al., 2021). Even porcine cases of human SARS-CoV have been reported indicating interspecies transmission which poses a threat to human population (Opriessnig & Huang, 2020). Since most of the animal coronaviruses have got the ability to shift the host and could lead to global pandemic in humans, preventing the virus spread at the animal level could reduce the global threat. Piglets were found to be highly protected with an inactivated vaccine possessing CV777 strain via passive transfer of antibodies from their sows (Ma et al., 1994). South Korea has developed two attenuated vaccines using SM98-1 and DR13 strains and Japan's commercially available 83P-5 strain (Sato et al., 2011; Kweon et al., 1999; Song et al., 2007). These vaccines controlled PEDV in China until highly virulent variants emerged in late 2010, leading to severe outbreaks and necessitating vaccines targeting G2 strains. Multivalent vaccines including trivalent (PEDV, TEGV, porcine rotavirus) and bivalent (TGEV and porcine rotavirus) vaccines have been officially licensed in China (Niu & Wang, 2022). Previous study revealed that a recombinant PDCoV spike protein vaccine could able to generate a neutralizing antibody against PDCoV (Zhang et al., 2022). In the USA, vaccines targeting the emerging non-S INDEL PEDV strains have been developed using alphavirus (Merck Animal Health) and also through inactivated strategy (Zoetis). mRNA lipid nanoparticle (mRNA-LNP) vaccine containing the complete PEDV spike protein elicited strong antibody response in piglets and also provided passive transfer of antibodies to neonatal piglets through the colostrum of immunized sows (Zhao et al., 2024). Surveillance among animals and humans for the emergence of new coronavirus is necessary to curb the transmission of virus across species and also helps in developing efficacious vaccines for the current strain of virus.

Bacterial Diseases

Brucellosis

Brucellosis is a globally significant zoonotic disease caused by *Brucella sps*, a Gram-negative, non-spore-forming, non-capsulated, and non-motile cocco-bacilli. *Brucella suis* is endemic in swine population worldwide, causing disease in both pigs and humans. It is categorized into five biovars, with biovars 1, 2, and 3 being zoonotic (Mailles et al., 2017). It causes abortions in sows, orchitis in boars, and undulant fever in humans (Wilson & Miles, 1955). Human infection typically arises from occupational exposure. Person-to-person transmission is extremely rare; therefore, eradicating the disease in animals significantly reduces human cases. Control measures in the OIE Manual include off-farm surveillance and managing infections in feral pigs. Preventing human infection is a priority, but no commercial vaccine for swine brucellosis is currently approved. Strategies include testing and selective depopulation. Brucellosis in livestock can be managed through vaccination, whereas human brucellosis is treated with antibiotics (Di et al., 2016). In the early stages, vaccines such as M5, H38, and 45/20 were utilized to prevent and control animal brucellosis. Currently, commonly used vaccines include S19, Rev.1, S2, RB51, and SR82. However, these vaccines have certain limitations, including residual virulence and interference with conventional serological tests (Hou et al., 2019). The *Brucella suis* S2 vaccine strain, characterized by reduced virulence, was first isolated from an aborted swine fetus in China in 1952. Through successive passages on media, the *B. suis* biovar 1 strain underwent natural attenuation, resulting in the development of *B. suis* S2, commonly referred to as the "strain 2" vaccine (Di et al., 2016). The S2 vaccine consists of the live attenuated *B. suis* strain S2, with no adjuvants added. It effectively protects swine from Brucella infection through oral administration, typically via drinking water containing the vaccine. Compared to other vaccines like S19 and Rev.1, S2 offers several benefits, including lower residual virulence, reduced production costs, and the simplicity of oral vaccination. These advantages have made it a widely adopted vaccine in China, where it has been used to immunize cattle, goats, sheep, and swine since 1971 (Xin, 1986; Mustafa & Abusowa, 1993). Studies by Blasco et al. (1993) and Verger et al. (1995) show that S19 and Rev.1 stains induce higher protection compared to S2 in large animals. Studies from mice revealed that S2 remains in the body for a short duration of time thereby inducing only short-term immunity (Bosseray & Plommet, 1990).

Leptospirosis

Leptospirosis is a widely distributed zoonotic disease caused by *Leptospira sps*, which poses a significant threat to both human and animal health worldwide (Haake & Levett, 2015; Ellis, 2015). *Leptospira interrogans* (serovars *pomona*, *icterohaemorrhagiae*, *canicola*, *hardjo*, *bratislava*), *L. borgpetersenii* (serovars *sejroe*, *tarassovi*), and *L. kirschneri* (serovar *grippotyphosa*) can infect pigs. Serovar *pomona* is primarily associated with reproductive diseases in pigs and presents a significant zoonotic risk. Developing vaccines for leptospirosis is challenging due to the fastidious growth requirements of spirochetes. Over the past five decades, a variety of leptospira vaccines, predominantly inactivated bacterins, have frequently proven ineffective at generating robust antibody responses, particularly in swine. For example, a single administration of a killed vaccine failed to elicit MAT (Microscopic Agglutination Test) titers in 96% of swine within 15 days. However, administering a booster on day 15 increased the titers to 1:100 by day 28 (Francois et al., 1995). Stalheim's studies showed protection in hamsters and swine vaccinated with irradiated or dihydrostreptomycin-exposed serovar *pomona*. Despite this, only 60% of vaccinated hamsters were protected from renal infection. However, leptospires were absent in the kidneys of pigs that were challenged 14 days post-vaccination (Stalheim, 1967). Hodges et al. (1985) reported that a commercial bivalent vaccine targeting *pomona* and *hardjo* serovars in New Zealand provided effective protection against infection in pigs and successfully prevented leptospiruria. Currently, the polyvalent Suileptovac TPCI vaccine for swine, containing serovars *tarassovi*, *canicola*, *pomona*, and *icterohaemorrhagiae*, could offer broad protection, but their efficacy against all included serovars is uncertain, with some reports indicating that vaccinated animals may not develop antibodies for every serovar (Danczig &Polner, 1997). In the 1970s, Fish and Kingscote (1973) demonstrated that a live, avirulent *pomona* vaccine effectively protected swine during a challenge, with vaccinated pigs showing only low and transient antibody titer. Despite higher titer from live vaccines, they are less popular due to storage issues and the risk of reversion to virulence. Previous research demonstrated that two commercial leptospiral vaccines were ineffective in preventing leptospiruria in more than 50% of pigs naturally exposed to the disease after receiving two doses (Hodges et al., 1976). However, an experimental bacterin prevented leptospiruria completely with multiple injections (Hodge et al., 1976). In New Zealand, a vaccine designed for cattle and sheep, which includes the serovars *pomona* and *hardjo*, was tested on pigs. The results demonstrated significant protection ($P < 0.005$) against leptospiruria in pigs naturally exposed to the disease on a commercial farm (Hodges et al., 1985). A pentavalent vaccine comprising Leptospira serovars *canicola*, *hardjo*, *pomona*, *icterohaemorrhagiae*, and *grippotyphosa* (0.2 mg per serovar per dose) is capable of eliciting a robust and effective antibody response. Challenge with serovar *canicola* revealed absence of leptospiremia or kidney infections in vaccinated swine compared to control swine (Bey & Johnson, 1983). The octavalent vaccine Porcilis Ery + Parvo + Lepto, which contains inactivated antigens of *Erysipelothrix rhusiopathiae*, Parvovirus, and six serovars of *L. interrogans* (*canicola*, *grippotyphosa*, *icterohaemorrhagiae*, *australis*, *pomona*, and *tarassovi*), provides cross-protection against all these serovars. It also plays a role in preventing renal infections and urinary shedding following exposure (Jacobs et al., 2015). Although commercial leptospira vaccines are available for cattle, swine, and dogs their effectiveness can be limited by serovar-specific immunity, and vaccinated animals may still become carriers.

Erysipelas

Erysipelas in animals and erysipeloid in humans are both caused by the Gram-positive bacterium belonging to the *Erysipelothrix* spp., with *E. rhusiopathiae* being the primary causative agent. This bacterium is ubiquitous and found worldwide (Wood, 1984; Ogawa et al., 2011). Pigs are the main natural reservoir, with approximately 30–50% of healthy pigs carrying the bacterium in their tonsils or lymphoid tissues (Stephenson & Berman, 1978). *Erysipelothrix* isolates have historically been classified into at least 28 serovars based on their unique polysaccharide complexes. Erysipelas vaccines are widely utilized in pig breeding herds across the globe, with the majority of herds in Europe, South America, and North America receiving vaccinations every 4–6 months. In the United States, between October 2018 and September 2019, approximately 10,683,595 doses of autogenous *E. rhusiopathiae* vaccines, 72,440,500 doses of attenuated vaccines, and 33,257,460 doses of bacterin vaccines were distributed across various animal species (Source: USDA, Dr. Paul Hauer, 2019). In the United Kingdom, around 1,359,120 doses of inactivated vaccines were sold in 2018 (Source: Kynetec, UK data, 2019). Erysipelas live-culture vaccines have been in use for pigs since 1955, with the introduction of the avirulent erysipelas vaccine (EVA) (Gray & Norden, 1955). The development of oral live vaccines in the 1960s (Ose et al., 1963; Lawson et al., 1966) provided a safe and effective solution, without creating carriers or shedders (Neumann et al., 2009), and they demonstrated stability in both dried and liquid forms (Lawson et al., 1966). The first bacterin, made from formalin-killed *E. rhusiopathiae* cultures with aluminum hydroxide gel, was introduced in East Germany in 1947 and licensed in the United States in 1953. These bacterins, typically derived from serovar 2 isolates, produce a glyco-lipoprotein in a serum-containing medium, which is the key immunogenic component (Wood, 1999). In the 1990s, this glyco-lipoprotein was identified as a 64–66 kDa protein, known as surface protective antigen (Spa) A (Sato et al., 1995; Makino et al., 1998). The original bacterin provided immunity for just 2–4 months, prompting the development of a water-in-oil emulsion bacterin (composed of manide mono-oleate and light mineral oil; bayol F) (Jungk & Murdock, 1957), which extended immunity to 7–8 months. Using ginseng as a coadjuvant can enhance the effectiveness of aluminum hydroxide-adjuvanted vaccines (Rivera et al., 2003). By 2004, autogenous vaccines accounted for 15–20% of the US pig vaccine market (Chase, 2004). These autogenous bacterins, derived from virulent strains isolated from farms experiencing clinical issues, are used exclusively on the same farms. Most commercial vaccines are based on serovar 1a, typically used in attenuated vaccines or serovar 2 typically used in bacterins. Attenuated *E. rhusiopathiae* vaccines, which express the P97 adhesin protein of *Mycoplasma hyopneumoniae*, have been shown to induce protective immunity against *E. rhusiopathiae* while also reducing mycoplasmal lesions when administered intranasally (Shimoji et al., 2002) or orally (Ogawa et al., 2009). These attenuated strains may also serve as vectors for delivering heterologous antigens. A recent mutant of *E. rhusiopathiae*, lacking the *tagF* gene, has demonstrated potential as a safe and effective candidate for both oral and subcutaneous vaccination (Shimoji et al., 2019a, b). Key protective antigens for *E. rhusiopathiae* include RspA (rhusiopathiae surface protein A) (Shimoji et al., 2003), CbpB (choline-binding protein) (Shi et al., 2013; Zhu et al., 2018), and GAPDH (glyceraldehyde-3-phosphate dehydrogenase) (Zhu et al., 2017), which contribute to immune responses through opsonophagocytic killing by macrophages. In Australia, issues with the efficacy of multivalent and bivalent vaccines have been reported. Additionally, an acriflavine-resistant *E. rhusiopathiae* vaccine strain in Japan has reverted to virulence, causing clinical disease (Shimoji et al., 2019a, b). As of 2019, in the United States, 62.2% of licensed erysipelas vaccines were attenuated, 28.6% were inactivated, and 9.2% were autogenous (USDA, Dr. Paul Hauer). Vaccination of breeding herds has been proven to increase the number of live-born pigs per litter, reduce farrowing intervals, and decrease periparturient vulval discharge, making it a standard practice in pig breeding (Hoffmann & Bilkei, 2002).

Streptococcosis

Streptococcus suis is a prominent pathogen in pigs, responsible for a range of serious diseases, including septicemia, meningitis, pneumonia, endocarditis, and arthritis. As a zoonotic agent, it is also capable of causing similar diseases in humans (Sanford & Tilker, 1982; Gottschalk et al., 2007). This bacterium is a gram-positive encapsulated coccus, with 35 distinct serotypes identified based on capsular polysaccharide antigenicity, with serotype 2 being the most prevalent (Higgins & Gottschalk, 2006). Vaccines, including commercial and autogenous bacterins made from heat- or formalin-killed bacteria, have been developed but their effectiveness remains limited (Lapointe et al., 2002; Gottschalk, 2012). An autogenous vaccine, which utilized sonicated bacteria from a *S. suis* capsular type 1/2 strain combined with Rehydragel® and Emulsigen® adjuvants, demonstrated significant improvements in antibody response when administered to piglets at 3 and 5 weeks of age (Lapointe et al., 2002). A live vaccine based on a non-encapsulated serotype 2 mutant offered only partial protection and failed to prevent clinical signs due to insufficient antibody production (Wisselink et al., 2002). Formalin-killed *S. suis* type 2, provided complete protection in piglets, although high doses or repeated injections were needed. The serotype 2 formalin-killed vaccine conferred protective immunity against homologous infections but showed no protection against heterologous serotype 9 infections. Serotype 9 bacterins elicited low or no opsonizing antibodies and were less protective than serotype 2 bacterins (Baums et al., 2009; Buttner et al., 2012). A vaccine incorporating Quil-A adjuvant successfully protected mice and pigs from serotype 2 infections, inducing all IgG subclasses and opsonizing activity (Garibaldi et al., 2010; Mandanici et al., 2010). A key virulence factor of *Streptococcus suis* is its cell-associated capsular polysaccharide (CPS), which helps the pathogen resist phagocytosis and evade the immune response (Fittipaldi et al., 2012; Roy et al., 2015; Segura, 2012). Antibodies targeting CPS have been shown to be particularly effective in providing protection (Bottomley et al., 2012; Song et al., 2013). Calzas et al. (2013) demonstrated that CPS stimulation of dendritic cells (DCs) did not induce cytokine production but increased CCL2 and CCL3. However, purified CPS from serotype 3, when combined with the adjuvant TiterMax Gold, induced strong IgG and IgM antibody responses, unlike other serotypes (Calzas et al., 2017). Administering two doses of a live, avirulent *S. suis* serotype 2 strain effectively protected both mice and pigs from virulent serotype 2 strains. Yao et al. (2015) isolated the avirulent serotype 2 strain (05HAS68) from the tonsil of a healthy pig, and when administered in two doses, it provided full protection against the highly virulent Chinese ST7 strain (Quessy et al., 1994; Busque et al., 1997; Yao et al., 2015). Subunit vaccines, incorporating conserved proteins from multiple serotypes, hold promise for offering better protection against heterologous strains. Proteins such as MRP, EF, and SLY have cross-protective potential (Vecht et al., 1991). A vaccine combining MRP and EF subunits effectively protected pigs against virulent serotype 2 strains, but effectiveness varied with adjuvants. Recombinant viruses expressing truncated MRP showed partial protection, while purified SLY, when combined with Diluvac Forte®, conferred full protection in mice but only partial protection in pigs (Jacobs et al., 1994). The *S. suis* type 2 glycoconjugate vaccine, which uses CPS linked to an immunogenic carrier protein such as tetanus toxoid, has shown promise in inducing functional and protective IgG antibodies in mice and pigs. The most immunogenic formulation, with a 2:1 ratio of CPS to tetanus toxoid, induced strong anti-CPS IgM and IgG responses, which were effective in both in vitro and in vivo tests (Goyette-Desjardins et al., 2016). CPS-OVA (chicken ovalbumin) elicited a stronger antibody response in pigs and provided comparable protection against *S. suis* infection, suggesting CPS-OVA as a viable alternative to CRM197 for vaccine development (Kralova et al., 2022). The development of effective vaccines remains challenging due to the multifactorial nature of *S. suis*'s virulence and its high phenotypic variability (Busque et al., 1997; Fittipaldi et al., 2007; Baums et al., 2010).

Colibacillosis

Swine Colibacillosis, caused by pathogenic strains of *Escherichia coli*, is a significant zoonotic bacterial disease. This Gram-negative bacterium includes both commensal strains residing in the gastrointestinal tract and pathogenic strains causing various diseases. Traditional treatments involve antibiotics or zinc oxide, but rising antimicrobial resistance requires an alternative method such as immunization. Vangroenweghe and Boone (2022) compared standard antimicrobial treatment with an oral live non-pathogenic *E. coli* vaccine in piglets for active immunization. The vaccinated groups showed improved performance, reduced mortality, and lower antimicrobial use, including fewer secondary infections by *Streptococcus suis*. Edema disease (ED), also referred to as "bowel edema" or "gut edema," is caused by specific pathotypes of *E. coli*. It primarily affects healthy, fast-growing nursery pigs and typically occurs 1–2 weeks after weaning (Kausche et al., 1992). Johansen et al. (1997) treated pigs infected with persistent post-weaning edema disease caused by VT2e-producing *E. coli* O139 with a VT2e-toxoid vaccine. Effective vaccines, including live attenuated and killed bacterins, target fimbrial adhesins (F4, F5, F6, F41) and enterotoxins to boost immunity in sows and piglets. Oral vaccines with non-pathogenic *E. coli* strains show promising results in preventing ED. Good hygiene practices and management strategies in farrowing areas reduce pathogen load, enhancing piglet immunity and reducing disease incidence.

Salmonellosis

Salmonella sp. is a genus of Gram-negative, rod-shaped, non-spore-forming enterobacteria distinguished by peritrichous flagella. In pigs, it may manifest as either a clinical disease or a subclinical, asymptomatic carrier state (Beltran et al., 1988). Salmonella infections in swine are significant due to their dual impact: causing clinical disease in pigs (salmonellosis) and contaminating pork products, which poses a considerable public health threat due to their zoonotic potential. Swine are susceptible to infection by a wide variety of Salmonella serotypes, with *S. choleraesuis* and *S. typhimurium* being historically notable. Control of diverse serovars remains a major challenge. In pigs, Salmonella infections are typically subclinical, though in rare instances, they may progress to enterocolitis or septicemia (Fosse et al., 2009). In a study conducted by Davies et al. (1997), several serotypes commonly found in swine were also identified as major contributors to human infections. A detailed systematic review and meta-analysis of 44 studies on Salmonella vaccines in swine show that both attenuated and inactivated vaccines significantly reduce Salmonella prevalence, aiding in public health risk reduction (Cruz et al., 2017). Recent strategies involving the mucosal presentation of antigens, live vaccines, and adjuvants to boost cell-mediated immunity have shown greater success. Vaccination, particularly with live vaccines stimulating cell-mediated immunity, has proven effective in controlling systemic salmonellosis (Wales & Davies, 2017). In some regions, addressing outbreaks of *S. choleraesuis* may require the use of an autogenous killed vaccine based on the specific strain causing the outbreak, especially if no commercial vaccine is available. This method, combined with other control measures, can be effective (Roesler et al., 2006; Barrow & Methner, 2013). Salmonella infections primarily evade humoral immunity by residing inside body cells (O'Brien, 1966). Despite this, a robust humoral response, which includes secretory IgA, plays a crucial role in preventing the initial invasion of mucosal surfaces. Effective immunity against Salmonella primarily relies on cell-mediated, especially through the activation of macrophages and cytotoxic lymphocytes. Live Salmonella vaccines, when delivered to mucosal surfaces, are believed to provide the best combination of antigen presentation and co-stimulatory signals, triggering both cell-mediated and mucosal immunity (Haesebrouck et al., 2004). Live attenuated Salmonella strains also offer the added benefit of non-parenteral administration in pigs, such as through drinking water or aerosol, which eliminates the need for handling and injecting individual animals. A robust mucosal IgA response is likely essential for effective protection. According to Lentsch et al. (2023), Evovax, a strategically designed oral inactivated *Salmonella typhimurium* vaccine, is highly safe and stimulates strong, long-lasting IgG responses in pigs. Additionally, vaccination with the live attenuated Salmoporc vaccine effectively controls *Salmonella typhimurium* in swine populations by triggering a strong $CD4^{+}$ T-cell response.

Parasitic Diseases

Taeniasis

Pig vaccinations are an effective way to lower human exposure to pigs that are diseased, which in turn lowers the risk of taeniasis. Animal vaccination development is less complicated and more affordable than that of human vaccines. Consequently, up until now, immunization against Taeniosis in humans has not been seen to be a viable control method. Although not yet commercially available in all endemic areas, an effective vaccination for *T. solium* cysticercosis has been produced in pigs; however, as of yet, no human vaccine is available for use. Various *T. solium* antigens, such as *T. solium* scolex (Nascimento et al., 1995), TSOL16, TSOL18, TSOL45-1A, TSOL45-1B (oncosphere protein) (Gauci et al., 2012; Jayashi et al., 2012), a muscle and tegument protein *T. solium* paramyosin (Vázquez-Talavera et al., 2001) have been investigated for their applicability in the production of pig vaccines. The most promising candidate for a recombinant vaccine development against PCC among those antigens is TSOL18. 99.5% protection against PCC can be obtained with this vaccine (Butala et al., 2021). Indian Immunologics (IIL), University of Melbourne, and GALVmed were the first companies to market the TSOL18 vaccine (Thomas, 2015). The vaccine was then granted an Indian license in 2016. A combination of both Oxfendazole (Paranthic 10%TM) medication and the TSOL18 vaccine (CysvaxTM) was tested in field trials against PCC in Cameroon (Assana et al., 2010) and Nepal (Poudel et al., 2019). Pigs with pre-existing cyst infections are treated with oxyfendazole and any subsequent *T. solium* infection is monitored by TSOL18. In endemic countries, the combination therapy significantly lowers the prevalence of PCC and increases protection to 99.7% of animals exposed to recurrent infection (Garnes et al., 2018; Kato, 2020; Kabululu et al., 2020). To far, the majority of *T. solium* vaccine research has mostly concentrated on developing candidate pig vaccines to manage PCC in endemic nations. A tegument protein that is necessary for oogenesis, spermiogenesis, and embryogenesis in *Taenia solium* parasite is calreticulin. Numerous studies have demonstrated decreased worm load in an experimental hamster model of taeniasis, and this protein has been investigated as a potential target for a vaccination (Leon-Cabrera et al., 2012; Salazar et al., 2013; Mendlovic et al., 2017). Pigs were immunized with native oncosphere antigens or recombinant antigens from *Taenia ovis*, resulting in 83% protection against viable cysticerci and 89% protection against total cysticerci. Recombinant antigens provided 93% and 74% protection, supporting the idea of creating a vaccine to prevent *T. solium* spread in pigs.

Trichinellosis

Trichinella spiralis is a global food-borne parasite that causes trichinellosis of zoonotic nature. Various methods have been employed to manage *T. spiralis* infections, such as vaccinations that enhance animal well-being and augment public health by impeding trichinellosis transmission between animals and humans. Regardless of the genotype of *Trichinella* sp., the predominant protective immunological response in pigs is thought to be elicited from the newborn larvae (Marinculic et al., 1991). To evaluate the protective impact against *T. spiralis* infection, a variety of potential antigens have been studied in rodent or swine models. These antigens were selected from functional proteins and excretory-secretory (ES) products involved in the process of developing infection. Nonetheless, not much study has been done on *T. spiralis* vaccinations in pigs, thus more studies required. According to Zhang et al. (2018), vaccinations offer a number of benefits over chemical treatment when it comes to preventing *T. spiralis* infection. For instance, vaccinations cure *T. spiralis* of drug resistance and offer long-term protection. According to Joachim (2016) and Sander et al. (2020), vaccinations also increase food safety by lowering medication residues in meat. Over the past few decades, a lot of work has been done to investigate the protective impact of *T. spiralis* vaccines using various approaches (Zhang et al., 2018). Live attenuated vaccines, recombinant protein vaccines, natural antigen vaccines, DNA vaccines, and synthetic peptide vaccines are the basic categories into which *T. spiralis* vaccine development is classified. The safety of live attenuated vaccination is questionable despite the fact that it provides a potent immune response and protective immunity. Although inactivated vaccines are safe and offer a high level of protection, the requirements of many animals limit the availability of antigen resources. Gu et al. (2020) showed that immunization of mice with MAP-containing CD4+ T cell and B cell epitopes (MAP-TB) induced a significantly higher protection against the *T. spiralis* larvae challenge (35.5% reduction in muscle larvae) than mice immunized with MAP-containing B cell epitope alone (MAP-B), which resulted in a 12.4% reduction in muscle larvae. Increased IgG1 and IgG2a antibody titers and mixed Th1/Th2 cytokine secretion released by inoculated mice's splenocytes were linked to the improved protection brought about by MAP-TB immunization (Gu et al., 2020). As to Xue et al. (2021) mice which received oral vaccination with invasive *L. plantarum* expressing pValac-SS1/pSIP409-FnBPA showed reduced intestinal damage and worm load, with the strongest immune response against *T. spiralis* infection. A unique method for preventing *T. spiralis* infection is offered by the DNA vaccine that the invasive *L. plantarum* delivers (Xue et al., 2021). *T. spiralis* burdens in mice were reduced by 75.2% and 68.2% with high and low *T. gondii* dosages. ROP18 and TsSP expressions were downregulated. IgG2a antibodies were elevated in coinfected mice. Th1-type immune response by *T. gondii* suppresses Th2 response to *T. spiralis* and other helminths, enabling the development of new vaccines and effective control measures (Hamed et al., 2023). Currently, available vaccinations against trichinellosis are effective, although they have limited immunogenicity and low antibody generation. Adjuvants have the power to boost vaccine immunogenicity and antibody levels. Therefore, creating a potent adjuvant for the *T. spiralis* vaccine is essential (Lu et al., 2024).

Ascariasis

One of the most prevalent intestinal parasitic diseases in developing nations is human ascariasis; recent estimates place the global infection rate at about 450 million (Metrics, 2020). This is closely linked to precarious health conditions, primarily in tropical and subtropical regions of sub-Saharan Africa, Southeast Asia, and South America (Disease, 2020). The DALY index, which calculates the total number of years lost to premature death and years lived with disability, indicates that ascariasis caused a loss of 0.754 million years worldwide in 2019 (Disease, 2020). Ascaris eggs are resilient, challenging to eradicate, and persist in the environment for years (Jourdan et al., 2018). Re-infection occurs when residents of endemic areas are frequently exposed to Ascaris eggs directly from their surroundings. Re-infection might occur as soon as 3 months after therapy. Communities with high Ascaris prevalence had a 95% re-infection rate 12 months after treatment, which is more proof that the existing eradication tactics are inadequate (Jia et al., 2012). World Health Organization has set an aim of ascariasis elimination by 2030 as a public health issue; however, the emergence of Ascaris anthelmintic resistance poses a risk to that goal. Preclinical research using an ASCVac-1 chimera showed marked protection against Ascaris infection linked to a Th2 dominant immune response and decreased lung inflammation brought on by *A. suum* larval movement, offering a potentially useful vaccination for the control group (Gazzinelli-Guimarães et al., 2021). Using a reverse vaccinology method, four additional potential immunization targets against ascariasis in humans and pigs were predicted. The four proteins, which include a protocadherin-like protein, two voltage-dependent calcium channels, and a piezo protein, are expressed in the ovaries and muscles of Ascaris species and have high-affinity epitopes for T and B cells. It is now possible to examine these targets further in vivo and in vitro experiments to demonstrate their efficacy in humans and pigs (Evangelista et al., 2022).

Type of vaccine	Vaccine target	Experimental group	Result	Authors
Lyophilized Ascaris larvae	L2 larval stage	Rabbits		Arean and Crandall (1962)
UV-attenuated	Infective eggs	Pigs	89.2%	Tromba (1978)
UV-attenuated	Infective eggs	Pigs	88%	Urban and Tromba (1982)
UV-attenuated	Infective eggs	Pigs	94%	Urban and Tromba (1984)
Purified fractions	(1) 97 kDa (2) 42 kDa (3) 14 kDa	Pigs	14 kDa and 42 kDa: 67–93%	Serrano et al. (2001)
Purified hemoglobin	AsHb	Piglets	28.7%	Vlaminck et al. (2011)
Chimeric protein	As37, As16, As14	BALB/c mice	73.54%	de Castro et al. (2021)

The challenge of choosing a suitable target to create protective immunity without also inducing an autoimmune response or IgE response in the human host is another barrier to the Ascaris vaccine development. An algorithmic pipeline for in-silico prediction of the most immunogenic and antigenic B- and T-cell epitopes from Ascaris parasites has been made possible by the rapid advancements in the disciplines of transcriptomics and proteomics (de Castro et al., 2021). We may be able to overcome obstacles to vaccine development and get closer to an Ascaris vaccine that is safe, effective, and reasonably priced with the help of new technology and worldwide investments in vaccine development.

Toxoplasmosis

An intracellular parasite *Toxoplasma gondi* which belongs to the Phylum Apicomplexa is responsible for Toxoplasmosis which infects all homeothermic animals (Dubey, 2016; Attias et al., 2020). The primary goal of implementing a control strategy against *Toxoplasma gondii* in pig is to decrease the establishment of *T. gondii* tissue cysts in pork, thereby reducing the risk of the parasite entering the human food chain, since clinical toxoplasmosis is not thought to be a problem in pigs. Burrells et al. (2015) examined the efficacy of vaccination (incomplete S48 strain) in reducing tissue cyst burden in pigs after oocyst (M4 strain) challenge using a mouse bioassay with *T. gondii* DNA molecular detection. In contrast to 51.1% of mice that received tissues from non-vaccinated and challenged pigs, 100% of mice that received porcine tissues from vaccinated and challenged pigs survived, according to the results of the mouse bioassay. These findings were also validated by the presence (or lack) of *T. gondii* DNA in individual mouse brains. This suggests that the number of live *T. gondii* tissue cysts in the tissues of pigs that received the S48 strain vaccination earlier has decreased. These optimistic results demonstrate the S48 strain tachyzoites' potential to decrease the number of *T. gondii* tissue cysts in pork thus enhancing the food safety.

Conclusion

Rapid globalization, population explosion, climate change, industrialization, and deforestation all appear to contribute to the spread of viruses into new regions. Most pathogenic diseases today are caused by emerging or re-emerging pathogens with more virulent strains or serovars. A One Health approach, which equally prioritizes animal and human health, is essential, with immunization being the most effective preventive measure. Ideal vaccines should be easy to administer, induce robust immune responses for broad protection, and work in the presence of maternal antibodies or active immunity. However, pharmaceutical companies are often discouraged from producing and procuring vaccines for seasonal diseases or outbreaks due to low demand outside of outbreak periods. To address this, the OIE World Fund manages, procures, and deploys vaccine banks for emergency situations. These vaccine banks help control disease outbreaks more rapidly. Additionally, surveillance among animals and humans for newer variant of pathogen, implementing strict biosecurity measures, therapeutic administration, and appropriate vaccine strategies are highly recommended to prevent future pandemics.

References

Alluwaimi, A. M., Alshubaith, I. H., Al-Ali, A. M., & Abohelaika, S. (2020). The coronaviruses of animals and birds: Their zoonosis, vaccines, and models for SARS-CoV and SARS-CoV2. *Frontiers in Veterinary Science, 7*, 582287. https://doi.org/10.3389/fvets.2020.582287

Arean, V. M., & Crandall, C. A. (1962). The effect of immunization on the fate of injected second stage *Ascaris lumbricoides* larvae in the rabbit. *The American Journal of Tropical Medicine and Hygiene, 11*, 369–379.

Assana, E., Kyngdon, C. T., Gauci, C. G., Geerts, S., Dorny, P., De Deken, R., et al. (2010). Elimination of *Taenia solium* transmission to pigs in a field trial of the TSOL18 vaccine in Cameroon. *International Journal of Parasitology, 40*(5), 515–519. https://doi.org/10.1016/j.ijpara.2010.01.006

Attias, M., Teixeira, D. E., Benchimol, M., Vommaro, R. C., Crepaldi, P. H., & De Souza, W. (2020). The life-cycle of *Toxoplasma gondii* reviewed using animations. *Parasites & Vectors, 13*, 1–13. https://doi.org/10.1186/s13071-020-04445-z

Barrow, P. A., & Methner, U. (Eds.). (2013). *Salmonella in domestic animals*. CABI.

Batchelor, P., & Petersen, K. (2015). Japanese encephalitis: A review of clinical guidelines and vaccine availability in Asia. *Tropical Diseases, Travel Medicine and Vaccines, 1*(1), 11. https://doi.org/10.1186/s40794-015-0013-6

Baums, C. G., Kock, C., Beineke, A., et al. (2009). *Streptococcus suis* bacterin and subunit vaccine immunogenicities and protective efficacies against serotypes 2 and 9. *Clinical and Vaccine Immunology, 16*(2), 200–208. https://doi.org/10.1128/CVI.00377-08

Baums, C. G., Brüggemann, C., Kock, C., Beineke, A., Waldmann, K.-H., & Valentin-Weigand, P. (2010). Immunogenicity of an autogenous *Streptococcus suis* bacterin in preparturient sows and their piglets in relation to protection after weaning. *Clinical and Vaccine Immunology, 17*(10), 1589–1597. https://doi.org/10.1128/CVI.00263-10

Beltran, P., Musser, J. M., Helmuth, R., Farmer, J. J., Frerichs, W. M., Wachsmuth, I. K., Ferris, K., McWhorter, A. C., Wells, J. G., & Cravioto, A. (1988). Toward a population genetic analysis of *Salmonella*: Genetic diversity and relationships among strains of serotypes *S. choleraesuis, S. derby, S. dublin, S. enteritidis, S. heidelberg, S. infantis, S. newport*, and *S. typhimurium. Proceedings of the National Academy of Sciences, 85*(20), 7753–7757. https://doi.org/10.1073/pnas.85.20.7753

Berger, A., Drosten, C., Doerr, H. W., Stürmer, M., & Preiser, W. (2004). Severe acute respiratory syndrome (SARS)–Paradigm of an emerging viral infection. *Journal of Clinical Virology, 29*(1), 13–22. https://doi.org/10.1016/j.jcv.2003.10.019

Bey, R. F., & Johnson, R. C. (1983). Leptospiral vaccines: Immunogenicity of protein-free medium cultivated whole cell bacterins in swine. *American Journal of Veterinary Research, 44*(12), 2299–2301.

Blasco, J. M., Marin, C., Jimenez de Bagues, M. P., & Barberan, M. (1993). Efficacy of *Brucella suis* strain 2 vaccine against *Brucella ovis* in rams. *Vaccine, 11*(13), 1291–1294. https://doi.org/10.1016/0264-410X(93)90187-X

Bosseray, N., & Plommet, M. (1990). *Brucella suis* S2, *Brucella melitensis* Rev. 1 and *Brucella abortus* S19 living vaccines: Residual virulence and immunity induced against three *Brucella* species challenge strains in mice. *Vaccine, 8*(5), 462–468. https://doi.org/10.1016/0264-410X(90)90055-X

Bottomley, M. J., Serruto, D., Sáfadi, M. A. P., & Klugman, K. P. (2012). Future challenges in the elimination of bacterial meningitis. *Vaccine, 30*(Suppl 2), B78–B86. https://doi.org/10.1016/j.vaccine.2012.05.045

Burchard, G. D., Caumes, E., Connor, B. A., Freedman, D. O., Jelinek, T., Jong, E. C., von Sonnenburg, F., Steffen, R., Tsai, T. F., Wilder-Smith, A., et al. (2009). Expert opinion on vaccination of travelers against Japanese encephalitis. *Journal of Travel Medicine, 16*(3), 204–216. https://doi.org/10.1111/j.1708-8305.2009.00330.x

Burrells, A., Benavides, J., Cantón, G., Garcia, J. L., Bartley, P. M., Nath, M., Thomson, J., Chianini, F., Innes, E. A., & Katzer, F. (2015). Vaccination of pigs with the S48 strain of *Toxoplasma gondii* – Safer meat for human consumption. *Veterinary Research, 46*(1). https://doi.org/10.1186/s13567-015-0177-0

Busque, P., Higgins, R., Caya, F., et al. (1997). Immunization of pigs against *Streptococcus suis* serotype 2 infection using a live avirulent strain. *Canadian Journal of Veterinary Research, 61*(4), 275–279.

Butala, C., Brook, T. M., Majekodunmi, A. O., & Welburn, S. C. (2021). Neurocysticercosis: Current perspectives on diagnosis and management. *Frontiers in Veterinary Science, 8*, 256. https://doi.org/10.3389/fvets.2021.615703

Buttner, N., Beineke, A., de Buhr, N., et al. (2012). *Streptococcus suis* serotype 9 bacterin immunogenicity and protective efficacy. *Veterinary Immunology and Immunopathology, 146*(1–2), 191–200. https://doi.org/10.1016/j.vetimm.2012.01.016

Calzas, C., Goyette-Desjardins, G., Lemire, P., Gagnon, F., Lachance, C., Van Calsteren, M. R., & Segura, M. (2013). Group B *Streptococcus* and *Streptococcus suis* capsular polysaccharides induce chemokine production by dendritic cells via Toll-like receptor 2- and MyD88-dependent and -independent pathways. *Infection and Immunity, 81*(8), 3106–3118. https://doi.org/10.1128/IAI.00444-13

Calzas, C., Taillardet, M., Fourati, I. S., Roy, D., Gottschalk, M., Soudeyns, H., Defrance, T., & Segura, M. (2017). Evaluation of the immunomodulatory properties of *Streptococcus suis* and Group B *Streptococcus* capsular polysaccharides on the humoral response. *Pathogens, 6*(1), 16. https://doi.org/10.3390/pathogens6010016

Chanthavanich, P., Limkittikul, K., Sirivichayakul, C., Chokejindachai, W., Hattasingh, W., Pengsaa, K., Surangsrirat, S., Srisuwannaporn, T., Kaewma, B., Yoksan, S., et al. (2018).

Immunogenicity and safety of inactivated chromatographically purified Vero cell-derived Japanese encephalitis vaccine in Thai children. *Human Vaccines & Immunotherapeutics, 14*(4), 900–905. https://doi.org/10.1080/21645515.2017.1414763

Chase, C. C. (2004). Autogenous vaccines: Current use in the field in the U.S. cattle and hog industry. *Developments in Biologicals, 117*, 69–71.

Chattopadhyay, A., & Rose, J. K. (2011). Complementing defective viruses that express separate paramyxovirus glycoproteins provide a new vaccine vector approach. *Journal of Virology, 85*(5), 2004–2011. https://doi.org/10.1128/JVI.01852-10

Chen, R., & Holmes, E. C. (2006). Avian influenza virus exhibits rapid evolutionary dynamics. *Molecular Biology and Evolution, 23*(11), 2336–2341. https://doi.org/10.1093/molbev/msl102

Dailey Garnes, N. J. M., White, A. C., & Serpa, J. A. (2018). *Taenia solium*, *Taenia asiatica*, and *Taenia saginata*. In *Principles and practice of pediatric infectious diseases* (pp. 1397–1404.e4). Elsevier. https://doi.org/10.1016/B978-0-323-40181-4.00280-2

Danczig, E., & Polner, A. (1997). Vaccination against leptospirosis in a pig herd. *Magyar Állatorvosok Lapja, 119*, 420–424.

Daszak, P., Zambrana-Torrelio, C., Bogich, T. L., Fernandez, M., Epstein, J. H., Murray, K. A., & Hamilton, H. (2013). Interdisciplinary approaches to understanding disease emergence: The past, present, and future drivers of Nipah virus emergence. *Proceedings of the National Academy of Sciences, 110*(Supplement 1), 3681–3688. https://doi.org/10.1073/pnas.1201243109

Davies, R. H., Nicholas, R. A. J., McLaren, I. M., Corkish, J. D., Lanning, D. G., & Wray, C. (1997). Bacteriological and serological investigation of persistent *Salmonella enteritidis* infection in an integrated poultry organization. *Veterinary Microbiology, 58*(2–4), 277–293. https://doi.org/10.1016/S0378-1135(97)00009-3

de Castro, J. C., de Almeida, L. V., Cardoso, M. S., Oliveira, F., Nogueira, D. S., Reis-Cunha, J. L., Magalhaes, L., Zhan, B., Bottazzi, M. E., Hotez, P. J., Bueno, L. L., Bartholomeu, D. C., & Fujiwara, R. T. (2021). Vaccination with chimeric protein induces protection in murine model against ascariasis. *Vaccine, 39*, 394–401.

de la Cruz, M. L., Conrado, I., Nault, A., Perez, A., Dominguez, L., & Alvarez, J. (2017). Vaccination as a control strategy against *Salmonella* infection in pigs: A systematic review and meta-analysis of the literature. *Research in Veterinary Science, 114*, 86–94. https://doi.org/10.1016/j.rvsc.2017.03.005

De Vleeschauwer, A., Qiu, Y., & Van Reeth, K. (2015). Vaccination-challenge studies with a Port Chalmers/73 (H3N2)-based swine influenza virus vaccine: Reflections on vaccine strain updates and on the vaccine potency test. *Vaccine, 33*(18), 2360–2366. https://doi.org/10.1016/j.vaccine.2015.03.031

Dhama, K., Khan, S., Tiwari, R., Sircar, S., Bhat, S., Malik, Y. S., Singh, K. P., Chaicumpa, W., Bonilla-Aldana, D. K., & Rodriguez-Morales, A. J. (2020). Coronavirus disease 2019-COVID-19. *Clinical Microbiology Reviews, 33*(4), e00028–e00020. https://doi.org/10.1128/CMR.00028-20

Di, D. D., Jiang, H., Tian, L. L., Kang, J. L., Zhang, W., Yi, X. P., Ye, F., Zhong, Q., Ni, B., He, Y. Y., & Xia, L. (2016). Comparative genomic analysis between newly sequenced *Brucella suis* vaccine strain S2 and the virulent *Brucella suis* strain 1330. *BMC Genomics, 17*(1), 1–12. https://doi.org/10.1186/s12864-016-2705-4

Disease, G. B. of. (2020). *Ascariasis – Level 4 cause | Institute for Health Metrics and Evaluation*. http://www.healthdata.org/results/gbd_summaries/2019/ascariasis-level-4-cause

Dubey, J. P. (2016). *Toxoplasmosis of animals and humans* (2nd ed.). CRC Press. https://doi.org/10.1201/9781420092370

Edwards, C. E., Yount, B. L., Graham, R. L., Leist, S. R., Hou, Y. J., Dinnon, K. H., Sims, A. C., Swanstrom, J., Gully, K., Scobey, T. D., et al. (2020). Swine acute diarrhea syndrome coronavirus replication in primary human cells reveals potential susceptibility to infection. *Proceedings of the National Academy of Sciences, 117*(43), 26915–26925. https://doi.org/10.1073/pnas.2001046117

Ellis, W. A. (2015). Animal leptospirosis. In B. Adler (Ed.), *Leptospira and leptospirosis* (Vol. 387, pp. 99–137). Springer. ISBN 978-3-662-45059-8.

Erlanger, T. E., Weiss, S., Keiser, J., Utzinger, J., & Wiedenmayer, K. (2009). Past, present, and future of Japanese encephalitis. *Emerging Infectious Diseases, 15*(1), 1–7. https://doi.org/10.3201/eid1501.080311

Evangelista, F. M. D., Van Vliet, A. H. M., Lawton, S. P., & Betson, M. (2022). A reverse vaccinology approach identifies putative vaccination targets in the zoonotic nematode *Ascaris*. *Frontiers in Veterinary Science, 9*. https://doi.org/10.3389/fvets.2022.1014198

Everett, H. E., Aramouni, M., Coward, V., Ramsay, A., Kelly, M., Morgan, S., et al. (2019). Vaccine-mediated protection of pigs against infection with pandemic H1N1 2009 swine influenza A virus requires a close antigenic match between the vaccine antigen and challenge virus. *Vaccine, 37*(19), 2288–2293. https://doi.org/10.1016/j.vaccine.2019.02.078

Fish, N. A., & Kingscote, B. (1973). Protection of gilts against leptospirosis by use of a live vaccine. *Canadian Veterinary Journal, 14*(1), 12–15.

Fittipaldi, N., Harel, J., D'Amours, B., Lacouture, S., Kobisch, M., & Gottschalk, M. (2007). Potential use of an unencapsulated and aromatic amino acid-auxotrophic *Streptococcus suis* mutant as a live attenuated vaccine in swine. *Vaccine, 25*(18), 3524–3535. https://doi.org/10.1016/j.vaccine.2007.01.060

Fittipaldi, N., Segura, M., Grenier, D., & Gottschalk, M. (2012). Virulence factors involved in the pathogenesis of the infection caused by the swine pathogen and zoonotic agent *Streptococcus suis*. *Future Microbiology, 7*(3), 259–279. https://doi.org/10.2217/fmb.12.1

Fosse, J., Seegers, H., & Magras, C. (2009). Prevalence and risk factors for bacterial food-borne zoonotic hazards in slaughter pigs: A review. *Zoonoses and Public Health, 56*(8), 429–454. https://doi.org/10.1111/j.1863-2378.2008.01182.x

Francois, S., Gualtiere, C., Drab, S., Creixell, B., Capelletti, G., & Anthony, I. (1995). Serological study after vaccination against leptospirosis in pigs. *Veterinaria Argentina, 12*, 530–533.

Garibaldi, M., Rodriguez-Ortega, M. J., Mandanici, F., et al. (2010). Immunoprotective activities of a *Streptococcus suis* pilus subunit in murine models of infection. *Vaccine, 28*(19), 3609–3616. https://doi.org/10.1016/j.vaccine.2010.03.010

Gauci, C. G., Jayashi, C. M., Gonzalez, A. E., Lackenby, J., & Lightowlers, M. W. (2012). Protection of pigs against *Taenia solium* cysticercosis by immunization with novel recombinant antigens. *Vaccine, 30*(540), 3824–3830. https://doi.org/10.1016/j.vaccine.2012.03.048

Gazzinelli-Guimarães, A. C., Nogueira, D. S., Amorim, C. C. O., Oliveira, F. M. S., Coqueiro-Dos-Santos, A., Carvalho, S. A. P., Kraemer, L., Barbosa, F. S., Fraga, V. G., Santos, F. V., De Castro, J. C., Russo, R. C., Akamatsu, M. A., Ho, P. L., Bottazzi, M. E., Hotez, P. J., Zhan, B., Bartholomeu, D. C., Bueno, L. L., & Fujiwara, R. T. (2021). ASCVac-1, a multi-peptide chimeric vaccine, protects mice against *Ascaris suum* infection. *Frontiers in Immunology, 12*. https://doi.org/10.3389/fimmu.2021.788185

Glennon, E. E., Restif, O., Sbarbaro, S. R., Garnier, R., Cunningham, A. A., Suu-Ire, R. D., Osei-Amponsah, R., Wood, J. L. N., & Peel, A. J. (2018). Domesticated animals as hosts of henipaviruses and filoviruses: A systematic review. *The Veterinary Journal, 233*, 25–34. https://doi.org/10.1016/j.tvjl.2017.12.024

Gottschalk, M. (2012). Streptococcosis. In J. J. Zimmerman, A. Ramirez, K. J. Schwartz, & G. W. Stevenson (Eds.), *Diseases of swine* (10th ed., pp. 841–855). Wiley-Blackwell.

Gottschalk, M., Segura, M., & Xu, J. (2007). *Streptococcus suis* infections in humans: The Chinese experience and the situation in North America. *Animal Health Research Reviews, 8*(1), 29–45. https://doi.org/10.1017/s1466252307001247

Goyette-Desjardins, G., Calzas, C., Shiao, T. C., Neubauer, A., Kempker, J., Roy, R., Gottschalk, M., & Segura, M. (2016). Protection against *Streptococcus suis* serotype 2 infection using a capsular polysaccharide glycoconjugate vaccine. *Infection and Immunity, 84*(7), 2059–2075. https://doi.org/10.1128/IAI.00292-16

Gray, C. W., & Norden, C. J., Jr. (1955). Erysipelas vaccine avirulent (EVA) a new agent for erysipelas control. *Journal of the American Veterinary Medical Association, 127*(964), 506–510.

Gu, Y., Sun, X., Huang, J., Zhan, B., & Zhu, X. (2020). A multiple antigen peptide vaccine containing CD4+ T cell epitopes enhances humoral immunity against *Trichinella spiralis* infection in mice. *Journal of Immunology Research, 2020*, 1–14. https://doi.org/10.1155/2020/2074803

Haake, D. A., & Levett, P. N. (2015). Leptospirosis in humans. In B. Adler (Ed.), *Leptospira and leptospirosis* (Vol. 387, pp. 65–97). Springer. ISBN 978-3-662-45058-1.

Haesebrouck, F., Pasmans, F., Chiers, K., Maes, D., Ducatelle, R., & Decostere, A. (2004). Efficacy of vaccines against bacterial diseases in swine: What can we expect? *Veterinary Microbiology, 100*(3–4), 255–268. https://doi.org/10.1016/j.vetmic.2004.02.006

Halpin, K., Young, P. L., Field, H. E., & Mackenzie, J. S. (2000). Isolation of Hendra virus from pteropid bats: A natural reservoir of Hendra virus. *Journal of General Virology, 81*(Pt 8), 1927–1932. https://doi.org/10.1099/0022-1317-81-8-1927

Hamed, E. F. A., Mostafa, N. H., Fawzy, E., Ibrahim, M. N., Ibrahim, B., Radwan, M., & Salama, M. A. (2023). *Toxoplasma gondii* suppresses Th2-induced by *Trichinella spiralis* infection and downregulates serine protease genes expression: A critical role in vaccine development. *Iranian Journal of Parasitology*. https://doi.org/10.18502/ijpa.v18i2.13183

Hameed, M., Wahaab, A., Nawaz, M., Khan, S., Nazir, J., Liu, K., Wei, J., & Ma, Z. (2021). Potential role of birds in Japanese encephalitis virus zoonotic transmission and genotype shift. *Viruses, 13*(3), 357. https://doi.org/10.3390/v13030357

Hegde, N. R., & Gore, M. M. (2017). Japanese encephalitis vaccines: Immunogenicity, protective efficacy, effectiveness, and impact on the burden of disease. *Human Vaccines & Immunotherapeutics, 13*(6), 1320–1337. https://doi.org/10.1080/21645515.2017.1285472

Higgins, R., & Gottschalk, M. (2006). Streptococcal diseases. In B. E. Straw, S. D'Allaire, W. L. Mengeling, & D. J. Taylor (Eds.), *Diseases of swine* (pp. 769–783). Iowa State University Press.

Hodges, R. T., Stocker, R. P., & Buddle, J. R. (1976). *Leptospira interrogans* serotype pomona infection and leptospiruria in vaccinated pigs. *New Zealand Veterinary Journal, 24*(2), 37–39. https://doi.org/10.1080/00480169.1976.34367

Hodges, R. T., Young, G. W., & Thomson, J. T. (1985). The efficacy of a leptospirosis vaccine in preventing leptospiruria in pigs. *New Zealand Veterinary Journal, 33*(3), 31–34. https://doi.org/10.1080/00480169.1985.35210

Hoffmann, C. W., & Bilkei, G. (2002). Case study: Chronic erysipelas of the sow–a subclinical manifestation of reproductive problems. *Reproduction in Domestic Animals, 37*(2), 119–120. https://doi.org/10.1046/j.1439-0531.2002.00339.x

Hou, H., Liu, X., & Peng, Q. (2019). The advances in brucellosis vaccines. *Vaccine, 37*(30), 3981–3988. https://doi.org/10.1016/j.vaccine.2019.05.032

Jacobs, A. A., Loeffen, P. L., van den Berg, A. J., et al. (1994). Identification, purification, and characterization of a thiol-activated hemolysin (suilysin) of *Streptococcus suis*. *Infection and Immunity, 62*(4), 1742–1748. https://doi.org/10.1128/IAI.62.4.1742-1748.1994

Jacobs, A., Harks, F., Hoeijmakers, M., & Segers, R. (2015). A novel octavalent combined Erysipelas, Parvo and Leptospira vaccine provides (cross) protection against infection following challenge of pigs with 9 different *Leptospira interrogans* serovars. *Porcine Health Management, 1*(1), 1–10. https://doi.org/10.1186/s40813-015-0011-0

Jayashi, C. M., Kyngdon, C. T., Gauci, C. G., Gonzalez, A. E., & Lightowlers, M. W. (2012). Successful immunization of naturally reared pigs against porcine cysticercosis with a recombinant oncosphere antigen vaccine. *Veterinary Parasitology, 188*(1–2), 261–265. https://doi.org/10.1016/j.vetpar.2012.02.003

Jia, T.-W., Melville, S., Utzinger, J., King, C. H., & Zhou, X.-N. (2012). Soil-transmitted helminth reinfection after drug treatment: A systematic review and meta-analysis. *PLoS Neglected Tropical Diseases, 6*(e1621). https://doi.org/10.1371/journal.pntd.0001621

Joachim, A. (2016). Vaccination against parasites – Status quo and the way forward. *Porcine Health Management, 2*, 30. https://doi.org/10.1186/s40813-016-0047-9

Johansen, M., Andresen, L. O., Jorsal, S. E., Thomsen, L. K., Waddell, T. E., & Gyles, C. L. (1997). Prevention of edema disease in pigs by vaccination with verotoxin 2e toxoid. *Canadian Journal of Veterinary Research, 61*(4), 280–285.

Jourdan, P. M., Lamberton, P., Fenwick, A., & Addiss, D. G. (2018). Soil-transmitted helminth infections. *The Lancet, 391*, 252–265. https://doi.org/10.1016/S0140-6736(18)30475-4

Jungk, N. K., & Murdock, F. M. (1957). An emulsion-type erysipelas bacterin. I. Duration of immunity in pigs vaccinated at weaning. *American Journal of Veterinary Research, 18*(68), 121–125.

Kabululu, M. L., Ngowi, H. A., Mlangwa, J. E. D., Mkupasi, E. M., Braae, U. C., Colston, A., et al. (2020). TSOL18 vaccine and oxfendazole for control of *Taenia solium* cysticercosis in pigs: A field trial in endemic areas of Tanzania. *PLoS Neglected Tropical Diseases, 14*, e0008785. https://doi.org/10.1371/journal.pntd.0008785

Kamthania, M., & Sharma, D. K. (2015). Screening and structure-based modeling of T-cell epitopes of Nipah virus proteome: An immunoinformatic approach for designing peptide-based vaccine. *3 Biotech, 5*(6), 877–882. https://doi.org/10.1007/s13205-015-0303-8

Kato, H. (2020). Mucosal vaccine for parasitic infections. In *Mucosal vaccines*. https://doi.org/10.1016/B978-0-12-811924-2.00050-X

Kausche, F. M., Dean, E. A., Arp, L. H., Samuel, J. E., & Moon, H. W. (1992). An experimental model for subclinical edema disease (*Escherichia coli* enterotoxemia) manifest as vascular necrosis in pigs. *American Journal of Veterinary Research, 53*(3), 281–287. https://doi.org/10.2460/ajvr.1992.53.281

Kitikoon, P., Gauger, P. C., Anderson, T. K., Culhane, M. R., Swenson, S., Loving, C. L., et al. (2013). Swine influenza virus vaccine serologic cross-reactivity to contemporary US swine H3N2 and efficacy in pigs infected with an H3N2 similar to 2011-2012 H3N2v. *Influenza and Other Respiratory Viruses, 7*(Suppl 4), 32–41. https://doi.org/10.1111/irv.12189

Kralova, N., Stepanova, H., Gebauer, J., Norek, A., Matiaskova, K., Zouharova, M., Nedbalcova, K., Babak, V., Jarosova, R., Makovicky, P., et al. (2022). Vaccine against *Streptococcus suis* infection in pigs based on alternative carrier protein conjugate. *Vaccine, 10*(10), 1620. https://doi.org/10.3390/vaccines10101620

Ksiazek, T. G., Erdman, D., Goldsmith, C. S., Zaki, S. R., Peret, T., Emery, S., et al. (2003). A novel coronavirus associated with severe acute respiratory syndrome. *The New England Journal of Medicine, 348*(20), 1953–1966. https://doi.org/10.1056/NEJMoa030781

Kumar, R., Tripathi, P., & Rizvi, A. (2009). Effectiveness of one dose of SA 14-14-2 vaccine against Japanese encephalitis. *New England Journal of Medicine, 360*(14), 1465–1466. https://doi.org/10.1056/NEJMc0808664

Kweon, C. H., Kwon, B. J., Lee, J. G., Kwon, G. O., & Kang, Y. B. (1999). Derivation of attenuated porcine epidemic diarrhea virus (PEDV) as vaccine candidate. *Vaccine, 17*(20–21), 2546–2553. https://doi.org/10.1016/S0264-410X(99)00062-4

Lapointe, L., D'Allaire, S., Lebrun, A., et al. (2002). Antibody response to an autogenous vaccine and serologic profile for *Streptococcus suis* capsular type 1/2. *Canadian Journal of Veterinary Research, 66*(1), 8–14.

Lawson, K. F., Pepevnak, F., Walker, V. C. R., & Crawley, J. F. (1966). Vaccination of swine with erysipelas vaccine (live culture-modified) by the oral route. *The Canadian Veterinary Journal, 7*(1), 13–17.

Lednicky, J. A., Tagliamonte, M. S., White, S. K., Elbadry, M. A., Alam, M. M., Stephenson, C. J., Bonny, T. S., Loeb, J. C., Telisma, T., Chavannes, S., et al. (2021). Independent infections of porcine deltacoronavirus among Haitian children. *Nature, 600*(7887), 133–137. https://doi.org/10.1038/s41586-021-04024-1

Lentsch, V., Aslani, S., Echtermann, T., Preet, S., Cappio Barazzone, E., Hoces, D., Moresi, C., Kümmerlen, D., & Slack, E. (2023). "EvoVax" – A rationally designed inactivated *Salmonella Typhimurium* vaccine induces strong and long-lasting immune responses in pigs. *Vaccine, 41*(38), 5545–5552. https://doi.org/10.1016/j.vaccine.2023.07.059

Leon-Cabrera, S., Cruz-Rivera, M., Mendlovic, F., Romero-Valdovinos, M., Vaughan, G., Salazar, A. M., et al. (2012). Immunological mechanisms involved in the protection against intestinal taeniosis elicited by oral immunization with *Taenia solium* calreticulin. *Experimental Parasitology, 132*, 334–340. https://doi.org/10.1016/j.exppara.2012.08.006

Lewis, N. S., Russell, C. A., Langat, P., Anderson, T. K., Berger, K., Bielejec, F., et al. (2016). The global antigenic diversity of swine influenza A viruses, *eLife, 5*, e12217. https://doi.org/10.7554/eLife.12217.019

Li, C., & Chen, H. (2014). Enhancement of influenza virus transmission by gene reassortment. *Current Topics in Microbiology and Immunology, 385*, 185–204. https://doi.org/10.1007/82_2014_389

Li, X., Ma, S. J., Liu, X., Jiang, L. N., Zhou, J. H., Xiong, Y. Q., Ding, H., & Chen, Q. (2014). Immunogenicity and safety of currently available Japanese encephalitis vaccines: A systematic review. *Human Vaccines & Immunotherapeutics, 10*(12), 3579–3593. https://doi.org/10.4161/21645515.2014.980197

Loving, C. L., Lager, K. M., Vincent, A. L., Brockmeier, S. L., Gauger, P. C., Anderson, T. K., et al. (2013). Efficacy in pigs of inactivated and live attenuated influenza virus vaccines against infection and transmission of an emerging H3N2 similar to the 2011-2012 H3N2v. *Journal of Virology, 87*(18), 9895–9903. https://doi.org/10.1128/JVI.01038-13

Lu, M., Yao, Y., Zhang, X., et al. (2023). Both chimpanzee adenovirus-vectored and DNA vaccines induced long-term immunity against Nipah virus infection. *npj Vaccines, 8*, 170. https://doi.org/10.1038/s41541-023-00762-3

Lu, H., Zhang, T., Zhao, Z., Wang, Z., Guan, J., Quan, Y., Zhu, Z., Pan, T., Huang, H., Shi, C., Yang, W., Jiang, Y., Wang, J., Zeng, Y., Cao, X., Wang, C., Wang, N., & Yang, G. (2024). *Lycium barbarum* polysaccharide promotes the immunoprotective effects of a recombinant *Lactobacillus plantarum* vaccine expressing the *Trichinella spiralis* cathepsin F-like protease 1 gene. *Microbial Pathogenesis, 186*, 106489. https://doi.org/10.1016/j.micpath.2023.106489

Ma, C. (1993). Bovine coronavirus. *British Veterinary Journal, 149*(1), 51–70.

Ma, S., Wang, M., Zhou, J., & Feng, L. (1994). Adaptation of porcine epidemic diarrhea virus to Vero cells and evaluation of the inactivated vaccine against porcine epidemic diarrhea virus. *Chinese Animal Infectious Diseases, 2*, 15–18.

Mailles, A., Ogielska, M., Kemiche, F., Garin-Bastuji, B., Brieu, N., Burnusus, Z., Creuwels, A., Danjean, M. P., Guiet, P., Nasser, V., Tourrand, B., Valour, F., Maurin, M., O'Callaghan, D., Mick, V., Vaillant, V., Jay, M., Lavigne, J. P., & De Valk, H. (2017). *Brucella suis* biovar 2 infection in humans in France: Emerging infection or better recognition? *Epidemiology and Infection, 145*(13), 2711–2716. https://doi.org/10.1017/S0950268817001704

Makino, S., Yamamoto, K., Murakami, S., Shirahata, T., Uemura, K., Sawada, T., et al. (1998). Properties of repeat domain found in a novel protective antigen, SpaA, of *Erysipelothrix rhusiopathiae*. *Microbial Pathogenesis, 25*(2), 101–109. https://doi.org/10.1006/mpat.1998.0202

Mandanici, F., Gomez-Gascon, L., Garibaldi, M., et al. (2010). A surface protein of *Streptococcus suis* serotype 2 identified by proteomics protects mice against infection. *Journal of Proteomics, 73*(11), 2365–2369. https://doi.org/10.1016/j.jprot.2010.03.011

Marinculic, A., Gamble, H. R., Urban, J. F., Rapic, D., Zivicnjak, T., Smith, H. J., & Murrell, K. D. (1991). Immunity in swine inoculated with larvae or extracts of a pig isolate and a sylvatic isolate of *Trichinella spiralis*. *American Journal of Veterinary Research, 52*, 754–758. https://doi.org/10.2460/ajvr.1991.52.754

Masic, A., Babiuk, L. A., & Zhou, Y. (2009). Reverse genetics-generated elastase-dependent swine influenza viruses are attenuated in pigs. *Journal of General Virology, 90*(Pt 2), 375–385. https://doi.org/10.1099/vir.0.005447-0

Masic, A., Pyo, H. M., Babiuk, S., & Zhou, Y. (2013). An eight-segment swine influenza virus harboring H1 and H3 hemagglutinins is attenuated and protective against H1N1 and H3N2 subtypes in pigs. *Journal of Virology, 87*(18), 10114–10125. https://doi.org/10.1128/JVI.01348-13

Mendlovic, F., Cruz-Rivera, M., Diaz-Gandarilla, J. A., Flores-Torres, M. A., Avila, G., Perfliev, M., et al. (2017). Orally administered *Taenia solium* calreticulin prevents experimental intestinal inflammation and is associated with a type 2 immune response. *PLoS One, 12*, e0186510. https://doi.org/10.1371/journal.pone.0186510. ed. F. Cominelli.

Metrics, G. H. (2020). Ascariasis – Level 4 cause (pp. 3–4).

Mustafa, A. A., & Abusowa, M. (1993). Field-oriented trial of the Chinese *Brucella suis* strain 2 vaccine on sheep and goats in Libya. *Veterinary Research, 24*(5), 422–429. https://doi.org/10.1051/vetres:19930501

Nascimento, E., Costa, J. O., Guimarães, M. P., & Tavares, C. A. P. (1995). Effective immune protection of pigs against cysticercosis. *Veterinary Immunology and Immunopathology, 45*, 127–137. https://doi.org/10.1016/0165-2427(94)05327-o

Nasveld, P. E., Ebringer, A., Elmes, N., Bennett, S., Yoksan, S., Aaskov, J., McCarthy, K., Kanesa-thasan, N., Meric, C., & Reid, M. (2010). Long-term immunity to live attenuated Japanese encephalitis chimeric virus vaccine: Randomized, double-blind, 5-year phase II study in healthy adults. *Human Vaccines, 6*(12), 1038–1046. https://doi.org/10.4161/hv.6.12.13057

Nelson, M. I., & Vincent, A. L. (2015). Reverse zoonosis of influenza to swine: New perspectives on the human-animal interface. *Trends in Microbiology, 23*(3), 142–153. https://doi.org/10.1016/j.tim.2014.12.002

Neumann, E. J., Grinberg, A., Bonistalli, K. N., Mack, H. J., Lehrbach, P. R., & Gibson, N. (2009). Safety of a live attenuated Erysipelothrix rhusiopathiae vaccine for swine. *Veterinary Microbiology, 135*(3–4), 297–303. https://doi.org/10.1016/j.vetmic.2008.09.069

Niu, X., & Wang, Q. (2022). Prevention and control of porcine epidemic diarrhea: The development of recombination-resistant live attenuated vaccines. *Viruses, 14*(6), 1317. https://doi.org/10.3390/v14061317

O'Brien, J. D. P. (1966). An outbreak of *Salmonella cholerae-suis* infection in a large pig fattening enterprise in Lancashire. *Veterinary Record, 78*(22), 558–561.

Ogawa, Y., Oishi, E., Muneta, Y., Sano, A., Hikono, H., Shibahara, T., et al. (2009). Oral vaccination against mycoplasmal pneumonia of swine using a live *Erysipelothrix rhusiopathiae* vaccine strain as a vector. *Vaccine, 27*(32), 4543–4550. https://doi.org/10.1016/j.vaccine.2009.04.081

Ogawa, Y., Ooka, T., Shi, F., Ogura, Y., Nakayama, K., Hayashi, T., et al. (2011). The genome of Erysipelothrix rhusiopathiae, the causative agent of swine erysipelas, reveals new insights into the evolution of firmicutes and the organism's intracellular adaptations. *Journal of Bacteriology, 193*(11), 2959–2971. https://doi.org/10.1128/JB.01500-10

Opriessnig, T., & Huang, Y. W. (2020). Coronavirus disease 2019 (COVID-19) outbreak: Could pigs be vectors for human infections? *Xenotransplantation, 27*(2), e12591.

Ose, E. E., Barnes, L. E., & Berkman, R. N. (1963). Experimental evaluation of an avirulent oral erysipelas vaccine. *Journal of the American Veterinary Medical Association, 143*(9), 1084–1089.

Parashar, U. D., Sunn, L. M., Ong, F., Mounts, A. W., Arif, M. T., Ksiazek, T. G., et al. (2000). Case-control study of risk factors for human infection with a new zoonotic paramyxovirus, Nipah virus, during a 1998-1999 outbreak of severe encephalitis in Malaysia. *Journal of Infectious Diseases, 181*(5), 1755–1759. https://doi.org/10.1086/315457

Peiris, J. S. M., Lai, S. T., Poon, L. L. M., Guan, Y., Yam, L. Y. C., Lim, W., et al. (2003). Coronavirus as a possible cause of severe acute respiratory syndrome. *The Lancet, 361*(9366), 1319–1325. https://doi.org/10.1016/S0140-6736(03)13077-2

Pickering, B. S., Hardham, J. M., Smith, G., Weingartl, E. T., Dominowski, P. J., Foss, D. L., et al. (2016). Protection against henipaviruses in swine requires both, cell-mediated and humoral immune response. *Vaccine, 34*(39), 4777–4786. https://doi.org/10.1016/j.vaccine.2016.08.028

Poudel, I., Sah, K., Subedi, S., Singh, D. K., Kushwaha, P., Colston, A., et al. (2019). Implementation of a practical and effective pilot intervention against transmission of *Taenia solium* by pigs in the Banke district of Nepal. *PLoS Neglected Tropical Diseases, 13*, e0006838. https://doi.org/10.1371/journal.pntd.0006838

Quessy, S., Dubreuil, J. D., & Higgins, R. (1994). Immunization of mice against *Streptococcus suis* serotype 2 infections using a live avirulent strain. *Canadian Journal of Veterinary Research, 58*(4), 299–301.

Ravichandran, L., Venkatesan, A., & Febin Prabhu Dass, J. (2018). Epitope-based immunoinformatics approach on RNA-dependent RNA polymerase (RdRp) protein complex of Nipah virus (NiV). *Journal of Cellular Biochemistry, 2018*. https://doi.org/10.1002/jcb.27979

Ricklin, M. E., Python, S., Vielle, N. J., Brechbuhl, D., Zumkehr, B., Posthaus, H., et al. (2017). Virus replicon particle vaccines expressing nucleoprotein of influenza A virus mediate enhanced inflammatory responses in pigs. *Scientific Reports, 7*(1), 16379. https://doi.org/10.1038/s41598-017-16419-w

Rivera, E., Daggfeldt, A., & Hu, S. (2003). Ginseng extract in aluminium hydroxide adjuvanted vaccines improves the antibody response of pigs to porcine parvovirus and *Erysipelothrix rhusiopathiae*. *Veterinary Immunology and Immunopathology, 91*(1), 19–27. https://doi.org/10.1016/S0165-2427(02)00276-2

Roesler, U., Heller, P., Waldmann, K. H., Truyen, U., & Hensel, A. (2006). Immunization of sows in an integrated pig-breeding herd using a homologous inactivated *Salmonella* vaccine decreases the prevalence of *Salmonella* Typhimurium infection in the offspring. *Journal of Veterinary Medicine, Series B, 53*(5), 224–228. https://doi.org/10.1111/j.1439-0450.2006.00977.x

Roy, D., Auger, J. P., Segura, M., Fittipaldi, N., Takamatsu, D., Okura, M., & Gottschalk, M. (2015). Role of the capsular polysaccharide as a virulence factor for *Streptococcus suis* serotype 14. *Canadian Journal of Veterinary Research, 79*(2), 141–146.

Saha, C. K., Mahbub Hasan, M., Saddam Hossain, M., Asraful Jahan, M., & Azad, A. K. (2017). In silico identification and characterization of common epitope-based peptide vaccine for Nipah and Hendra viruses. *Asian Pacific Journal of Tropical Medicine, 10*(6), 529–538. https://doi.org/10.1016/j.apjtm.2017.06.016

Said, A., Lange, E., Beer, M., Damiani, A., & Osterrieder, N. (2013). Recombinant equine herpesvirus 1 (EHV-1) vaccine protects pigs against challenge with influenza A(H1N1)pmd09. *Virus Research, 173*(2), 371–376. https://doi.org/10.1016/j.virusres.2013.01.004

Sakib, M. S., Islam, M. R., Hasan, A. K., & Nabi, A. H. (2014). Prediction of epitope-based peptides for the utility of vaccine development from fusion and glycoprotein of Nipah virus using in silico approach. *Advances in Bioinformatics, 2014*, 402492. https://doi.org/10.1155/2014/402492

Salazar, A. M., Mendlovic, F., Cruz-Rivera, M., Chávez-Talavera, O., Sordo, M., Avila, G., et al. (2013). Genotoxicity induced by *Taenia solium* and its reduction by immunization with calreticulin in a hamster model of taeniosis. *Environmental and Molecular Mutagenesis, 54*, 347–353. https://doi.org/10.1002/em.21782

Sandbulte, M. R., Spickler, A. R., Zaabel, P. K., & Roth, J. A. (2015). Optimal use of vaccines for control of influenza A virus in swine. *Vaccine, 3*(1), 22–73. https://doi.org/10.3390/vaccines3010022

Sander, V. A., Sanchez Lopez, E. F., Mendoza Morales, L., Ramos Duarte, V. A., Corigliano, M. G., & Clemente, M. (2020). Use of veterinary vaccines for livestock as a strategy to control foodborne parasitic diseases. *Frontiers in Cellular and Infection Microbiology, 10*, 288. https://doi.org/10.3389/fcimb.2020.00288

Sanford, S. E., & Tilker, M. E. (1982). *Streptococcus suis* type II-associated diseases in swine: Observations of a one-year study. *Journal of the American Veterinary Medical Association, 181*(6), 673–676.

Sato, H., Hirose, K., & Saito, H. (1995). Protective activity and antigenic analysis of fractions of culture filtrates of *Erysipelothrix rhusiopathiae*. *Veterinary Microbiology, 43*(2–3), 173–182. https://doi.org/10.1016/0378-1135(94)00118-L

Sato, T., Takeyama, N., Katsumata, A., Tuchiya, K., Kodama, T., & Kusanagi, K.-I. (2011). Mutations in the spike gene of porcine epidemic diarrhea virus associated with growth adaptation in vitro and attenuation of virulence in vivo. *Virus Genes, 43*(1), 72–78. https://doi.org/10.1007/s11262-011-0614-4

Satterfield, B. A., Dawes, B. E., & Milligan, G. N. (2016a). Status of vaccine research and development of vaccines for Nipah virus. *Vaccine, 34*(26), 2971–2975. https://doi.org/10.1016/j.vaccine.2015.12.075

Satterfield, B. A., Geisbert, T. W., & Mire, C. E. (2016b). Inhibition of the host antiviral response by Nipah virus: Current understanding and future perspectives. *Future Virology, 11*(5), 331–344. https://doi.org/10.2217/fvl-2016-0027

Schuller, E., Jilma, B., Voicu, V., Golor, G., Kollaritsch, H., Kaltenböck, A., Klade, C., & Tauber, E. (2008). Long-term immunogenicity of the new Vero cell-derived, inactivated Japanese encephalitis virus vaccine IC51: Six and 12 month results of a multicenter follow-up phase 3 study. *Vaccine, 26*(34), 4382–4386. https://doi.org/10.1016/j.vaccine.2008.05.081

Segura, M. (2012). Fisher scientific award lecture: The capsular polysaccharides of group B *Streptococcus* and *Streptococcus suis* differently modulate bacterial interactions with dendritic cells. *Canadian Journal of Microbiology, 58*(3), 249–260. https://doi.org/10.1139/w2012-003

Serrano, F. J., Reina, D., Frontera, E., Roepstorff, A., & Navarrete, I. (2001). Resistance against migrating ascaris suum larvae in pigs immunized with infective eggs or adult worm antigens. *Parasitology, 122*(06). https://doi.org/10.1017/s0031182001007806

Shi, F., Ogawa, Y., Sano, A., Harada, T., Hirota, J., Eguchi, M., et al. (2013). Characterization and identification of a novel candidate vaccine protein through systematic analysis of extracellular proteins of *Erysipelothrix rhusiopathiae*. *Infection and Immunity, 81*(11), 4333–4340. https://doi.org/10.1128/IAI.00549-13

Shimoji, Y., Oishi, E., Kitajima, T., Muneta, Y., Shimizu, S., & Mori, Y. (2002). *Erysipelothrix rhusiopathiae* YS-1 as a live vaccine vehicle for heterologous protein expression and intranasal immunization of pigs. *Infection and Immunity, 70*(1), 226–232. https://doi.org/10.1128/IAI.70.1.226-232.2002

Shimoji, Y., Ogawa, Y., Osaki, M., Kabeya, H., Maruyama, S., Mikami, T., et al. (2003). Adhesive surface proteins of *Erysipelothrix rhusiopathiae* bind to polystyrene, fibronectin, and type I and IV collagens. *Journal of Bacteriology, 185*(9), 2739–2748. https://doi.org/10.1128/JB.185.9.2739-2748.2003

Shimoji, Y., Bito, M., Shiraiwa, K., Ogawa, Y., Nishikawa, S., & Eguchi, M. (2019a). Disassociation of Spa type and serovar of an *Erysipelothrix rhusiopathiae* serovar 6 strain isolated from a diseased pig. *Journal of Veterinary Diagnostic Investigation, 31*(4), 488–491. https://doi.org/10.1177/1040638719835883

Shimoji, Y., Ogawa, Y., Tsukio, M., Shiraiwa, K., Nishikawa, S., & Eguchi, M. (2019b). Genome-wide identification of virulence genes in *Erysipelothrix rhusiopathiae*: Use of a mutant deficient in a tagF homolog as a safe oral vaccine against swine erysipelas. *Infection and Immunity, 87*(2), e00673–e00619. https://doi.org/10.1128/IAI.00673-19

Singh, A., Mitra, M., Sampath, G., Venugopal, P., Rao, J. V., Krishnamurthy, B., Gupta, M. K., Sri Krishna, S., Sudhakar, B., Rao, N. B., et al. (2015). A Japanese Encephalitis vaccine from India induces durable and cross-protective immunity against temporally and spatially wide-ranging global field strains. *Journal of Infectious Diseases, 212*(5), 715–725.

Solomon, T. (2004). Flavivirus encephalitis. *New England Journal of Medicine, 351*(4), 370–378. https://doi.org/10.1056/NEJMra030476

Solórzano, A., Webby, R. J., Lager, K. M., Janke, B. H., García-Sastre, A., & Richt, J. A. (2005). Mutations in the NS1 protein of swine influenza virus impair anti-interferon activity and confer attenuation in pigs. *Journal of Virology, 79*(12), 7535–7543. https://doi.org/10.1128/JVI.79.12.7535-7543.2005

Song, D. S., Oh, J. S., Kang, B. K., Yang, J. S., Moon, H. J., Yoo, H. S., Jang, Y. S., & Park, B. K. (2007). Oral efficacy of Vero cell attenuated porcine epidemic diarrhea virus DR13 strain. *Research in Veterinary Science, 82*(1), 134–140. https://doi.org/10.1016/j.rvsc.2006.08.005

Song, J. Y., Moseley, M. A., Burton, R. L., & Nahm, M. H. (2013). Pneumococcal vaccine and opsonic pneumococcal antibody. *Journal of Infection and Chemotherapy, 19*(3), 412–425. https://doi.org/10.1007/s10156-012-0545-0

Stalheim, O. H. (1967). Vaccination against leptospirosis: Protection of hamsters and swine against renal leptospirosis by killed, intact, gamma irradiated or dihydrostreptomycin exposed *Leptospira pomona*. *American Journal of Veterinary Research, 28*(124), 1671–1676.

Stephenson, E. H., & Berman, D. T. (1978). Isolation of Erysipelothrix rhusiopathiae from tonsils of apparently normal swine by two methods. *American Journal of Veterinary Research, 39*(1), 187–188.

Tandan, J. B., Ohrr, H., Sohn, Y. M., Yoksan, S., Ji, M., Nam, C. M., & Halstead, S. B. (2007). Single dose of SA 14-14-2 vaccine provides long-term protection against Japanese encephalitis: A case-control study in Nepalese children 5 years after immunization. *Vaccine, 25*(27), 5041–5045. https://doi.org/10.1016/j.vaccine.2007.04.052

Taubenberger, J. K., & Kash, J. C. (2010). Influenza virus evolution, host adaptation, and pandemic formation. *Cell Host & Microbe, 7*(5), 440–451. https://doi.org/10.1016/j.chom.2010.05.009

Thomas, L. F. (2015). *Landscape analysis: Control of Taenia solium*. World Health Organization. WHO

Tromba, F. G. (1978). Immunization of pigs against experimental *Ascaris suum* infection by feeding ultraviolet-attenuated eggs. *Journal of Parasitology, 64*, 651–656.

U.S. Food and Drug Administration. (2018). *Ixiaro: Japanese Encephalitis vaccine [package insert]*. FDA.

Urban, J. F., & Tromba, F. G. (1982). Development of immune responsiveness to *Ascaris suum* antigens in pigs vaccinated with ultraviolet-attenuated eggs. *Veterinary Immunology and Immunopathology, 3*, 399–409.

Urban, J. R., & Tromba, F. G. (1984). An ultraviolet-attenuated egg vaccine for swine ascariasis: Parameters affecting the development of protective immunity. *American Journal of Veterinary Research, 45*, 2104–2108.

Van Reeth, K., & Vincent, A. L. (2019). Influenza viruses. In J. J. Zimmerman, L. A. Karriker, A. Ramirez, K. J. Schwartz, G. W. Stevenson, & J. Zhang (Eds.), *Diseases of swine* (pp. 480–504). Wiley.

Vandali, V., & Biradar, R. B. (2018). Nipah virus (NiV) infection: A systematic review. *JOJ Nursing & Health Care, 8*(1), 555729. https://doi.org/10.19080/JOJNHC.2018.08.555729

Vangroenweghe, F. A. C. J., & Boone, M. (2022). Vaccination with an *Escherichia coli* F4/F18 vaccine improves piglet performance combined with a reduction in antimicrobial use and secondary infections due to *Streptococcus suis*. *Animals, 12*(17), 2231. https://doi.org/10.3390/ani12172231

Vázquez-Talavera, J., Solís, C. F., Terrazas, L. I., & Laclette, J. P. (2001). Characterization and protective potential of the immune response to *Taenia solium* paramyosin in a murine model of cysticercosis. *Infection and Immunity, 69*(9), 5412–5416. https://doi.org/10.1128/IAI.69.9.5412-5416.2001

Vecht, U., Wisselink, H. J., Jellema, M. L., et al. (1991). Identification of two proteins associated with virulence of *Streptococcus suis* type 2. *Infection and Immunity, 59*(10), 3156–3162. https://doi.org/10.1128/IAI.59.10.3156-3162.1991

Verger, J. M., Grayon, M., Zundel, E., Lechopier, P., & Olivier-Bernardin, V. (1995). Comparison of the efficacy of *Brucella suis* strain 2 and *Brucella melitensis* Rev. 1 live vaccines against a *Brucella melitensis* experimental infection in pregnant ewes. *Vaccine, 13*(2), 191–196. https://doi.org/10.1016/0264-410X(94)00080-C

Vincent, A. L., Ma, W., Lager, K. M., Janke, B. H., & Richt, J. A. (2008). Swine influenza viruses: A north American perspective. *Advances in Virus Research, 72*, 127–154. https://doi.org/10.1016/S0065-3527(08)00403-X

Vlaminck, J., Martinez-Valladares, M., Dewilde, S., Moens, L., Tilleman, K., Deforce, D., Urban, J., Claerebout, E., Vercruysse, J., & Geldhof, P. (2011). Immunizing pigs with *Ascaris suum* haemoglobin increases the inflammatory response in the liver but fails to induce a protective immunity. *Parasite Immunology, 33*, 250–254.

Wales, A. D., & Davies, R. H. (2017). *Salmonella* vaccination in pigs: A review. *Zoonoses and Public Health, 64*(1), 1–13. https://doi.org/10.1111/zph.12256

Walpita, P., Cong, Y., Jahrling, P. B., Rojas, O., Postnikova, E., Yu, S., Johns, L., & Holbrook, M. R. (2017). A VLP-based vaccine provides complete protection against Nipah virus challenge following multiple-dose or single-dose vaccination schedules in a hamster model. *npj Vaccines, 2*(1), 21. https://doi.org/10.1038/s41541-017-0023-7

Weingartl, H. M., Berhane, Y., Caswell, J. L., Loosmore, S., Audonnet, J. C., Roth, J. A., & Czub, M. (2006). Recombinant Nipah virus vaccines protect pigs against challenge. *Journal of Virology, 80*(16), 7929–7938. https://doi.org/10.1128/JVI.00263-06

Wilson, G. S., & Miles, A. A. (1955). *Topley and Wilson's principles of bacteriology and immunity* (Vol. 1, pp. 939–943). Edward Arnold.

Wisselink, H. J., Stockhofe-Zurwieden, N., Hilgers, L. A., et al. (2002). Assessment of protective efficacy of live and killed vaccines based on a non-encapsulated mutant of *Streptococcus suis* serotype 2. *Veterinary Microbiology, 84*(2), 155–168. https://doi.org/10.1016/S0378-1135(01)00332-7

Wood, R. L. (1984). Swine erysipelas–A review of prevalence and research. *Journal of the American Veterinary Medical Association, 184*(8), 944–949.

Wood, R. L. (1999). Erysipelas. In E. B. Straw, S. D'Allaire, W. L. Mengeling, & D. J. Taylor (Eds.), *Diseases of swine* (pp. 419–430). Iowa State University Press.

Xin, X. (1986). Orally administrable brucellosis vaccine: *Brucella suis* strain 2 vaccine. *Vaccine, 4*(2), 212–216. https://doi.org/10.1016/0264-410X(86)90030-1

Xue, Y., Yang, K., Quan, Y., Jiang, Y., Wang, N., Huang, H., Lu, H., Zhu, Z., Zhang, B., Li, J., Pan, T., Shi, C., Yang, G., & Wang, C. (2021). Oral vaccination with invasive *Lactobacillus plantarum* delivered nucleic acid vaccine co-expressing SS1 and murine interleukin-4 elicits protective immunity against *Trichinella spiralis* in BALB/c mice. *International Immunopharmacology, 101*, 108184. https://doi.org/10.1016/j.intimp.2021.108184

Yang, L., Xiao, A., Wang, H., Zhang, X., Zhang, Y., Li, Y., Wei, Y., Liu, W., & Chen, C. (2022). A VLP-based vaccine candidate protects mice against Japanese encephalitis virus infection. *Vaccine, 10*(2), 197. https://doi.org/10.3390/vaccines10020197

Yao, X., Li, M., Wang, J., et al. (2015). Isolation and characterization of a native avirulent strain of *Streptococcus suis* serotype 2: A perspective for vaccine development. *Scientific Reports, 5*, 9835. https://doi.org/10.1038/srep09835

Yun, K. W., Lee, H. J., Kang, J. H., Eun, B. W., Kim, Y. J., Kim, K. H., Kim, N. H., Hong, Y. J., Kim, D. H., Kim, H. M., et al. (2015). Safety and immunogenicity of a freeze-dried, Vero cell culture-derived, inactivated Japanese encephalitis vaccine (KD-287, ENCEVAC®) versus a mouse brain-derived inactivated Japanese encephalitis vaccine in children: A phase III, multicenter, double-blinded, randomized trial. *BMC Infectious Diseases, 15*, 7.

Zhang, N., Li, W., & Fu, B. (2018). Vaccines against *Trichinella spiralis*: Progress, challenges and future prospects. *Transboundary and Emerging Diseases, 65*(6), 1447–1458. https://doi.org/10.1111/tbed.12917

Zhang, K., Lin, S., Li, J., Deng, S., Zhang, J., & Wang, S. (2022). Modulation of innate antiviral immune response by porcine enteric Coronavirus. *Frontiers in Microbiology, 13*, 845137. https://doi.org/10.3389/fmicb.2022.845137

Zhao, Y., Fan, B., Song, X., Gao, J., Guo, R., Yi, C., He, Z., Hu, H., Jiang, J., Zhao, L., et al. (2024). PEDV-spike-protein-expressing mRNA vaccine protects piglets against PEDV challenge. *MBio, 15*(1), e02958–e02923. https://doi.org/10.1128/mbio.02958-23

Zhu, W., Zhang, Q., Li, J., Wei, Y., Cai, C., Liu, L., et al. (2017). Glyceraldehyde-3-phosphate dehydrogenase acts as an adhesin in *Erysipelothrix rhusiopathiae* adhesion to porcine endothelial cells and as a receptor in recruitment of host fibronectin and plasminogen. *Veterinary Research, 48*(1), 16. https://doi.org/10.1186/s13567-017-0421-x

Zhu, W., Wu, C., Kang, C., Cai, C., Wang, Y., Li, J., et al. (2018). Evaluation of the protective efficacy of four newly identified surface proteins of *Erysipelothrix rhusiopathiae*. *Vaccine, 36*(50), 8079–8083. https://doi.org/10.1016/j.vaccine.2018.10.071

Zumla, A., Dar, O., Kock, R., Muturi, M., Ntoumi, F., Kaleebu, P., Eusebio, M., Mfinanga, S., Bates, M., Mwaba, P., et al. (2016). Taking forward a 'one health' approach for turning the tide against the Middle East respiratory syndrome coronavirus and other zoonotic pathogens with epidemic potential. *International Journal of Infectious Diseases, 47*, 5–9. https://doi.org/10.1016/j.ijid.2016.06.012

Diagnostic Techniques for Detection of Swine Zoonoses

Prachand Pratap Singh, Ravi Dabas, Prem Kumar, and Kritika Dhial

Abstract

Swine zoonoses which are diseases transmitted to pigs from humans are a major cause of concern to both veterinary as well as public health. These illnesses and the prevention of their occurrence require early diagnosis and treatment. Diagnostic methods for swine zoonoses are as diverse as the zoonoses themselves and include sample testing to advanced molecular techniques. We have used routine diagnosis methods for the identification of pathogens such as histopathology of tissues, culture techniques of the sample and ELISA test. However, these techniques may be time-consuming and require a lot of workforces and they can sometimes be too general. Molecular diagnostics do therefore become a potent technique to overcome these limitations. Quick and precise identification of zoonotic disease diagnosis and effective treatment of these diseases are possible because of methods such as real-time PCR, Next Generation Sequencing (NGS), PCR, etc. It also looks into other new technologies such as the CRISPR-Cas systems that have brought about labelled point-of-care testing. These meth-

P. P. Singh
Division of Parasitology, ICAR-Indian Veterinary Research Institute, Izatnagar, Bareilly, U.P., India

R. Dabas
Division of Medicine, ICAR-Indian Veterinary Research Institute, Izatnagar, Bareilly, U.P., India

P. Kumar
Division of Physiology and Climatology, ICAR-Indian Veterinary Research Institute, Izatnagar Bareilly, U.P., India

K. Dhial (✉)
Department of Veterinary Microbiology, Apollo College of Veterinary Medicine, Jaipur, Rajasthan, India

R. Deb et al. (eds.), *Emerging Zoonotic Threats from Swine*, https://doi.org/10.1007/978-981-96-7407-7_18

ods give rapid, reliable, and portable results needed in identifying, and containing early and prevalent diseases affecting swine, thus reducing human exposure.

Keywords

Swine Zoonoses · Molecular diagnostics · ELISA · Next-generation sequencing · CRISPR-Cas system · Public health

Introduction

According to the 20th Livestock Census in 2019, the current animal population in our country is 535.78 million, reflecting a 4.6% increase since the 19th Census in 2012. However, the pig population is 9.06 million which has declined by 12.03% from the previous census and constitutes approximately 1.7% of the total livestock (BAHS, 2023).

Zoonotic diseases that are hosted in both commercial and wildlife have been a menace to many countries because of the large population that resides and is employed in rural areas. The consequences of zoonotic and parasitic diseases and linked food-borne illness to health and the economy are progressively increasing and limiting the burgeoning forum nations significantly. Among them, they have a negative impact on food production, agricultural productivity, distribution of trade in the world and the population's health and life expectancy. Zoonoses are conceived as a problem that has increased significantly from isolated rural focus areas toward regional and, at times, global outbreaks. This arises from the changes that have taken place in the social-economic fabric of societies in the past few decades mainly the rise of urbanization which is most of the time inadequately managed. Zoonotic diseases have also had a rise due to massive migration, the opening of new needed areas for agriculture, commerce in meat, milk among other products derived from animals, increased number and speed of means of transport, and tourism. We know that the production of pigs has important economic importance in several parts of the world (Solaymani & Petri, 2006).

Pigs are vulnerable to a number of parasitic and infectious diseases. Some of them are zoonotic diseases and affect only pigs while others affect other domestic livestock and wild animals as well. Judging by the increased numbers and the expanding geographical distribution of both the domestic cattle and the wild pigs it can be expected that the interactions between the two are bound to increase. They also purported that there will be an increased likelihood of human exposure to swine diseases whether through contact or ingestion (Solaymani & Petri, 2006).

Pig farming goes back to at least 9000 B.C. when wild boars were already being tamed. Since then, pork has become an important and popular part of people's diets. The general consumption of pork and the total market of pig products have been on the rise within the last half a century. At the same time, it is possible to compare the pigs and humans by the similar organization of the digestive, circulatory, ophthalmic, cutaneous, and dental systems. Although they promote the total enhancement of human and pig health, they are capable, at times, of permitting infections to jump species and change human organs with pig organs. It has been known for some time that pigs can be potential carriers of viruses although the exact ecology of zoonotic diseases in pigs is still unknown. Consequently, while many swine diseases are well regulated other zoonotic organisms have taken root in swine production units and are a source of disease and a drain on finances. Some of the viruses, bacteria, and parasites are coming back or are present in the wild while others may be present intermittently; or can only infect humans under certain circumstances. Malting these illnesses in humans and animals often calls for the interventions of primary or secondary preventive measures, or both. However, this entails understanding husbandry practices, environmental conditions, high-risk human activities, and the pattern of transmission of swine-associated zoonoses (Uddin Khan et al., 2013).

Zoonoses are diseases that occur in pigs naturally are transmissible to human beings and are caused by pathogen agents that comprise bacteria, viruses, and parasites. Pigs and humans have close and multiple contacts as these animals are also used for agriculture, and food processing and can even be homes, thus these illnesses pose severe threats to public health. Swine zoonoses are of significant concern since they are potentially zoonotic with some of them having disastrous effects on world health as evidenced by the H1N1 influenza pandemic in 2009 (Smith et al., 2009).Swine zoonoses have been considered an important source of public health infection burdens for a long time. For example, detection of the parasite illness Trichinellosis a species of Roundworm (*Trichinella* spp.) after their discovery in humans has been traced to thousands of years ago (Pathak and Chabra, 2010). Likewise, in the late nineties, new swine zoonotic infections emerged and some of these include which pointed to the fact that these sicknesses are menacing to the health of both humans and animals. The global trade in animal products, environmental conditions/features, and the systems of animal farming are other factors that explain the diverse and dynamic epizootiology of swine zoonoses (Long et al., 2015) (Table 1).

Table 1 Important zoonotic disease of swine

Viral disease	Causative agent
Swine influenza	H1N1, H3N2
Hepatitis E (HEV)	Hepatitis E virus
Nipah virus disease	Nipah virus
Bacterial disease	
Erysipeloid	*Erysipelothrix rhusiopathiae*
Brucellosis	*Brucella suis*
Leptospirosis	*Leptospira spp*
Streptococcus suis infection	*Streptococcus suis*
Salmonellosis	*Salmonella spp*
Yersiniosis	*Yersinia enterocolitica*
Listeriosis	*Listeria monocytogenes*
Parasitic disease	
Toxoplasmosis	*Toxoplasma gondii*
Taeniasis/Cysticercosis	*Taenia solium*
Trichinellosis	*Trichinella spiralis*

The Importance of Early Detection

Due to the consequences of swine zoonoses on the health of the population of the country as well as the economy, early diagnosis should be applied. Zoonotic diseases that originate from swine have the tendency to affect many people within the shortest time possible thus leading to a high mortality rate, high losses in trade because of bans on imports and exports, animal demolition, and other cost of treatment (Brown et al. 2018). For instance; the 2009 H1N1 flu is reported to have led to the death of 284,000 people globally implying the importance of identifying the unfamiliar disease and hoping to stop its spread before it infects many people (Dawood et al., 2012).

Therefore, it can be stated that the role of early diagnosis in risk assessment and prevention of zoonotic diseases is inestimable. This means that when an impairment is identified at an early stage there are the right interventions, vaccines and quarantine measures which are useful in controlling the spread of infection. In addition, early detection significantly contributes to the formulation of surveillance systems because it is an effective way of identifying and evaluating possibly new-emerging viruses that may affect humans once they have spread through their communities. The previous records of similar epidemics such as the Nipah virus in Malaysia revealed that delayed diagnosis would cause catastrophic effects, which include many cases of death among the affected humans and animals (Bruno et al., 2022).

Traditional Diagnostic Techniques

To date, the basic approach to disease diagnosis for swine zoonoses has relied on traditional diagnostic tools. A great number of these procedures involve culture-based methods that develop the infection in the lab for identification and serological tests which detect a certain number of antibodies in an animal's blood. Many tests such as the ELISA serologic test are commonly used in diagnosing pig diseases for instance brucellosis and leptospirosis. On the same note, the greatest method of differentiating bacterial pathogens such as *Salmonella* spp. from clinical samples has in the past identified only culture-based intervention (Chiu and Ou, 1996). In fact, there are some problems and limitations when it comes to traditional diagnostic techniques that have been widely used. While beneficial, there is a tendency of higher chance of cross-reacting hence serological tests give instances of false results. Also, despite the fact that methods based on cultural parameters are rather accurate, they are time-consuming and need specific equipment which may be absent at times. Furthermore, the sensitivity of these techniques could be slightly lower than they would otherwise be, particularly when subculturing fastidious organisms or organisms that are difficult to cultivate such as those that require complex growth media or when examining samples with low pathogen concentrations (Levett et al., 2001).

Understanding Swine Zoonoses

Epidemiology and Pathogenesis of Swine Zoonoses

A disease of pigs known as swine zoonoses can be transmitted from pigs to humans directly and or in an indirect manner with the surroundings. Preparation for detailed diagnosis and controlling these diseases is possible only if pathophysiology of such illnesses is understood.

Swine Influenza

Swine influenza is caused by influenza A viruses, these include H1N1, H3N2, and H1N2 subtypes of the virus. These viruses are zoonotic, which means they can be transmitted from pigs directly to humans, and more often cause flu-like illnesses at other times severe respiratory diseases. The invention of the flu vaccine and diagnostic tools is an effort that is not easily achieved. Major factors that make the invention of influenza vaccine and diagnostic tools challenging include the fact that the virus mutates at a high rate as explained by Bouvier et al. (2008).

Brucellosis

Caused by Brucella species, brucellosis in pigs affects people through consumption of raw dairy products and handling infected animals. It may cause flu-like symptoms and if the infection remains long-term, possible complications include endocarditis and arthritis (Pappas et al., 2006).

Trichinellosis

The common type of Trichinella that is responsible for the occurrence of Trichinellosis in pigs belongs to *Trichinella spiralis*. Transmission of this occurs when one consumes raw pork that contains larvae. In people, it may cause intestinal signs and symptoms that are accompanied by fever, muscle swelling as well as other signs of body affection (Soulsby, 1982) (Fig. 1).

Leptospirosis

Leptospira spp. causes a disease known as leptospirosis, which can get transmitted to humans through contaminated soil and water. They are likely to get infected through direct contact with contaminated soil or water. In pigs, it may cause no clinical signs at all or have an impact on the reproductive system. It can also cause flu-like symptoms in men and if not treated can lead to some complications like kidney and liver complications (Levett et al., 2001).

Economic and Public Health Effects

There is a heavy impact of disease on the swine industry besides the Health Issues, The Swine zoonoses and Swine Disease. A decreased rate of producing animals, high costs of employing the services of a veterinarian, and restrictions on the

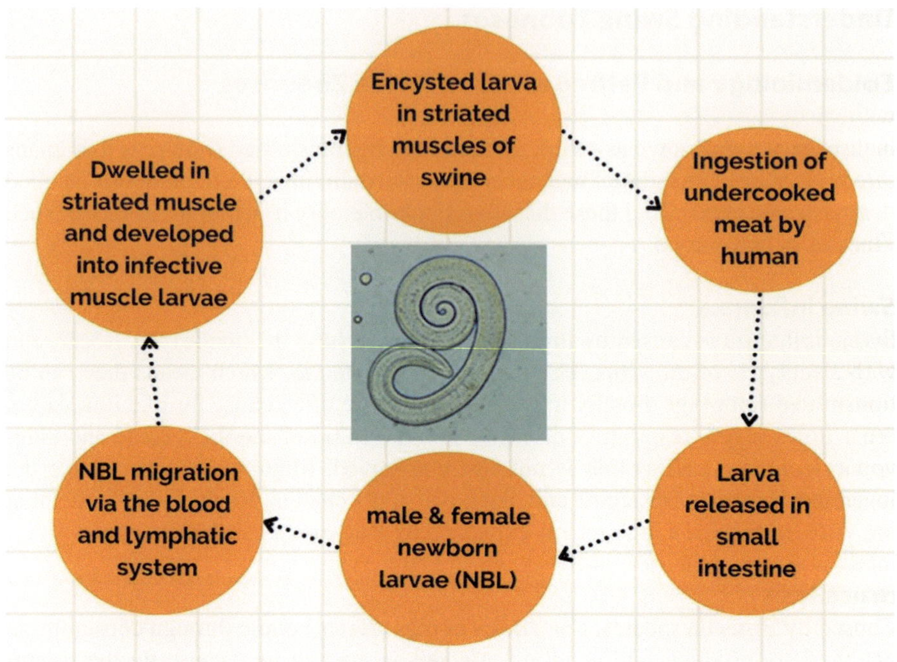

Fig. 1 Flow chart for the life cycle of Trichinella

exportation of animals lead to losses. Diseases such as Trichinellosis and other diseases may have severe economic effects; the economic loss due to swine influenza is estimated to be billions of US$ dollars due to the quarantine of diseased animals and restrictions on trade (Long et al., 2015).

People are prone to zoonotic diseases that may be mere illnesses or severe issues leading to death. Outbreaks and pandemics are still possible as evidenced by the case of swine influenza and thus diagnosis and monitoring systems should be strong (Libera, et al., 2022).

Difficulties Encountered in the Management of Swine Zoonoses

Asymptomatic Carriers: Some of the zoonotic diseases are quite difficult to diagnose during the early stages of the outbreak since most of them have very mild effects on pigs and therefore difficult to note. Inapparent infections may transmit disease to persons and other animals, thus serving as bridges for the sick. Zoonotic diseases are accounted for, diagnostics are lacking in reliability, and timeliness in their detection is also essential (Morris, 2005).

Traditional Diagnostic Techniques

The preliminary work necessary for the detection of swine zoonoses has been laid with conventional diagnostic techniques. There are several of them some of which include microscopy, culture procedures, and serological testing.

Techniques for Serology

Various methods of testing serology are useful when diagnosing diseases in pigs that affect the public. These techniques point out antibodies or antigens associated with some pathogens and provide valuable information on the presence of infections as well as the immune response of the host. Due to these qualities, such tests are easily implementable, relatively cheap and capable of handling a large sample volume, thus they are employed. Here we provide an exhaustive account of serological techniques including basic principles, application, advantages, limitations, and examples with reference to swine zoonoses. The immune system's reaction to infections is the foundation of serological techniques. An organism's immune response involves the production of certain antibodies in response to a disease. Through the use of serum or blood samples, serological assays can identify these antibodies (or the antigens they target) which indicate exposure to or infection by the pathogen.

Antibodies are proteins that the immune system produces in reaction to foreign substances known as antigens. Antibodies can reveal past or present infections as well as, in certain situations, the disease's stage based on their kind and quantity. Antigens are pathogen molecules that the immune system can identify. Antigen detection may be a sign of a continuing infection. Agglutination tests, immunofluorescence assays, and enzyme-linked immunosorbent assays (ELISA) are among the serological procedures that are grouped according to how they are detected (Fig. 2).

Enzyme-Linked Immunosorbent Assay (ELISA)

ELISA is a popular serological test that uses enzyme-labelled antibodies and a colorimetric substrate to quantify the number of antigens or antibodies in a sample. The fundamental steps are:

Coating: Particular antigens or antibodies are applied to the wells of a microtiter plate. Target antibodies or antigens from the sample can now bind to the plate as a result.

Blocking: A blocking solution is injected into the wells to stop non-specific binding.

Sample Addition: Antibodies or antigens in the sample can attach to the coated antigens or antibodies when serum or other sample types are introduced to the wells.

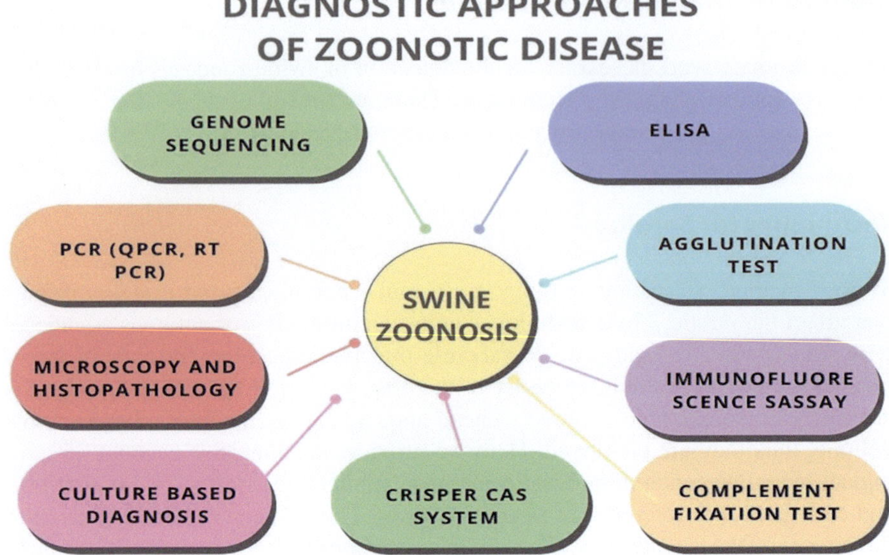

Fig. 2 Flow chart for the diagnosis of zoonotic diseases

Detection: An enzyme-conjugated secondary antibody is added. This secondary antibody binds to the primary antibody or antigen and is coupled with an enzyme that reacts with a substrate to produce a detectable signal.

Substrate Reaction: The substrate is added, which reacts with the enzyme to produce a colorimetric change. The intensity of the colour is proportional to the amount of antigen or antibody present.

Reading: The colour intensity is measured using a spectrophotometer (Clark et al., 1986).

Applications in Swine Zoonoses

Swine Influenza: ELISA is used to detect antibodies against various strains of swine influenza viruses. This helps in determining exposure and vaccination status (Buehler et al., 2014).

Brucellosis: ELISA is employed to detect Brucella-specific antibodies in swine. It is effective for screening and epidemiological studies (Paulo et al., 2000).

Leptospirosis: ELISA can detect antibodies against Leptospira spp., helping in diagnosing and monitoring leptospirosis in swine (Monahan et al., 2009).

Agglutination Tests

The principles of agglutination testing are based on the fact that interacting antigens and antibodies matter ads cause the particles to stick together. The fundamental actions are:

Preparation: Suspensions of Antigens coated-particles like Latex beads are prepared.
Mixing: The antigen-coated particles are mixed with the serum samples.
Observation: When certain antibodies are present in the serum these antibodies fix on the antigens existing on the particles of the preparation and cause clumping or agglutination of the particles which can be observed easily.

Agglutination procedures can detect specific Salmonella antigens in the blood or feces of pigs, in conditions of salmonellosis. These assays assist in the identification as well as the differentiation of the serotype of Salmonella infections (Bonardi et al., 2003).

Applications in Brucellosis

There is a test known as the Rose Bengal test and it is a form of agglutination test that is used to test pigs for possible Brucella infections. It identifies Brucella antigens that have been coated with specific antibodies (Gusi et al., 2019).

Immunofluorescence Assays

In immunofluorescence assays, the secondary reagents are antibodies conjugated with fluorochromes that are used to detect specific antigens in the tissue or cell preparations. The fundamental actions are:

Incubation: The samples are incubated with primary antibodies that have a high affinity for the target antigen and do not cross-react with other proteins.
Secondary Antibody: A fluorescein-labelled secondary antibody is then applied. This links up to the principal antibody linking to an antigen.
Visualization: Fluorescent microscope is used to study the samples. This is usually the case when the target antigen is present as evidenced by any fluorescence (Bayer et al., 2001).

Applications in Swine Zoonoses

Trichinellosis: Muscle tissue contains Trichinella larvae detecting using immunofluorescence assays that are useful in Trichinellosis identification (Sofronic et al., 2017).

Leptospirosis: *Leptospira* spp. In clinical samples or tissue sections may be identified using immunofluorescence gives diagnostic information about leptospirosis (Levett et al., 2001).

Compliment Fixation Test

As a diagnostic test, the complement fixation test is the ability of an antibody to bind complement proteins during an antigen-antibody reaction. The fundamental actions are:

Antigen-Antibody Reaction: The sample is mixed with an antigen and left for a certain period.

Addition of Complement: The mixture is then supplemented with proteins which are known as complement proteins. Among the organs/organisms whose embryonic morphogenesis can be considered as an indication system, one ought to mention red blood cells. The process of complement fixation inhibits the reaction of red blood cell haemolysis.

Observation: To know whether the complement was fixed, the extent of haemolysis is determined (Sam-Yellowe & Sam-Yellowe, 2021).

Applications in Swine Zoonoses

Brucellosis: Although it is less common to be applied than now there are a variety of more complex assays, Complement Fixation Test is still used in the diagnostics of Brucella-specific antibodies in pigs (Meirelles-Bartoli et al., 2020).

Trichinellosis: Muscle tissues contain Trichinella larvae which can be located by immunofluorescent methods that are used in the diagnosis of Trichinellosis (Sofronic et al., 2017).

Leptospirosis: Leptospira spp. In clinical samples including tissues or tissue sections the above-said proteins may be detected by immunofluorescence that provides diagnostic data on leptospirosis (Levett et al., 2001).

Culture-Based Techniques

Culture techniques are used in the isolation and growth of pathogens from clinical samples with direct identification being possible.

Bacterial Cultures: One of the methods for the recognition of bacterial zoonoses is the isolation of bacterial agents from such objects as faeces and tissues. For instance, selective media and biochemical assays may be involved in the detection of *Campylobacter* spp. from pig faeces (Mughini-Gras et al., 2016).

Viral Cultures: In infections such as swine influenza, viral isolation from clinical samples that may include tissue biopsy or nasal swab may be challenging however it is an indispensable tool. The first one is the adaptation of the virus, growth and identification using cell cultures or embryonated eggs (Janke, 2014).

Microscopy and Histopathology

For tissue alterations associated with zoonotic diseases and for the identification of parasites, microscopy and histopathological examination is very important.

Light microscopy: Originally described to visualize parasites in muscle tissues for example; *Trichinella* spp. Some of them are staining and using a microscope to examine a piece of muscle or a tissue slide (Nöckler et al., 2005).

Histopathology: This entails searching for changes related to infections in the tissues retrieved from patients. Leptospirosis and other infections can be detected with the help of immunohistochemical staining of the tissues in which certain types of pathogens are present (Sykes et al., 2022).

Molecular Diagnostic Techniques

Advanced diagnostic technology at the molecular level has brought very efficient and precise methods of detecting pathogens and is widely used in diagnosing swine zoonoses.

Polymerase Chain Reaction (PCR)

It is a highly sensitive form of molecular biology that has been applied extensively in the diagnosis of pathogen, especially, in swine zoonoses. The strength in using PCR is centred on the capacity to identify particular sections in DNA or RNA for detection of pathogens even in low concentrations.

Conventional PCR

The first and basic type of PCR is the conventional PCR which is often used for amplifying the genetic material of a pathogen. Standard PCR focuses on amplifying one or the other DNA or RNA sequence to a level at which it will be easily observed. For instance, in the analysis of swine zoonoses, conventional PCR as a method for diagnosis is used to amplify RNA sequences of Swine influenza viruses. According to Bastien et al. (2008), PCR is very effective for identifying the existence of these viruses especially when they are in low concentrations and therefore should be applied when there is suspicion of an outbreak of the disease.

Quantitative PCR (qPCR)

Standard PCR is seemingly plain compared to qPCR which serves a similar function to standard PCR but is capable of determining the quantity of DNA or RNA in a given sample. This quantification is necessary in explaining the viral load which is the amount or volume of the virus in the host. In diseases such as swine influenza, the technique proves very useful in studying the copy number and rate of replication of the virus within the host. Richt et al. (2004) pointed out that, qPCR specifically, offers not only a simple identification of ASF but comprehensive data as well on the viral load which is extremely essential for therapeutic intervention and planning.

Reverse Transcription PCR (RT-PCR)

RT-PCR as a method is mainly used for RNA viruses and is in fact a sub-type of PCR. PCR specifically works on DNA and therefore RNA has to undergo reverse transcription whose enzyme is reverse transcriptase. The RNA once reverse transcribed into cDNA can be amplified using standard PCR methods such as

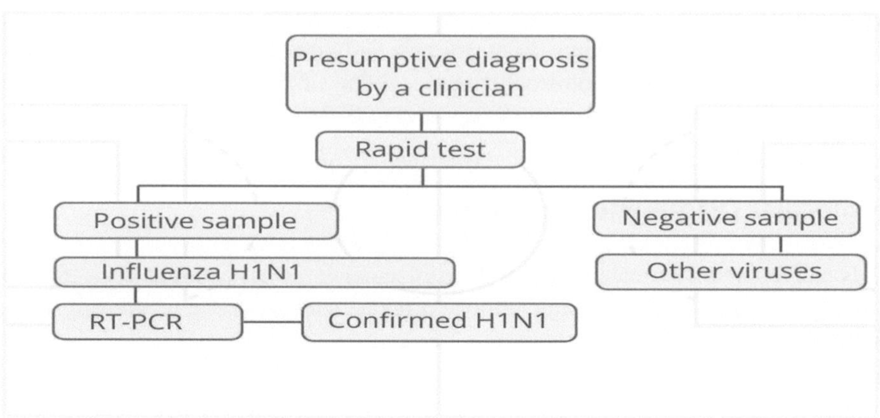

Fig. 3 Flow chart for the diagnosis of swine influenza

semi-quantitative PCR. It is widely used in the diagnosis of RNA virus which include Swine Influenza. As stated by Chiapponi et al. (2012), the RT-PCR method is valuable for the identification of these viruses; it is characterised by high sensitivity and specificity. This makes it one of the best methods of diagnosing RNA-based zoonotic diseases in swine (Fig. 3).

Next-Generation Sequencing (NGS)

The technological advancement that has come in handy which offers a broad perspective of the genetic structure of pathogens is the Next-Generation Sequencing (NGS). Such an approach provides insight into the sequence determination of the pathogen, including new zoonotic diseases and an understanding of pathogen genomics. As an approach, NGS is very useful for uncovering the genetic variability of organisms and for the identification of new viruses, and therefore should be considered as a fundamental tool for the study and management of zoonoses in swine.

Metagenomics

One of the most important applications of NGS is metagenomics is the identification of all microbial DNA in a given sample. Metagenomic sequencing is much different from the traditional methods that are used for the recognition of known pathological microbes; metagenomic sequencing implements a worldview of the microbial community, which allows identifying new, unusual pathogens. This is especially important for discovering new zoonotic viruses that may not be easily detected by other diagnostic processes.

For instance, through meta-genomic analysis of such mosquitoes, the following viruses have been detected; parvoviruses, circoviruses, flaviviruses, rhabdoviruses, as well as seadornaviruses where the mosquito feed on animal with viremia. As stated by Hameed et al. (2020), these identification findings reveal Mosquito's role as vectors of such viruses thus underlining the utility of metagenomics in the surveillance and study of zoonotic diseases. Through integration of metagenomics, a comprehensive view of microbial systems is achieved thus enabling identification and control of compelling zoonoses hence promoting public and animal health.

Whole Genome Sequencing (WGS)

Whole Genome Sequencing (WGS) is yet another important application of NGS which comprises of information concerning the whole genome of a pathogen. While other sequencing techniques centre on specific genes or niche sections of the genome, WGS encompasses the whole genome, thus enabling the evaluation of the pathogen's traits in their entirety. It is very useful in epidemiological studies as it helps in identifying disease occurrence trends and patterns of spread of infections. In the context of swine zoonoses, the study has contributed to the understanding of genetic variation and transmission dynamics of pathogens including the swine influenza. According to Revez et al. (2017), WGS is useful in the identification of the variations within the Influenza virus genome and the help the world has been able to achieve for monitoring the spread of the virus and developing strategies to control outbreaks. Since WGS provides better understanding of the pathogens' evolution and distribution, it proves to be helpful in disease control and prevention.

CRISPR-Cas Systems

CRISPR-Cas systems that were initially designed for genome editing have shown high specificity and sensitivity in recognition and binding of the target nucleic acids, therefore, are applied in diagnostics. Two most well-known diagnostic systems from the CRISPR technology are named SHERLOCK (Specific High-Sensitivity Enzymatic Reporter UnLOCKing) and DETECTR (DNA Endonuclease-Targeted CRISPR Trans Reporter).**SHERLOCK** (CRISPR-Cas13-Based Diagnostic Tool).

SHERLOCK utilizes the CRISPR-Cas13 techniques to identify certain RNA sequences within a sample. Cas13 is an RNA-guided RNA endonuclease which implies that Cas13 targets RNA not DNA as in the articles. In the SHERLOCK diagnostic platform, CRISPR-Cas13 is guided by a chosen guide RNA that targets an RNA sequence bases with a corresponding pathogen. Upon recognition, a structural change occurs in the Cas13, which enhances its collateral cleavage activity. Using this activity, the enzyme is able to cut whatever RNA molecule is within its vicinity, including a reporter RNA which was introduced to the reaction. The reporter RNA is labelled by a fluorescent moiety and when cleaved by the activity of the target enzyme, an easily measurable signal is generated. This signal indicates the presence of the target RNA, confirming the presence of the pathogen.

Several studies have reported the use of SHERLOCK for the detection of various viral RNA sequences including those consisting of swine influenza virus, with high sensitivity and specificity. Similarly, in the study by Mustafa and Makhawi (2021), SHERLOCK was proven to correctly detect swine influenza RNA from clinical samples pointing to its uses in veterinary medicine. The platform is highly beneficial especially in field applications since it can provide quick results without much need for sophisticated laboratory instruments.

DETECTR (Efficient CRISPR-Cas12 Based Diagnostic Tool).

DETECTR is based on the CRISPR-Cas12 system in which target DNA sequences are identified. Cas12 is a DNA-target DNA cleavage enzyme, further, shows off-target activity that occurs in the presence of guide DNA and the targeted DNA sequence. This property is used in the DETECTR platform to identify DNA pathogens. When the Cas12 complex associates with target DNA with the help of the specific RNA molecule, the Cas12 complex turns, cuts close single-stranded DNA as well as the reporter DNA containing a fluorescence or enzymatic label. The cleavage of the reporter forms a product that can be visualized by the naked eye or using simple fluorescence detectors making it easy to realize the presence of the target pathogen DNA.

DETECTR has been used in the detection of several DNA pathogens; some of them are the swine influenza Virus which affects pigs in a fatal way through a disease which is also fatal in pigs. The method has been observed to be highly specific in its detection and has short turnaround time, hence will be suitable for point-of-care diagnosis. In the research done by Mann and Pitts in 2022, the authors pointed out that DETECTR works as an efficient tool to diagnose the influenza Virus in field samples with high sensitivity. This is especially important in dealing with epidemic situations when early and accurate diagnosis is vital to containing the diseases.

Molecular Epidemiology

In molecular epidemiology, distribution and causes of diseases are studied using molecular approaches and provide time series of incidence and aetiology of diseases and pathogens.

Molecular Typing: Methods like genotyping and sequencing are used to monitor the transmission of zoonotic infections and locate the origins of outbreaks. For example, patterns of transmission between pigs and humans can be shown by molecular typing of strains of Salmonella and E. coli (Sokurenko, 2017).

Integration with Monitoring Systems: Since it provides detailed information regarding the genetics of pathogens and the spread of diseases in different regions molecular epidemiology aids in the monitoring of diseases across the globe. New techniques of molecular diagnostics, that include high specificity, sensitivity, and working speed, have completely altered the methods of identifying swine zoonoses. These methods are based on detection and analysis of nucleic acids namely the DNA or RNA associated with the infection. They can be used for case identification, monitoring, as well as disease control with relation to the swine-related zoonosis. Several molecular diagnostic procedures have been outlined in detail in this section alongside details of the advantages, limitations, uses and examples involving swine zoonoses.

New and Creative Technologies Relative to Diagnosis

Non-Laboratory-Based Testing of HIV/AIDS

POCT refers to point-of-care testing or point-of-care diagnostic testing, that is, tests that can be done quickly. POCT equipment for zoonotic illnesses includes the portable PCR machines and lateral flow tests. These gadgets are designed to be used in places that are far from the laboratory, or areas that have limited or no access to laboratory equipment. There are some advantages to adopting POCT such as rapid testing, ease to use, and minimal sample processing. However, there are limitations which include lower sensitivity and specificity in comparison to lab-based approaches, and the need for validation in different settings (Bora et al., 2022).

Biosensors and Nanotechnology

Biosensors can also be described as analytical instruments that contain a biological sensing element and a physicochemical transducer which help in the identification of specific pathogens and the conversion of this identification into an analytically measurable signal. These sensors employ biomolecules including enzymes, antibodies, nucleic acids, whole cells or other receptor molecules that can selectively recognize desired pathogenic organisms. In capturing, a signal is generated when the receptor is bound and this is transformed into an electrical, optical or thermal signal which can be quantified.

One of the most promising areas is the use of biosensors in diagnostics of zoonotic infections. For example, electrochemical biosensors allow a determination of the presence of a particular viral protein or nucleic acids such as those characteristics of swine influenza through the changes in the electrical signals after binding to pathogen. Likewise, optical biosensors make use of alteration in the condition of light in terms of fluorescence or absorbance in order to detect the existence of pathogens. It stated that these biosensors have high sensitivity and specificity together with fast response time and real-time monitoring, which are useful when it comes to disease detection and management (Castillo-Henríquez et al., 2020).

Nanotechnology involves manipulation of Nano particularity and Nano materials in the improvement of sensitivity and specificity of tests. Some types of nanoparticles include gold nanoparticles, quantum dots and magnetic nanoparticles; these are important in diagnostic assays since they possess improved sensitivity and specificity. Such nanomaterials can be designed to selectively attach to the pathogen and increase the signal that is produced from the presence of a relatively small number of target organisms. Several benefits derive from the use of nanotechnology-based methods of diagnostics as compared to regular techniques. For instance, gold nanoparticles coated with antibodies or nucleic acid can specifically bind to pathogens. Once anchored to the target analyte; these nanoparticles cause a colour change or amplify a signal that can easily be measured spectroscopically. Likewise, the magnetic nanoparticles can be used for the concentrating of pathogens from the sample matrices enhancing the sensitivity of the subsequent methods (Thwala et al., 2023).

Moreover, using nanotechnology makes it possible to create diagnostics equipment that are small, easy to transport and can be used at location where the test is to be conducted. These devices allow for on-site testing thus ensuring a quick answer that may help to prevent the spread of disease. Nanotechnology-based assays have the ability to detect the presence of pathogens at extremely low levels of sensitivity thus playing a major role in early detection and prevention of disease transmission.

Artificial Intelligence and Digital Diagnostics

One of the most emerging technologies in the field of veterinary diagnostics especially concerning the diagnosis and control of the swine zoonoses is artificial intelligence (AI). They are used to enhance diagnostic speed and precision in zoonotic diseases in swine thereby altering the general approach towards disease identification, surveillance as well as prevention. The info-processing power, pattern identification and future pandemics forecasting make advanced contributions to the veterinary medicine, which allows early and accurate identification of diseases and timely preventive efforts both for animals and humans.

AI in Recognizing Weak Patterns and Disease Outbreak Prediction

Another factor that makes AI systems desirable is that they are usually adept in identifying patterns, including those used in diagnostics and in making other predictions concerning diseases and their occurrence. Concerning swine zoonoses, AI can work through huge datasets from diverse sources, such as patient's histories, lab tests, environmental information, etc. to determine whether there are signs of a zoonotic disease. By virtue of this capability, the likelihood of an outbreak can be predicted in advance and so steps can be taken by the veterinarian or public health officials to minimize on it. Shafi & Parwani, 2023 state that the integration of information derived from a variety of diagnostic tests makes the chances of misdiagnosis hard hence optimizing the efficiency of disease control techniques. In diagnostics of swine zoonosis, the use of AI has been seen to be useful in image analysis of microscopic images. Small pictures produced through a lens can be scrutinized by an AI algorithm, and the presence of pathogens or other signs of diseases may be tough to single out with the naked eye. This technology is of special value in diseases that call for examination under the microscope such as bacterial or parasitic diseases. Scholars established that with the use of AI for analysis, the rate at which diagnosis is conducted increases while the chances of errors increase hence making the results precise. This application is very important in veterinary practice especially when diagnosis is done early and accurately in order to prevent or control the spread of diseases.

Integration with Molecular Diagnostics

The next shift in the detection of swine zoonoses is AI's incorporation into molecular diagnostics that uses DNA, RNA, or proteins to detect pathogens involved in zoonotic diseases. However, the usage of these techniques is relatively complicated and the results obtained may have to be analysed with the help of other analytical tools to arrive at appropriate conclusions. This can be made easy through use of AI where data analysis and interpretation is done in shorter time and results produced. Advanced molecular diagnostic tools implemented through artificial intelligence can reduce the time of diagnosing diseases hence fasten the execution of control measures (Wang et al., 2022).

Immunoassays and Novel Biotechnologies

Advances in biotechnology as well as immunoassays are constant and further extending diagnostic capabilities. Sequential infections can also be identified by new immunoassay approaches such as multiplex technologies. These techniques improve the diagnostics, and are useful in cases of zoonotic diseases which have complex profiles (Huang et al., 2020).

Some of the diagnostic reagents which are central to identification of zoonotic illnesses in pigs include monoclonal antibodies (mAbs) and recombinant proteins. What these biotechnology instruments provide are very specific, precise measurements that help in the early diagnosis and management of diseases that may be transmitted from pigs to human beings. Virus of Swine Influenza (SIV): In diagnostic tests HA and NA proteins of the recombinant SIV are used to detect antibodies that are formed during the infection. For example, recombinant HA proteins prove useful for subtype-specific diagnosis (Zhao et al., 2013).

Challenges and Limitations in Diagnostic Techniques

Possible issues related to diagnostic practices and particular difficulties in apparatus utilization. However, following the development of diagnostic technologies some several issues and limitations can be identified.

Technical and Operational Challenges

Sensitivity and Specificity: The biopsy analysis must therefore yield high sensitivity as well as high specificity to enable an accurate diagnosis to be made. Failure to treat diseases, missing the illness' symptoms, or providing wrong diagnosis arises from false positive/negative findings (Trevethan, 2017).

Standardization: This might be due to the fact that most of the diagnostic techniques used may not have been standardized and therefore may produce varying results.

For developing reliable diagnostics, it is necessary to define the steady procedures for diagnosing and validating (Maunder & Punt, 2004).

Diagnostics Accessible in Low-Resource Environments

Barriers to Access: Availability of cost, infrastructure, and training can all be the barriers towards adoption and utilization of modern diagnostic technology in low-resourced settings. Decreasing illness in such regions has to overcome these challenges of improving the management of such conditions. T. solium zoonoses that affect swine can be controlled and even improve by enhancing local capacity to detect diseases in improving the use of cheap diagnostic tools.

Ethical and Regulatory Considerations

Ethical Issues: Some of the ethical issues arising from diagnostic testing for zoonotic diseases include animal rights, privacy, and consent. These problems need to be addressed for maintaining the research & clinical ethical practice foreseen in the current world. Diagnostic tools have to go through a certain set of specifications that include accuracy, safety and efficacy as per the existing regulations. The FDA and EMA and similar authorities have the challenging task of making sure that the diagnostic tests meet these standards (Buikstra, et al., 2020).

Integration into Surveillance Systems

Integration Challenges: Combination of these diagnostic methods to the national and international surveillance systems is also a complex process due to the aspect of coordination and sharing of information. It is important that diagnostic data are used well in decision-making as far as public health is concerned. In this case, One Health concept which focuses on human and animal health as well as the environment plays a role in disease diagnosis and prevention. Some of the ethical consideration observed when diagnosing zoonotic diseases include privacy, informed consent, and animal rights. The above concerns have to be addressed in order to maintain ethical standards in both clinical practice and research. For the purpose of regulating, diagnostics equipment should be accurate, safe, and efficient. As for the diagnostics, those regulatory organizations such as the U.S. Food and Drug Administration (FDA) and the European Medicines Agency (EMA) should ensure that diagnostics abide by these guidelines (Buikstra et al., 2020). This means that there must be integration of diagnostic procedures into National and International surveillance networks and this has to involve coordination and data exchange, if need be. Special attention needs to be paid to the fact that diagnostic information should be used effectively when considering issues related to the population's health. An important principle for a fast and effective detection and control of diseases is the One Health concept that integrates the environmental, animal, and human health. Coordinating efforts across sectors can enhance the detection and management of zoonotic diseases (Latinne et al., 2023).

Case Studies

Case Study 1: The 2009 H1N1 Pandemic

The 2009 H1N1 influenza pandemic highlighted the importance of rapid diagnostic techniques in managing widespread outbreaks.

Role of Diagnostics In the course of the pandemic PCR and serological tests were helping to detect and track the cases. The increase in the speed of the development and deployment of diagnostic tests did help towards controlling the spread of the. The Covid-19 pandemic was a reminder of the preparedness and the ability to adapt with diagnostic technologies when threatened (Tamerius et al., 2011).

Case Study 2: Nipah Virus Outbreak

The short and emerging Zoonotic disease outbreak like Nipah virus in Bangladesh and South India reveal the diagnostic and knowledge gap, as well as control strategies.

Diagnostic Challenges: It highlighted the importance of enhanced molecular testing for the allele of the virus and its pattern of transmission The outbreak that struck during the world influenza season of 2009–2010 identified the efficacy of rapid diagnostic tools in containing widespread pandemics like H1N1.

The Diagnostics Role: PCR and antibodies were crucial from the identification and follow-up of the patients came into enactment throughout the epidemic. This virtually means that diagnostic tests need to be invented and deployed before they can be STOPPED from proliferating. Tamerius et al. (2011) have also stated that the gold standard also needs to be ready for the threats of the pandemic and has also quickened the readiness of diagnostic tools.

Control Strategies: Due to the epidemic, more efficient technology in surveillance and diagnostics has been enhanced along with the diagnostic tests such as the timely tests are the improved public health contingencies plans (Chowdhury et al., 2014).

Future Directions in Diagnostic Techniques for Swine Zoonoses

Innovation and Research Priorities

Key Research Areas: Subsequent researchers should focus their efforts on designing a diagnostic test that is more accurate and sensitive, optimization of point-of-care devices and integrating modern technologies in diagnostics such as artificial intelligence and nanotechnology.

Potential Breakthroughs: Several enhanced diagnostics that can lead to the enhanced recognition of illnesses and their management include the CRISPR-based method and next-generation sequencing.

International Collaboration's Role in Global Collaboration

Q Paradoxically, coordinating illness surveillance and developing diagnostic technologies are today's global activities. It is derived that through cooperation; international health security can be achieved, diagnostic practices can be made more uniform, and Information sharing can also be enhanced.

Future Standards and Protocols: To control and minimize the inconsistencies and/or inaccuracies in the diagnosis of illness, it will be crucial to have and implement standard and procedures that are universally recognized.

Adoption of Emerging Technologies

Adoption Prospects: There are a lot of potentials that new technologies hold in enhancing diagnostic procedures including biosensors and digital diagnostics. The objectives should be to increase and eliminate implementation barriers so that these technologies could be applied.

Implementation problems: When it comes to the introduction of new diagnostic technologies to various healthcare facilities, it would be critical to note that implementation difficulties in regard to infrastructure, cost, and training warrant further attention.

Conclusions

Effective diagnostics are crucial for managing and controlling swine zoonoses, which pose major risks to the health of both humans and animals. The advancement of diagnostic techniques from traditional methods to advanced molecular technology has improved our ability to recognize and treat many diseases. However, there are still challenges to be addressed, including issues with accessibility, technological limitations, and the need for international cooperation. Future advancements in diagnostic technologies might enhance the detection and treatment of illnesses. By addressing current problems and making use of new advancements, it is possible to protect animal and public health around the world and effectively control swine zoonoses.

References

BAHS. (2023). *Basic animal husbandry statistics, AHS series 13*. Department of Animal Husbandry, Dairying and Fisheries, Government of India.

Bastien, P., Procop, G. W., & Reischl, U. (2008). Quantitative real-time PCR is not more sensitive than "conventional" PCR. *Journal of Clinical Microbiology, 46*(6), 1897–1900.

Bayer, P. M., Fabian, B., & Hübl, W. (2001). Immunofluorescence assays (IFA) and enzyme-linked immunosorbent assays (ELISA) in autoimmune disease diagnostics-technique, benefits, limitations and applications. *Scandinavian Journal of Clinical and Laboratory Investigation, 61*(235), 68–76.

Bonardi, S., Brindani, F., Pizzin, G., Lucidi, L., D'incau, M., Liebana, E., & Morabito, S. (2003). Detection of salmonella spp., Yersinia enterocolitica and verocytotoxin-producing Escherichia coli O157 in pigs at slaughter in Italy. *International Journal of Food Microbiology, 85*(1–2), 101–110.

Bora, M., Mathew, D. D., Das, H., Bora, D. P., & Barman, N. N. (2022). Point of care diagnostics and non-invasive sampling strategy: A review on major advances in veterinary diagnostics. *Acta Veterinaria Brno, 91*(1), 17–34.

Bouvier, N. M., Lowen, A. C., & Palese, P. (2008). Oseltamivir-resistant influenza a viruses are transmitted efficiently among Guinea pigs by direct contact but not by aerosol. *Journal of Virology, 82*(20), 10052–10058.

Brown, V. R., Bowen, R. A., & Bosco-Lauth, A. M. (2018). Zoonotic pathogens from feral swine that pose a significant threat to public health. *Transboundary and Emerging Diseases, 65*(3), 649–659.

Bruno, L., Nappo, M. A., Ferrari, L., Di Lecce, R., Guarnieri, C., Cantoni, A. M., & Corradi, A. (2022). Nipah virus disease: Epidemiological, clinical, diagnostic and legislative aspects of this unpredictable emerging zoonosis. *Animals, 13*(1), 159.

Buehler, J., Lager, K., Vincent, A., Miller, C., Thacker, E., & Janke, B. (2014). Issues encountered in development of enzyme-linked immunosorbent assay for use in detecting influenza a virus subtype H5N1 exposure in swine. *Journal of Veterinary Diagnostic Investigation, 26*(2), 277–281.

Buikstra, S., Bernice, B., & Elsbeth, S. (2020). Ethical decision-making in zoonotic disease control. *Journal of Agricultural and Environmental Ethics, 33*(2), 239–259.

Castillo-Henríquez, L., Brenes-Acuña, M., Castro-Rojas, A., Cordero-Salmerón, R., Lopretti-Correa, M., & Vega-Baudrit, J. R. (2020). Biosensors for the detection of bacterial and viral clinical pathogens. *Sensors, 20*(23), 6926.

Chiapponi, C., Moreno, A., Barbieri, I., Merenda, M., & Foni, E. (2012). Multiplex RT-PCR assay for differentiating European swine influenza virus subtypes H1N1, H1N2 and H3N2. *Journal of Virological Methods, 184*(1–2), 117–120.

Chiu, C. H., & Ou, J. T. (1996). Rapid identification of salmonella serovars in feces by specific detection of virulence genes, invA and spvC, by an enrichment broth culture-multiplex PCR combination assay. *Journal of Clinical Microbiology, 34*(10), 2619–2622.

Chowdhury, S., Khan, S. U., Crameri, G., Epstein, J. H., Broder, C. C., Islam, A., et al. (2014). Serological evidence of henipavirus exposure in cattle, goats and pigs in Bangladesh. *PLoS Neglected Tropical Diseases, 8*(11), e3302.

Clark, M. F., Lister, R. M., & Bar-Joseph, M. (1986). ELISA techniques. In *Methods in enzymology* (Vol. 118, pp. 742–766). Academic Press.

Dawood, F. S., Iuliano, A. D., Reed, C., Meltzer, M. I., Shay, D. K., Cheng, P. Y., et al. (2012). Estimated global mortality associated with the first 12 months of 2009 pandemic influenza a H1N1 virus circulation: A modelling study. *The Lancet Infectious Diseases, 12*(9), 687–695.

Gusi, A. M., Bertu, W. J., Jesús de Miguel, M., Dieste-Pérez, L., Smits, H. L., Ocholi, R. A., et al. (2019). Comparative performance of lateral flow immunochromatography, iELISA and rose Bengal tests for the diagnosis of cattle, sheep, goat and swine brucellosis. *PLoS Neglected Tropical Diseases, 13*(6), e0007509.

Hameed, M., Liu, K., Anwar, M. N., Wahaab, A., Li, C., Di, D., et al. (2020). A viral metagenomic analysis reveals rich viral abundance and diversity in mosquitoes from pig farms. *Transboundary and Emerging Diseases, 67*(1), 328–343.

Huang, C., Wang, Y., Li, X., Ren, L., Zhao, J., Hu, Y., et al. (2020). Clinical features of patients infected with 2019 novel coronavirus in Wuhan, China. *The lancet, 395*(10223), 497–506.

Janke, B. H. (2014). Influenza a virus infections in swine: Pathogenesis and diagnosis. *Veterinary Pathology, 51*(2), 410–426.

Latinne, A., Nga, N. T. T., Long, N. V., Ngoc, P. T. B., Thuy, H. B., PREDICT Consortium, et al. (2023). One health surveillance highlights circulation of viruses with zoonotic potential in bats, pigs, and humans in Viet Nam. *Viruses, 15*(3), 790.

Levett, P. N., Branch, S. L., Whittington, C. U., Edwards, C. N., & Paxton, H. (2001). Two methods for rapid serological diagnosis of acute leptospirosis. *Clinical Diagnostic Laboratory Immunology, 8*(2), 349–351.

Libera, K., Konieczny, K., Grabska, J., Szopka, W., Augustyniak, A., & Pomorska-Mól, M. (2022). Selected livestock-associated zoonoses as a growing challenge for public health. *Infectious Disease Reports, 14*(1), 63–81.

Long, S. R., Tian, X. Y., Wang, Z. Q., Liu, R. D., Liu, L. N., Jiang, P., et al. (2015). Serodiagnosis of trichinellosis by ELISA using recombinant nudix hydrolase of Trichinella spiralis. *Tropical Biomedicine, 32*, 669–675.

Mann, J. G., & Pitts, R. J. (2022). PrimedSherlock: A tool for rapid design of highly specific CRISPR-Cas12 crRNAs. *BMC Bioinformatics, 23*(1), 428.

Maunder, M. N., & Punt, A. E. (2004). Standardizing catch and effort data: A review of recent approaches. *Fisheries Research, 70*(2–3), 141–159.

Meirelles-Bartoli, R. B., de Alvarenga Cruz, C., de Moraes, R. S., Oliveira, R. A., de Paula, E. M. N., de Sousa, D. B., et al. (2020). Comparison of four serological tests for the diagnosis of swine brucellosis. *Research, Society and Development, 9*(7), e493974418.

Monahan, A. M., Miller, I. S., & Nally, J. E. (2009). Leptospirosis: Risks during recreational activities. *Journal of Applied Microbiology, 107*(3), 707–716.

Morris, R. S. (2005). Disease control challenges for the pig industry–what will the future bring. Manipulating pig. *Production, X*, 23.

Mughini-Gras, L., Penny, C., Ragimbeau, C., Schets, F. M., Blaak, H., Duim, B., et al. (2016). Quantifying potential sources of surface water contamination with campylobacter jejuni and campylobacter coli. *Water Research, 101*, 36–45.

Mustafa, M. I., & Makhawi, A. M. (2021). SHERLOCK and DETECTR: CRISPR-Cas systems as potential rapid diagnostic tools for emerging infectious diseases. *Journal of Clinical Microbiology, 59*(3), 10–1128.

Nöckler, K., Serrano, F. J., Boireau, P., Kapel, C. M., & Pozio, E. (2005). Experimental studies in pigs on Trichinella detection in different diagnostic matrices. *Veterinary Parasitology, 132*(1–2), 85–90.

Pappas, G., Papadimitriou, P., Akritidis, N., Christou, L., & Tsianos, E. V. (2006). The new global map of human brucellosis. *The Lancet Infectious Diseases, 6*(2), 91–99. Rosenberg, D., et al. (2020). Future directions in diagnostic research. *Journal of Clinical Pathology, 73*(7), 387–393.

Pathak, K. M. L., & Chhabra, M. B. (2010). Parasites and parasitic diseases of the camel in India: A review. *Indian Journal of Animal Sciences, 80*(8), 699–706.

Paulo, P. S., Vigliocco, A. M., Ramondino, R. F., Marticorena, D., Bissi, E., Briones, G., et al. (2000). Evaluation of primary binding assays for presumptive serodiagnosis of swine brucellosis in Argentina. *Clinical Diagnostic Laboratory Immunology, 7*(5), 828–831.

Revez, J., Espinosa, L., Albiger, B., Leitmeyer, K. C., Struelens, M. J., & ECDC National Microbiology Focal Points and Experts Group. (2017). Survey on the use of whole-genome sequencing for infectious diseases surveillance: Rapid expansion of European national capacities, 2015–2016. *Frontiers in Public Health, 5*, 347.

Richt, J. A., Lager, K. M., Clouser, D. F., Spackman, E., Suarez, D. L., & Yoon, K. J. (2004). Real–time reverse transcription–polymerase chain reaction assays for the detection and differentiation of north American swine influenza viruses. *Journal of Veterinary Diagnostic Investigation, 16*(5), 367–373.

Sam-Yellowe, T. Y., & Sam-Yellowe, T. Y. (2021). Exercise 19: Complement fixation assays. In *Immunology: Overview and laboratory manual* (pp. 381–386).

Shafi, S., & Parwani, A. V. (2023). Artificial intelligence in diagnostic pathology. *Diagnostic Pathology, 18*(1), 109.

Smith, G. J., Vijaykrishna, D., Bahl, J., Lycett, S. J., Worobey, M., Pybus, O. G., et al. (2009). Origins and evolutionary genomics of the 2009 swine-origin H1N1 influenza a epidemic. *Nature, 459*(7250), 1122–1125.

Sofronic-Milosavljevic, L., Ilic, N., & Gruden-Movsesijan, A. (2017). Trichinella. In *Laboratory models for foodborne infections* (pp. 793–808). CRC Press.

Sokurenko, E. (2017). Pathoadaptive mutations in uropathogenic Escherichia coli. In *Urinary tract infections: Molecular pathogenesis and clinical management* (pp. 331–357).

Solaymani-Mohammadi, S., & Petri, W. A., Jr. (2006). Zoonotic implications of the swine-transmitted protozoal infections. *Veterinary Parasitology, 140*(3–4), 189–203.

Soulsby, E. J. L. (1982). *Helminths, arthropods and protozoa of domesticated animals* (7th ed.). Affiliated East-West Press Private Limited.

Sykes, J. E., Reagan, K. L., Nally, J. E., Galloway, R. L., & Haake, D. A. (2022). Role of diagnostics in epidemiology, management, surveillance, and control of leptospirosis. *Pathogens, 11*(4), 395.

Tamerius, J., et al. (2011). Lessons from the 2009 H1N1 influenza pandemic. *Journal of Infectious Diseases, 204*(6), 807–814.

Thwala, L. N., Ndlovu, S. C., Mpofu, K. T., Lugongolo, M. Y., & Mthunzi-Kufa, P. (2023). Nanotechnology-based diagnostics for diseases prevalent in developing countries: Current advances in point-of-care tests. *Nanomaterials, 13*(7), 1247.

Trevethan, R. (2017). Sensitivity, specificity, and predictive values: Foundations, pliabilities, and pitfalls in research and practice. *Frontiers in Public Health, 5*, 307.

Uddin Khan, S., Atanasova, K. R., Krueger, W. S., Ramirez, A., & Gray, G. C. (2013). Epidemiology, geographical distribution, and economic consequences of swine zoonoses: A narrative review. *Emerging Microbes & Infections, 2*(1), 1–11.

Wang, S., Jiang, H., Qiao, Y., Jiang, S., Lin, H., & Sun, Q. (2022). The research progress of vision-based artificial intelligence in smart pig farming. *Sensors, 22*(17), 6541.

Zhao, N., Lange, E., Kubald, S., Grund, C., Beer, M., & Harder, T. C. (2013). Distinction of subtype-specific antibodies against European porcine influenza viruses by indirect ELISA based on recombinant hemagglutinin protein fragment-1. *Virology Journal, 10*, 1–12.

Biosecurity Measures for Swine Farms and Zoonotic Disease Mitigation

Nitin M. Attupuram, K. Meera, Rajib Deb, and Vivek Kumar Gupta

Abstract

The emergence and incidence of zoonotic pathogens represent a formidable challenge to both the veterinary and public health sectors, particularly in the context of swine husbandry. The chapter delineates critical biosecurity interventions necessary to restrict and control disease transmission within swine production systems, with a special emphasis on zoonotic diseases. A systematic implementation of stringent hygiene protocols, enforced bio-access controls, and the establishment of comprehensive animal health protocols are fundamental components in curtailing the incidence and spread of infectious agents. Additionally, epidemiological surveillance and capacity building regarding biosecurity among stakeholders are indispensable for fortifying farm resilience against zoonotic diseases. The chapter elaborates on the infrastructural requirements and operational biosecurity protocols necessary for effective disease prevention and control. It critically examines potential challenges and constraints in the implementation of these measures, providing a basis for formulating a robust and adaptable biosecurity strategy. These strategies are designed to minimize the risks associated with zoonotic pathogens, thereby enhancing animal health and welfare. Furthermore, they contribute to the economic sustainability of swine farming systems by reducing disease outbreaks, improving productivity, and supporting public health.

Keywords

Biosecurity · Pig health · Swine husbandry · Porcine diseases

---

N. M. Attupuram (✉) · K. Meera · R. Deb · V. K. Gupta
National Research Centre on Pig, Indian Council of Agricultural Research, Guwahati, Assam, India

R. Deb et al. (eds.), *Emerging Zoonotic Threats from Swine*,
https://doi.org/10.1007/978-981-96-7407-7_19

Introduction

The pig, as a domesticated animal, exhibits remarkable anatomical, physiological, and immunological similarities to humans. Given that nearly two-thirds of human pathogens are of animal origin, zoonotic diseases of porcine origin need critical attention. Among zoonoses, some diseases associated with pigs like Japanese encephalitis virus (JEV), hepatitis E virus (HEV), Nipah virus (NiV), Streptococcus suis, Swine influenza virus (SIV), Brucella spp., Leptospira spp., Salmonella spp., Trichinella spiralis, etc. have been reported (Lin et al., 2023; Augustyniak & Pomorska-Mól, 2023). Notably, pigs serve as amplifier hosts for JEV and NiV, which emphasize their zoonotic potential. In recent times, antimicrobial resistance (AMR) has emerged as a significant global public health threat, which also require adequate attention from policymakers and farm administrators. Consequently, preventing disease occurrence in pigs can be identified as the most critical step towards mitigating challenges related to zoonosis, pathogen amplification, and AMR resulting from antibiotic use during a disease outbreak. In this context, implementing biosecurity measures on pig farms represents the most effective and economical solution towards achieving disease prevention. Implementing robust biosecurity measures reduces disease occurrence on farms, improves productivity, and reduces the need for antibiotics.

Biosecurity may be defined as the adoption of a set of management protocols that minimize the risk of disease-causing agents being introduced and spread (FAO, 2010) into a pig farm. Practically, it requires adopting a set of attitudes & behaviours by people and implementation of operational protocols for restricting the entry of disease-causing pathogens into a pig farm and minimize the occurrence of various risk factors. In fact, farm biosecurity is the only proven management strategy to limit, reduce, and remove infectious pathogens from a farm in case of emerging pathogenic outbreaks, especially when vaccines are not available. Two essential elements of farm biosecurity are bio-insulation and bio-containment. Bio-insulation procedures, as the name indicates, insulate the farm from disease outbreaks in nearby farms by minimizing the probability of exposure to pathogens or disease-causing organisms. Bio-containment methods are employed to prevent diseases from spreading from sick animals to healthy ones in a farm and to prevent infectious agents from spilling to other farms or nearby pig sheds.

Significance of Biosecurity

In recent years, the farm managers, veterinarian, and policymakers are increasingly conscious about the vital significance of pig health in relation to the biosecurity, particularly with the diseases such as Porcine Epidemic Diarrhoea and African Swine Fever (Alarcón et al., 2021). The transboundary transmission of emerging and remerging diseases is another major concern. These diseases will continue to pose a serious threat to the livestock industry, farmer livelihoods, food security, and public health as globalization deepens the interconnectedness between nations, economies, and industries (Beltran-Alcrudo et al., 2019). For example, the phylogenetic analysis of the UK isolates of the Foot and Mouth Disease (FMD) epidemic in 2001 showed the greatest similarity to a South African strain (Pharo, 2002), while strains of Porcine Epidemic Diarrhoea (PED) in the United States was reported to have maximum similarity with Chinese strains (Huang et al., 2013). It may also be noted that Classical Swine Fever (Moennig et al., 2003) and African Swine Fever (Zhou et al., 2018) also have transboundary origins.

A general understanding of the risk factors will be of much significance at this point. Most diseases spread through the animal movement, air, pig-derived pork products, semen, manure, embryos, hides, etc. Moreover, fomites such as contaminated vehicles, veterinarians, and clothes of farm staff also play a role in disease transmission. Leakage of suspected biological samples on transit and improper disposal of contaminated carcass are also critical risk factors. The international trade of semen, animals, pork, and feed ingredients, which are potentially contaminated with substantial concentrations of pathogens poses a significant risk for the transboundary transmission of swine diseases through viable pathogens. In fact, the viral particles can persist for several weeks to months in contaminated fomites. Non-existence of a global disease surveillance, traceability, and monitoring system to assess the presence and/or concentrations of pathogens in feed materials is a public health concern (Shurson et al., 2023a, b).

As mentioned earlier, the recent emergence and re-emergence of transboundary and zoonotic diseases underscore the importance of adopting strategies that prioritize "prevention rather than cure." This approach is particularly critical given that vaccines are not available for all diseases, and the use of therapeutic agents can have significant economic implications, as well as adverse effects on production performance. The effective implantation and success of every biosecurity protocols depend on adapting management practices within pig farms to minimize the exposure of both humans and animals to risk factors. This emphasis on behavioural upgradations and farm management is particularly crucial, as human actions are often the underlying cause of most health emergencies in livestock production practices (Beltran-Alcrudo et al., 2019).

Principle of Biosecurity

An underlying principle of epidemiology is that diseases do not occur randomly in a population, but are more likely to happen when a pathogen, a susceptible host, and an environment that facilitates the pathogen-host interaction, occur simultaneously. If the co-occurrence of these three factors simultaneously at a place at a time can be averted, by adopting management measures, the disease can be prevented. "Preventing the exposure of susceptible hosts (pig) to the pathogen by suitable environmental interventions" is the key principle of biosecurity (Attupuram et al., 2023). Thus, biosecurity relies on the interrelated processes of bio-insulation, constant surveillance, and bio-containment. Balaban et al. (2023) rightly pointed out that biosecurity involves implementing a set of organizational and technical measures in order to prevent the introduction, spread and persistence of pathogens. In simple terms it involves measures to reduce the probability of effective transmission, either between farms or within the farm. Biosecurity involves minimizing or diluting the risk factors. Thus, understanding the epidemiology of a specific disease is a key component in devising successful biosecurity protocols (FAO, 2010).

The knowledge of disease epidemiology is an important part is an important part of biosecurity because it helps to understand the complex interactions between disease determinants, and to optimally allocate resources to control infectious diseases. Veterinarians need to have a deep understanding of the risk factors, mitigation strategies, and modes of disease transmission in order to efficiently develop a biosecurity program. According to Alarcón et al. (2021), a farm manager or a veterinarian is supposed to be competent to evaluate biosecurity at all levels and implement customized improvisations, regularly in a farm. It requires knowledge on potential source of infection and disease transmission. An infected animal is the most common source of a disease. In addition to identifying the pathogenic source, comprehensive data on pathogen shedding dynamics, host range, mode of transmission, and associated husbandry practices are critical determinants for effective epidemiological assessment and formulating suitable strategies.

A farm-to-farm transmission occurs through (a) Animal movement from outside, e.g., in the case of finisher farms when new stocks of weaners or growers are brought from breeder farms for rearing purposes, (b) Anthropogenic routes like visitors, animal attendants, or veterinarians who have attended to a diseased animal or animal in carrier status, before entering the farm, (c) Fomites like clothes, shoes, and even vehicle tyres, (d) Contaminated feedstuffs, soiled roughages or Swill feeding, (e) Stray/Wild animals like wild boars, bovines, stray animals, rodents, migratory birds, (f) Ectoparasites like soft ticks of the *Ornithodoros* spp. as in the case of African Swine Fever, (g) Air and water as in the case of Foot and mouth disease, etc.

Within the farm transmission happens through (a) Pig to Pig contact when infected animals act as a potent source of infection to pen mates and pigs of nearby pens, (b) Farm staff: Attendants, who attended infected animals, may carry pathogens through their clothing and utensils, (c) Body fluids like secretions, excretions, semen, etc., of infected animals, (d) Carcass and slaughter wastes of improperly disposed of carcass materials and slaughterhouse wastes are a potent source of infection, (e) Poor shed design resulting in overcrowding, poor ventilation, insufficient space allocation, poor housing plan, and (f) mixing of animals of different age are risk factors favouring the spread of diseases.

Biosecurity Measures

Biosecurity measures in a farm should be designed to maintain external biosecurity to prevent farm-to-farm disease transmission and internal biosecurity to prevent within-the-farm transmission of diseases. The biosecurity measures adaptable at the field level depend on the type of production system (viz., intensive production system or backyard piggery), type of stock maintained (viz., breeder unit or finisher unit), and epidemiological factors. In addition to the practices in a conventional piggery, implementation of biosecurity measures may include infrastructural improvisations, amendments in the farm operation, and imparting training to human resources (Attupuram et al., 2023). Every biosecurity programme requires a regular reassessment of the risks at fixed intervals. This is of much significance as our knowledge of epidemiology of emerging diseases may have important gaps that need to be filled. Another important point is prioritization of the biosecurity measures based on its potential efficacy (Alarcón et al., 2021). This requires precise information on the role of each route of pathogen entry or impact of various risk factors in the transmission of the infection. Moreover, implementation of the selected biosecurity measures should also consider economic, sociological, and even psychological aspects. A comprehensive biosecurity plan ought to be a hierarchy of conceptual, structural, and procedural elements aimed at eliminating the chances of a potential spread of infectious disease not only within and between farms, but also between regions, nations, and continents (Torremorell, 2021).

Conceptual Biosecurity of Animals

Conceptual biosecurity, the primary level of biosecurity, concerns the location of animal facilities and their various components. Location significantly influences the occurrence of disease outbreaks, such as Foot and Mouth Disease (FMD), African Swine Fever, Classical Swine Fever, Swine Enzootic Pneumonia, and Porcine Reproductive and Respiratory Syndrome (Attupuram et al., 2023). Physical isolation is the most effective strategy for risk reduction and should be a key consideration when constructing new farms or confinement facilities. Ideally, facilities should be located away from other farms, public roads, slaughterhouses, live-animal markets, agricultural fairs, or animal exhibits. Isolation measures should also include restricting the use of shared vehicles and facilities, limiting access to personnel not directly involved in operations, and preventing the spread of disease by vermin, wild animals, and wind (Torremorell, 2021). It is important to note that high-density, intensive pig production, either on a single farm or in clusters of nearby farms, poses a greater risk of epidemic outbreaks, particularly those spread through air and water.

Biosecurity Infrastructure

Biosecurity Zones in a Pig Farm

Zoning is the division of farms into separate areas based on the level of biosecurity that is needed to minimize the possibility of pests and diseases from coming onto and moving around the farm. For a pig farm, the tetra-zone biosecurity concept has evolved as a result of efforts to minimize exposure to biological risks. The concept envisages classification into four zones viz., Risk zone, Zone I (entry zone), Zone II (buffer zone), and Zone III (core zone). The area outside the outer perimeter of the farm may be considered a Risk zone, from where most of the biological risks arise. Within the boundaries of the farm area, the entry zone (Zone I) is conditionally open to visitors, and staff and for delivery access. Farmhouses/offices, parking lots/garages, slurry/manure pits, fodder cultivation plots, etc., should be in this area. Roadways for essential vehicles for the on-farm supply of feed, livestock, and fuel and facilities for storage and processing of feed may be located in the buffer zone. Monitored entry is allowed to this area. The change room should be located in the buffer zone. It is preferred that the livestock and feed movement across the separation between the buffer zone and core zone be allowed through loading ramps. Animals will be sheltered in core zone where strict adherence to the biosecurity plan will be implemented.

Layout

The sheds are located inside the core biosecurity zone of a pig farm. The design of a farm is also very important. Overcrowding and poor ventilation resulting in stress render the animal more susceptible to diseases. It should also be noted that older pigs have greater resistance and immunity to diseases than younger pigs. Therefore, the different age groups must be kept separately. The layout of the sheds should be such that boar pens or mating area should be farthest from the entry gate, followed by sow sheds, farrowing sheds, weaner sheds, and grower-finisher sheds in decreasing order of distance from the farm gate. This will reduce the exposure of more precious stock from extrinsic risk factors. Holding pens for market-age pigs should be the nearest to the loading ramp or fence. Loading ramp should facilitate animal movement across the core zone to the buffer zone without entry of vehicles or buyers from outside. The office should be near the loading ramp. This will keep transactions easy with minimum interaction with outsiders (drivers of vehicles or buyers).

Fencing or Boundary Wall

A biosecurity plan requires external perimeter fences and internal fences separating various units of the farm. Pig farms require strong fences that are built close to the ground to prevent animal movement and to provide protection against pests and invaders. Barbed wire along the ground helps prevent rooting. Fences of height 1–1.2 meters will be sufficient for a pig farm. Permanent fences should be well constructed using high-quality materials so they will last a long time with minimum repairs. Fences may be erected with woven wire, barbed wire, electric, or a combination of any of these. In the case of woven wire fences, several horizontal lines of smooth wires will be held apart by vertical wires called stays. Stay wires should be spaced 15 cm apart. Thickness of 12-to-14-gauge size may be used. Barbed wire fences are made of two or more strands of smooth, galvanized-coated, steel wire twisted together with two or four barbs spaced every 10–12 centimetres. Standard barbed wire fences usually have three to five strands of barbed wire stretched between posts that are spaced between 5 and 7 meters apart. Farms located near forest areas can also install electric fences and they can be used for the control of feral and wild animals. It must be well designed and there should be provisions to ensure adequate power for the length of fencing (Attupuram et al., 2023).

Water Supply and Drainages

Drinking water distribution systems within buildings on pig farms have critical elements of their design and management that impact water provision to pigs, water quality, the efficacy of in-water antimicrobial dosing, and, thus, pig health and performance. Similarly, the system of drainages has an important role in securely disposing of the contaminated water/effluents from the sheds. Ensure potable drinking water supply, and avoid chances of mixing with contaminated water. Regular cleaning of pipelines, drinkers, or pans should be included in the operational biosecurity plan. Farm drainages should be designed in such a way that the effluents should flow from more biosecure areas to less biosecure areas. Effluents from the isolation shed/sick animal shed should never be allowed to pass through the healthy animal shed areas.

Foot Dips and Tyre Dips

The tyre washing facility and tyre dip should be located at the farm gate. Tyre dip should have sufficient length to facilitate at least two tyre rotations while passing through it. The width should be more than the width of the road to avoid the chances of bypassing. Depth should be sufficient to facilitate disinfection of all treaded areas of the tyre. A facility for draining off the disinfectant solution should be provided in the dip.

Change Rooms/Anterooms

The location of change rooms should be before reaching up to the core biosecurity area or well before the main shed area. The change room/anteroom plays a critical role in nullifying the contamination from man-material movement. It serves as the single point of entry for all staff, workers, visitors, and others. It should have (a) Structures for an acceptable entry and exit sequence, (b) Provisions for keeping external clothing and personal accessories, (c) Facilities for personal hygiene like toilets, bathrooms, wash basins, etc., (d) Facilities for cleaning and laundering clothing and footwear. A suggestive layout for constructing change room/anteroom for a pig farm is indicated in Fig. 1. Changing rooms may have a definite barrier, which divides the external side of the changing room from the clean farm area. This barrier can be a bench that operators can sit on when applying footwear cover before

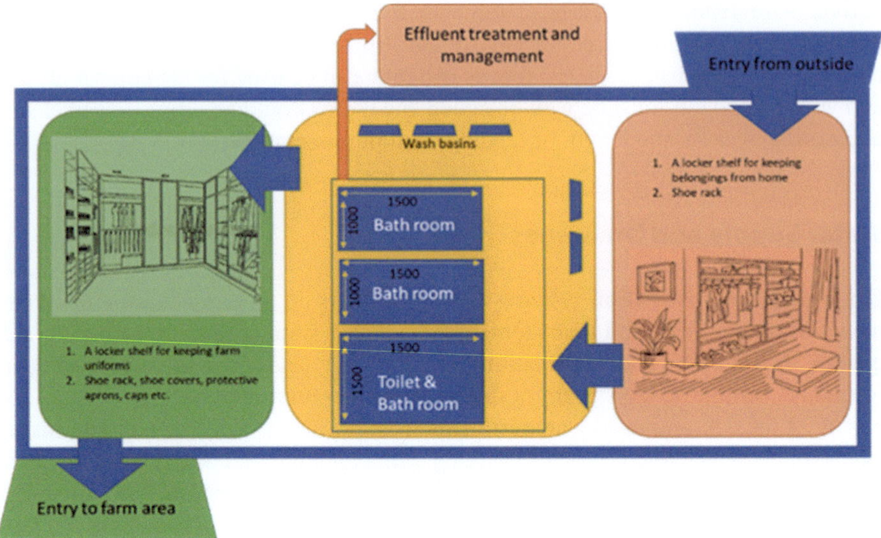

Fig. 1 Layout of a change room

swinging their legs over into the next area. The employees, managers, office staff, veterinarians, and visitors should enter the farm only through the same single entrance after following the same changing and hygiene procedures.

Procedural Biosecurity

Manpower Management

The list of porcine zoonoses having occupational risk for farmers and veterinarians includes Swine influenza, Nipah, Japanese encephalitis, Corona viruses, Erysipelothrix rhusiopathiae, etc. (McLean & Graham, 2022; Augustyniak & Pomorska-Mól, 2023). Conversely, farm personnels and fomites like shoes, clothes, etc., are potential risk factors that can carry various pathogens causing ailments in pigs (Kim et al., 2017; Filippitzi et al., 2018; Hampson & Burrough, 2019). To eliminate this concern, zonal classification of farm areas into various biosecurity zones has been designed which will restrict the manpower movement. In a zone-wise classification system, the farm area will be clearly segregated into clean and dirty areas. Clean areas are those inside the farm perimeter, including all the structures that are in contact with live pigs. While everything outside of the clean areas can be considered a dirty area. Way forward, the clean area may also be further segregated into entry zone, buffer zone and core biosecurity zone based on the expected exposure to risk factors. Work routines must be organized to minimise any movement of farm staff from zones of higher risk zones to cleaner areas. Farm workers are required to take bathe, change into clean clothes, and wear gumboots before entering the pig farm. Separate changing rooms are preferred for storing personal belongings carried from their residence. Veterinary doctors must sanitize instruments which were used on other pig farms. Normally visitors should not be allowed to enter the core biosecurity zone. In conditions that warrant authorization of a farm visit by a visitor, strict adherence to biosecurity protocols is required. Although some reports indicate that the longer viability of pathogens *like Mycoplasma hyopneumoniae* on various surfaces for up to 8 days at 4 °C (Browne et al., 2017), most pathogens are inactivated within 24 h (Kim et al., 2017; Oma et al., 2018). Considering the emerging epidemiology, a window period of 24–48 h to permit entry of a visitor who has a history of previous visit to another farm is recommended (Alarcón et al., 2021). The format for visitors' self-declaration as provided in Table 1 will be useful to assess the biosecurity risk.

Movement of Vehicles

A review of recent literature indicates that truck wheels, driver footwear, clothes, bags, etc., are the most critical biosecurity risk (Galvis et al., 2022; Gebhardt et al., 2022). Farm operations require vehicle movements into the farm area for tasks such as delivering feed, removing manure, and collecting dead animals. Proper infrastructure design, such as positioning feed silos, manure pits, sick animal sheds, and finisher sheds near a perimeter will help to minimize risks of exposure of precious stock to outside. It is always recommended to minimize the number of entry points. Vehicles requiring their delivery up to the farm area may be cautiously and selectively directed to the farm and that too, only after performing the required sanitization procedures. The procedures should include mandatory tyre dipping, pressure washing, disinfectant spraying, etc. If the vehicle has been used for transporting other animals in recent days a thorough disinfection protocol should be initiated. If the truck driver or loading personnels were exposed to any biosecurity risk in the preceding days, the entry of such personnel may be avoided.

Animal Movement

Procurement of replacement stock or new animals is another risk factor causing introduction of diseases to a pig farm (Corzo et al., 2010; Maes et al., 2016). In farms practising external replacements through purchase of replacement stock from other breeder farms, especially the finisher farms, the higher frequency of new entries inflates the probability of pathogen entry. Similarly, if breeding using a male from other farms is practised or the use of semen doses from outside is routinely done, they may also be considered as risk factors for the introduction of pathogens. Internal replacements may be convenient for farms maintaining a closed breeding system and relying on their own males or semen doses. However, internal replacement has limitations in genetic improvement and eradication of endemic diseases.

Table 1 Self-declaration format for visitors at the farm gate

	Farm Biosecurity – Visitor's Declaration		
1	Have you visited any farms, livestock premises, livestock fairs and abattoirs during the last 7 days	Yes	No
2	Are you rearing any animals in my home (Yes/No)		
	If yes, do your herd have any incidence of diseases during the past 30 days	Yes	No
3	Has your vehicle/equipment contacted livestock or materials of animal origin during the last 7 days	Yes	No
4	Have you visited or travelled any overseas country in the past 30 days	Yes	No
5	If Yes, did you visit any livestock farm or abattoir or livestock fairs during the overseas travel	Yes	No

I declare that the information provided above are true to the best of my knowledge.

Signature
Name

Details of the visitor:
Contact number:
In time :
Out time:
Purpose of visit:

Instruction

Visitors who answered "Yes" to any of the above questions may be redirected to the farm manager for assessment of the biosecurity risks associated with their entry.

(Adopted from Attupuram *et al.*, 2023)

For procurement of replacements, the biosecurity measure should invariably include disease testing based on a list that classifies diseases based on the risk they pose to the farm. This will help the farm manager to discard the stock at the supplier's end itself (Alarcón et al., 2021), if the animal is infected. The following points need to be followed during the procurement of replacement stock. (1) All purchases should be made from a quality-assured reliable source; (2) Procure vaccinated stock, if possible; (3) Perform disease testing; (4) New stock may be purchased from the same source rather than sourcing from multiple or unknown vendors; (5) Request records of treatments, vaccinations etc.; (6) Obtain a health certification by an authorized veterinarian at the source; and (7) Ensure comfort and welfare throughout the transportation of pigs.

Quarantine

Quarantine facilities must be designed as bio-containment units to prevent the spillover of pathogens from incoming animals (Alarcón et al., 2021). The quarantine involves the isolation and acclimatization of incoming stock from other animals on the farm. This process entails isolating and acclimatizing incoming stock to prevent disease spread, as pathogens may remain asymptomatic during their incubation period (Attupuram et al., 2023). During this time, vaccination against endemic diseases, deworming, and testing for infections such as African swine fever (ASF), brucellosis, porcine circovirus type 2 (PCV2), porcine reproductive and respiratory syndrome (PRRS), and porcine parvovirus (PPV) may be performed. Animal management in the quarantine facility requires maintaining strict separation between the main herd and quarantined animals to prevent disease transmission. Ideally, the quarantine shed/sty should be situated at least 1000 meters away from the main pig farm (Alarcón et al., 2021). This is considered a safe distance for most pathogens and for transmission by rodents, flies, etc. (Desrosiers, 2011). However, pathogens causing diseases such as foot and mouth disease virus, aujeszky's disease virus, *Mycoplasma hyopneumoniae*, porcine reproductive and respiratory virus 2 (PRRSV2), etc., can potentially be transmitted by air to even longer distances (Christensen et al., 1990; Otake et al., 2010).

The duration of the quarantine depends on the incubation period of the diseases concerned, the duration of the contagious period for such diseases, and the time needed to establish a diagnosis (Dewulf & Van Immerseel, 2019). In any case the quarantined animals must be retained for a minimum of 21 days. During this period, disease testing, vaccinations, and deworming must be performed, and animals should be monitored for any signs of illness. Implementing an all-in, all-out strategy will ensure that new animals are grouped together while purchase to facilitate uniform entry and are moved out collectively at the end of the quarantine period. This will enable adherence to proper disinfection protocols between the quarantine cycles. Staff should use separate clothing and equipment to reduce contamination risks. Effective labour management in a quarantine facility necessitates the establishment of a controlled access point equipped with footbaths and hand-washing facilities. Entry should be restricted to authorized personnel only, with proper records maintenance.

Feed Supply

The major swine viruses of concern for potential transmission through global feed supply chains are classical swine fever virus (Kim et al., 2008), African swine fever virus (Gebhardt et al., 2022), Seneca Valley A virus, porcine respiratory and reproductive syndrome virus (Leme et al., 2019; Dee et al., 2022), and foot and mouth disease virus. Biosecurity protocols for feed supply chains are often overlooked in most biosecurity plans, despite the fact that feed constitutes a significant external input. It carries an inherent risk for pathogen contamination and transmission to pig populations (Shurson et al., 2023a, b). Cochrane et al. (2016) outlined essential components for developing biosecurity plans for feed mills. Their methodology involved (1) hazard analysis: identifying and evaluating potential hazards in process steps used in the production of feed ingredients; (2) hazard mitigation: steps to prevent hazard entry during receiving, entry due to people, feed loading and delivery;

(3) use of thermal treatment; and (4) use of approved chemical treatments such as formaldehyde, essential oils, and medium-chain fatty acids. Several studies have identified truck wheels, driver footwear, clothes, bags, etc., as the primary routes of pathogen transmission related to feed (Bowman et al., 2015; Gebhardt et al., 2022; Galvis et al., 2022). Therefore, the cleaning and disinfection of trucks and trailers utilized for transporting pigs and feed between loads should be integral components of biosecurity protocols within the feed supply chain.

The standard operating procedure for feed-biosecurity and surveillance programs should also take note on the ingredient sourcing, receiving, processing, and storage. Key actions for implementing biosecurity into practice in feed production facilities were delineated by Shurson et al. (2023a, b): (1) Ensure that suppliers of feed ingredients adhere to safety and quality standards thorough auditing and verification; (2) Establish personal hygiene protocols for employees, visitors and truck drivers entering the facility; (3) Implement routine housekeeping practices that effectively minimize pathogen risks; (4) Cleaning and disinfection protocols for facilities; (5) Keep records of storage conditions and duration for each lot of feed ingredient; and (6) Conduct regular training and regular upgradation through the adoption of corrective measures.

Most small-scale low-input pig production systems rely on food waste/refuse or agro by-products especially in geographical areas where majority of pig farmers are located and hence guidelines should address the biosecurity measures concerning the use of non-conventional nutritional sources of plant or animal origin. Moreover, in the process of up-scaling the food wastes into high-quality animal protein, pig husbandry could be a game changer (Shurson et al., 2023a, b). The potential pathogen transmission associated with byproduct feeding requires specific biosecurity interventions. While some nations prohibit feeding of food waste containing meat of animal origin, several countries have established legal frameworks to facilitate the recycling of biomass, including kitchen and animal waste, into animal protein through pork production. For example, Japan's Promotion of Utilization of Recyclable Food Waste Act permits the recycling of food waste for animal feed, while South Korea's Wastes Control Act (Ministry of Environment, 2010) and the Control of Livestock and Fish Feed Act (Ministry of Agriculture, Food, and Rural Affairs, 2010) authorize the recycling of all food waste as animal feed. A comprehensive biosecurity plan should include mandatory pretreatment protocols to effectively inactivate potential pathogens in these materials. Research indicates that food waste containing meat is safe for animal consumption if heated to 70 °C for 30 min or 80 °C for 3 min (Sugiura et al., 2009).

Water Supply

Leptospirosis and other diseases associated with fecal-oral transmission cycles can be transmitted through drinking water used on farms (Losinger et al., 1998). All water sources must be safeguarded from places where manure and carcasses of animals are disposed of. Water tanks and troughs should be cleaned on a regular basis since biofilm can harbour bacteria that can infect pigs (Dewulf & Van Immerseel, 2019). Furthermore, water tanks must be disinfected at least twice a year, and the water's bacteriological quality must be examined at least once a year (Roman et al. 2006). According to Silva et al. (2018), source water treatment is a crucial instrument for the management of risks associated with herd health.

Biosecurity During Outbreaks

Once an infectious aetiology is identified in a pig farm, effective measures to control the spread of disease from infected to healthy animals is a crucial step. At that juncture, a farm manager should promptly initiate biosecurity measures for bio-containment. The first line of intervention is segregation, followed by cleaning and disinfection. Briefly, segregation involves the isolation of an infected animal, while cleaning aims at removal of all contagious materials in the shed. Disinfection will be done to eliminate all the pathogens that adhere on the surfaces. The instant at which a diseased animal has been identified; it is highly advisable to invoke the standard operation plan for a disease contingency with stern adherence strictly followed. Ensure to segregate the unhealthy animal. Alert the veterinarian in charge of the farm within no time to assure early treatment and monitor animals in close contact. Proceed to initiate a comprehensive cleaning and disinfection drive within the pig farm, including all relevant areas, animal sheds, premises, equipment, and personal protective clothing. All these measures are meant to ensure that the health of the whole herd population is protected and to prevent further spread of the disease.

Discharge materials, effluents, or faecal discharge from the sick animals and also from the nearby sites must be disposed of separately. The disposal method should take an account of the possible options to completely eliminate the potential of its exposure to healthy animals. Sick animals may be moved to isolation sheds, if the condition warrants. In those conditions, biosecurity in the isolation shed should also be maintained: (1) disinfecting foot baths at entry point, (2) separate farm uniforms/dress for workers with personal protective apparels, (3) all utensils of isolation shed may be exclusively used for the purpose only, and (4) all wastes must be properly disposed of. Ideally, dedicated attendants may be assigned to isolation sheds, depending upon the availability of manpower. In the absence of such dedicated attendants, the isolated animals may be attended after all healthy animals have been attended to, thus preventing the chances of pathogen spillover through farm attendants. Isolated pigs must remain housed in isolation sheds for at least 21 days. Disinfection and cleaning are major activities to decrease the pathogen load and prevent the transmission of disease.

Once sick animals are moved to isolation shed, the cleaning and disinfection of normal sty where they stayed before is also desired. Overall disinfection of the premises and materials needs to be done. Dispose of manure, feeds, and wastes by burial or through incineration. Thoroughly scrape the floors and other equipment before proceeding to spraying the disinfectant. Spraying disinfectants including 2% sodium hypochlorite are effective over contaminated surfaces. For liquid wastes such as blood or urine, a 30% suspension of chloride of lime is adequate. Equipment should also be submerged in a 2% sodium hypochlorite solution for 48 hours, and metal structures can be disinfected with a flame gun. Vehicles entering the affected areas must be disinfected using the appropriate chemical agents, and all personnel must observe strict hygiene measures, including hand and foot washing with approved disinfectants. Direct application of disinfectants to animals should only be practised when the disinfectant is specifically labelled for that purpose.

Evaluation of Farm Biosecurity

Every biosecurity plan requires constant upgradation at regular intervals. Several biosecurity evaluation systems have been developed to finetune the existing biosecurity programme by identifying the loopholes. Assessing biosecurity includes collection of information on biosecurity practices using questionnaires that evaluate the external and internal biosecurity measures. Ghent University developed the Biocheck.UGent™ biosecurity scoring system where biosecurity practice is recorded and multiplied by a weight factor which is fixed according to their relative significance, thus arriving at a risk-based weighted scoring of the biosecurity protocol in a farm (Gelaude et al., 2014). BioAsseT is a similar biosecurity assessment tool (Sasaki et al., 2020). Swine Sureksha App and Biosecurity Integrity Assessment Score Sheet are also questionnaire-based direct scoring system to evaluate biosecurity integrity in pig farms, which are designed to deliver tailored advisories for optimization of biosecurity practises (Atttupuram et al., 2023). Interestingly, some researches applied statistical methods to develop biosecurity scores based on the rank of biosecurity practices according to their importance. For example, Zang et al. (2012) used a multi-criteria Decision Analysis (MCDA), a method that assesses the relative importance of biosecurity practices by pair-wise comparison of measures in order to estimate how many times more important is one measure in relation to other. Silva et al. (2018) used the item response theory in their effort to develop a general biosecurity scoring system suited to pig farms and the biosecurity vulnerability scores for PRRS. Such evaluations often pinpoint the possible biosecurity breaches, like the findings of Silva et al. (2018) which suggested that events related to pathogen transmission by water and air, and by animal and human movements should be prioritized in pig husbandry.

Conclusion

The pressure to combat emerging, re-emerging, and transboundary diseases has reinforced biosecurity as the most effective protective measure in pig farming. As biosecurity becomes integral to farm operations, developing a sustainable and effective biosecurity plan demands continual optimization and strategic allocation of resources. A deeper understanding of pig disease epidemiology will further enhance the design of these programs. Routine evaluation and upgradation of biosecurity protocols by addressing vulnerabilities in current systems are crucial to ensuring their long-term success and resilience in disease prevention.

References

Alarcón, L. V., Allepuz, A., & Mateu, E. (2021). Biosecurity in pig farms: A review. *Porcine Health Management, 7*, 5. https://doi.org/10.1186/s40813-020-00181-z

Attupuram, N. M., Pegu, S. R., De, K., Das, P. J., Meera, K., Thomas, R., Islam, R., Deb, R., Doley, J., Paul, S., Rajkhowa, S., & Gupta, V. K. (2023). *Package of practices: Biosecurity measures in pig production* (1st ed.). ICAR-National Research Centre on Pig.

Augustyniak, A., & Pomorska-Mól, M. (2023). An update in knowledge of pigs as the source of zoonotic pathogens. *Animals, 13*(20), 3281. https://doi.org/10.3390/ani13203281

Balaban, A., Ştefan, G., & Bărăităreanu, S. (2023). Biosecurity measures to prevent African swine fever in pig fattening farms. *Practica Veterinara, 4*, 50–52.

Beltran-Alcrudo, D., Falco, J. R., & Raizman, E. (2019). Transboundary spread of pig diseases: The role of international trade and travel. *BMC Veterinary Research, 15*, 64. https://doi.org/10.1186/s12917-019-1800-5

Bowman, A. S., Krogwold, R. A., Price, T., Davis, M., & Moeller, S. J. (2015). Investigating the introduction of porcine epidemic diarrhea virus into an Ohio swine operation. *BMC Veterinary Research, 11*, 1–7.

Browne, C., Loeffler, A., Holt, H. R., Chang, Y. M., Lloyd, D. H., & Nevel, A. (2017). Low temperature and dust favour in vitro survival of mycoplasma hyopneumoniae: Time to revisit indirect transmission in pig housing. *Letters in Applied Microbiology, 64*(1), 2–7.

Christensen, L. S., Mousing, J., Mortensen, S., Soerensen, K. J., Strandbygaard, S. B., Henriksen, C. A., & Andersen, J. B. (1990). Evidence of long distance airborne transmission of Aujeszky's disease (pseudorabies) virus. *The Veterinary Record, 127*(19), 471–474.

Cochrane, R. A., Dritz, S. S., Woodworth, J. C., Stark, C. R., Huss, A. R., Cano, J. P., & Jones, C. K. (2016). Feed mill biosecurity plans: A systematic approach to prevent biological pathogens in swine feed. *Journal of Swine Health and Production, 24*(3), 154–164.

Corzo, C. A., Mondaca, E., Wayne, S., Torremorell, M., Dee, S., Davies, P., & Morrison, R. B. (2010). Control and elimination of porcine reproductive and respiratory syndrome virus. *Virus Research, 154*(1–2), 185–192.

Dee, S., Havas, K., & Spronk, G. (2022). Detection of Senecavirus A in pigs from a historically negative national swine herd and associated with feed imports from endemically infected countries. *Transboundary and Emerging Diseases, 69*(6), 3147.

Desrosiers, R. (2011). Transmission of swine pathogens: Different means, different needs. *Animal Health Research Reviews, 12*(1), 1–13.

Dewulf, J., & Van Immerseel, F. (Eds.). (2019). *Biosecurity in animal production and veterinary medicine*. CAB International.

FAO, Food and Agriculture Organization of the United Nation. (2010). Good practices for biosecurity in the pig sector – Issues and options in developing and transition countries. FAO Animal Production and Health Paper No. 169. Rome, FAO

Filippitzi, M. E., Brinch Kruse, A., Postma, M., Sarrazin, S., Maes, D., Alban, L., & Dewulf, J. (2018). Review of transmission routes of 24 infectious diseases preventable by biosecurity measures and comparison of the implementation of these measures in pig herds in six European countries. *Transboundary and Emerging Diseases, 65*(2), 381–398.

Galvis, J. A., Corzo, C. A., & Machado, G. (2022). Modelling and assessing additional transmission routes for porcine reproductive and respiratory syndrome virus: Vehicle movements and feed ingredients. *Transboundary and Emerging Diseases, 69*(5), e1549–e1560.

Gebhardt, J. T., Dritz, S. S., Elijah, C. G., Jones, C. K., Paulk, C. B., & Woodworth, J. C. (2022). Sampling and detection of African swine fever virus within a feed manufacturing and swine production system

Gelaude, P., Schlepers, M., Verlinden, M., Laanen, M., & Dewulf, J. (2014). Biocheck. UGent: A quantitative tool to measure biosecurity at broiler farms and the relationship with technical performances and antimicrobial use. *Poultry Science, 93*(11), 2740–2751.

Hampson, D. J., & Burrough, E. R. (2019). Swine dysentery and Brachyspiral colitis. In *Diseases of swine* (pp. 951–970).

Huang, Y. W., Dickerman, A. W., Pineyro, P., Li, L., Fang, L., Kiehne, R., & Meng, X. J. (2013). Origin, evolution, and genotyping of emergent porcine epidemic diarrhea virus strains in the United States. *MBio, 4*(5), e00737–e00713.

Kim, B., Song, J. Y., Tark, D. S., Lim, S. I., Choi, E. J., Kim, J., & Kang, M. I. (2008). Feed contaminated with classical swine fever vaccine virus (LOM strain) can induce antibodies to the virus in pigs. *Veterinary Record, 162*(1), 12–17.

Kim, Y., Yang, M., Goyal, S. M., Cheeran, M. C., & Torremorell, M. (2017). Evaluation of biosecurity measures to prevent indirect transmission of porcine epidemic diarrhea virus. *BMC Veterinary Research, 13*, 1–9.

Leme, R. A., Miyabe, F. M., Dall Agnol, A. M., Alfieri, A. F., & Alfieri, A. A. (2019). Seneca Valley virus RNA detection in pig feed and feed ingredients in Brazil. *Transboundary and Emerging Diseases, 66*(4), 1449–1453.

Lin, C. N., Okabayashi, T., Tummaruk, P., & Ooi, P. T. (2023). Editorial: Zoonotic diseases among pigs. *Frontiers in Veterinary Science, 9*, 1122679. https://doi.org/10.3389/fvets.2022.1122679

Losinger, W. C., Bush, E. J., Hill, G. W., Smith, M. A., Garber, L. P., Rodriguez, J. M., & Kane, G. (1998). Design and implementation of the United States national animal health monitoring system 1995 national swine study. *Preventive Veterinary Medicine, 34*(2–3), 147–159.

Maes, D., Van Soom, A., Appeltant, R., Arsenakis, I., & Nauwynck, H. (2016). Porcine semen as a vector for transmission of viral pathogens. *Theriogenology, 85*(1), 27–38.

McLean, R. K., & Graham, S. P. (2022). The pig as an amplifying host for new and emerging zoonotic viruses. *One Health, 14*, 100384.

Moennig, V., Floegel-Niesmann, G., & Greiser-Wilke, I. J. T. V. J. (2003). Clinical signs and epidemiology of classical swine fever: A review of new knowledge. *The Veterinary Journal, 165*(1), 11–20.

Oma, V. S., Klem, T., Tråvén, M., Alenius, S., Gjerset, B., Myrmel, M., & Stokstad, M. (2018). Temporary carriage of bovine coronavirus and bovine respiratory syncytial virus by fomites and human nasal mucosa after exposure to infected calves. *BMC Veterinary Research, 14*, 1–8.

Otake, S., Dee, S., Corzo, C., Oliveira, S., & Deen, J. (2010). Long-distance airborne transport of infectious PRRSV and mycoplasma hyopneumoniae from a swine population infected with multiple viral variants. *Veterinary Microbiology, 145*(3–4), 198–208.

Pharo, H. J. (2002). Foot-and-mouth disease: An assessment of the risks facing New Zealand. *New Zealand Veterinary Journal, 50*(2), 46–55.

Roman, A. V., Lukešová, D., Novak, P., & Žižlavský, M. (2006). Biosecurity in pig breeding herds. *Agricultura Tropica et Subtropica, 39*, 120–123.

Sasaki, Y., Furutani, A., Furuichi, T., Hayakawa, Y., Ishizeki, S., Kano, R., & Otake, S. (2020). Development of a biosecurity assessment tool and the assessment of biosecurity levels by this tool on Japanese commercial swine farms. *Preventive Veterinary Medicine, 175*, 104848.

Shurson, G. C., Dierenfeld, E. S., & Dou, Z. (2023a). Rules are meant to be broken–rethinking the regulations on the use of food waste as animal feed. *Resources, Conservation and Recycling, 199*, 107273.

Shurson, G. C., Urriola, P. E., & Schroeder, D. C. (2023b). Biosecurity and mitigation strategies to control swine viruses in feed ingredients and complete feeds. *Animals, 13*(14), 2375.

Silva, G. S., Corbellini, L. G., Linhares, D. L., Baker, K. L., & Holtkamp, D. J. (2018). Development and validation of a scoring system to assess the relative vulnerability of swine breeding herds to the introduction of PRRS virus. *Preventive Veterinary Medicine, 160*, 116–122.

Sugiura, K., Yamatani, S., Watahara, M., & Onodera, T. (2009). Ecofeed, animal feed produced from recycled food waste. *Veterinaria Italiana, 45*(3), 397–404.

Torremorell, M. (2021). The three levels of biosecurity of animals. MSD Veterinary Manual. https://www.msdvetmanual.com/public-health/biosecurity/the-three-levels-of-biosecurity-of-animals. Assessed on 12 Mar 2024

Zang, Y. T., Tan, Y. P., Hu, Y. N., & Lu, C. H. (2012). Construction of index system for external risk factors of disease on large-scale farm based on the analytic hierarchy process. *Procedia Engineering, 37*, 274–280.

Zhou, X., Li, N., Luo, Y., Liu, Y. E., Miao, F., et al. (2018). Emergence of African swine fever in China, 2018. *Transboundary and Emerging Diseases, 65*(6), 1482–1484.

Risk Communication and Education: Raising Awareness About Swine Zoonoses

Shruti Shaurya and Abhishek Pathak

Abstract

Swine zoonoses are the diseases which are transmissible from pigs to humans. They are a major global public health concern due to their potential to cause widespread illness, especially in regions of frequent human-pig interaction. These zoonotic diseases like Swine Influenza, Brucellosis, and Trichinosis can have severe health consequences and significant socio-economic impacts. Communicating risks and educating the public about these diseases are crucial to prevent their transmission and outbreaks. Swine influenza has been responsible for several human pandemics, while Brucellosis remains a resolute problem in parts of Europe, Asia, and Africa. Trichinosis, though less common today, still poses a threat in areas where traditional pork consumption practices are prevalent. A variety of risk communication and educational strategies along with community engagement have been employed to combat these zoonotic diseases. Educating the public and encouraging preventative measures can reduce the transmission of these diseases and protect human and animal health.

Keywords

Education · Public health · Risk Communication · Swine Zoonoses

S. Shaurya
Division of Medicine, ICAR-Indian Veterinary Research Institute, Izatnagar, UP, India

A. Pathak (✉)
Department of Veterinary Pharmacology & Toxicology, MJF College of Veterinary & Animal Sciences, Jaipur, Rajasthan, India

R. Deb et al. (eds.), *Emerging Zoonotic Threats from Swine*,
https://doi.org/10.1007/978-981-96-7407-7_20

Introduction

Swine zoonoses are the diseases which are transmissible from pigs to humans. These zoonotic diseases pose significant public health risks due to the close interactions between humans and pigs, especially in the farming environments. The zoonotic pathogens can be transmitted from pigs to humans through direct contact, ingestion of contaminated pork products, or indirect contact via environmental exposure (Centers for Disease Control and Prevention, 2018). The global burden of zoonotic diseases, in particular those linked to the livestock like pigs, punctuates the critical importance of effective risk communication and educational strategies.

One of the most well-known swine zoonoses is Swine influenza, a respiratory disease caused by influenza A viruses. Swine influenza viruses can occasionally infect humans, leading to outbreaks of ailment, as seen in the 2009 H1N1 pandemic (Karabatsos et al., 2009). This interspecies transmission underscores the importance of monitoring and controlling influenza viruses in pig populations to prevent future pandemics (Webster et al., 1992).

In addition to the viral zoonoses, bacterial infections such as Brucellosis, Leptospirosis, and Salmonellosis are concerning as well. Leptospirosis, caused by bacteria of the genus Leptospira, can be transmitted from pigs to humans by contact with contaminated water or soil (Ganter, 2015). Salmonellosis, caused by Salmonella spp., is often connected to the consumption of contaminated pork products, highlighting the need for strict food safety measures (Clifford & Morton, 2019).

Swine trichinosis, a zoonotic disease, is caused by consuming undercooked or raw pork containing the nematode parasite *Trichinella spiralis* larvae. These larvae invade human muscle tissues, leading to symptoms like gastrointestinal distress, muscle pain, and severe neurological issues. The disease is common in areas where raw or undercooked pork is traditionally consumed (Centers for Disease Control and Prevention, 2018). Prevention involves proper cooking practices to eliminate the larvae (Clifford & Morton, 2019). However, cultural practices and global pork trade complicate control efforts, underscoring the need for public education and rigorous pork industry monitoring (Brookes et al., 2014; Ganter, 2015).

Changes in farming practices, environmental changes, and globalization all contribute to the emergence and spread of swine zoonoses (Brookes et al., 2014). At the human-animal-environment interface, it is critical to improve biosecurity, surveillance, and public health measures to reduce the hazards associated with swine zoonoses (Gibbs & Anderson, 2009; Balbus & Malina, 2009).

Public awareness campaigns and educational programs are vital tools in preventing the spread of these diseases by informing the at-risk populations about transmission modes, symptoms, and preventive measures (Greger, 2007). During the 2009 H1N1 pandemic, public health authorities used extensive communication campaigns to educate the public on the virus, its transmission, and preventive actions like vaccination and better hygiene practices, which played a crucial role in controlling the spread of virus (Smith, 2009).

However, the effectiveness of these communication strategies can significantly vary across different geographical regions due to cultural differences, health literacy levels, and access to reliable information. In many low- and middle-income countries, where resources are limited and with inadequate healthcare infrastructure, the dissemination of accurate and timely information about swine zoonoses presents a considerable challenge (Kleczkowski et al., 2015). Traditional communication channels such as radios and communal meetings may be more effective than digital platforms, which require internet access and a certain level of digital literacy (Paton & McLaughlin, 2008).

What people think and do about the risk of zoonotic illnesses is greatly influenced by cultural practices and beliefs. There are certain cultures where pigs are regarded as dirty or suspicious, which can cause stigma and make people reluctant to consult doctors or report illnesses (MacLachlan et al., 2007). Misunderstandings exist in certain regions of Sub-Saharan Africa regarding the origins of illnesses such as Brucellosis, which impede the efficacy of public health measures (Mutua et al., 2011). A balanced strategy that honors regional customs and delivers factual, scientific knowledge is needed to overcome these cultural obstacles. The public's knowledge of swine zoonoses can be improved by addressing these obstacles and utilizing culturally appropriate communications in conjunction with community leaders (Brookes et al., 2014).

Another major obstacle to risk communication is misinformation, especially in the social media age when inaccurate or misleading information can spread quickly. Misinformation regarding the origins of the virus and the safety of vaccines caused uncertainty and reluctance among the public during the H1N1 pandemic in certain localities (VanderWaal & Deen, 2018). Public health officials need to be proactive in dispelling false information by using precise, unified messaging across all media. This entails dispelling myths and educating the public in advance about swine zoonoses in addition to responding to untrue allegations (Bibard et al., 2024).

Utilizing a variety of communication channels and tactics, a multifaceted strategy is necessary to improve the efficacy of risk communication and education initiatives. It is still essential to use mass media, such as radio, television, and internet platforms, to provide timely and reliable information to large audiences (Brookes et al., 2014). At times of outbreak, media outlets can disseminate information on preventive measures, public health recommendations, and outbreak updates. The efficacy of mass media campaigns, however, may be diminished if community-based interventions are not also implemented (Fasina et al., 2012).

Digital channels, especially in urban and technologically advanced areas, present new avenues for risk communication in addition to traditional means. Real-time information sharing and interactive engagement between public health authorities and the public are facilitated by social media, websites, and mobile applications (Martinez-Lopez et al., 2009). The target audience's accessibility and level of digital knowledge, however, determine how effective digital communication is. In order to make vital information accessible to all sectors of the population, including those with limited internet connection or technical abilities, efforts should be taken to ensure that digital tools are user-friendly (Paton & McLaughlin, 2008).

Public health authorities can improve their efforts to curb the spread of these zoonotic illnesses by incorporating digital platforms, mass media, community participation, and tackling cultural obstacles and disinformation. In the constantly shifting field of global health, communication tactics must be evaluated and adjusted on a regular basis to maintain their efficacy.

Swine Zoonoses: Transmission Mechanisms, Signs, and Health Consequences

Swine zoonoses are naturally transmitted from pigs to humans and can pose serious health concerns to the population, especially in locations where human-livestock contacts are frequent. These zoonotic illnesses, which can affect people as well as pigs, might be parasitic, bacterial, or viral in origin. They can have a serious negative impact on health. To effectively prevent and control swine zoonoses, it is imperative to comprehend their transmission mechanisms, symptoms, and effects.

Swine Influenza

Influenza A is the virus that causes swine influenza, a respiratory illness that affects both humans and pigs. Given that this zoonosis has the potential to spread like a pandemic—as evidenced by the 2009 H1N1 influenza outbreak—it is especially worrying. When pigs or humans with the virus cough or sneeze, the virus is released into the air and spreads throughout the environment, mainly by airborne droplets. Additionally, direct contact with pigs that have the virus or contaminated surfaces can expose humans to it (Choi et al., 2003; Ellison et al., 2016).

Swine influenza commonly causes fever, coughing, sore throats, body aches, and exhaustion in humans, these symptoms are similar to those of seasonal influenza. When it gets serious, it can cause pneumonia, respiratory failure, or even death. People with compromised immune systems or underlying medical disorders are more susceptible to this (Centers for Disease Control and Prevention, 2018). Pigs affected by the disease may experience abrupt fever, coughing, nasal discharge, and lethargic behavior. Due to lower growth rates, higher veterinary expenses, and decreased productivity, swine influenza can have a major negative effect on the swine business (Karabatsos et al., 2009).

The influenza virus's propagation between species and the ability of a virus to engage in genetic reassortment facilitate the creation of novel strains that carry the potential to spread globally. This emphasizes how crucial it is to keep an eye on influenza viruses in swine and human populations in order to identify and contain possible outbreaks (Webster et al., 1992).

Swine Brucellosis

Brucella species, mainly *Brucella suis* in pigs, is the source of the bacterial zoonosis known as brucellosis. Because they frequently come into touch with sick animals, farmers, veterinarians, and workers in slaughterhouses are particularly vulnerable to contracting the disease, which is endemic in many regions of the world. Direct contact with infected animals or their bodily fluids, such as blood, urine, or reproductive secretions, is the means by which Brucellosis is spread. Human infection can potentially result from consuming tainted animal products, especially unpasteurized milk (Centers for Disease Control and Prevention, 2018; Díaz, 2019).

Numerous nonspecific symptoms, such as fever, sweating, joint pain, muscular aches, and exhaustion, are indicative of human brucellosis. If left untreated, the illness can become chronic and result in more serious side effects including arthritis, endocarditis, and neurological issues. Brucellosis mostly affects the reproductive system in pigs, leading to lower litter sizes, abortions, and stillbirths. Due to decreased reproductive efficiency and the need to cull diseased animals, the presence of Brucellosis in a swine herd can result in severe economic losses (Gibbs, 2005).

A comprehensive strategy is needed to control and prevent Brucellosis, which includes immunizing livestock, regularly testing and eliminating affected animals, and enforcing stringent biosecurity protocols on farms. Public health education programs are also necessary to encourage safe handling techniques among individuals who may be exposed to Brucellosis and to increase awareness of the disease's hazards (Brookes et al., 2014).

Swine Trichinosis

Consumption of raw or undercooked pork that contains the infectious larvae of the worm *Trichinella spiralis* can expose people to the parasitic zoonosis known as trichinosis. According to the Centers for Disease Control and Prevention (2018), the disease is particularly common in areas where consuming raw or undercooked pork products, such as sausages and cured meats, is a customary culinary habit.

Following ingestion, the larvae leave their stomach cysts and go into the intestines, where they develop into adult worms. The female worms give birth to larvae that eventually migrate to muscle tissues where they encyst after passing through the intestinal wall and into the bloodstream. Depending on how many larvae are consumed and the stage of the illness, different people have different symptoms of trichinosis. In the early stages, there are gastrointestinal distress symptoms including nausea, vomiting, and diarrhea. These are followed by fever, facial swelling, muscle discomfort, and in more serious cases, brain problems such as meningitis or encephalitis (Díaz, 2019; Clifford & Morton, 2019).

Trichinosis in pigs is commonly undetected because, in cases of mild illness, afflicted pigs may not exhibit any clinical symptoms. Pigs may, however, display symptoms like diminished weight gain, weakness, and stiffness in their muscles in extreme cases. Due to the serious health risk that Trichinella larvae provide in pork, the pig industry is required to implement stringent controls, such as routine testing and inspection of meat products and public education about safe cooking techniques (Ganter, 2015; Brookes et al., 2014).

Swine Salmonellosis

Salmonella bacteria are the cause of swine salmonellosis, and humans can contract the infection by eating contaminated pork or by coming into close contact with sick pigs. Salmonella may persist in a range of environmental circumstances, making it difficult to control the disease, which makes it more problematic. Human cases of salmonellosis usually present with fever, cramping in the abdomen, and diarrhea. Dehydration may result from severe cases, particularly in small infants, the elderly, and people with impaired immune systems (Centers for Disease Control and Prevention, 2018; Brookes et al., 2014).

Pigs infected with Salmonellosis may present with a variety of symptoms, ranging from carriers who show no signs to severe enteritis, septicemia, and fatality. A serious risk to the public's health exists when Salmonella is found in swine herds, particularly when it comes to foodborne transmission. Strict pig farming hygiene regulations, routine surveillance, and thorough cooking of pork products to eradicate the germs are all necessary to stop the spread of salmonellosis (Clifford & Morton, 2019).

Swine Leptospirosis

Leptospira pomona are the cause of swine leptospirosis, a bacterial zoonosis that affects both humans and pigs. Usually, the bacteria are spread by direct contact with polluted water, soil, or the urine of diseased animals. Leptospirosis in people can manifest as a variety of symptoms, ranging from minor flu-like symptoms to serious illnesses like renal impairment, liver failure, and respiratory distress. Leptospirosis can cause jaundice, fever, and renal failure in pigs, as well as reproductive failures such as miscarriages and stillbirths (Centers for Disease Control and Prevention, 2018; Ganter, 2015).

In tropical and subtropical areas, where the conditions favor the bacteria's survival and spread, leptospirosis is more common. Enhancing sanitation, managing rodent populations—which are frequent carriers of leptospirosis—and immunizing livestock are all necessary for effective leptospirosis control (Clifford & Morton, 2019).

Transmission Mechanisms of Swine Zoonoses

Pork zoonoses can spread through a number of routes, such as direct contact, foodborne, and airborne contact. To reduce the danger of zoonotic disease outbreaks and design targeted preventative methods, it is imperative to comprehend different mechanisms of transmission.

1. Direct Contact: Direct contact with diseased animals or their bodily fluids is a typical way for diseases like leptospirosis and brucellosis to spread. Workers in slaughterhouses, veterinary clinics, and farms are more likely to have these illnesses. Wearing protective clothing, maintaining proper hygiene, and putting biosecurity procedures in place on farms are examples of preventive measures (Collins & Acha, 1989; Ganter, 2015).
2. Foodborne Transmission: Eating contaminated pork products is the main way that zoonoses like Trichinosis and Salmonellosis are spread. Public health initiatives include encouraging safe meat handling practices, teaching people about the significance of properly cooking pigs, and making sure that the pork sector follows the right procedures for meat inspection and certification (Fasina et al., 2012; Clifford & Morton, 2019).
3. Airborne Transmission: Human or pig infections spread by the airborne droplets of swine influenza. In places where humans and animals are in close proximity, such as farms and markets, airborne transmission poses a serious risk. In order to stop the virus from spreading, preventive strategies include immunization, better ventilation in animal housing, and urging sick people to wear masks (Webster et al., 1992).
4. Environmental Contamination: Contact with water or soil tainted by an infected animal's urine is a frequent way for leptospirosis to spread. Enhancing cleanliness, managing rodent populations, and guaranteeing that animals have access to clean water are necessary for effective control (Centers for Disease Control and Prevention, 2018; Ganter, 2015).

Health Impacts on Human and Swine

Human and pig health are significantly impacted by swine zoonoses, which can result in a variety of clinical complaints as well as financial ramifications.

1. Health Impacts on Humans: Swine zoonoses can produce a wide range of symptoms in people, from minor to severe. For instance, in susceptible groups, swine influenza may cause respiratory symptoms that are potentially fatal. If left untreated, brucellosis can result in crippling, persistent symptoms that last for months or even years. While salmonellosis can cause significant gastrointestinal irritation, especially in high-risk individuals, leptospirosis can cause serious complications such as kidney damage and liver failure. Medical expenses, lost productivity from disease and the strain on healthcare systems during outbreaks

Table 1 Swine zoonoses with transmission pathways and symptoms

Disease	Causative agent	Transmission	Symptoms in humans	Symptoms in swine
Swine Influenza	Influenza A virus	Airborne	Fever, cough, sore throat	Cough, fever, anorexia
Swine Brucellosis	*Brucella suis*	Direct contact	Fever, joint pain, fatigue	Abortions, infertility
Swine Trichinosis	*Trichinella spiralis*	Foodborne	Diarrhea, muscle pain	Muscle stiffness
Swine Leptospirosis	*Leptospira pomona*	Direct contact, contaminated water	Fever, headache, jaundice, kidney damage	Abortions, jaundice, renal failure
Swine Salmonellosis	*Salmonella* spp.	Foodborne, direct contact	Diarrhea, fever, abdominal cramps	Enteritis, septicemia, asymptomatic carriers

are some of the financial effects of swine zoonoses (Centers for Disease Control and Prevention, 2018; Díaz, 2019).

2. Health Impacts on Swine: These zoonoses in pigs can cause a range of health problems, from minor ones like decreased weight gain to serious ones like reproductive failure and mortality. Significant respiratory distress might result from swine influenza, which lowers productivity all around. Because of their primary effects on the reproductive systems—decreased fecundity and the requirement to cull affected animals—brucellosis and leptospirosis cause economic losses. Salmonellosis in swine herds is a risk to food safety and animal welfare; hence management methods must be strict to stop the disease from spreading (Brookes et al., 2014; Gibbs, 2005).

Notable zoonotic diseases in swine along with their transmission pathways, symptoms, and prevention strategies are depicted in Table 1 and Fig. 1 respectively.

Risk Communication Strategies

Public health requires effective risk communication, especially when dealing with zoonotic diseases—diseases that can spread from animals to people. Effective risk communication is essential when it comes to swine zoonoses in order to prevent and control outbreaks, safeguard the public's health, and make sure people who come into direct contact with pigs are aware of any potential hazards and how to avoid them.

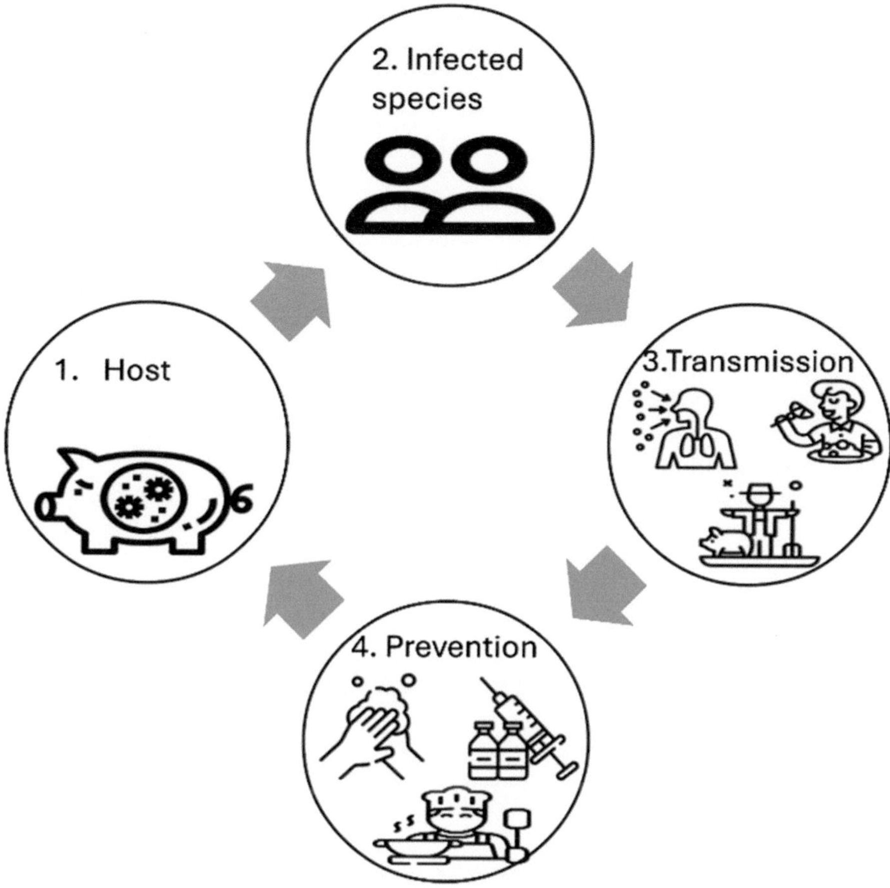

Fig. 1 Transmission and prevention of swine zoonoses

Mass Media

The mass media, which includes radio, newspapers, and television, has long been a vital component of public health communication. Its rapid mass communication capability makes it a vital tool for spreading knowledge about swine zoonoses.

Information delivery to a wide range of audiences is a strength of the mass media. Mass media can quickly disseminate information, precautions, and warnings during a zoonotic disease outbreak, possibly reaching millions of individuals in a short amount of time. This broad reach is especially useful in cities with high media consumption rates and is essential for prompt response.

However, a number of variables limit the efficiency of mass media. Making sure the information being shared is accurate is one of the biggest challenges. Confusion and a decline in public confidence in health authorities might result from inaccurate or insufficient information (Ferreira Caceres et al., 2022). Furthermore, traditional media lacks interactivity due to its one-way character, which can impede public response and involvement.

Community Engagement

Working directly with the community to distribute health information in a way that is both accessible and appropriate for their culture is known as community engagement. This approach works especially well in underserved and rural areas where access to mainstream media may be limited or where cultural circumstances may require public health messages to be properly understood and accepted (Khan et al., 2022).

Building relationships and fostering trust between local people and public health officials are two benefits of community participation. Public health communications can be adapted to suit particular local issues and cultural customs by working with community leaders and health professionals. This strategy can result in the more successful application of preventative measures by improving the acceptability and relevance of health messaging.

The primary obstacle to community engagement is the process's resource-intensive nature. It takes patience, persistence, and consistent engagement to develop trust and comprehend local situations. Moreover, the reliability of the intermediaries and their capacity to provide accurate information are key factors influencing this strategy's efficacy.

Digital Platforms

The increased involvement and reach of digital platforms like as social media, mobile apps, and websites makes them ideal for risk communication. Engaging younger groups and those with greater internet connectivity is made especially effective by these platforms.

Digital platforms provide a number of advantages, such as interactive features, real-time updates, and the capacity to target particular groups. Social media networks, for instance, can provide direct user-to-user connection, enabling prompt feedback and interaction. Mobile apps can also encourage users to take preventive action and offer individualized information to them.

The dissemination of false information is a serious problem for internet platforms. False information spreads quickly on social media, undermining attempts to promote public health and causing confusion. Active monitoring, fact-checking, and the promotion of trustworthy sources are necessary to combat misinformation (Emre, 2024).

Integration of Communication Methods

A successful risk communication plan frequently incorporates a variety of techniques to maximize each one's advantages and minimize its disadvantages. Mass media can be used to spread alarms and broad messages, while community participation can offer information that is more locally relevant and culturally appropriate. These initiatives can be strengthened via digital platforms which provide interactive, real-time communication.

To guarantee accuracy and consistency in the information delivered, rigorous coordination is needed when integrating various methods. The goal of public health authorities should be to develop a unified communication plan that addresses the unique problems of each approach while capitalizing on its advantages (WHO, 2017).

Table 2 highlights a set of advantages and challenges of each communication method, which must be carefully managed to achieve the desired public health outcomes; Fig. 2 further outlines the key strategies for public awareness, illustrating the importance of coordinated efforts across different communication platforms.

Educational Programs and Tools for Controlling Swine Zoonoses

The prevention and control of zoonotic diseases, particularly those like swine zoonoses that can have a serious negative effect on the health of both humans and animals, depend heavily on educational initiatives. Raising awareness, enhancing biosecurity procedures, and promoting preventive measures among farmers, veterinarians, meat processors, and the general public are the objectives of these educational programs. In addition to conventional teaching techniques, community-based learning initiatives and the use of digital resources have grown in significance, allowing for more targeted and extensive outreach.

Targeted Educational Programs

People who come into direct contact with pigs, such as farmers, slaughterhouse workers, and veterinarians, are at serious danger of contracting pig-related diseases such as swine influenza, brucellosis, leptospirosis, salmonellosis, and trichinosis.

Table 2 Comparison of risk communication methods

Method	Target audience	Advantages	Challenges
Mass media	General public	Wide reach, fast dissemination	Risk of misinformation
Community engagement	Local communities	Personal interaction, trust-building	Time-consuming, resource-intensive
Social media campaigns	Younger population	Interactive, viral potential	Echo chambers, misinformation spread

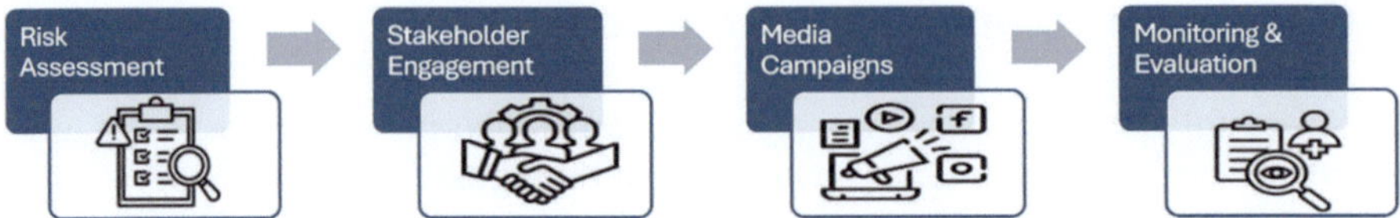

Fig. 2 Risk communication strategies for public awareness

These groups are the target of educational programs that emphasize biosecurity, hygiene, illness detection, and responsible handling of animals and meat products (Rizvi, 2022).

Due to their frequent interactions with livestock, farmers are leading the charge in the fight against zoonotic illnesses. Swine farmers are the target of educational initiatives that highlight biosecurity measures that lower the possibility of disease transfer from animals to humans and vice versa. Modules on good cleanliness, safe handling practices, and animal health management are commonly included in these programs. In order to stop the spread of illnesses, farmers should be educated how important it is to keep pig housing clean and contained. The correct use of personal protective equipment (PPE) when working with pigs and how to keep an eye on animal health in order to spot early illness symptoms are also covered in training.

Workers in slaughterhouses and meat processing plants are also more vulnerable to zoonotic illness exposure. The proper handling and processing of pork products is the main topic of educational programs for these groups. Lessons frequently stress the significance of fully boiling food to stop the spread of foodborne zoonoses such as Trichinosis, which is contracted by eating undercooked pork contaminated with the parasite Trichinella spiralis. Within this framework, instructional materials offer comprehensive guidelines regarding the proper cooking temperatures for pig as well as the significance of avoiding cross-contamination between raw and cooked meat.

Veterinary Education

Due to their responsibility for recognizing and treating animal illnesses, veterinarians are essential to the management of swine zoonoses. Courses on diagnosing zoonotic diseases, treatment procedures, and biosecurity measures are available through veterinary colleges and continuing education initiatives. With the help of specialized training, veterinarians can advise farmers on preventing disease outbreaks by gaining the skills necessary to oversee large-scale swine operations.

Education on zoonotic diseases is included in curriculum related to public health and animal health at veterinary colleges. Pupils are taught to identify signs of zoonotic illnesses such as brucellosis, leptospirosis, and swine flu, as well as the effects these illnesses have on human health. Veterinary practitioners can receive updates on the most recent approaches to disease prevention and management through continuing education programs. In order to control zoonotic infections, these programs also emphasize how crucial it is for veterinarians, farmers, and public health officials to work together (Leggett et al., 2011).

Digital Tools for Public Health Education

As digital technology has grown, websites and smartphone applications have become useful resources for enlightening the general public and medical professionals about zoonotic illnesses. Real-time information dissemination, interactive learning possibilities, and the facilitation of updated guidelines for disease prevention and management are all made possible by these platforms.

Mobile Apps

The general public and farmers are being educated about zoonotic illnesses through mobile apps. These apps provide a number of interactive features, including quizzes, video instructions on caring for pigs, and tools for identifying diseases. For instance, a smartphone app may give farmers information on when to vaccinate their pigs, how to increase farm biosecurity, and how to spot swine flu or other zoonotic disease symptoms.

Apps can also connect users with veterinary services in addition to offering instructional information. This enables farmers to report sick animals and receive prompt guidance. A community forum is another feature of certain programs that allows farmers to interact with one another and exchange experiences. Peer-to-peer education is particularly beneficial in remote locations where there may be limited access to veterinary care.

Websites and Online Portals

Websites and online portals are excellent instructional tools that offer comprehensive details on zoonotic disease prevention, treatment choices, and related topics. Reaching a larger audience, such as veterinarians, public health officials, and the general public, is made especially easy using these platforms. Articles, videos, and downloadable resources are frequently available on educational websites for users to access whenever it's convenient for them.

These internet resources can give farmers and veterinarians the most recent information on new infections, biosecurity guidelines, and government legislation related to swine zoonoses. Both the World Health Organization (WHO) and the Centers for Disease Control and Prevention (CDC) have a wealth of information available online about zoonotic illnesses, including fact sheets, disease bulletins, and protocols for controlling and avoiding outbreaks.

In order to offer continuous education for professionals, numerous public health and veterinary schools have created e-learning platforms. Focused on zoonotic

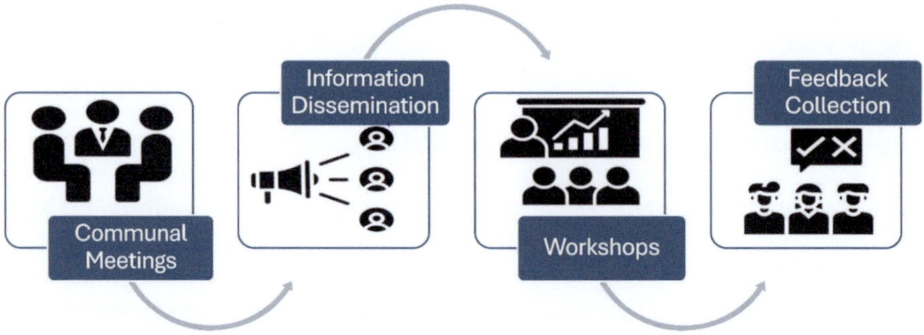

Fig. 3 Community-based educational programs for swine zoonoses

disease control, these platforms provide webinars, certification programs, and online courses. By using these platforms, professionals may remain up to date on the most recent advancements in the prevention of zoonotic diseases without having to physically attend training sessions.

Community-Based Educational Programs

Community-based initiatives continue to be essential to the prevention of zoonotic diseases, particularly in rural regions, even as digital tools have made educational programs more widely accessible. Through seminars, demonstrations, and the distribution of instructional materials like pamphlets, posters, and flyers, these initiatives engage the public directly. Public health officials can address regional issues and customize educational initiatives to the unique requirements of the populace by interacting with the community.

Figure 3 demonstrates how community-based educational programs focus on swine zoonoses, emphasizing direct participation and practical prevention strategies that resonate with locals. This direct engagement not only helps raise awareness but also empowers communities to take active roles in their health, making these programs an essential part of public health strategies in zoonotic disease control.

Workshops and Demonstrations

Farmers can learn about biosecurity and disease protection through workshops and practical demonstrations. Farmers can practice the skills necessary to apply biosecurity measures on their farms, such as using PPE when handling livestock, cleaning and disinfecting properly, and quarantining sick animals, during these events. These systems guarantee that farmers retain the knowledge and are more likely to apply it in their daily operations by making the learning process interactive and practical.

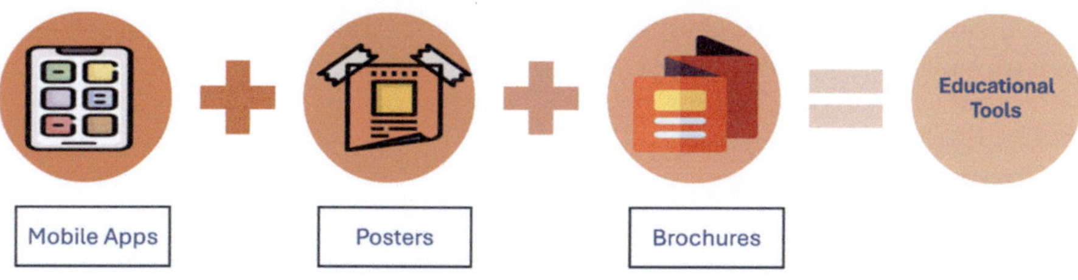

Fig. 4 Educational tools for raising awareness

In these instructional initiatives, community health workers and veterinarians frequently work together to answer farmers' questions and offer professional advice. The fact that the workshops are frequently conducted in nearby farming villages guarantees that everyone may access the material. Farmers who attended these workshops were more likely to take preventive action, which decreased the number of zoonotic disease outbreaks.

Educational Materials

Spreading informational materials like pamphlets and posters is another practical strategy for increasing public knowledge about zoonotic illnesses. These resources, which farmers and other community members can use as a reference, are frequently given out at community gatherings or workshops. Brochures usually include information on how to prevent diseases, how to handle livestock and meat products properly, and signs of various diseases. Veterinary clinics and other high-traffic locations frequently have posters up to warn farmers and the general public of crucial health precautions.

When educational resources are customized for the local environment, they can be especially successful. Content that addresses particular community issues, uses regional languages, or includes imagery that is culturally appropriate, is more likely to strike a chord with the intended audience. Visual aids, such as diagrams or videos, can be utilized to convey important lessons about disease prevention in areas with poor literacy rates. Figure 4 illustrates several educational tools designed to raise awareness about zoonotic diseases, showcasing how visual aids like diagrams and videos can be particularly useful in areas with low literacy rates.

Challenges in Risk Communication and Education

Education and risk communication are essential parts of maintaining public health and safety. These regions do, however, confront a number of important obstacles that limit their efficacy. It is crucial to comprehend and tackle these obstacles in order to improve public responsiveness and improve health outcomes. This investigation highlights the challenges faced by lawmakers and health professionals as it digs into the nuances of risk education and communication.

Information Overload

The sheer amount of data that is available to people in the current information age can be overwhelming. Confusion can arise during health emergencies like pandemics due to the deluge of information from several sources, such as news outlets, social media platforms, and official announcements. Controlling loudness is important, but so is ensuring that important messages are clearly heard over background noise. People may find it difficult to discern what is most important when they are inundated with information, which could result in selective attention or misunderstanding. The impact of important health messages may be lessened by this overload and risk communication initiatives may become less effective overall (Casal et al., 2007).

Misinformation and Disinformation

Effective risk communication is seriously hampered by misinformation and disinformation. The quick dissemination of these falsehoods, especially on social media, makes it more difficult to distribute accurate information. Disinformation and false information have the power to sow doubt, anxiety, and uncertainty, which eventually undermines public health programs. Fighting false narratives without unintentionally making them more prevalent is the difficult part. Proactive approaches are needed to combat disinformation, such as fact-checking, openness, and enlisting the help of reputable local leaders to refute misleading statements (Elbers et al., 2006).

Cultural and Language Barriers

The various linguistic and cultural needs of various communities must be taken into account in effective risk communication. The way that individuals view and react to health threats is influenced by cultural norms and beliefs. Health messages that conflict with cultural norms or beliefs could be disregarded or interpreted incorrectly. Communication attempts are further complicated by language difficulties, especially in multicultural settings where non-native speakers may find it difficult to obtain reliable information. To ensure diversity and comprehension, health communicators need to modify their messaging to appeal to a variety of cultural groups and offer resources in many languages (Crump et al., 2001).

Low Health Literacy

Effective risk communication depends heavily on health literacy or the capacity to comprehend and apply health information. Many people lack health literacy, which can make it difficult for them to understand complicated medical information, adhere to recommendations, or make wise decisions. People with low literacy levels might not be able to understand health messages that are extremely complicated or technical. Risk communication techniques should make use of visual aids, simple language, and messages that are easier to understand in order to get beyond this obstacle. Enhancing health knowledge across demographics should be another goal of educational initiatives.

Trust and Credibility Issues

Effective risk communication is based on trust. The impact of risk messaging can be greatly reduced when public confidence in government or health authority is undermined. Inconsistent message, perceived conflicts of interest, and prior mistakes in handling health emergencies are some of the factors that lead to trust problems. Consistent, open, and fact-based communication is necessary for establishing and preserving confidence. Building trust and credibility requires interacting with communities, being transparent about uncertainty, and exhibiting expertise.

Uncertainty in Risk Assessment

Information on dangers may be ambiguous or lacking during rising health emergencies, such as new infectious diseases. It is difficult to give the public clear, practical information when there is uncertainty. Risk communication needs to strike a balance between giving precise information and admitting the gaps in our current understanding. An emphasis on updating information as new evidence becomes available and appropriate message framing is important to communicate uncertainty without unnecessarily inciting panic. Clear communication regarding how dangers are changing can help control public expectations and lower anxiety.

Behavioral Responses to Risk

Human conduct frequently deviates from making logical decisions due to psychological influences like denial, optimism bias, or fear. These actions can have an impact on how people view and react to danger information. Fear-based communication may increase anxiety or cause avoidance, but optimism bias may cause one to underestimate one's own danger. It is imperative for effective risk communication to take into account these psychological dynamics and utilize tactics that encourage adaptive behaviors. Public behavior can be influenced to conform to suggested health practices by utilizing a combination of factual information, reassurance, and motivating tactics.

Digital Divide

Disparities in risk communication may result from the digital divide or the difference in access to digital technology between rich and poor. People without digital literacy or internet connection may not be able to get timely and accurate health information as digital tools become more and more integral to information distribution. This disparity has the potential to worsen already-existing health disparities, especially for vulnerable groups like the elderly and people living in rural regions. To meet this problem, information must be disseminated using a variety of platforms, such as community outreach and traditional media, in order to guarantee that everyone has access to crucial risk communication.

Consistency Across Platforms

Maintaining uniformity across traditional media, social media, and government websites is essential for effective risk communication. Confusion and a loss of public trust in health authority can result from inconsistent communications. To retain clarity and reinforce important ideas, messaging must be cohesive and synced across several mediums. The overall effectiveness of risk communication can be improved and consistency can be achieved by coordinating communication efforts and setting clear criteria for message delivery.

Community Engagement and Participation

In order to promote cooperation and trust, communities must be included in risk communication. Involving communities, meanwhile, can be difficult, particularly when there is mistrust or disinterest. Establishing connections, being aware of the needs in the community, and incorporating community leaders in the communication process are all necessary for effective community engagement. The applicability and acceptance of risk messaging can be increased by implementing strategies that take into account community input, resolve issues, and involve local stakeholders. Engaging in active engagement ensures that communication efforts are in line with the priorities and values of the community.

Conclusion

Swine zoonoses continue to offer a noteworthy threat to global public health, particularly in regions with high levels of pig-human interaction. Effective risk communication and public health education are essential tools in alleviating these risks. While mass media, community engagement, and digital platforms offer promising avenues for diffusing information, challenges such as cultural barriers, misinformation, and resource constraints must be addressed. A collaborative, versatile approach involving public health agencies, veterinary services, and community organizations is crucial to enhancing public understanding and preventing the spread of zoonotic diseases. Continued efforts are needed to improve communication strategies, fabricate messages to specific audiences, and ensure accuracy in the information reaching those at risk.

References

Balbus, J. M., & Malina, C. (2009). Identifying vulnerable subpopulations for climate change health effects in the United States. *Journal of Occupational and Environmental Medicine, 51*(1), 33–37.

Bibard, A., Martinetti, D., Picado, A., Chalvet-Monfray, K., & Porphyre, T. (2024). Assessing the risk of windborne dispersal of Culicoides midges in emerging epizootic hemorrhagic disease virus outbreaks in France. *Transboundary and Emerging Diseases*.

Brookes, V. J., Hernández-Jover, M., Black, P. F., & Ward, M. P. (2014). Preparedness for emerging infectious diseases among veterinarians in Australia. *Preventive Veterinary Medicine, 117*(3–4), 392–398.

Casal, J., Mateu, E., Mejía, W., & Martín, M. (2007). Biosecurity measures on swine farms in Spain: Perceptions by farmers and their relationship to current on-farm measures. *Preventive Veterinary Medicine, 82*(1–2), 138–150.

Centers for Disease Control and Prevention. (2018). *Zoonotic diseases*.

Choi, Y. K., Goyal, S. M., & Joo, H. S. (2003). Retrospective analysis of etiologic agents associated with respiratory diseases in pigs. *The Canadian Veterinary Journal, 44*(9), 735–737.

Clifford, A. B., & Morton, L. (2019). Communicating risks and benefits in food safety: The case of pork. *Journal of Food Protection, 82*(4), 617–625.

Collins, J. E., & Acha, P. N. (1989). Zoonoses and communicable diseases common to man and animals. *Journal of the American Veterinary Medical Association, 195*(11), 1588–1591.

Crump, J. A., Murdoch, D. R., & Baker, M. G. (2001). Emerging infectious diseases in an island ecosystem: The New Zealand perspective. *Emerging Infectious Diseases*, *7*(5), 767–772.14.

Díaz, J. H. (2019). Swine zoonoses and public health: A comprehensive review. *International Journal of Infectious Diseases, 89*, 20–30.

Elbers, A. R. W., Stegeman, J. A., de Jong, M. F., & Vos, J. H. (2006). The classical swine fever epidemic 1997–1998 in The Netherlands: Descriptive epidemiology. *Preventive Veterinary Medicine, 35*(3), 117–139.

Ellison, L. T., Delgado, A. H., & Harder, T. C. (2016). Insights into the epidemiology of porcine influenza: A worldwide perspective. *Transboundary and Emerging Diseases, 63*(2), 127–135.

Emre, T. (2024). Active monitoring and promotion of trustworthy sources: Necessary tools to combat misinformation. *Journal of Information and Media Studies, 42*(1), 15–28.

Fasina, F. O., Lazarus, D. D., Spencer, B. T., Makinde, A. A., & Bastos, A. D. S. (2012). Cost implications of African swine fever in smallholder farrow-to-finish units: Economic benefits of disease prevention through biosecurity. *Transboundary and Emerging Diseases, 59*(3), 244–255.

Ferreira Caceres, M. M., Sosa, J. P., Lawrence, J. A., Sestacovschi, C., Tidd-Johnson, A., Rasool, M. H. U., Gadamidi, V. K., Ozair, S., Pandav, K., Cuevas-Lou, C., Parrish, M., Rodriguez, I., & Fernandez, J. P. (2022). The impact of misinformation on the COVID-19 pandemic. *AIMS Public Health, 9*(2), 262–277.

Ganter, M. (2015). Zoonotic risks from small ruminants. *Veterinary Microbiology, 181*(1–2), 53–65.

Gibbs, E. P. J. (2005). Emerging zoonotic epidemics in the interconnected global community. *Veterinary Record, 157*(21), 673–679.

Gibbs, E. P. J., & Anderson, T. C. (2009). One world – One health: The evolutionary concept and reality. *Veterinary Record, 164*(7), 203–204.

Greger, M. (2007). The human/animal interface: Emergence and resurgence of zoonotic infectious diseases. *Critical Reviews in Microbiology, 33*(4), 243–299.

Karabatsos, N., Needham, L. L., & Saracci, R. (2009). Swine influenza: Zoonotic transmission and epidemiology. *Influenza Research and Treatment, 2009*, 1–7.

Khan, S., Mishra, J., Ahmed, N., Onyige, C. D., Lin, K. E., Siew, R., & Lim, B. H. (2022). Risk communication and community engagement during COVID-19. *International Journal of Disaster Risk Reduction, 74*, 102903.

Kleczkowski, A., Hoyle, A., & McMenemy, P. (2015). One model to rule them all? Modelling approaches across OneHealth for human, animal and plant epidemics. *Philosophical Transactions of the Royal Society B: Biological Sciences, 370*(1666), 20140291.

Leggett, F. E. D., Like, B., Vigneau, D. L., Jarvin, L., & Lindenmayer, J. M. (2011). Education of veterinary medical and other public health providers: Linking interventions with health outcomes. *Journal of Veterinary Medical Education, 38*(2), 160–167.

Martínez-López, B., Perez, A. M., & Sánchez-Vizcaíno, J. M. (2009). Social network analysis. Review of general concepts and use in preventive veterinary medicine. *Transboundary and Emerging Diseases, 56*(4), 109–120.

McLachlan, R. I., Rajpert-De Meyts, E., Hoei-Hansen, C. E., de Kretser, D. M., & Skakkebaek, N. E. (2007). Bluetongue: History, global epidemiology, and pathogenesis. *Preventive Veterinary Medicine, 102*(2), 107–111.

Mutua, M. K., Kimani-Murage, E., & Ettarh, R. R. (2011). Childhood vaccination in informal urban settlements in Nairobi, Kenya: Who gets vaccinated? *BMC Public Health, 11*, 6.

Paton, R. A., & McLaughlin, S. (2008). Services innovation: Knowledge transfer and the supply chain. *European Management Journal, 26*(1), 77–83.

Rizvi, D. S. (2022). Health education and global health: Practices, applications, and future research. *Journal of Education and Health Promotion, 11*, 262.

Smith, J. (2009). Public awareness campaigns in zoonoses. *Journal of Health Communication, 12*(3), 215–225.

VanderWaal, K., & Deen, J. (2018). Global trends in infectious diseases of swine. *Proceedings of the National Academy of Sciences, 115*(45), 201806068.

Webster, R. G., Bean, W. J., Gorman, O. T., Chambers, T. M., & Kawaoka, Y. (1992). Evolution and ecology of influenza A viruses. *Microbiological Reviews, 56*(1), 152–179.

WHO. (2017). *Risk communication and community engagement: Preparedness and response to public health emergencies: A WHO guide*. World Health Organization.

Prevention and Control Strategies for Swine Zoonoses

Devendra Singh, Pratishtha Sharma, Ashok Gaur, and Lakshmi Kant

Abstract

Swine zoonoses, caused by pathogens such as bacteria, viruses, and parasites, pose significant public health and economic risks, particularly in regions with intensive pig farming. Key zoonotic diseases include brucellosis, leptospirosis, salmonellosis, and influenza. Despite advancements in pathogen control, the persistence of zoonotic pathogens and increasing antimicrobial resistance necessitate robust biosecurity, vaccination, and surveillance measures. Biosecurity practices, including controlled farm access, visitor management, and quarantine protocols, are critical for preventing disease transmission and reducing antibiotic use. Vaccination complements these measures by preserving herd health and minimizing zoonotic outbreaks. Surveillance systems enable early detection and effective management of diseases, supported by diagnostic tools, comprehensive health screenings, and accurate record-keeping. Additionally, vector control strategies targeting rodents, insects, and other carriers are essential to mitigate pathogen transmission. These integrated approaches align with the One Health framework, emphasizing the interconnectedness of animal, human, and environmental health, to ensure sustainable swine production and protect public health. Preventing disease in pig farms requires vector control, sanitation, biosecurity, and waste management. Key measures include integrated pest management, proper hygiene, manure handling, and regular cleaning. Biosecurity protocols and staff training ensure early disease detection and control. Effective waste management and compliance with environmental regulations minimize health risks and promote sustainability.

D. Singh (✉) · P. Sharma · A. Gaur · L. Kant
Department of Veterinary Pharmacology and Toxicology, College of Veterinary and Animal Science, Bikaner, Rajasthan, India

Rajasthan University of Veterinary and Animal Sciences, Bikaner, Rajasthan, India

R. Deb et al. (eds.), *Emerging Zoonotic Threats from Swine*,
https://doi.org/10.1007/978-981-96-7407-7_21

Keywords

Zoonoses · Swine health · Biosecurity · Vaccination · Disease surveillance · Vector control · One health · Sustainable farming

Zoonoses are diseases and infections that are naturally transmitted between vertebrate animals and humans. These diseases can be caused by a variety of pathogens, including bacteria, viruses, parasites, and fungi. Zoonotic agents can be transmitted through direct contact with animals, their secretions, or their excretions, along with the consumption of contaminated food or water and exposure to vectors such as mosquitoes or ticks. The term "zoonosis" is derived from the Greek words "zoon," meaning "animal," and "nosos," meaning "ailment" or "disease." Zoonotic diseases can spread through multiple pathways, such as direct contact with animals, ingestion of contaminated food or water, exposure to vectors like mosquitoes or ticks, and inhalation of airborne particles.

Significance of Swine Zoonoses

Pig farming traces its roots to around 9000 BC, likely originating from the domestication of wild boars in Eurasia (Bökönyi, 1974). Since then, pork has been a vital contributor to human nutrition. Over the past 50 years, both the consumption of pork and the demand for various pig-derived products have witnessed a notable increase. The pig sector is experiencing rapid growth within the agricultural landscape, ranking as the fastest-growing livestock subsector alongside poultry. On a global scale, pork consumption is increasing, rising from 9.1 kg per capita in 1964 to a projected 15.1 kg per capita in 2030 (FAO, 2003), and projected that by 2030, pork consumption will represent approximately 33% of the overall increase in meat consumption (FAO, 2021). This expansion is particularly pronounced in low and middle-income countries, where semi-commercial and backyard farmers constitute the majority of pig production (Kenya, 2012; Bettencourt et al., 2015). However, this growth is not without its challenges. In certain instances, livestock, including pigs, can serve as intermediate or amplifying hosts, potentially leading to disease outbreaks in humans. This phenomenon underscores the intricate link between animal and human health. Notably, viruses endemic in pig populations pose a significant threat to public health, necessitating vigilant monitoring and control measures. Therefore, despite effective control measures for numerous swine pathogens, certain zoonotic pathogens have established themselves in swine populations, contributing to health and economic challenges. The continuous expansion of the human population, coupled with a simultaneous surge in the demand for animal protein, has resulted in increased proximity between people, livestock, and wild animals. This phenomenon is especially prevalent in lower and middle-income countries (Muehlenbein, 2013).

Pigs share similarities with humans in terms of anatomy and physiology, including skin, ocular structures, dentition, digestive system, kidneys, and cardiovascular system (Pond and Houpt, 1978). While pigs have long been recognized as reservoirs for zoonotic pathogens, our knowledge of zoonotic disease ecology in swine remains limited. Thus, while many swine pathogens are effectively managed, certain zoonotic pathogens have established themselves in swine populations, leading to health and economic challenges. The increasing intensity of these interactions highlights concerns about the risk of disease transmission between animals and humans, underscoring the need for strong biosecurity measures, effective disease surveillance, and targeted public health interventions in the pig farming sector.

As the pig industry continues to grow, sustainable and responsible practices become paramount to mitigate the risks associated with zoonotic diseases and ensure the health and well-being of both animals and humans in these evolving agricultural landscapes. Most human transmission routes of zoonoses are linked to close interaction with infected pigs or the intake of raw or undercooked pork products. Furthermore, antimicrobial resistance has emerged as a worldwide public health concern over the past two decades, encompassing resistance in zoonotic species. Hence, there is a necessity to emphasize zoonotic diseases in livestock, including pigs.

Overview of Major Swine Zoonotic Diseases

A zoonotic disease refers to an infectious ailment that can be spread between animals and humans. Nearly two-thirds of the pathogens that cause human diseases are known to originate from animals. Unfortunately, the majority of emerging infectious diseases identified in pigs over the past four decades have been associated with zoonoses. Diseases linked with swine encompass brucellosis, erysipelas, leptospirosis, ringworm, salmonellosis, cryptosporidiosis, campylobacterosis, balantidiasis, giardiasis, influenza, infections by pathogenic *E. coli*, and streptococcosis. Several of these zoonoses were previously unidentified diseases, including examples such as coronavirus disease 2019 (COVID-19), swine-origin H1N1 (2009), and Nipah virus (1999). Some of the common zoonotic diseases associated with swine are shown in Fig. 1 and their preventive measures in man and swine are presented in Table 1.

A. Biosecurity Measures

1. **Importance of Biosecurity on Swine Farms:** Biosecurity involves safeguarding agricultural animals against various infectious agents, including viruses, bacteria, fungi, and parasites. The absence of biosecurity measures is evident as agricultural fairs in the USA have been identified as hotspots for swine-human transmission (Baudon et al., 2017; Nelson et al., 2016; Watson et al., 2015). So, It is critically important on swine farms for several reasons:
   (a) **Disease Prevention:** A key reasons for implementing biosecurity measures on swine farms is to avoid the introduction and transmission of

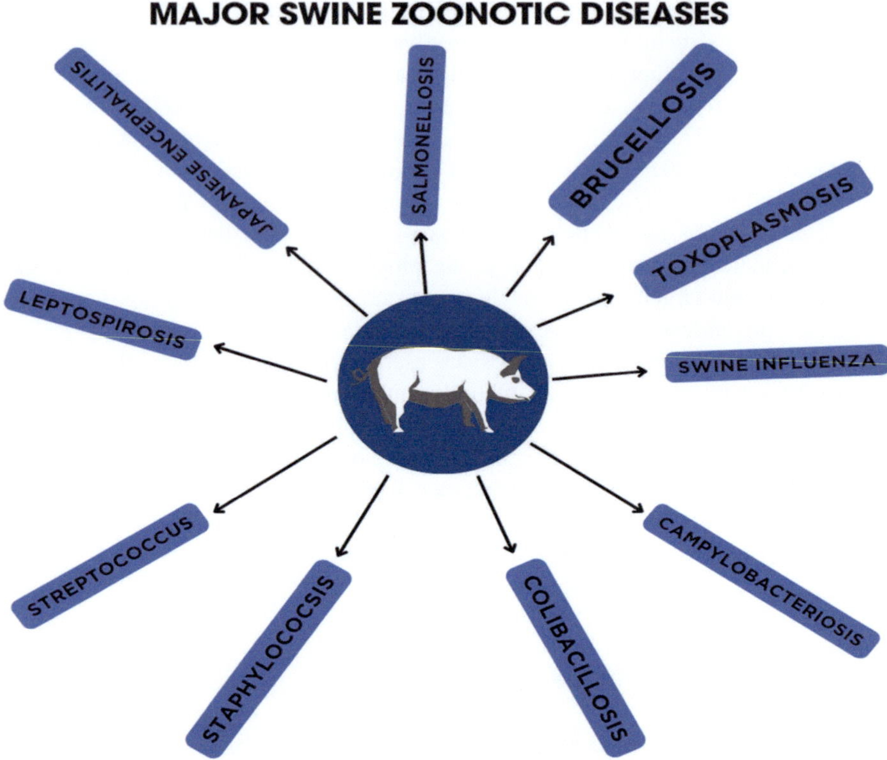

Fig. 1 Common zoonotic diseases of swine

diseases. Swine farms can be susceptible to various pathogens, including viruses, bacteria, and parasites, which can cause substantial economic losses through decreased productivity, increased mortality, and treatment costs. Instinctively, introducing an infected animal to a susceptible herd is a main source of infection. Therefore, once a pathogen-free status is achieved, the goal is to avoid reintroducing the pathogen. To minimize the risk of zoonotic diseases spreading to a vulnerable population through new arrivals, it is advisable to quarantine them before integrating them with the existing herds. This is because clinical symptoms often appear after the peak period of viral shedding.

(b) **Protection of Animal Health:** Maintaining high levels of biosecurity helps protect the health and welfare of the swine herd. Diseases such as African swine fever, foot-and-mouth disease, and porcine reproductive and respiratory syndrome (PRRS) can devastate pig populations and have significant economic consequences. Strict biosecurity protocols help minimize the chances of these diseases reaching the farm. Overall, all-in-all-out systems would decrease the chances of new arrivals getting infected. However, the operational intricacies and dynamic nature of

Table 1 Major swine zoonotic diseases and their preventive measures in man and swine

Disease	Pathogen	Transmission	Preventive measures (swine)	Preventive measures (man)
Swine influenza	Influenza A virus (H1N1, H3N2)	Aerosolized droplets, direct contact, contaminated surfaces	Vaccination, isolate sick pigs, improve ventilation, biosecurity	Wear PPE, practice good hygiene, avoid close contact with infected pigs, vaccinate at-risk individuals
Brucellosis	*Brucella suis*	Physical contact with infected tissues, ingestion, inhalation	Test and cull infected animals, proper disposal of aborted materials	Use PPE, avoid handling infected materials, ensure good hygiene, avoid raw dairy or meat
Campylobacteriosis	Campylobacter species	Fecal-oral route, contaminated food/water	Clean water supply, sanitation, biosecurity	Avoid raw/undercooked pork, wash hands, prevent cross-contamination during food preparation
Leptospirosis	Leptospira bacteria	Contact with urine, contaminated water/soil	Vaccination, rodent control, provide clean water, biosecurity	Avoid contaminated water, use PPE, wash hands thoroughly, maintain environmental sanitation
Streptococcosis	*Streptococcus suis*	Close contact with pigs or their secretions	Proper sanitation, isolate infected pigs, regular veterinary checks	Use PPE, practice good hygiene, seek early medical attention for cuts or wounds after pig contact
Erysipelas	*Erysipelothrix rhusiopathiae*	Close interaction with infected animals or environments	Vaccination, sanitation, and biosecurity	Wear PPE, avoid exposure to infected pigs or contaminated environments, wash hands properly

(continued)

Table 1 (continued)

Disease	Pathogen	Transmission	Preventive measures (swine)	Preventive measures (man)
Cysticercosis	*Taenia solium* larvae	Ingestion of eggs via contaminated food, water, or feces	Deworm pigs, proper disposal of feces, cook pig feed thoroughly	Avoid raw/unprepared pork, maintain proper sanitation, wash hands before eating, improve food safety
Salmonellosis	Salmonella species	Fecal-oral route, contaminated food/water	Maintain clean pens, provide uncontaminated feed and water, rodent control	Wash hands after handling pigs, cook pork thoroughly, avoid cross-contamination during food preparation
Hepatitis E	Hepatitis E virus (HEV)	Consumption of undercooked pork, direct contact with infected pigs	Improve hygiene in farms, ensure clean feed and water	Avoid undercooked pork, use clean water, maintain good hygiene
Colibacillosis	*Escherichia coli* (ETEC strains)	Fecal-oral route, contaminated feed, water, or environment	Ensure clean water and feed, sanitation, vaccination	Avoid raw pork, practice good food hygiene, ensure clean drinking water
Staphylococcosis	*Staphylococcus aureus*	Interaction with infected pigs or contaminated equipment	Sanitation, isolate infected pigs, biosecurity	Wear PPE, wash hands, avoid handling of infected animals or materials
Japanese encephalitis	Japanese encephalitis virus (JEV)	Mosquito bites (vectors from infected pigs or birds)	Control mosquito breeding, vaccination of pigs in endemic areas	Use mosquito repellents, wear protective clothing, vaccination in endemic areas

swine breeding make this approach impractical. If the pathogen status of the breeding farms is determined, destination farms can either have confidence or implement appropriate mitigation strategies.

(c) **Preservation of Production Efficiency:** Disease outbreaks can lead to reduced growth rates, decreased feed efficiency, increased mortality, and reproductive problems in pigs. By implementing effective biosecurity measures, farmers can safeguard the productivity and efficiency of their operations, ultimately ensuring a more sustainable and profitable swine production system.

(d) **Minimization of Antibiotic Use:** Disease outbreaks often demand the administration of antibiotics to treat affected animals. However, overuse of antibiotics can lead to antimicrobial resistance, posing a threat to both animal and public health. The prevalence of zoonotic diseases arises from the complex interplay of numerous factors, including biological, genetic, social, ecological, political, physical, and environmental influences. Over 60% of human infectious diseases stem from zoonotic pathogens. Among them, antibiotic-resistant bacteria are the most widespread zoonotic pathogens found commonly in the environment (Daffale et al., 2020).

Antibiotic use in agriculture should be minimized promptly to prevent the rise of bacterial resistance and to maintain the effectiveness of antibiotics, especially for treating human infections. Some of the most hopeful alternatives to antibiotics comprise antimicrobial proteins, bacteriophages, probiotics, and plant-derived compounds. The ideal antimicrobial agents must target a specific range of pathogens and minimize the risk of serious side effects. Enhanced biosecurity can decrease the need for antibiotic treatments by preventing diseases from entering the farm in the first place.

(e) **Protection of Human Health:** Biosecurity measures should extend beyond pigs, as workers on swine farms can transmit zoonotic diseases between pigs and humans. If an employee or pig contracts both a species-specific strain and a zoonotic strain, genomic reassortment may occur. Limiting pig farm access to essential personnel, ensuring vaccinations for employees and their families, and maintaining good hygiene practices can reduce the risk of bidirectional transmission and the emergence of new strains through zoonoses (Ramirez et al., 2006). Stringent inspection and quarantine measures for pig-derived products should be implemented at customs departments in shipping terminals, international airports, and railway stations to prevent international travelers from importing any type of pork products. By preventing the introduction and spread of these diseases on swine farms, biosecurity measures help protect the health and safety of farm workers, veterinarians, and others involved in pig production.

(f) **Compliance with Regulations:** Many countries have regulations and biosecurity standards in place to control the transmission of diseases in livestock populations. Adhering to these regulations not only safeguards swine herd health but also ensures compliance with legal requirements, avoiding potential penalties or restrictions on trade.

2. **Controlled Access and Visitor Management:** Controlled access and visitor management are crucial components of biosecurity protocols on pig farms to minimize the risk of disease introduction and transmission. It is recognized that other businesses requiring access to the farm or with which the farm

must interact, such as slaughterhouses, slurry disposal services, feed suppliers, animal by-product collectors/renderers, and roads used by pig transporters, pose potential risks (Pritchard et al., 2005). Hence, the farm should be situated at a reasonable distance from these potential hazards. Some commonly implemented measures are given below:

(a) **Designated Entry Points:** Establish designated entry points for farm personnel, visitors, and vehicles. Limit access to the farm to only essential personnel and authorized visitors.
(b) **Signage:** Clearly post signage at entry points outlining biosecurity protocols, like requirements for protective clothing, disinfection procedures, and restricted access areas.
(c) **Visitor Registration:** Humans are believed to act as both mechanical and biological vectors, spreading pathogens between farms when biosecurity measures are inadequately enforced (Amas, 2005b). Require all visitors to register upon arrival, providing information such as their name, contact details, purpose of visit, and any recent exposure to other pig farms or livestock.
(d) **Health Screening:** Implement health screening measures for all visitors before entry to the farm. This may include checking for symptoms of illness and recent travel history to areas with disease outbreaks.
(e) **Vehicle Disinfection:** Vehicles, especially pig transport trucks, can transfer pathogens between farms when biosecurity measures are not followed. Since these vehicles and drivers often interact with different farms and slaughterhouses, they pose a significant risk. To reduce this risk, vehicles should be prohibited from entering clean areas, disinfected before entering the farm, and avoid picking up animals from different farm (Amas, 2005b). Hence, creating a "permitted transports and actions" list for each truck, coupled with carefully planned route designs, should be the initial step. Subsequently, truck cleaning and disinfection should be conducted systematically and diligently.
(f) **Restricted Access Areas:** Limit access to sensitive areas, such as farrowing units, nursery barns, and isolation facilities, to authorized personnel only.
(g) **Supervised Visits:** Assign farm staff to accompany and supervise visitors during their time in the farm to ensure compliance with biosecurity protocols.
(h) **Training and Education:** Provide training to all personnel and visitors on the significance of biosecurity and the specific protocols to follow when entering pig farm premises.
(i) **Record Keeping:** Maintain records of all visitors, including their contact information, the date and time of entry and exit, and any areas of the farm they accessed. Such data can be valuable for traceability purposes during a disease outbreak.

(j) **Regular Review and Updates:** Periodically review and update biosecurity protocols and visitor management procedures based on changes in disease risks, industry best practices, and regulatory requirements.

3. **Dedicated Clothing and Footwear:** Provide and enforce the use of clothing specific to the farm, such as coveralls, boots, gloves, and hairnets, for all visitors entering pig housing areas. These items should be properly washed and sanitized both before and after use. Having an area designated for changing into protective clothing and footwear before entering pig housing is commonly considered good practice, and it is linked to a decreased prevalence of zoonotic diseases. Providing dedicated clothing and footwear for pig farm workers is essential for maintaining biosecurity and preventing the transmission of diseases between swine and humans. Here are some key considerations:
   (a) **Coveralls:** Workers should wear dedicated coveralls or overalls when working with pigs. These coveralls should be made of durable, easy-to-clean material that can withstand frequent washing and disinfection. Coveralls should be worn over regular clothing to avoid contamination.
   (b) **Boots:** Farm workers should wear dedicated boots that are only worn on the farm grounds. These boots should have non-porous surfaces that are easy to wash and sanitize. Ideally, boots should be made of rubber or other waterproof materials to prevent the absorption of liquids and contaminants.
   (c) **Gloves:** Disposable or reusable gloves should be provided to workers for tasks that involve direct contact with pigs or their environment. Gloves should be changed regularly, and hands should be washed thoroughly after glove removal.
   (d) **Hairnets and Head Coverings:** Workers with long hair should wear hairnets or other head coverings to prevent hair from contaminating the pig environment. This is particularly important in areas where pigs are housed or fed.
   (e) **Protective Eyewear:** In some situations, such as during cleaning or handling of chemicals, protective eyewear may be essential to prevent eye injuries and exposure to hazardous substances.
   (f) **Regular Cleaning and Sterilization:** All dedicated apparel and footwear should be cleaned and sterilized regularly to remove any potential pathogens. Washing machines and disinfectant solutions specifically designed for farm clothing should be utilized to ensure effective decontamination.
   (g) **Storage Facilities:** Provide designated storage areas for farm protective wear and boots to prevent cross-contamination with personal clothing and belongings. These storage areas should be kept clean and organized to minimize the risk of contamination.
   (h) **Training and Education:** Ensure that all farm workers are properly trained on the importance of using dedicated clothing and footwear, as well as proper procedures for cleaning and disinfection. Regular remind-

ers and refresher training sessions may be necessary to reinforce these practices.

(i) **Regular Inspection:** Conduct regular inspections of farm clothing and footwear to check for signs of wear and tear, damage, or contamination. Replace worn or damaged items promptly to maintain biosecurity standards.

4. **Quarantine Procedures for New Animals:** Quarantine procedures for new animals at a pig farm are crucial to avoid the introduction and transmission of diseases. A suggested strategy to mitigate the elevated risk associated with these imports is to isolate or quarantine the pigs for a specified period. During this time, they should be closely monitored to detect any signs of infectious diseases during the incubation phase and examined for the signs of chronic illnesses. Quarantines should be structured as bio-containment facilities, specifically designed to prevent the introduction of any unwanted pathogens from incoming animals. As such, there should be no direct link between the quarantine unit and the main farm. Here's a step-by-step guide on implementing effective quarantine protocols:
   (a) **Designated Quarantine Area**: Establish a designated quarantine area separate from the main pig population. This area should have its own facilities, including housing, feeding, and waste management systems, to prevent any physical interaction with existing pigs on the farm. For the quarantine to be effective, it should operate as a completely isolated unit separate from the rest of the farm. Furthermore, the quarantine should operate on a strict all-in/all-out basis to prevent the potential spread of pathogens between different batches of gilts. The risk linked with introducing gilts can be reduced by decreasing the rate of new batch entries (Alarcón et al., 2021).
   (b) **Preparation of Quarantine Facilities**: Ensure that the quarantine facilities are thoroughly washed and disinfected prior to introduction of new animals. Remove any remaining bedding or debris, and disinfect all surfaces, equipment, and water sources to diminish the risk of disease communication. Regarding the location of quarantine areas, it is generally advised that they be situated at least 1000 meters away from any other pig facility. This distance is deemed safe for the airborne spread of majority of pathogens (though not all types) and reducing transmission via rodents, flies, and other vectors (Stark, 1999; Desrosiers, 2011).
   (c) **Health Assessment**: Conduct a comprehensive health evaluation of the new animals before placing them in quarantine. This assessment should include a physical examination by a veterinarian, along with testing for common pig diseases, including swine fever, PRRS (porcine reproductive and respiratory syndrome), and respiratory pathogens.
   (d) **Isolation Period**: Implement a mandatory isolation period for new animals in quarantine. The length of the isolation period may vary based on the specific disease risks and farm protocols, but it typically ranges from 30 to 60 days. During this time, closely monitor the health status of the

animals for any signs of illness. The isolation period should be adjusted based on the specific pathogen(s) of concern, taking into account their maximum shedding period (Amass 2005a).

(e) **Restricted Access**: Restrict access to the quarantine area to essential personnel only. Implement strict biosecurity measures, including dedicated clothing and footwear, hand hygiene protocols, and sterilization procedures, to prevent the transmission of pathogens between the quarantine area and other parts of the farm. Proper hygiene practices encompass wearing Personal Protective Equipment (PPE) and enforcing a strict policy that prevent sick employees from attending farms.

(f) **Separate Equipment**: Use separate equipment and tools for handling animals in quarantine to avoid cross-contamination with existing pigs at the facility. Equipment used in the quarantine area should be carefully sanitized and disinfected after each use.

(g) **Regular Monitoring**: Monitor the health and behavior of animals in quarantine regularly. Keep detailed records of any observations, including temperature, appetite, fecal consistency, and respiratory rate, to detect any signs of illness promptly. Farm personnel attending to quarantined animals should do so at the completion of their working day, wearing separate protective clothing, and minimizing direct interaction with the animals.

(h) **Veterinary Oversight**: Engage a veterinarian in overseeing the quarantine process. A veterinarian can provide guidance on health assessments, diagnostic testing, treatment protocols, and any necessary adjustments to quarantine protocols in accordance with the health conditions of the animals.

(i) **Gradual Introduction**: After the finalization of the isolation period and confirmation of good health, gradually introduce the new animals to the existing pig population. Monitor them closely for any signs of illness during this transition period.

(j) **Post-Quarantine Monitoring**: Continue to monitor the health of new animals after they are introduced to the main pig population. Conduct regular health checks and remain vigilant for any signs of disease outbreaks, particularly in the weeks following integration.

B. **Vaccination Program:**

(a) **Role of Vaccination in the Prevention of Zoonotic Diseases:** Vaccination plays a crucial role in controlling zoonotic diseases, which are illnesses, that spread from animals to humans. With the growing demand for pork products, pig production has expanded, leading to an increased adoption of vaccination to mitigate zoonotic diseases. Following Swine Flu outbreak in 2009, vaccine adoption increased as pork producers sought to counteract the threat of future zoonotic event. This highlighted the vulnerability of consumer confidence in pork products and the financial repercussions of a swine-origin influenza A virus outbreak (Pappaioanou and Gramer, 2010; Verikios et al., 2011). Here is how vaccination helps prevent zoonosis:

(b) **Disrupt the Transmission Chain:** When accessible, vaccination is unquestionably the most economical method for preventing, controlling, and potentially eradicating infectious diseases. Vaccination can reduce the infection cycle on farms by increasing the threshold required for an infection to spread. Vaccines can be developed for many zoonotic pathogens, targeting the specific bacteria, virus, or parasite that causes the disease. Vaccinating animals against these pathogens can disrupt the transmission cycle, preventing the transmission of disease from animals to humans.

(c) **Protect Animal Health**: Vaccinating animals not only prevents them from contracting zoonotic diseases but also helps maintain their overall health and well-being. Healthy animals are less likely to shed pathogens in their environment, reducing the chances of transmission to humans.

(d) **Reduce Human Exposure**: Vaccinating animals lowers the chance of humans being exposed to infectious agents transmitted by animals. This is especially important in settings where humans and animals coexist closely, such as farms, slaughterhouses, and wildlife habitats.

(e) **Prevent Outbreaks in Animal Populations**: Zoonotic diseases can cause outbreaks within animal populations, leading to economic losses and health risks to the public. Vaccination programs can help prevent these outbreaks by reducing the prevalence of disease-causing agents in animal groups.

(f) **Protect Public Health**: By reducing the occurrence of zoonotic diseases in animals, vaccination programs ultimately protect human health. Vaccines help prevent outbreaks of diseases like rabies, brucellosis, and avian influenza, which can have serious consequences for public health and well-being. Veterinary vaccines can potentially address several of these challenges. A prime illustration of a veterinary vaccine employed for public health objectives is the immunization of wildlife against rabies. The main aim was not to safeguard wildlife from rabies but to avert human exposure and the transmission of the disease within human communities (Brochier et al., 1991; Pinard-Van Der Laan and Gay, 2008).

(g) **One Health Approach**: Vaccination aligns with the One Health framework, which recognizes the interconnectedness of animal, human, and environmental health. By vaccinating animals against zoonotic diseases, we not only protect human and animal health but also contribute to the overall health of ecosystems.

(h) **Control Emerging Diseases**: Vaccination can be an important tool in controlling emerging zoonotic diseases. Rapid development and deployment of vaccines can help contain outbreaks and prevent the passage of newly emerging pathogens from animals to humans. For example, when confronted with an occurrence of African swine fever and lacking a vaccine, the only recourse is to promptly euthanize the infected animals and dispose of the carcasses to prevent further spread of infection to unaffected locations. In some cases, vaccination is the most effective solution, particularly for infections caused by arthropod-borne viruses.

1. **Implementation of Effective Vaccination Strategies:** Implementing effective vaccination strategies in swine is crucial for maintaining herd health, preventing disease outbreaks, and minimizing the risk of zoonotic spread to humans. Here's how to execute such strategies effectively:
   (a) **Disease Surveillance and Risk Assessment**: Surveillance data, when optionally collected, assists in understanding the epidemiology and progression of zoonotic diseases and can guide policy decisions. Conduct regular surveillance of prevalent diseases in swine, including zoonotic pathogens like influenza viruses and hepatitis E. Assess the risk factors contributing to disease transmission within pig populations, including herd density, biosecurity practices, and exposure to wild animals.
   (b) **Vaccine Selection and Development**: Choose vaccines that target specific pathogens known to affect pigs, including zoonotic agents. Vaccines against diseases like swine influenza, porcine reproductive and respiratory syndrome (PRRS), and leptospirosis are commonly used in swine production. Work with veterinarians and vaccine manufacturers to ensure appropriate selection and availability of vaccines.
   (c) **Vaccination Schedule and Regimen**: Develop a vaccination schedule tailored to the needs of the pig herd, taking into account factors like age, production stage, and disease prevalence. Administer vaccines according to recommended dosages and intervals, and consider the use of booster doses to maintain long-term immunity. Vaccination schedule of important zoonotic diseases in swine is presented in Table 2.
   (d) **Vaccine Delivery and Administration**: Ensure proper storage, handling, and administration of vaccines to maintain their efficacy. Train farm personnel in vaccine administration techniques, including proper injection site preparation and dosage calculation. Use sterile needles and syringes for each pig to prevent cross-contamination.
   (e) **Herd Health Management**: Integrate vaccination into comprehensive herd health management practices, including biosecurity measures, nutrition, and housing. Implement strict biosecurity protocols to avoid the emergence and spread of diseases within the herd, complementing vaccination efforts.
   (f) **Monitoring and Surveillance**: Monitor vaccine efficacy and disease prevalence through regular health assessments, serological testing, and disease monitoring. Collect and analyze data on vaccination coverage, disease incidence, and performance indicators to assess the effectiveness of vaccination strategies and identify areas for improvement.
   (g) **Education and Training**: Educate farm personnel about the importance of vaccination in maintaining porcine health and preventing disease outbreaks. Provide training on proper vaccination techniques, biosecurity protocols,

Table 2 Vaccination schedule of important zoonotic diseases in swine

Disease	Causative agent	Available vaccines	Initial vaccination	Booster
Swine influenza	Influenza A virus (H1N1, H3N2)	Inactivated or modified live vaccines	3–4 weeks of age	3–4 weeks after the first dose
Hepatitis E	Hepatitis E virus	Inactivated vaccine	6–8 weeks of age	3–4 weeks after the first dose
Leptospirosis	Leptospira species	Bacterin or killed vaccine	6–8 weeks of age	3–4 weeks after the first dose
Porcine reproductive and respiratory syndrome	PRRS virus (Arteri virus)	Modified live or inactivated vaccines	3–4 weeks of age	3–4 weeks after the first dose
Erysipelas	*Erysipelothrix rhusiopathiae*	Inactivated vaccines	6–8 weeks of age	3–4 weeks after the first dose
Classical swine fever	Classical swine fever virus (Pesti virus)	Live attenuated or inactivated vaccines	3–4 months of age	1 year after initial dose
Salmonellosis	Salmonella species	Live attenuated or inactivated vaccines	6–8 weeks of age	3–4 weeks after the first dose
Streptococcosis	*Streptococcus suis*	Inactivated vaccines	4–6 weeks of age	3–4 weeks after the first dose

and early disease detection to empower staff to contribute to herd health management effectively.

(h) **Collaboration and Communication**: Collaborative fieldwork involving multidisciplinary teams, supported by expert staff scientists and advanced laboratories equipped with molecular biology and immunology techniques, is crucial for investigating new and emerging zoonotic diseases. Share information and best practices within the porcine farming community through workshops, conferences, and industry publications. Highly trained field epidemiologists, ecologists, and environmentalists, particularly those with a veterinary background, will play essential roles in these efforts. The need for interdisciplinary collaboration is crucial in identifying new zoonotic agents.

(i) **Adaptation and Continuous Improvement**: Continuously evaluate and adapt vaccination strategies response to evolving disease threats, changes in herd dynamics, and advancements in vaccine technology. Stay updated on vaccine recommendations and guidelines from regulatory agencies and veterinary authorities.

C. **Surveillance and Monitoring:**

1. **Establishment of Surveillance Systems:** The economic success of a pig farm hinges on the well-being and health of its pigs (Benjamin and Yik, 2019). As a result, all participants in pig farming strive to confirm that pigs exhibit healthy behavior and physiological functions, free from injuries, diseases, or malnutrition. Establishing surveillance systems at pig farms is crucial for prompt identification, monitoring, and control of diseases. On a pig farm, continuously monitoring the health and well-being of all animals presents a significant challenge for the farm caretaker throughout the day. Here's how to establish effective surveillance systems:
   (a) **Identify Objectives**: Determine the objectives of the surveillance system, such as monitoring disease prevalence, detecting emerging pathogens, or evaluating the effectiveness of control measures. Clear objectives will guide the design and execution of the surveillance system.
   (b) **Define Target Diseases**: Identify the specific diseases of interest for surveillance, including both endemic and newly arising pathogens that threaten pig health and productivity. Consider zoonotic diseases that can potentially affect human health.
   (c) **Select Surveillance Methods**: Choose appropriate surveillance methods according to the objectives, target diseases, resources available, and farm-specific characteristics. Common surveillance methods include passive surveillance (reporting of clinical cases), active surveillance (systematic sampling of animals), syndromic surveillance (monitoring of clinical symptoms), and serological testing.
   (d) **Establish Case Definitions**: Develop clear and standardized case definitions for the target diseases to ensure consistency in disease reporting and data collection. Define criteria for suspect cases, confirmed cases, and non-cases based on clinical signs, laboratory results, or epidemiological factors.
   (e) **Train Personnel**: Provide training to farm personnel involved in surveillance activities, including veterinarians, livestock health technicians, and farm workers. Ensure that staff understand their roles and responsibilities in disease surveillance, data collection, and reporting procedures.
   (f) **Implement Data Collection Protocols**: Establish standardized protocols for data collection, including procedures for sample collection, handling, and transport. Use appropriate sampling techniques and tools to collect specimens for laboratory testing, like blood samples, nasal swabs, or fecal samples. Unlike systems designed for collecting production data, the tools required for effective monitoring of infectious diseases demanded significant advancements in diagnostic medicine. Diagnostic technology is continually evolving, and it is recommended to periodically review new commercially available tests and their performance to stay updated with innovations.

   (g) **Laboratory Testing**: Preventing and controlling emerging zoonotic diseases requires the use of increasingly advanced diagnostic tools. Local investigators must have access to reference laboratories that are fully equipped with molecular biology instruments. Partner with accredited veterinary diagnostic laboratories to conduct laboratory testing of collected samples. Ensure that laboratories follow standardized procedures for sample processing, testing methodologies, and result reporting to maintain the quality and reliability of diagnostic data.
   (h) **Data Management and Analysis**: Set up systems for managing, storing, and analyzing data to efficiently organize surveillance information. Use electronic databases or software tools to record and analyze surveillance data, generate reports, and identify trends or patterns in disease occurrence.
   (i) **Communication and Reporting**: Establish communication channels for prompt reporting of surveillance data to relevant stakeholders, including farm management, veterinary authorities, and health regulatory bodies. Ensure transparency and collaboration in sharing surveillance findings and addressing disease threats.
   (j) **Feedback and Evaluation**: Provide feedback to farm personnel and stakeholders on surveillance findings, trends, and outcomes. Evaluate the efficiency of the surveillance system regularly by assessing its capability to detect diseases, inform decision-making, and contribute to disease control efforts. In swine production, herd immunity is optimized to minimize clinical losses, biosecurity measures are put in place to block pathogen entry, and surveillance is conducted to verify that herd immunity and biosecurity are operating effectively.
   (k) **Continuous Improvement**: Continuously review and update the monitoring system by incorporating feedback, applying lessons learned, and adapting to changes in disease dynamics. Adapt surveillance strategies and methods to address emerging threats, enhance data quality, and improve the overall efficiency of the system such as individual pig detection and tracking system, electronic sensor system, etc.
2. **Health Screenings and Diagnostic Tests**: Health screenings and diagnostic tests at pig farm are essential for maintaining animal health and welfare while ensuring a safe and reliable food supply. Listed below are typical screenings and tests performed at pig farms:
   (a) **Physical Examinations**: Regular physical examinations by trained veterinarians or animal health professionals are crucial for detecting any signs of illness or injury in pigs.
   (b) **Parasite Checks**: Pigs can be prone to various parasites such as worms, lice, and mange. Routine checks for parasites and appropriate treatment measures are necessary to prevent infestations.
   (c) **Blood Tests**: Blood tests are used to detect various diseases, including swine fever, porcine reproductive and respiratory syndrome (PRRS), and other viral or bacterial infections.

(d) **Fecal Tests**: Fecal examinations are conducted to identify internal parasites such as roundworms, whipworms, and coccidia.
(e) **Respiratory Health Checks**: Monitoring respiratory health is crucial in pigs, especially in intensive farming systems where respiratory diseases can quickly spread. Diagnostic tests like PCR (polymerase chain reaction) may be used to detect respiratory pathogens.
(f) **Reproductive Health**: Regular reproductive health checks, including ultrasound examinations, are often performed on breeding sows to monitor pregnancy status and identify any reproductive disorders.
(g) **Zoonotic Disease Surveillance**: Surveillance of zoonotic diseases, those transmissible between animals and humans, is vital for protecting public health. Examples include monitoring for salmonella and *E. coli* infections.
(h) **Diagnostic Imaging**: In certain situations, diagnostic imaging techniques such as X-rays or ultrasound are utilized to diagnose injuries or internal health issues in pigs.
(i) **Mastitis Checks**: Mastitis checks are essential for lactating sows to maintain udder health and prevent infections that could impact milk production and piglet well-being.
(j) **Nutritional Assessments**: Regular assessment of feed quality and nutritional balance is crucial for maintaining the overall health and productivity of the pigs.
(k) **Post-Mortem Examinations**: In cases of sudden deaths or unexplained illnesses, post-mortem examinations (necropsies) may be performed to determine the cause of death or illness and prevent future occurrences.
(l) **Health Record Keeping**: Accurate record-keeping of health screenings, treatments, and observations is essential for tracking the health status of individual animals and the overall herd, as well as for compliance with regulatory requirements.

D. **Vector Control**

1. **Identification of Disease Vectors:** Identifying disease vectors related to pigs is crucial for implementing effective management and mitigation strategies. Disease vectors are organisms that can carry and spread pathogens (such as bacteria, viruses, or parasites) from one host to another. Rodents, birds, insects, feral animals, dogs, and cats are capable of spreading pathogens mechanically (Amass 2005b). Among these, rodents are especially significant. Although pests are often thought to introduction of diseases to the herd, they are more likely to act as reservoirs for farm-resident strains, sustaining infections between successive groups of animals. In pig farming, various vectors can play a role in disease transmission. Figure 2 illustrates the role of critical vectors in the transmission of diseases between swine and human. Here are some common disease vectors related to pigs:

(a) **Flies (*Musca domestica*)**: House flies are known vectors for various pathogens, including bacteria (Salmonella and *E. coli*) and parasites

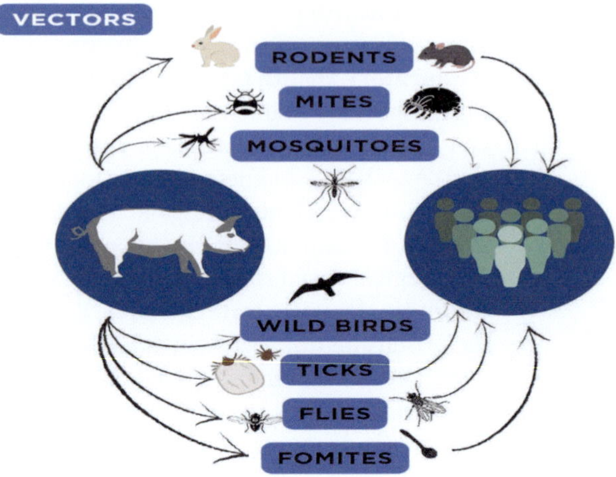

Fig. 2 Vectors of disease transmission between swine and human

(roundworm eggs). Flies can transmit these pathogens by landing on contaminated surfaces and then transferring them to pigs or their environment.

(b) **Ticks**: Ticks can transmit a range of pathogens to pigs, including bacteria (*Borrelia* spp., which causes Lyme disease) and viruses (African swine fever virus). Ticks may either attach directly to pigs or infest the environment where pigs are kept, depending on the species.

(c) **Mosquitoes**: Mosquitoes can transmit several viral pathogens to pigs, including West Nile virus and Japanese encephalitis virus. Mosquito-borne diseases can present a major threat to pig health, particularly in areas where these viruses are endemic.

(d) **Mites**: Mites like *Sarcoptes scabiei*, the causative agent of sarcoptic mange, can infest pigs, leading to skin lesions and severe itching. Mites can quickly spread within pig herds and facilitate the transmission of other pathogens through skin abrasions.

(e) **Rodents (Rats and Mice)**: Rodents can carry and transmit various diseases to pigs, including leptospirosis, salmonellosis, and pseudorabies. Rodents can contaminate pig feed and water supplies with their urine, feces, and hair, leading to disease transmission.

(f) **Wild Birds**: Certain species of wild birds, such as starlings and pigeons, can carry and shed pathogens that are harmful to pigs. For instance, avian influenza viruses can spread from wild birds to pigs, posing a risk of disease outbreaks.

(g) **Fomites**: Inanimate objects or surfaces (fomites) can also act as disease vectors by harboring and transmitting pathogens. Common fomites in pig environments include equipment, vehicles, and clothing that may become contaminated with infectious agents and transfer them to pigs.

(h) **Humans**: People handling pigs can unintentionally spread diseases to the animals via contaminated hands, clothing, or equipment. Similar to pigs, mere exposure to a pathogen doesn't necessarily lead to infection. Individuals with compromised immune systems require special attention, and minimizing contact rates is a primary preventive measure. Direct contact remains the most probable transmission route, with farmworkers and slaughterhouse employees facing the greatest risks. Strict biosecurity measures, including hand hygiene and personal protective equipment, are essential to reduce the risk of disease communication from humans to pigs.

2. **Use of Insecticides and Rodenticides:** Applying insecticides and rodenticides on pig farm is a common practice to control populations of insects and rodents, which can carry diseases and threaten both pig health and farm hygiene. Here's how insecticides and rodenticides are typically used and some considerations for their application:
   (a) **Selection of Insecticides**: Select insecticides that effectively target the pests while ensuring safety for pigs. Some common insecticides used on farms that raise pigs include pyrethroids, organophosphates, and insect growth regulators.
   (b) **Application Methods**: Insecticides can be administered using various methods, including sprays, dusts, baits, and fogging. The choice of application method depends on the type of insecticide, the target pests, and the layout of the farm facilities.
   (c) **Targeted Application**: Apply insecticides directly to areas prone to pest harboring or breeding, such as pig housing units, feed storage areas.
   (d) **Minimize Non-target Exposure:** Minimize the risk of non-target exposure to rodenticides by using bait stations and securing bait placements in areas inaccessible to pigs and other livestock. Remove spilled bait and rodent carcasses promptly to prevent accidental ingestion by non-target species.
   (e) **Compliance with Regulations:** Comply with local regulations and guidelines governing the use of rodenticides, including restrictions on active ingredients, application methods, and disposal of unused products or rodent carcasses.
   (f) **Environmental Considerations:** Consider the potential environmental impact of rodenticide use, particularly in areas near water bodies or sensitive habitats. Choose rodenticides with lower risks of bioaccumulation and persistence in the environment.
   (g) **Alternative Control Methods:** Explore non-chemical methods of rodent control, such as exclusion measures (e.g., sealing entry points), trapping, and habitat modification, as part of an integrated pest management approach.

3. **Preventing Vector-Mediated Disease Transmission**

Preventing vector-mediated disease transmission in a pig farm is essential for maintaining the health and welfare of the pigs and minimizing the risk of disease outbreaks. Here are some strategies to prevent vector-borne diseases:

(a) **Vector Control Measures**:
- Implement integrated pest management (IPM) strategies to control vectors such as flies, mosquitoes, ticks, and mites. This may include the use of insecticides, traps, biological control agents, and habitat modification to reduce vector populations.
- Regularly inspect and maintain facilities to identify and eliminate potential breeding sites for vectors, such as standing water, organic debris, and areas with poor sanitation.
- Install physical barriers like screens on windows and doors to prevent entry of flying insects into pig housing units.
- Use rodent-proofing measures to restrict access of rodents to feed storage areas and buildings, minimizing the risk of rodent-borne diseases.

(b) **Sanitation Practices**:
- Maintain high standards of cleanliness and hygiene throughout the farm to minimize the attraction of vectors and lower the risk of disease transmission.
- Implement proper manure management practices to reduce fly breeding sites and avoid the contamination of feed and water with pathogens.
- Clean and disinfect equipment, housing units, and common areas regularly to remove organic matter that may attract vectors and harbor pathogens.

(c) **Animal Husbandry Practices**:
- Implement biosecurity protocols to prevent the introduction and transmission of diseases on the farm. These measures include controlling visitor access, quarantining new animals, and maintaining strict hygiene practices.
- Rotate pastures and resting areas to reduce exposure of pigs to vectors and minimize the buildup of harmful microorganisms in the environment.
- Provide appropriate housing and bedding materials to minimize contact of pigs to vectors and ensure their comfort and well-being.

(d) **Education and Training**:
- A frequent situation with emerging diseases in swine populations is a significant delay between identification and subsequent control measures. Provide education and training to farm workers on vector-borne diseases, their transmission routes, and preventive measures. Encourage prompt reporting of any symptoms of illness or unusual behavior in pigs to enable early detection and response.

(e) **Environmental Management**:
- Manage vegetation and landscaping near the farm to minimize habitats for vectors and reduce their presence near pig facilities.
- Consider environmental factors including temperature, humidity, and rainfall that may influence vector populations and disease transmission dynamics.

E. **Hygiene and Sanitation**

1. **Sanitation and Disinfection Protocols:** Sanitation and disinfection protocols are critical components of biosecurity measures at a pig farm. Disinfection is a specific procedure designed to minimize disease transmission by addressing contamination on protective clothing, particularly boots, vehicles, and equipment. These protocols help preventing disease spread, maintain hygiene standards, and ensure the health and well-being of the pigs. Strict All In, All Out policies should be enforced for all groups of quarantined animals, and thorough sanitation and disinfection carried out between batches (Wong et al., 2004). The following is an overview of standard sanitation and disinfection protocols practiced on a swine farm:

(a) **Preparation and Planning**: Develop a written sanitation and disinfection protocol tailored to the specific needs and layout of the swine farm. Identify high-risk areas including pig housing units, feeding areas, water sources, and equipment storage areas. Allocate sufficient time, resources, and personnel for sanitation and disinfection tasks.

(b) **Personal Protective Equipment (PPE)**: Provide appropriate PPE to farm workers involved in cleaning and disinfection activities, including gloves, goggles, coveralls, and respirators as necessary. Train workers on the proper use and disposal of PPE to reduce the risk of exposure to chemicals and pathogens.

(c) **Cleaning Procedures**: Proper cleaning of buildings and equipment should be conducted beforehand. After washing, they should be allowed to dry, and disinfectant should be applied until saturation is reached. It is necessary to ensure thorough application, including the undersides of equipment, and care should be taken to avoid recontaminating surfaces that have been recently disinfected. Eliminate all organic matter (e.g., manure, feed residues) from surfaces using water, brushes, and high-pressure washers. Use detergent or alkaline cleaners to break down and remove stubborn dirt and grease from surfaces. Pay particular attention to areas where organic matter can accumulate, such as corners, crevices, and floor drains.

(d) **Rinsing and Flushing**: Thoroughly rinse all surfaces with clean water to remove residual detergent and loosened debris. Flush drains and gutters with water to remove any remaining organic matter and prevent clogging.

(e) **Disinfection Procedures**: Disinfection utilizes physical or chemical agents to destroy infectious organisms. Select an appropriate disinfectant according to the target pathogens, surface materials, and environmental conditions. Prepare disinfectant solutions following the manufacturer's guidelines and recommended dilution rates. Apply disinfectant to all surfaces using sprayers, foggers, or foamers, ensuring complete coverage. Allow sufficient contact time as specified on the product label to ensure effective disinfection. Generally, regular disinfection should be conducted in areas where the pig farm comes into contact with the external environment, such as sales barns, stockyards, staff entrances, gilt pick-up areas, and the like. Thorough cleaning prior to disinfection is a vital component of the disinfection process (Block, 2001). On swine farms, disinfection is often ineffective when animals cannot be relocated. Therefore, adopting an all-in/all-out feeding system to reduce pathogen spread within the facility, combined with disinfecting the barn during idle periods, is a more efficient and reliable approach (Kahrs, 1995).

(f) **Ventilation and Drying**: Ensure adequate ventilation during cleaning and disinfection activities to minimize exposure to chemical fumes and facilitate drying. Allow surfaces to air dry completely before reintroducing pigs or equipment to the cleaned area.

(g) **Equipment and Tools**: Sanitize and disinfect all equipment, tools, and vehicles used in pig housing units and common areas. Store sanitized and disinfected equipment in designated areas away from contaminated zones.

(h) **Monitoring and Validation**: Regularly monitor the effectiveness of cleaning and disinfection protocols through visual inspections and microbial testing. Validate the efficacy of disinfectants by periodically conducting surface swabbing and testing for residual pathogens.

(i) **Record Keeping**: Maintain detailed records of cleaning and disinfection activities, including dates, locations, products used, and any observations or corrective actions taken. Keep records readily accessible for inspection purposes and to track trends in cleanliness and biosecurity compliance over time.

2. **Training and Education**: Provide comprehensive training to farm workers on proper cleaning and disinfection techniques, safety procedures, and the critical role of biosecurity. Conduct regular refresher training sessions to reinforce protocols and address any emerging issues or challenges. Expanded and more extensive research on the behavior of swine workers concerning precautions for influenza and other zoonotic diseases, along with the evaluation of task-specific risks associated with influenza and other pathogen exposures could enhance this initiative. This could identify opportunities to improve the prevention of zoonotic influenza virus transmission with pandemic potential.
3. **Waste Management Strategies:** Waste management at a pig farm is crucial for maintaining hygiene, managing environmental impacts, and preventing the spread of diseases. Waste management systems should be separate from the primary farm operations, and equipment designated for quarantine area must never be used anywhere else on the farm under any circumstances. Here are several waste management strategies commonly employed at pig farms:

(a) **Manure Handling**: Manure can serve as a significant source of various infections, including classical swine fever, swine dysentery, foot and mouth disease, porcine reproductive and respiratory syndrome virus, *S. suis, Escherichia coli*, and Salmonella spp., among others. The risk is especially elevated when the manure originates from other pig farms. It is recommended to avoid spreading, spraying, or injecting manure from other swine facilities within a 3.2 km radius of pig farms (Amass 2005b). Develop a systematic plan for the collection, storage, and disposal of pig manure. Utilize manure pits or storage facilities to contain and store pig waste, minimizing runoff and leaching into the surrounding environment. When dealing with liquid slurry, it is advised to have flowing channels from the pig buildings leading to an external pit. The slurry level in the pit should be maintained well below that of the channels to prevent any backflow. Implement regular removal and disposal of manure to prevent buildup and reduce odor emissions.
(b) **Composting**: Implement composting systems to process pig manure into a valuable organic fertilizer. Establish designated composting areas with proper drainage, aeration, and moisture control. Monitor compost piles regularly to ensure proper decomposition and temperature management.
(c) **Anaerobic Digestion**: Install anaerobic digesters to convert pig manure into biogas and organic fertilizer. Anaerobic digestion helps generate renewable energy while reducing methane emissions and odor from manure storage. Proper management of anaerobic digesters includes monitoring temperature, pH levels, and gas production.
(d) **Land Application**: Apply treated pig manure to agricultural land as a nutrient-rich fertilizer, following appropriate application rates and timing. Conduct soil testing to determine nutrient requirements and minimize the risk of nutrient runoff or groundwater contamination. Implement practices such as injection or incorporation of manure into the soil to reduce odor and nutrient losses.
(e) **Nutrient Management Planning**: Develop nutrient management plans to optimize the use of pig manure as a fertilizer while minimizing environmental impacts. Consider factors such as soil type, crop nutrient requirements, and weather conditions when planning manure application. Monitor nutrient levels in soil and water bodies to assess the effectiveness of nutrient management practices and identify potential risks.
(f) **Water Management**: Implement runoff control measures like vegetative buffers, terracing, and contouring to minimize erosion and avoid contamination of water bodies with pig waste. Install drainage systems to manage excess water and prevent waterlogging in pig housing units and manure storage facilities. Regularly monitor water quality in surface water and groundwater sources to detect any contamination from pig waste.

(g) **Odor Control**: Implement measures to mitigate odor emissions from pig waste, such as covering manure storage facilities, using odor-neutralizing additives, and incorporating manure into the soil. Utilize vegetative buffers and windbreaks to reduce the spread of odors to neighboring properties.
(h) **Regulatory Compliance**: Ensure compliance with local regulations and environmental permits governing waste management practices at pig farms. Maintain accurate records of waste handling and disposal activities to demonstrate compliance with regulatory requirements.
(i) **Education and Training**: Train farm workers on proper waste management practices, covering handling, storage, and disposal procedures. Raise awareness among farm staff about the significance of waste management for environmental stewardship and regulatory compliance.

Summary and Conclusion

Swine zoonoses are diseases transferable from pigs to humans, posing significant public health risks due to potential outbreaks and epidemics Swine zoonoses result from pathogens like bacteria, viruses, parasites, and fungi in pigs and their environments, posing transmission risks to humans through direct or indirect contact. Mitigating and managing swine zoonoses requires comprehensive strategies targeting transmission pathways. These include enforcing strict biosecurity protocols on farms, maintaining proper hygiene and sanitation during pork production and processing, educating stakeholders about zoonotic risks, and establishing surveillance and monitoring systems to detect and manage outbreaks effectively. Furthermore, vaccinating swine against specific zoonotic pathogens and implementing regulatory measures to ensure food safety can help reduce the risk of transmission to humans.

References

Alarcón, L. V., Allepuz, A., & Mateu, E. (2021). Biosecurity in pig farms: A review. *Porcine Health Management, 7*(1), 5.

Amass, S. F. (2005a). *Biosecurity: Stopping the bugs from getting in* (pp. 104–114).

Amass, S. F. (2005b). *Biosecurity: Reducing the spread* (p. 87).

Baudon, E., Peyre, M., Peiris, M., & Cowling, B. J. (2017). Epidemiological features of influenza circulation in swine populations: A systematic review and meta-analysis. *PLoS One, 12*(6), e0179044.

Benjamin, M., & Yik, S. (2019). Precision livestock farming in swine welfare: A review for swine practitioners. *Animals, 9*(4), 133.

Bettencourt, E. M. V., Tilman, M., Narciso, V., Carvalho, M. L. D. S., & Henriques, P. D. D. S. (2015). The livestock roles in the wellbeing of rural communities of Timor-Leste. *Revista de Economia e Sociologia Rural, 53*, 63–80.

Block, S. S. (Ed.). (2001). *Disinfection, sterilization, and preservation*. Lippincott Williams & Wilkins.

Bökönyi, S. (1974). *History of domestic mammals in central and Eastern Europe*. Akadémiai Kiadó.

Brochier, B., Kieny, M. P., Costy, F., Coppens, P., Bauduin, B., Lecocq, J. P., et al. (1991). Large-scale eradication of rabies using recombinant vaccinia-rabies vaccine. *Nature, 354*(6354), 520–522.

Dafale, N. A., Srivastava, S., & Purohit, H. J. (2020). Zoonosis: An emerging link to antibiotic resistance under "one health approach". *Indian Journal of Microbiology, 60*, 139–152.

Desrosiers, R. (2011). Transmission of swine pathogens: Different means, different needs. *Animal Health Research Reviews, 12*(1), 1–13.

FAO. (2003). *World agriculture: Towards 2015/2030: An FAO perspective*. FAO.

Food and Agriculture Organization. (2021). 6. Meat. Available online: https://www.oecd-ilibrary.org/sites/cf68bf79en/index.html?itemId=/content/component/cf68bf79 en. Accessed on 1 May 2024.

Kahrs, R. F. (1995). General disinfection guidelines. *Revue scientifique et technique (International Office of Epizootics), 14*(1), 105–163.

Kenya, F. P. S. (2012). *FAO animal production and health livestock country reviews* (p. 3). FAO.

Muehlenbein, M. P. (2013). *Human-wildlife contact and emerging infectious diseases* (pp. 79–94). Current and future directions.

Nelson, M. I., Wentworth, D. E., Das, S. R., Sreevatsan, S., Killian, M. L., Nolting, J. M., et al. (2016). Evolutionary dynamics of influenza a viruses in US exhibition swine. *The Journal of Infectious Diseases, 213*(2), 173–182.

Pappaioanou, M., & Gramer, M. (2010). Lessons from pandemic H1N1 2009 to improve prevention, detection, and response to influenza pandemics from a one health perspective. *ILAR Journal, 51*(3), 268–280.

Pinard-Van Der Laan, M. H., & Gay, C. G. (2008). The future impact of animal genomics in animal health research. *Animal Genomics Animal Health, 132*, 3–11.

Pond, W. G., & Houpt, K. A. (1978). *The biology of the pig* (p. 371). Comstock Pub. Associates.

Pritchard, G., Dennis, I., & Waddilove, J. (2005). Biosecurity: Reducing disease risks to pig breeding herds. *Practice, 27*(5), 230–237.

Ramirez, A., Capuano, A. W., Wellman, D. A., Lesher, K. A., Setterquist, S. F., & Gray, G. C. (2006). Preventing zoonotic influenza virus infection. *Emerging Infectious Diseases, 12*(6), 997.

Stärk, K. D. C. (1999). The role of infectious aerosols in disease transmission in pigs. *The Veterinary Journal, 158*(3), 164–181.

Verikios, G., Sullivan, M., Stojanovski, P., Giesecke, J. A., & Woo, G. (2011). *The global economic effects of pandemic influenza*. Centre of Policy Studies (CoPS).

Watson, S. J., Langat, P., Reid, S. M., Lam, T. T. Y., Cotten, M., Kelly, M., et al. (2015). Molecular epidemiology and evolution of influenza viruses circulating within European swine between 2009 and 2013. *Journal of Virology, 89*(19), 9920–9931.

Wong, D. L. F., Dahl, J., Stege, H., Van Der Wolf, P. J., Leontides, L., Von Altrock, A., & Thorberg, B. M. (2004). Herd-level risk factors for subclinical salmonella infection in European finishing-pig herds. *Preventive Veterinary Medicine, 62*(4), 253–266.

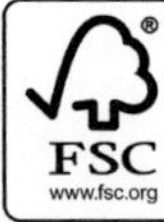

MIX
Papier aus verantwortungsvollen Quellen
Paper from responsible sources
FSC® C105338

If you have any concerns about our products,
you can contact us on
ProductSafety@springernature.com

In case Publisher is established outside the EU,
the EU authorized representative is:
Springer Nature Customer Service Center GmbH
Europaplatz 3, 69115 Heidelberg, Germany

Printed by Libri Plureos GmbH
in Hamburg, Germany